Tobacco and Public Health

Selections from the
American Journal of Public Health

Introduction by
Lyndon Haviland, DrPH
Cheryl G. Healton, DrPH

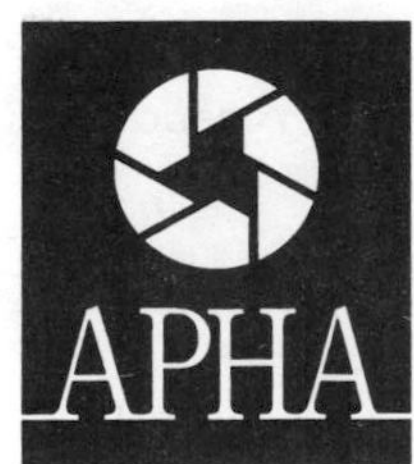

Promoting public health research, policy, and practice is the mission of the *American Journal of Public Health.* As we widen our scope to embrace global issues, we also sharpen our focus to support the needs of public health practitioners. We invite contributions of original unpublished research, opinion and commentary, departments, and letters to the editor.

American Public Health Association
800 I St., NW
Washington, DC 20001-3710

Georges Benjamin, MD, FACP
Executive Vice President

Printed and bound in the United States of America

Printing and Binding: Omnipress

ISBN 0-87553-031-1

IN MEMORY OF

JOHN SLADE, MD

vii Introduction | *L. Haviland and C. G. Healton*

SECTION I
Tobacco & Public Health Policy

1 **Effect of the tobacco price support program on cigarette consumption in the United States: an updated model** | *P. Zhang, C. Husten, and G. Giovino*

7 **Lessons learned from the tobacco industry's efforts to prevent the passage of a workplace smoking regulation** | *C. V. Mangurian and L. A. Bero*

12 **Failure to defend a successful state tobacco control program: policy lessons from Florida** | *M. S. Givel and S. A. Glantz*

18 **Tobacco industry allegations of "illegal lobbying" and state tobacco control** | *S. A. Bialous, B. J. Fox, and S. A. Glantz*

24 **Implications for Tobacco Control of the Multistate Tobacco Settlement** | *R. A. Daynard, W. Parmet, G. Kelder, and P. Davidson*

29 **Simulated effect of tobacco tax variation on population health in California** | *R. M. Kaplan, C. F. Ake, S. L. Emery, and A. M. Navarro*

35 **The new battleground: California's experience with smoke-free bars** | *S. Magzamen and S. A. Glantz*

43 **Constructing "Sound Science" and "Good Epidemiology": Tobacco, Lawyers, and Public Relations Firms** | *E. K. Ong and S. A. Glantz*

52 **Strange bedfellows: the history of collaboration between the Massachusetts Restaurant Association and the tobacco industry** | *W. A. Ritch and M. E. Begay*

58 **Louisiana Tobacco Control: Creating Momentum With Limited Funds** | *S. Moody Thomas, E. B. Schuler-Adair, S. Cunningham, M. Celestin, and C. Brown*

59 **Local Enactment of Tobacco Control Policies in Massachusetts** | *W. J. Bartosch and G. C. Pope*

62 **The Institute of Medicine Report on Smoking: A Blueprint for a Renewed Public Health Policy** | *G. Batta Gori*

63 **Tobacco Industry Surveillance of Public Health Groups: The Case of STAT and INFACT** | *R. E. Malone*

69 **Independent Evaluation of the California Tobacco Control Program: Relationships Between Program Exposure and Outcomes, 1996–1998** | *L. A. Rohrbach, B. Howard-Pitney, J. B. Unger, C. W. Dent, K. Ammann Howard, T. Boley Cruz, K. M. Ribisl, G. J. Norman, H. Fishbein, and C. Anderson Johnson*

78 **Evaluating the Tobacco Settlement Damage Awards: Too Much or Not Enough?** | *M. Coller, G. W. Harrison, and M. Morgan McInnes*

84 **Is Smoking Delayed Smoking Averted?** | *S. Glied*

88 **A Balanced Tobacco Control Policy** | *S. D. Sugarman*

SECTION II
Tobacco Advertising & Marketing

93 **Influence of a counteradvertising media campaign on initiation of smoking: the Florida "truth" campaign** | *D. F. Sly, R. S. Hopkins, E. Trapido, and S. Ray*

99 **The Relation Between Community Bans of Self-Service Tobacco Displays and Store Environment and Between Tobacco Accessibility and Merchant Incentives** | *R. E. Lee, E. C. Feighery, N. C. Schleicher, and S. Halvorson*

102 **Counteracting tobacco motor sports sponsorship as a promotional tool: is the tobacco settlement enough?** | *M. Siegel*

109 **Getting to the Truth: Evaluating National Tobacco Countermarketing Campaigns** | *M. C. Farrelly, C. G. Healton, K. C. Davis, P. Messeri, J. C. Hersey, and M. L. Haviland*

116 **Smooth Moves: Bar and Nightclub Tobacco Promotions That Target Young Adults** | *E. Sepe, P. M. Ling, and S. A. Glantz*

122 **Why and How the Tobacco Industry Sells Cigarettes to Young Adults: Evidence From Industry Documents** | *P. M. Ling and S. A. Glantz*

131 **Tobacco Industry Marketing at Point of Purchase After the 1998 MSA Billboard Advertising Ban** | *M. A. Wakefield, Y. M. Terry-McElrath, F. J. Chaloupka, D. C. Barker, S. J. Slater, P. I. Clark, and G. A. Giovino*

SECTION III
Tobacco & the Environment

137 **The Smoke You Don't See: Uncovering Tobacco Industry Scientific Strategies Aimed Against Environmental Tobacco Smoke Policies** | *M. E. Muggli, J. L. Forster, R. D. Hurt, and J. L. Repace*

142 **Boards of Health as Venues for Clean Indoor Air Policy Making** | *J. V. Dearlove and S. A. Glantz*

151 **Clean Indoor Air: Advances in California, 1990–1999** | *E. A. Gilpin, A. J. Farkas, S. L. Emery, C. F. Ake, and J. P. Pierce*

158 **Science, Politics, and Ideology in the Campaign Against Environmental Tobacco Smoke** | *R. Bayer and J. Colgrove*

SECTION IV
Tobacco & Maternal and Child Health

167 **Tobacco marketing and adolescent smoking: more support for a causal inference** | *L. Biener and M. Siegel*

172 **Variation in youthful risks of progression from alcohol and tobacco to marijuana and to hard drugs across generations** | *A. Golub and B. D. Johnson*

180 **Are the Sales Practices of Internet Cigarette Vendors Good Enough to Prevent Sales to Minors?** | *K. M. Ribisl, A. E. Kim, and R. S. Williams*

182 **Cigar Use in New Jersey Among Adolescents and Adults** | *C. D. Delnevo, E. S. Pevzner, M. B. Steinberg, C. W. Warren, and J. Slade*

184 **Validation of School Nurses to Identify Severe Gingivitis in Adolescents** | *D. Cappelli and J. P. Brown*

186 **Maternal Smoking During Pregnancy and Severe Antisocial Behavior in Offspring: A Review** | *L. S. Wakschlag, K. E. Pickett, E. Cook, Jr, N. L. Benowitz, and B. L. Leventhal*

195 **Tobacco Industry Youth Smoking Prevention Programs: Protecting the Industry and Hurting Tobacco Control** | *A. Landman, P. M. Ling, and S. A. Glantz*

209 **Coverage of Tobacco Dependence Treatments for Pregnant Women and for Children and Their Parents** | *J. K. Ibrahim, H. Halpin Schauffler, D. C. Barker, and C. T. Orleans*

SECTION V
Disparities in Tobacco Use

215 **Smoking Among Chinese Americans: Behavior, Knowledge, and Beliefs** | *E. S. H. Yu, E. H. Chen, K. K. Kim, and S. Abdulrahim*

221 **Prevalence and Predictors of Tobacco Use Among Asian Americans in the Delaware Valley Region** | *G. X. Ma, S. Shive, Y. Tan, and J. Toubbeh*

229 **Do Sex and Ethnic Differences in Smoking Initiation Mask Similarities in Cessation Behavior?** | *G. A. McGrady and L. L. Pederson*

234 **Burning Love: Big Tobacco Takes Aim at LGBT Youths** | *H. A. Washington*

244 **African American Women and Smoking: Starting Later** | *J. Moon-Howard, DrPH*

INTRODUCTION

TOBACCO USE REMAINS THE leading cause of preventable death and disease in the United States.[1] The World Bank estimates that by year 2030, tobacco use will be the leading cause of death worldwide.[2] This timely volume presents critical evidence on both the progress to date and the remaining challenges to reducing tobacco use globally. That is, it offers evidence of public health interventions that have proven successful in diverse populations, notwithstanding the ongoing challenges of an aggressive industry that continues to expand its marketing and promotional activities. Using research that delves into tobacco industry documents, this volume also provides evidence of the tobacco industry's strategies and policies to promote and sell tobacco despite clear knowledge of the adverse health consequences of tobacco use.

Successful public health and population-based strategies for reducing tobacco use offer important lessons for other emerging public health challenges, including the epidemic of childhood obesity. Both youth tobacco use and childhood obesity have social dimensions with far-reaching health and societal consequences. Many of the medical sequelae of both tobacco use and obesity in children continue into adulthood and later life. Therefore, it is essential to both develop a strong scientific evidence base for policies and prevention programs that work, while also advancing the science of treatment, in order to meaningfully improve the health of the public.

The public health response to tobacco control has been multidisciplinary and mulifactorial, incorporating epidemiology, health policy, legal advocacy, legislation, behavioral modification, pharmaceutical interventions, counter-marketing, and health communication. In the United States overall, the prevalence of tobacco use has decreased[3] and the social norms regarding tobacco use have changed following the successful implementation of a combination of policy interventions, notably clean indoor air policies, tax increases, public education campaigns, increased surveillance, effective public education, and youth prevention programs. Despite these gains, tobacco use remains unacceptably high, resulting in 440 000 deaths each year in the United States,[1] and approximately 4 million deaths each year worldwide.[4]

A comprehensive program of policy, science, and practice is needed to prevent tobacco initiation among the young and other vulnerable populations, break the progression from initiation to addiction, limit exposure to second hand smoke, and help smokers to quit. In 2001, the independent, nonfederal Task Force on Community Preventive Services (TFCPS) published a review of the evidence on interventions to reduce tobacco use and exposure to environmental tobacco smoke (ETS).[5] The TFCPS recommendations are important because they stress interventions meant to achieve tobacco use prevention and control in the general population. These population-based interventions afford an opportunity to reach broad populations, in contrast to clinical interventions, which are more narrowly focused on those seeking treatment. The major TFCPS recommendations include community education to reduce ETS exposure at home and mass media campaigns. The TFCPS also supports strategies to reduce tobacco use initiation (such as increasing the unit price for tobacco products), smoking bans, and restrictions as a way of both reducing exposure to second hand smoke and inducing smokers to quit, and supporting smokers in their quit attempts.

For public health practitioners and policymakers, the prevention, reduction, and eventual elimination of tobacco use are critical in building healthier futures for everyone. Indeed, the US Department of Health and Human Services' *Healthy People 2010* (*HP 2010*) includes 27 specific objectives related to the reduction of tobacco use by increasing cessation, reducing initiation, and reducing exposure to ETS.[6]

This volume is organized into five sections: (1) Tobacco and Public Health Policy, (2) Tobacco Advertising and Marketing, (3) Tobacco and the Environment, (4) Tobacco and Maternal and Child Health, and (5) Disparities in Tobacco Use. Each of these sections is discussed in turn below.

I

Section one is focused on **Tobacco and Public Health Policy**. As recommended by the TFCPS, public health policy encompasses the effects of workplace and second hand smoking restrictions, as well as increases in taxation on smoking initiation and prevalence. Also included is a discussion of the 1998 Master Settlement Agreement (MSA) and the ongoing opposition by the tobacco industry to the

TFCPS recommendations. From a public policy perspective, the MSA between 46 state attorneys general and the tobacco industry provided a historic opportunity to fund comprehensive tobacco control in each of 46 states, and to ensure that all Americans are informed about the medical and social consequences of tobacco use. The MSA will bring more than $200 billion dollars to the states over 25 years, and could conceivably assist the nation in achieving all of the *HP 2010* objectives on tobacco control. Unfortunately, the MSA did not require states to spend these funds on tobacco control or public health. It is therefore possible that the MSA will be remembered as a missed opportunity to advance public health. In this volume, Daynard et al. and Coller et al. provide detailed analyses of both the provisions and inherent limitations of the MSA.

The litigation that resulted in the MSA, notably the pre-MSA litigation in Minnesota, also produced millions of pages of previously secret tobacco industry documents. Public health researchers have begun to utilize these documents not only to expose the tobacco industry's marketing tactics, but also to expose their actions to obfuscate legitimate science. Ong and Glantz charge Philip Morris with supporting a "coalition of bad science"[7] in condemning their "junk science" tactics intended to derail policy interventions meant to protect the public from the harmful effects of second hand smoke. These formerly secret tobacco industry documents are critical to deconstructing the strategies and actions of the tobacco industry as they relate to thwarting public health policies intended to address the tragedy of tobacco use worldwide. Millions of pages of tobacco industry documents can now be searched and analyzed online through the *American Legacy Foundation Tobacco Documents Archive* at the University of California at San Francisco. Better understanding of the strategies, actions, and tactics of the tobacco industry is desperately needed to counteract its marketing techniques especially their efforts outside the United States where the tobacco epidemic is expanding. Public health researchers from diverse disciplines are encouraged to take full advantage of this rich resource.

II

The second section of this volume, **Tobacco Advertising and Marketing**, provides a critical look at both the actions of the tobacco industry to market its products, and the response of states and national organizations that are trying to "unmarket" them. Counter-marketing is strongly recommended by both the Centers for Disease Control and Prevention (CDC) and the TFCPS. Evidence to date suggests that—when conducted well—counter-marketing can be highly successful and cost-effective. Research presented in this volume by Sly at the state level in Florida and Farrelly at the national level in the United States demonstrates that teens can be reached and influenced by tailored messages. Both the Florida and United States "truth" campaigns are highly sophisticated, grounded in the science of public health, and committed to excellence in advertising. Upon careful evaluation, it was found that exposure to the "truth" campaign changes teen knowledge and attitudes at both the state and national levels. In addition, the Florida campaign which had been tracked for a longer period of time was effective in decreasing use of tobacco products among teens. These findings signal the importance of tailored messages designed to reach highly targeted audiences, and may hopefully lead to cost-effective intervention strategies for the prevention and amelioration of other chronic health conditions.

The tobacco advertising section also provides ample evidence of the ongoing actions of the tobacco industry to market its products. The Ling and Glantz article highlights the new focus of the tobacco industry on young adults. The tobacco industry continues to promote smoking as an adult choice, and places its advertisements and promotions in key venues for young adults, including bars and nightclubs. Understanding the tobacco industry strategies and adopting their tactics of, for example, segmenting the market, will be invaluable in replicating the success of the Florida "truth" campaign in decreasing tobacco use, and in expanding this success to the national "truth" campaign.

In 2001, the tobacco industry spent 11.22 billion dollars on marketing and promotions in the United States.[8] Certain strategies such as cartoon advertising and give-aways of items like branded T-shirts and hats, "trinkets and trash" were restricted after the MSA, yet in-store promotions and "2 for 1" sales have continued. Increased restrictions on self-serve displays and increases in tobacco excise taxes have helped propel the tobacco industry to explore new venues for tobacco sales, including the Internet. In this volume, Biener and Siegel provide a critical analysis of the impact of promotional items on adolescent smoking. They conclude that adolescents who own promotional items—especially gear—remain open to smoking and are more likely to progress to established smoking than adolescents who do not own promotional items. National studies have found that use of the Internet by teens to purchase cigarettes is currently low. Still, Ribisil and colleagues warn that the Internet offers few protections against underage purchases, and may become an increasingly important source of tobacco for youth, especially as prices rise and the digital divide among low income households narrows.

As a result of the MSA, the tobacco industry has also begun sponsoring a series of youth smoking prevention programs. These programs provide an opportunity for the tobacco industry to promote tobacco use as an adult choice, and position the industry as a partner in youth prevention programs. A critical article in this volume by Landma et al. documents the results of these programs, including positive public relations for the industry and positive youth attitudes toward the companies and smoking.

III

Section three of this volume deals with **Tobacco and the Environment**. Strategies to reduce exposure to second hand smoke, including smoking bans and restrictions on tobacco use in public places, are strongly recommended by the TFCPS. As discussed by Bayer and Colgrove, the public health community has used public restrictions on exposure to second hand smoke to change the political and ideological climate of tobacco use. The promotion of the rights of nonsmokers has resulted in widespread changes, including the banning of smoking on airplanes, in state and federal office buildings, and increasingly, in bars and restaurants. These policies have limited the opportunities for smokers to smoke, and have changed the perception of smoking from "normal" to "stigmatized." The focus on the rights of innocent bystanders has also changed the terms of the debate from the rights of adults to choose to smoke, to the rights of others to be protected from second hand smoke.

IV

The fourth section of this volume is devoted to **Tobacco and Maternal and Child Health**. The 2001 *Report of the Surgeon General on Women and Smoking* clearly documents that poor reproductive health outcomes can be attributed to smoking during pregnancy, including increased rates of low birth weight deliveries, miscarriage, sudden infant death syndrome (SIDS), and infant mortality due to perinatal disorders.[9] New research by Wakschlag and colleagues suggests potential long-term consequences of maternal smoking during pregnancy, including increased prevalence of severe anti-social behavior among the children of mothers who smoked throughout their pregnancies. Supporting pregnant women in quitting smoking and designing programs to meet their specific needs are critical to the health of both children and mothers, and make good fiscal sense.

V

The fifth and final section in this volume is devoted to **Disparities in Tobacco Use**. In the United States today, tobacco use is decidedly *not* an equal opportunity habit. While public health interventions including prevention programs and cessation services have expanded, disparities in access to culturally tailored programs have continued to increase. As a result, tobacco use is increasingly concentrated in low income and marginalized communities. The papers by Moon-Howard, Washington, Yu and Ma compellingly demonstrate that the tobacco industry has developed tailored marketing programs to encourage smoking in diverse communities and subcultures, including for African Americans, Hispanics, Asian/Pacific Islanders, lesbian, gay, bisexual, and transgender (LGBT) populations, and the homeless. Tobacco industry documents reveal the strategies and programs designed to encourage tobacco use and brand switching, and to market tobacco use as a glamorous lifestyle choice.

Tobacco use remains the leading cause of preventable death and disease in the United States today. This volume provides ample evidence that the tobacco industry, through its marketing practices, continues to promote tobacco use and work against the implementation of prevention programs and public policies that would limit death and disease for all of us. Better understanding of the tobacco industry strategies through close examination of their documents can help to write a public health success story. It would have a real-life ending of a world where the tobacco industry is prohibited from marketing its deadly and addictive products, and where the health of people everywhere is protected and promoted. This volume provides compelling evidence of the work of tobacco control to stem the tide of a deadly epidemic, challenging public health professionals across the globe to find the political will to implement the programs to protect and improve the health of the public.

Lyndon Haviland, DrPH
Cheryl G. Healton, DrPH

About the Authors

Lyndon Haviland is Chief Operating Officer and Cheryl Healton is President/Chief Executive Officer, American Legacy Foundation.

References

1. Centers for Disease Control and Prevention (CDC). Annual Smoking-Attributable Mortality, Years of Potential Life Lost and Economic Costs- United States, 1995-1999. *MMWR* 2002;51: 300–303.

2. The World Bank. Curbing the Epidemic: Governments and the Economics of Tobacco Control. 1999. The International Bank for Reconstruction and Development, The World Bank, Washington DC.

3. Johnston LD, O'Malley PM, Bachman JG. Monitoring the Future national survey results on drug use, 1975–2002. Volume 1: Secondary school students (NIH Publication No. 03-5375). Bethesda, MD: National Institute on Drug Abuse. 2003.

4. The World Health Organization. The Tobacco Atlas. 2002. Eds Mackay & Eriksen. Geneva, Switzerland.

5. Task Force on Community Preventive Services. Recommendations regarding interventions to reduce tobacco use and exposure to environmental tobacco smoke. *American Journal of Preventive Medicine.* 2001;20(2S):10–15.

6. U.S. Department of Health and Human Services. *Healthy People 2010.* 2nd ed. With Understanding and Improving Health and Objectives for Improving Health. 2 vols. Washington, DC: U.S. Government Printing Office, November 2000.

7. Ong, Elisa K, Glantz, S Constructing "Sound Science" and "Good Epidemiology": Tobacco, Lawyers, and Public Relations Firms. AJPH 2001. Vol. 91. 11. 43–51.

8. Federal Trade Commission. Federal Trade Commission Cigarette Report for 2001. 2003.

9. U.S. Department of Health and Human Services. Women and Smoking. A Report of the Surgeon General. Rockville, MD. U.S. Department of Health and Human Services, Public Health Service, Centers for Disease Control, Center for Chronic Disease Prevention and Health Promotion, Office on Smoking and Health, 2001.

| SECTION I |

Tobacco & Public Health Policy

Effect of the Tobacco Price Support Program on Cigarette Consumption in the United States: An Updated Model

Ping Zhang, PhD, Corinne Husten, MD, MPH, and Gary Giovino, PhD

ABSTRACT

Objectives. This study evaluated the direct effect of the tobacco price support program on domestic cigarette consumption.

Methods. We developed an economic model of demand and supply of US tobacco to estimate how much the price support program increases the price of tobacco. We calculated the resultant increase in cigarette prices from the change in the tobacco price and the quantity of domestic tobacco contained in US cigarettes. We then assessed the reduction in cigarette consumption attributable to the price support program by applying the estimated increase in the cigarette price to assumed price elasticities of demand for cigarettes.

Results. We estimated that the tobacco price support program increased the price of tobacco leaf by $0.36 per pound. This higher tobacco price translates to a $0.01 increase in the price of a pack of cigarettes and an estimated 0.21% reduction in cigarette consumption.

Conclusion. Because the tobacco price support program increases the price of cigarettes minimally, its potential health benefit is likely to be small. The adverse political effect of the tobacco program might substantially outweigh the potential direct benefit of the program on cigarette consumption. (*Am J Public Health.* 2000;90:746–750)

The US government has intervened in the tobacco market through a price support program since the 1930s.[1] Some have argued that this program is beneficial to public health because it reduces tobacco consumption by increasing prices,[2,3] but others have claimed that it hurts efforts to control tobacco because it has undesirable political consequences.[4,5] How much the price support program directly affects tobacco consumption is therefore an important policy issue; in this report, we consider this question for cigarettes only, which accounted for 90% of US tobacco use in 1996.[6]

In 1984, Sumner and Alston[7] reported their analysis of the consequences of eliminating the price support program; these researchers concluded that eliminating it would lead to a 3% decrease in cigarette prices and about a 1% increase in domestic sales. These estimates should now be recalculated for several reasons.

First, more up-to-date information on production, consumption, and prices is available. Second, empirically based estimates of the elasticity of demand and supply for US tobacco have been published.[8,9] (Sumner and Alston used a range of hypothetical elasticities.) Finally, the estimated effect of the tobacco price support program on domestic cigarette consumption depends on the share of domestic tobacco in US cigarettes. From 1983 to 1991, domestic tobacco declined as a percentage of the value of US-made cigarettes because of increased tobacco imports, greater expenses for items such as cigarette promotion, and larger gross markup by manufacturers.[10,11] However, a 1993 law establishing the minimum content of US-grown tobacco in cigarettes manufactured in the United States, as well as a 1995 law setting the amount of tobacco that each major supply country can export to the United States under a normal tariff rate, should help keep domestic share from falling much further.[1]

Tobacco Price Support Program

Marketing quotas, price support, and import restrictions form the core of the current tobacco price support program.[12]

Marketing Quotas

Marketing quotas specify the number of pounds of tobacco a grower can market that are eligible for price support; sales above this quota are subject to prohibitive penalties. Each grower's marketing quota is a share of the national quota, which is set annually by the US Department of Agriculture (USDA) on the basis of 3 criteria[12]: (1) intended purchases by cigarette manufacturers, (2) annual export for the 3 preceding years, and (3) the amount of tobacco needed to attain a specific level of reserve stock. The US secretary of agriculture can adjust this national quota by ±3%.

When the program began in 1938, the determination of individual marketing quotas was based on historical production.[12] Entry has been liberalized by changing the original rule that persons without a quota could grow tobacco only if they purchased or rented land with an attached quota. Since 1962, farmers can simply rent or purchase a quota and begin growing tobacco; they need not rent or purchase land from the quota owner.[12]

Ping Zhang is with the Department of Agricultural Economics, Kansas State University, Manhattan. Corinne Husten and Gary Giovino are with the Office on Smoking and Health, Centers for Disease Control and Prevention, Atlanta, Ga.

Correspondence and requests for reprints should be sent to Ping Zhang, PhD, Department of Agricultural Economics, 331D Waters Hall, Kansas State University, Manhattan, KS 66502-4011 (e-mail: pzhang@agecon.ksu.edu).

This article was accepted November 5, 1999.

Price Support

Each year, the USDA sets the tobacco price supports by announcing the "loan rate" (actually a minimum price per pound) for the domestic action market,[12] which varies by type and grade of tobacco leaf. This price is effectively guaranteed to the grower by the Commodity Credit Corporation, a USDA agency.[1] The tobacco farmer sells cured tobacco to the highest bidder at auction; if this bid is below the loan rate, the farmer is paid the support price by a producer cooperative with money borrowed from the Commodity Credit Corporation. The newly purchased tobacco is then consigned to the cooperative, which redries, packs, and stores it as collateral for the Commodity Credit Corporation loan. The cooperative, acting as an agent for the Commodity Credit Corporation, later sells the tobacco and uses the proceeds to repay the Commodity Credit Corporation loan principal and interest; sometimes this process ends in a loss for the cooperative.[13] The federal government, however, is reimbursed from an escrow account for any losses resulting from its operation of the price support program; this account is funded by tobacco farmers and buyers.[13]

Import Restrictions

Tobacco imports are restricted to limit replacement of domestic tobacco by cheaper imported tobacco.[1] In September 1995, legislation (tariff rate quota) was enacted to set for each major supplier country the amount of tobacco it could export to the United States under a normal tariff rate. Excess shipments are subjected to a 350% duty; most of the duty may be refunded, however, if the tobacco imported is used to manufacture cigarettes for export by the United States.[14]

Methods

To assess the direct effect of the tobacco price support program on cigarette consumption, we estimated 3 variables: (1) tobacco price increases due to the program, (2) changes in cigarette prices resulting from the higher tobacco prices, and (3) changes in cigarette consumption resulting from the higher cigarette prices.

Tobacco Price Increases Due to the Price Support Program

The primary purpose of controlling the tobacco supply is to raise and stabilize the price of tobacco.[12] If demand for tobacco does not change, prices will rise as the supply of tobacco declines. A simple model of demand and supply with the support program in place illustrates this point (Figure 1). Without the support program, the tobacco market would be in equilibrium at price (P_e) and quantity (Q_e). Marketing quotas, however, limit market supply to Q_f, in turn increasing the tobacco price from P_e to P_s (tobacco price with the quota). P_s can be observed from market data, but P_e must be estimated, which we did with a simple demand and supply model (Figure 2).

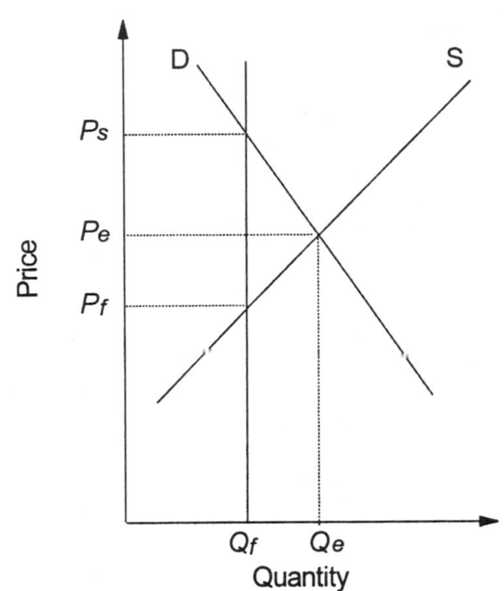

Note. D = demand curve for tobacco; S = supply curve of tobacco; P_e = tobacco price without the tobacco program; Q_e = quantity of tobacco demanded without the tobacco program; Q_f = quantity of tobacco supplied; P_s = tobacco price with quota; P_f = net price received by tobacco farmers.

FIGURE 1—Demand and supply of tobacco with the tobacco price support program.

Equations 1 and 2 in Figure 2 represent demand and supply in the tobacco leaf market, respectively. Equation 3 describes the relation between the market price of tobacco and the net prices received by tobacco farmers. This equation shows that tobacco farmers pay an amount up to L to quota owners for renting their quotas. The rent paid by tobacco farmers to quota owners also represents the program benefit created by the government price support to tobacco. Because quota owners acquire all the program benefit, the tobacco price support program "subsidizes" the tobacco quota owner rather than the tobacco farmer. Equation 4 describes the market-clearing condition at which the quantity of tobacco demanded equals the quantity of tobacco supplied; these quantities both equal the national tobacco quota.

To estimate P_e (the tobacco price in the absence of the support program), we first estimated the values for α and β. To do this, we first collected information on Q_d, P_s, L, η, and ξ from the observed market data and previous literature (Table 1). Q_d and Q_f averaged 1613 million pounds per year between 1990 and 1994, and the average P_s was \$1.76 per pound during the same period.[15] Results from previous studies indicated a value of −2 for η and a value of 7 for ξ.[8,9] L was \$0.45 per pound based on a survey in the major tobacco production area.[1]

P_f was \$1.31 per pound by applying the values of P_s and L to equation 3. We then applied the obtained values of Q_d, P_s, and η to equation 1 to solve for α and the obtained values of Q_f, P_f, and ξ to equation 2 to solve for β.

We used the estimated values on α and β and the values for η and ξ obtained from the previous literature to estimate P_e. The value for P_e was obtained by estimating P_s and P_f, because P_s and P_f were both equal to P_e when the tobacco market was at equilibrium. Q_d also was equal to Q_f at the market equilibrium. Applying those 2 market equilibrium conditions and the values for α, β, η, and ξ to equations 1 and 2 and solving the 2 equations for P_s and P_f yielded the value for P_e.

Changes in Cigarette Prices Resulting From Higher Tobacco Prices

The US cigarette manufacturing industry is oligopolistic; 5 manufacturers control almost the entire market.[16] As oligopolists, the manufacturers have substantial market power to influence the cigarette price. A recent study[17] showed that a state tax increase of \$0.10 resulted in an average price increase of \$0.11. We assumed that tobacco price increases resulting from the price support program would be fully (100%) passed on to the cigarette price at the retail level. If the actual increase in cigarette prices was more than the increase in tobacco prices, our calculation would underestimate the true increase in cigarette prices and the resultant reduction in cigarette consumption.

For a given unit of cigarettes (e.g., 1000), the change in its price attributable to a higher domestic tobacco price would equal the increase in the price of domestic tobacco per pound multiplied by the pounds of domestic tobacco used to produce that unit. The quantity of tobacco required to produce 1000 cigarettes declined from 2.3 pounds in 1960 through 1964 to about 1.7 pounds in 1980 through 1984 for several reasons: filter-tipped and smaller-diameter cigarettes became more popular, new technologies allowed tobacco stems to be blended into cigarettes, and tobacco sheets were used more efficiently.[10] Because the amount of tobacco for 1000 cigarettes has been stabilized at 1.7 pounds since 1984,[15] we used this ratio in the present study.

US cigarette manufacturers use both domestic and foreign tobacco. Foreign tobacco can be blended into a cigarette to make it more desirable to consumers and to reduce production costs. The shares of domestic tobacco without the price support program would be higher than those with the program because of the lower price of domestic tobacco in the absence of the program. We decided to use an estimate of the domestic share without the program to obtain a more conservative estimate of the cigarette price increase resulting from the price support program.

Predicting with reasonable accuracy what the share of domestic tobacco in US-produced cigarettes would be without the price support program presents substantial problems. In 1994, imported tobacco accounted for about 37% of US tobacco use (imported oriental tobacco constituted 12% of that use; imported flue-cured and burley tobacco constituted 25%). We assumed that oriental tobacco would continue to be imported if a price support program did not exist because the United States does not produce this type of tobacco. We also assumed that importation of flue-cured and burley tobacco would decrease without the price support program because of the decrease in the prices of these types of domestic tobacco. Still, foreign flue-cured and burley tobacco would probably continue to cost less than the domestic variety, and, thus, imports of these tobaccos would surely not end altogether. In addition, removal of the tobacco price support program might be combined with an import tariff reduction, in which case tobacco imports would be expected to increase.

(1) $$Q_d = \alpha \times P_s^{-\eta}$$

(2) $$Q_f = \beta \times P_f^{\xi}$$

(3) $$P_f = P_s - L$$

(4) $$Q_d = Q_f = \bar{Q}$$

Note. Q_d = quantity of tobacco demanded; Q_f = quantity of tobacco supplied; $\bar{Q}$ = tobacco quota; P_s = market price of tobacco; P_f = minimum price of tobacco to cover farmers' marginal costs of production; L = lease rate of tobacco quota; η = price elasticity of demand for US tobacco; and ξ = price elasticity of supply for US tobacco. α and β are constant parameters to be estimated.

FIGURE 2—A market equilibrium model for US tobacco leaf.

After considering these factors, and after a discussion with an expert at USDA (T. Capehart, oral communication, August 1997), we decided to use 75% as the value of domestic share of US tobacco use in the absence of the price support program for this analysis.

Changes in Cigarette Consumption Resulting From Higher Cigarette Prices

We estimated the percentage of reduction in cigarette consumption resulting from higher cigarette prices by multiplying the percentage of change in the cigarette price by the price elasticity of demand for cigarettes. Estimates of the price elasticity of demand for cigarettes at the retail level range from –0.28 to –0.80.[18–24] An expert panel of the National Cancer Institute recommended using –0.4 as the short-run price elasticity for such demand,[25] and we used this value in our study. We assumed that the long-run price elasticity of demand for cigarettes is about 1.5 times the short-run price elasticity[18–24] and thus used a value of –0.6 for this measure. We also converted the annual percentage of decrease in cigarette consumption resulting from the price support program into the decrease in the number of packs of cigarettes consumed per year.

Sensitivity Analysis

Values of the parameters used in the analysis still could be associated with uncertainties in spite of our efforts to incorporate the most likely value. We conducted a sensitivity analysis to address those uncertainties. Our sensitivity analysis focused on 2 scenarios—the maximum and the minimum effect of the tobacco price support program on domestic cigarette use.

We applied the following assumptions in estimating the maximum effect: (1) increasing or decreasing the values of price elasticities of demand and supply for tobacco leaf and price elasticities of demand for cigarettes by 50% in the direction favoring the maximum effect, (2) assuming that no tobacco imports would occur without the tobacco price support program, and (3) using the upper bound of the rent value for tobacco quota (\$0.50 per pound).[1] In estimating the minimum effect, we (1) increased or decreased price elasticities of demand and supply for tobacco leaf and price elasticities of demand for cigarettes by 50% in the direction favoring the minimum effect, (2) assumed that tobacco imports would increase up to 40% of the total tobacco use, and (3) applied the lower bound of the rent value for tobacco quota (\$0.40 per pound).[1] The parameter values used for the sensitivity analysis are presented in Table 1.

TABLE 1—Parameter Values Used in Estimating the Direct Effect of the Tobacco Price Support Program on US Cigarette Consumption

Parameters and Measuring Units	For Deriving the Most Likely Effect	For Sensitivity Analysis: Maximum Effect	For Sensitivity Analysis: Minimum Effect
Quantity of tobacco demanded and supplied, and tobacco quota (Q_d, Q_f, and $\bar{Q}$), million lbs	1613[a]	1613[a]	1613[a]
Market price of tobacco (P_s), \$/lb	1.76[a]	1.76[a]	1.76[a]
Lease rate of tobacco quota (L), \$/lb	0.45	0.50	0.40
Price elasticity of demand for tobacco leaf (η)	−2.00	−1.00	−3.00
Price elasticity of supply for tobacco leaf (ξ)	7.00	10.50	3.50
Tobacco leaf required for producing 1000 cigarettes, lbs	1.70	1.70	1.70
Importing share of total tobacco use	0.25	0	0.40
Short-run price elasticity of demand for cigarettes	−0.40	−0.20	−0.60
Long-run price elasticity of demand for cigarettes	−0.60	−0.30	−0.9
Price of cigarettes, \$/pack	1.76	1.76	1.76
Cigarette consumption, billion packs	24.25	24.25	24.25

[a]Average values between 1990 and 1994.

Results

We estimated that the price of tobacco at market equilibrium level without the tobacco price support program was \$1.40 per pound—\$0.36 less than the average \$1.76 per pound received by farmers between 1990 and 1994.[15]

We used a \$0.36 decrease in the tobacco price in the absence of the price support program, the estimate that 1.7 pounds of tobacco yield 1000 cigarettes, and a 75% market share value for domestic tobacco to estimate that the price support program increases the price of 1000 cigarettes by \$0.46, or \$0.009 per pack. The average retail price for a pack of cigarettes was \$1.76 in 1994,[26] so this represents a 0.52% increase in the price.

We estimated that this 0.52% increase, if short-run price elasticity is −0.4, reduces cigarette consumption by 0.21%. In 1994, 24.25 billion packs of cigarettes were consumed in the United States.[26] If this represents 99.79% of what consumption would be without the price support program, total consumption in 1994 without the program would have been 24.30 billion packs. On the basis of this level of consumption, a 0.21% reduction in cigarette consumption per year due to the direct effect of the system-induced price increase of the tobacco support program is equivalent to an annual cigarette reduction of 51 million packs, or just a pack per smoker per year. In the long run, the reduction in cigarette consumption resulting from the direct price effect of the program is 76 million packs per year, or fewer than 2 packs per smoker per year, according to our model.

Results from the sensitivity analysis showed that under the assumptions of the maximum effect, the tobacco price support program increases the price of a pound of tobacco leaf by \$0.46 and the price of a pack of cigarettes by \$0.016. Cigarette consumption is reduced by 0.53% in the short run and by 0.80% in the long run as a result of the program. In contrast, under the assumptions of the minimum effect, the tobacco program increases the price of a pound of tobacco leaf by \$0.20 and the price of a pack of cigarettes by just \$0.004. Cigarette consumption is reduced by only 0.05% in the short run and by 0.07% in the long run as a result of the tobacco price support program.

Discussion

This study suggests that the tobacco price support program increases the price of tobacco leaf by \$0.36 per pound, which was 21% of the tobacco price in 1994. This result is consistent with that in the earlier report of Sumner and Alston.[7]

This higher tobacco price translates to a 0.52% increase in cigarette prices. The fact that a relatively large percentage increase in tobacco prices has led to a small percentage increase in cigarette prices suggests that tobacco prices received by farmers and retail cigarette prices are very weakly related.

The small increase in cigarette prices may or may not have a real effect on reducing smoking, depending on the sensitivity of smokers to a small price change. Assuming that smokers are price-sensitive to a small price change, the higher cigarette prices resulting from the price support program would reduce both smoking prevalence and the number of cigarettes that continuing smokers consume. Previous studies indicated that at least one half of the reduction in consumption from an increase in cigarette prices results from a decrease in smoking prevalence, and that the other half is from the reduced number of cigarettes consumed by continuing smokers.[22,24,27] In 1994, on average, a smoker consumed 23.19 cigarettes per day,[28,29] a value adjusted for underreporting.[29] If 50% of the reduction in cigarette consumption were due to the reduced number of cigarettes smoked per smoker, a reduction of 51 million packs would be a decrease of 11 cigarettes per year (0.13%) per smoker. Similarly, if one half of the reduction in cigarette consumption were due to the decrease in smoking prevalence, there would be a reduction of 0.13% (60 000) in the number of US smokers.[28]

The reduction in cigarette consumption accruing from the tobacco price support program could have a health benefit, particularly if smoking prevalence is reduced.[30] The health benefit from reducing the number of cigarettes consumed by a smoker is less clear, because smokers may compensate by increasing the depth of inhalation or by smoking more of the cigarette.[31] In any case, the very modest reductions in cigarette consumption that we found suggest that any health benefit that might result from the tobacco price support program is likely to be quite small.

The potential health benefit of the tobacco price support program from reducing cigarette consumption is minimal compared with that of virtually all tobacco policy measures.[4] For example, a \$0.02 per pack increase in federal excise taxes would reduce cigarette consumption more than the price support program currently does. This is true even when the most conservative estimate under the maximum-effect scenario is used.

For proponents of tobacco control, this small direct effect of the tobacco price support program on cigarette consumption also must be weighed against the potential indirect adverse political effect of the program on reducing tobacco use. The tobacco price support program creates an additional political force (quota owners) that is likely to oppose tobacco control measures, and the program also changes the political influence of tobacco farmers by keeping many tobacco farmers in tobacco production.[32] The increase in potential opposition to tobacco control measures resulting from the additional political force created by the tobacco price support program could block policies such as a cigarette tax increase or other tobacco control initiatives.[4] Thus, it is very likely that the indirect political effect of the tobacco price support program on tobacco control far outweighs the direct program effect on reducing cigarette consumption.[4,32] □

Contributors

P. Zhang planned the study, conducted the analysis, and wrote the paper. C. Husten contributed to the analysis and the writing of the paper. G. Giovino contributed to the writing of the paper.

Acknowledgments

We gratefully acknowledge Anne Haddix of the Epidemiology Program Office, Centers for Disease Control and Prevention, Atlanta, Ga; Fred Gale and Tom Capehart of the Economic Research Service, US Department of Agriculture, Washington, DC; Ayda Yurekli of the World Bank, Washington, DC; and T. R. Owens of the Department of Agricultural and Applied Economics, Texas Tech University, Lubbock, for reviewing an earlier version of this paper and providing useful suggestions.

References

1. Grise VN. *Tobacco: Background for 1995 Farm Legislation.* Washington, DC: US Dept of Agriculture; 1995. Agricultural Economic Report 709.
2. Altman GD, Levine DW, Howard G, Hamilton H. Tobacco farmers and diversification: opportunities and barriers. *Tob Control.* 1996;5:182–198.
3. Manning WG, Keeler EB, Newhouse JP, Sloss EM, Wasserman J. *The Costs of Poor Health Habits.* Cambridge, Mass: Harvard University Press; 1991.
4. Warner KE. Tobacco subsidy: does it matter? *J Natl Cancer Inst.* 1988;80:81–83.
5. Northup A. U.S. agricultural policy on tobacco. In: *Tobacco Use: An American Crisis: Final Report and Recommendations From the American Health Community.* Washington, DC: US Dept of Health and Human Services; 1993.
6. *Tobacco Situation and Outlook Report.* Washington, DC: US Dept of Agriculture, Economic Research Service; September 1996. TBS-236.
7. Sumner DA, Alston JM. *Consequence of Elimination of the Tobacco Program.* Raleigh: North Carolina State University; 1984. Agricultural Research Service Bulletin 469.
8. Sumner DA, Alston JM. Substitutability for farm commodities: the demand for US tobacco in cigarette manufacturing. *Am J Agric Econ.* 1987;69:258–265.
9. Fulginiti LE, Perrin RK. The theory and measurement of producer response under quotas. *Rev Econ Stat.* 1993;75:97–106.
10. Grise VN. The changing tobacco user's dollar. In: *Tobacco Situation and Outlook Report.* Washington, DC: US Dept of Agriculture, Economic Research Service; June 1992:35–37. TBS-219.
11. Howell G, Congelio F, Yatsko R. Pricing practices for tobacco products, 1980–94. In: *Monthly Labor Review.* Washington, DC: Bureau of Labor Statistics, US Dept of Labor; December 1994;117:47–55.
12. Capehart T. Tobacco program—a summary and update. In: *Tobacco Situation and Outlook Report.* Washington, DC: US Dept of Agriculture, Economic Research Service; April 1997: 29–34. TBS-238.
13. Womach J. *Tobacco Price Support: An Overview of the Program.* Washington, DC: Congressional Research Service; 1995. CRS Report for Congress, 95-129 ENR.
14. *Tobacco Situation and Outlook Report.* Washington, DC: US Dept of Agriculture, Economic Research Service; September 1995. TBS-232.
15. *Tobacco Situation and Outlook Report.* Washington, DC: US Dept of Agriculture, Economic Research Service; December 1995. TBS-233.
16. *The 1995 Maxwell Tobacco Fact Book.* Raleigh, NC: Speccomm International Inc; 1996.
17. Keeler TE, Hu TW, Barnett PG, Manning PG, Sung HY. Do cigarette producers price-discriminate by state? An empirical analysis of local cigarette pricing and taxation. *J Health Econ.* 1996;15:499–512.
18. Batagi BH, Levin D. Estimating dynamic demand for cigarettes using panel data: the effect of bootlegging, taxation, and advertising reconsidered. *Rev Econ Stat.* 1986;68:148–155.
19. Becker GS, Gossman M, Murphy KM. An empirical analysis of cigarette addiction. *Am Econ Rev.* 1994;84:396–418.
20. Chaloupka F. Rational addictive behaviors and cigarette smoking. *J Polit Econ.* 1991;99: 722–742.
21. Coate D, Lewit EM. *The Potential for Using Excise Taxes to Reducing Smoking.* Washington, DC: National Bureau of Economic Research; 1994. Working Paper Series, No. 764.
22. Hu TW, Ren QF, Keeler TE, Bartlett J. The demand for cigarettes in California and behavioral factors. *Health Econ.* 1995;4:7–14.
23. Lewit EM, Coate D, Grossman M. The effects of government regulations on teenage smoking. *J Law Econ.* 1981;24:545–570.
24. Wasserman J, Manning WJ, Newhouse JP, Winkler JD. The effect of excise taxes and regulation on cigarette smoking. *J Health Econ.* 1991;10:43–64.
25. *The Impact of Cigarette Excise Taxes on Smoking Among Children and Adults: Summary Report of a National Cancer Institute Expert Panel.* Bethesda, Md: National Cancer Institute; 1993.
26. The Tobacco Institute. *The Tax Burden on Tobacco.* Vol 29. Washington, DC: Tobacco Institute; 1994.
27. Lewit EM, Coate D. The potential for using excise taxes to reduce smoking. *J Health Econ.* 1982;1:121–145.
28. *CDC National Tobacco Databook—1997.* Atlanta, Ga: Centers for Disease Control and Prevention. In press.
29. Hatziandreu EJ, Pierce JR, Fiore MC, Grise VN, Novotny TE, Davis RM. The reliability of self-reported cigarette consumption in the United States. *Am J Public Health.* 1989;79: 1020–1023.
30. *The Health Benefits of Smoking Cessation.* Washington, DC: US Dept of Health and Human Services; 1990.
31. *The Health Consequences of Smoking: Nicotine Addiction.* Washington, DC: US Dept of Health and Human Services; 1989.
32. Zhang P, Husten C. Impact of the tobacco price support program on tobacco control in the United States. *Tob Control.* 1998;7:176–182.

Lessons Learned From the Tobacco Industry's Efforts to Prevent the Passage of a Workplace Smoking Regulation

Christina V. Mangurian, BA, and Lisa A. Bero, PhD

ABSTRACT

Objectives. This study assessed the implementation of tobacco industry strategies to prevent a workplace smoking regulation.

Methods. Tobacco industry internal documents were identified; hearing transcripts for the affiliations, arguments, and positions regarding the regulation of testifiers were coded; and media coverage was analyzed.

Results. Tobacco industry strategies sought to increase business participation and economic discussions at public hearings and to promote unfavorable media coverage of the reugulation. The percentage of business representatives opposing the regulation grew from 18% (5 of 28) to 57% (13 of 23) between the hearings. Economic arguments opposing the regulation rose from 25% (7 of 28) to 70% (16 of 23). Press coverage was neutral and did not increase during the period of the regulatory hearings.

Conclusions. The tobacco industry was successful in implementing 2 of its 3 strategies but was not able to prevent passage of the comprehensive workplace regulation. (*Am J Public Health.* 2000; 90:1926–1930)

In the past, tobacco control researchers without access to tobacco industry internal documents could only speculate on the industry's strategies.[1–5] In this report, we identify specific tobacco industry strategies from internal industry documents and then determine whether implementation of these strategies was successful. Specifically, we assess the implementation of tobacco industry strategies to prevent passage of the Maryland Occupational Safety and Health (MOSH) regulation prohibiting smoking in enclosed workplaces.[6] Workplace smoking is of regulatory interest because environmental tobacco smoke is associated with lung cancer and heart and respiratory diseases.[7–11] Furthermore, smoking restrictions protect nonsmokers from environmental tobacco smoke and decrease tobacco use.[12] Proposed in November 1993, the Maryland regulation was one of the earliest workplace smoking regulations in the United States. If the Maryland legislature had not amended the regulation to exempt restaurants and bars,[13] it would have been the nation's most comprehensive workplace smoking regulation.[14]

We initiated this study while working on a comparative case study of federal and state workplace smoking regulations. We searched the Internet for references to each regulation and found tobacco industry internal documents that outlined strategies to oppose the Maryland regulation. The documents described 3 strategies to increase the tobacco industry's effectiveness at a final public hearing held by the Maryland commissioner of labor and industry: (1) develop a coalition of businesses to oppose the regulation at the hearing, (2) increase economic discussions at the hearing, and (3) increase unfavorable media coverage of the regulation. Therefore, we examined transcripts of the public hearings conducted before and after the tobacco industry internal documents were drafted, as well as press coverage of the regulation, to determine whether the strategies had been successfully implemented. Our findings could help public health advocates counteract industry efforts to prevent or weaken future indoor air regulations.

Methods

Data Sources

Our data sources were (1) tobacco industry internal documents, (2) regulatory hearing transcripts, and (3) the lay press.

Tobacco industry internal documents. Between March 8 and 15, 1999, we searched 3 tobacco industry document Web sites,[15–17] using the terms "MOSH" and "Maryland." Details of the search, inclusion and exclusion criteria, and search results are available at our Web site (http://itsa.ucsf.edu/~tobacco), copies of tobacco industry internal documents are available from the corresponding author. The authors, working independently, identified strategies from 10 documents that described tobacco industry plans to prevent the passage of the Maryland regulation.[18–27]

Public hearings. The MOSH advisory board, composed of individuals representing the local community, held 2 public hearings about the regulation (December 9 and 16, 1993) and prepared a recommendation for the commissioner of labor and industry in March 1994. Before publication of the final regulation,[28] an additional public hearing (May 3, 1994) was held by the commissioner. We obtained transcripts of the MOSH hearings and the subsequent commissioner's hearing from the Maryland Department of Licensing and Regulation, Division of Labor and Industry.

Two of the tobacco industry strategies were to increase the representation of the business community and to increase economic discussions in the period between the MOSH hearings and the commissioner's hearing. Therefore, we combined the 2 MOSH hearings and compared them with the commissioner's hearing to determine if there were differences between the hearings in the testifiers' affiliations or in the arguments presented.

We recorded the affiliation of all hearing presenters and whether they favored or opposed the regulation. The affiliation of each testifier was coded into mutually exclusive categories: (1) tobacco industry (e.g., Philip Morris), (2) business (e.g., National Restaurant Association, small business owner), (3) government (e.g., the Environmental Protection Agency),

Christina V. Mangurian is with the Department of Clinical Pharmacy and Lisa A. Bero is with the Department of Clinical Pharmacy and the Institute for Health Policy Studies, University of California, San Francisco.

Requests for reprints should be sent to Lisa A. Bero, PhD, Department of Clinical Pharmacy and the Institute for Health Policy Studies, University of California, San Francisco, 3333 California St, Suite 420, San Francisco, CA 94118.

This brief was accepted April 3, 2000.

(4) nonsmokers' lay organizations (e.g., Action on Smoking and Health), (5) labor (e.g., AFL-CIO), (6) health organization/private nonprofit organization (e.g., American Public Health Association, American Cancer Society), (7) private consulting/university affiliated (e.g., air quality consultant, University of California), or (8) private citizen.

Each testimony was coded for (1) economic arguments (e.g., cost to government, cross-border sales, cost/benefit to the employer, tobacco product production, and local/state economy), (2) scientific arguments (e.g., dose–response, study selection, bias, confounding, biological plausibility), (3) political arguments (e.g., jurisdiction, legal issues), (4) ideological arguments (e.g., freedom of choice, government intrusion, prohibition), and (5) building concerns (e.g., management, ventilation). These categories were based on previous work[29,30] and were derived from the data. We compared the number of individuals mentioning specific arguments between the hearings. Data were coded with QSR NUD*IST version 4.0 (Qualitative Solutions and Research Pty Ltd, Melbourne, Australia).

Media coverage. Because increasing unfavorable media coverage of the regulation was a stated goal in 6 tobacco industry documents,[18,19,21,23,25,26] we analyzed coverage of the Maryland regulation over time. We identified television and radio transcripts, newspaper and magazine news stories, letters, editorials, and other articles on the Maryland regulation between May 1, 1993 (6 months before the regulation was proposed) and September 30, 1995 (6 months after the regulation became state law), using the phrase "Maryland AND Workplace Smoking" to search the LEXIS-NEXIS electronic database. Search details and results are available on our Web site.

We coded the 187 identified media items as (1) in favor of, (2) against, or (3) neutral toward the regulation.

Analysis

We used χ^2 analysis to determine whether, between the MOSH and commissioner's hearings, there was a difference in (1) the number of presenters from the business community or (2) the relative frequency with which individuals presented economic arguments in favor of and opposed to the regulation. Descriptive statistics were used to show the frequency and content of media coverage over time.

Results

Three main strategies to prevent the regulation were to (1) develop a coalition of business interests to oppose the regulation,[18,22,23,25–27] (2) increase economic arguments between hearings,[18,23,25,26] and (3) increase media coverage.[18,19,21,23,25,26]

A document entitled "Strategy Outline for Maryland Occupational Safety and Health Regulations" noted that the industry wanted to increase opposition to the regulation between the MOSH and commissioner's hearings: "However, two major groups were not as vocal as desired [at the MOSH hearings]: the hospitality industry and individuals. A coalition against the proposed regulation needs to be further developed to provide deep grassroots opposition and greater press potential."[18] The document continued: "Major organizations have opposed the regulations, but additional depth must be given from individual businesses, hospitality groups, individuals who work in their home, and allies associated with the tobacco industry. Opposition to the proposal must be actively promoted to the press."[18]

A memo from APCO Associates (a public relations consulting firm that had several tobacco industry clients) entitled "Campaign Against State OSHA Anti-Smoking Regulations" described the following action items:

> build broadbased coalitions to:
> enable credible, new spokespeople to fight proposed regulations
> fight issue on economic grounds rather than to defend tobacco use
> Tactic: build new or adapt existing coalitions stressing individual or business rights[25]

The APCO Associates memo went on to list 65 types of business to attract to the coalition, in the fields of construction (n=11 types of business), building owners/managers (n=3), hospitality (n=18), lumber and wood products (n=5), real estate (n=2), retail outlets (n=20), and transportation (n=6). Membership organizations (e.g., churches or homeowner organizations) and tobacco-related businesses (e.g., tobacco dealers or warehouses) were also to be recruited for the coalition.

A document entitled "Media Plan for Maryland Citizens for Individual Rights" described the types of testimony that would be presented by the diverse coalition:

> As soon as a sufficient number of members are signed up, hold a press conference to announce the group and its goals. The coalition chairman would be the spokesman. He should be flanked by 15–20 members of the coalition to create the visual that this isn't one person and the tobacco industry, but a broad group opposed to these regulations. . . . The group needs to be diverse . . . we also need to personalize the story. This can be done through anecdotal stories by some 15 to 20 people with the chairman. For example: A bowling house proprietor explains, based on his own experience and accounting, what the regulation will cost his business . . .[19]

Other examples of anecdotes that were to be presented included stories from a restaurant owner, marina owner, boat owner, and homeowner.

An interoffice Philip Morris memo listed additional types of businesses to be sought for the coalition:

> The service station operators are also intending to express opposition, as are representatives of the restaurant association. I wish to add to the list representatives of other business groups, such as steamship companies, construction companies, and other specific labor groups, such as the International Longshoreman's Association, as we are currently soliciting those organizations. We will have a subsequent meeting to organize and coordinate the actual testimony to be presented at the hearings by those groups.[21]

The tobacco industry also considered shifting the debate from a regulatory proceeding to a court challenge or legislative debate.[20,22,25] For example, a Philip Morris memo stated:

> One option is pursuing a legislative track, the goal of which would be to issue a clear legislative intent on smoking in the workplace. While legislative leaders generally support that idea, they say politically it would be very difficult to pass. . . . Therefore, they recommend a more viable, judicial route. This alternative response would be to file suit against the state asking for an injunction on the ban.[22]

The state of Washington was also considering a workplace smoking regulation, and some of the tobacco industry internal documents referred to common strategies to prevent the regulations in both states. Three internal documents included references to developing a budget to defeat the regulations in both Maryland and Washington.[23,25,26] These documents included budgets for (1) coalition development, (2) an economic impact study, and (3) media relations in Maryland and Washington.[23,25,26] A memo from APCO Associates to a Philip Morris official stated: "I have collapsed Md and Wash into one plan based on my conversations with Pat and Dan."[25]

Strategy no. 1—Increase representation of the business community between the MOSH hearings and the commissioner hearing. Table 1 shows the affiliations of testifiers at the 2 hearings. Business representatives opposing the regulation grew from 18% (5 of 28) to 57% (13 of 23) between the hearings ($P < .002$, $df = 1$).

Strategy no. 2—Increase economic arguments between the MOSH hearings and the commissioner hearing. As shown in Table 1, the number of individuals against the regulation who used economic arguments rose from 25% (7 of 28) to 70% (16 of 23) between the hearings ($P < .05$, $df = 1$). These shifts were not seen among those in favor of the regulation.

TABLE 1—Affiliation of Individuals Who Testified and Arguments Used at Hearings on Maryland Workplace Smoking Regulation

	MOSH Hearing (December 1993)		Commissioner's Hearing (May 1994)	
	No. in Favor (%) (n=40)	No. Against (%) (n=28)	No. in Favor (%) (n=23)	No. Against (%) (n=23)
Affiliation				
Tobacco industry	1 (3)	18 (64)	0	8 (35)
Business	1 (3)	5 (18)	4 (17)	13 (57)
Government	8 (20)	0	3 (13)	0
Nonsmokers' lay organization	12 (30)	0	6 (26)	0
Labor	1 (3)	3 (11)	0	2 (9)
Health organization/private nonprofit organization	3 (8)	0	4 (17)	0
Private consulting/university affiliated	5 (12)	1 (4)	6 (26)	0
Private citizen	9 (23)	1 (4)	0	0
Arguments				
Economic	17 (43)	7 (25)	12 (52)	16 (70)
Scientific	12 (30)	7 (25)	8 (35)	5 (22)
Political	28 (70)	18 (64)	10 (43)	12 (52)
Ideological	25 (63)	20 (71)	10 (43)	19 (83)
Building-related	14 (35)	11 (39)	6 (26)	4 (17)

Note. MOSH = Maryland Occupational Safety and Health.

Economic arguments used by those against the regulation included (1) increased cross-border sales (4 and 26 arguments employed at MOSH hearings and commissioner's hearing, respectively), (2) cost to employers (7 and 52 arguments), (3) declining income from tobacco product production (11 and 9 arguments), (4) detriment to the local and state economy (4 and 30 arguments), and (5) increased cost to government (11 and 4 arguments). The arguments were mostly rhetorical and anecdotal and contained little data, as illustrated by the following examples (taken from testifiers at the commissioner's hearing on May 4, 1994):

"It takes away a loss [sic] of revenue from the state from sales tax and any other tax."
"It's going to create an unfair competition trying to compete with other states that allow smoking."

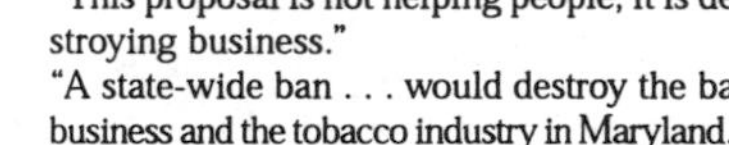
"This proposal is not helping people, it is destroying business."
"A state-wide ban . . . would destroy the bar business and the tobacco industry in Maryland."
"I don't think this is creating a very good economic impact for Maryland."

Strategy no. 3—Increase media coverage between the MOSH hearings and the commissioner hearing. Media coverage did not increase between the 2 hearings (see Figure 1). However, after the commissioner's hearing, there were 2 peaks of coverage: (1) the tobacco industry's challenge to the Maryland regulation in the Talbot County Circuit Court[31] and (2) the legislative debates that eventually exempted the hospitality industry from the workplace smoking restriction.[13] Eighty-two percent (154 of 187) of all media articles were neutral toward the regulation; 12% were in favor and 6% were opposed.

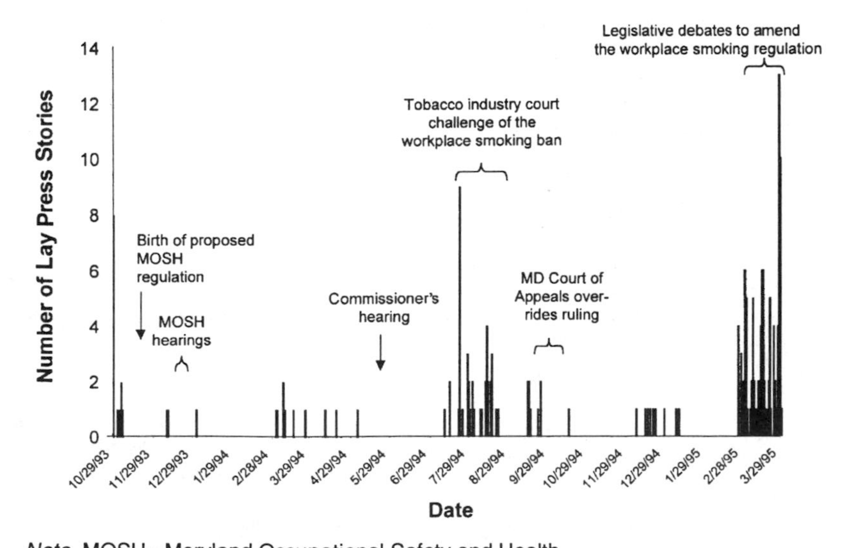

Note. MOSH = Maryland Occupational Safety and Health.

FIGURE 1—Media coverage in Maryland of hearings on Maryland workplace smoking regulation.

Conclusion

The tobacco industry was successful in implementing 2 of its 3 strategies to prevent the Maryland workplace smoking regulation. The industry successfully implemented the strategies to increase business representation and economic arguments at public hearings; it was not successful in its efforts to increase unfavorable media coverage during the regulatory hearing period. It was also not able to prevent passage of the comprehensive workplace regulation.

The Maryland legislature eventually amended the regulation and exempted the hospitality industry (March 1995).[13] The tobacco industry may have contributed to weakening the regulation through its long-term strategy of shifting the debate away from a regulatory procedure to a court challenge or legislative debate. Tobacco industry legal challenges that caused a 7-month delay in implementing the regulation[31,32] may have given the tobacco industry time to mobilize its effort at the legislative level, where it has more power.[33]

As illustrated by the examples provided, the economic arguments presented by those opposed to the regulation were often rhetorical and anecdotal and did not include economic data. This could represent an attempt by the tobacco industry to shift arguments away from the strong body of scientific research on the health effects of passive smoking to areas where the evidence is currently weak. Tobacco control advocates involved in regulatory proceedings should increase their use of economic data and continue to focus on the strong evidence of adverse health effects.

Although the tobacco industry was successful in implementing its strategy of developing a coalition including diverse types of small-business owners, it was not able to stimulate uniform opposition to the regulation in the business community. For example, the restaurant association of Maryland was 1 of the 4 business organizations that testified at the commissioner's hearing in support of the regulation. The association supported the regulation because it would apply equally to all establishments and therefore neither help nor harm specific types of businesses.[34] The association's presentation at the public hearings may have helped the commissioner to decide to include restaurants and bars in the final notice.[28] Public health advocates should continue to urge business owners to contest the tobacco industry's assertion that the business community is unanimously opposed to workplace smoking regulations.

Our finding that internal tobacco industry documents suggested common strategies and budgets for defeating workplace smoking regulations in the only 2 states then considering them—Maryland and Washington—suggests consistency in tobacco industry strategies to combat workplace smoking regulations. The public health community can expect that similar strategies of coalition formation, economic arguments, and media coverage will be used against future workplace smoking policies. □

Contributors

C. V. Mangurian collected the data, analyzed the results, and wrote the first draft of the paper. L. A. Bero aided in analysis, developed different methods to acquire pertinent information, and was involved with the writing of the final product; she is also the primary investigator of the larger study from which this project is derived.

Acknowledgments

This work was funded by the American Cancer Society (RPG9714301) and the California Tobacco-Related Disease Research Program (6RT0025).

We thank Marieka Schotland, BA, Katherine Bryan-Jones, BA, Theresa Montini, MSA, PhD, and Anke Schulz, MPA, for their comments on the paper and for generating useful ideas. Thanks to Paul Marvy for helping us unravel the NUD*IST mystery. Also, thanks to Vivian Weinberg for statistical analysis. We are also grateful to Glenn E. Schneider for providing invaluable tobacco industry documents and insight into the politics surrounding the Maryland regulation. Also thanks to the Maryland Department of Licensing and Regulation, Division of Labor and Industry, for providing us with the hearing transcripts. Finally, we thank the writing seminar at the Institute for Health Policy Studies at the University of California, San Francisco, for reviewing the draft.

References

1. Glantz SA, Barnes DE, Bero L, Hanauer P, Slade J. Looking through a keyhole at the tobacco industry. The Brown and Williamson documents. *JAMA.* 1995;274:219–224.
2. Chapman S. Tobacco industry memo reveals passive smoking strategy. *BMJ.* 1997;314:1569.
3. Chapman S. "Vast sums of money . . . to keep the controversy alive"—the 1988 BAT memo. *Tob Control.* 1997;6:236–239.
4. Traynor MP, Begay ME, Glantz SA. New tobacco industry strategy to prevent local tobacco control. *JAMA.* 1993;270:479–486.
5. Rabin RL, Sugarman SD. *Smoking Policy: Law, Politics, and Culture.* New York, NY: Oxford University Press; 1993.
6. Md Regs Code tit 9, §§ 12.23.01–12.23.05 (1995).
7. *Respiratory Health Effects of Passive Smoking: Lung Cancer and Other Disorders.* Washington, DC: Office of Health and Environmental Assessment, Office of Research and Development, US Environmental Protection Agency; 1992.
8. *Environmental Tobacco Smoke: Measuring Exposures and Assessing Health Effects.* Washington, DC: National Academy Press; 1986.
9. *The Health Consequences of Involuntary Smoking: A Report of the Surgeon General, 1986.* Rockville, Md: Centers for Disease Control, Office on Smoking and Health; 1986.
10. Glantz SA, Parmley WW. Passive smoking and heart disease. Epidemiology, physiology, and biochemistry [see comments]. *Circulation.* 1991;83:1–12.
11. Steenland K. Passive smoking and the risk of heart disease [see comments]. *JAMA.* 1992;267:94–99.
12. Chapman S, Borland R, Scollo M, Brownson RC, Dominello A, Woodward S. The impact of smoke-free workplaces on declining cigarette consumption in Australia and the United States. *Am J Public Health.* 1999;89:1018–1023.
13. Act of March 27, 1995, ch 5, 1995 Md Laws 350 (section 1 codified at Md Code Ann, Bus Reg § 2-105 [Supp 1995]; Md Code Ann, Lab & Empl §§ 2-106, 5-314 [Supp 1995]).
14. Patrick E. Maryland restricts workplace smoking. *Md Med J.* 1995;44:800–804.
15. US House of Representatives. Chairman Tom Bliley releases subpoenaed tobacco documents to the American people Available at: http://www.house.gov/commerce/tobaccodocs/documents.html. Accessed August 19, 1998.
16. Blue Cross and Blue Shield of Minnesota. Reducing tobacco usage. Available at: http://www.mnbluecrosstobacco.com. Accessed August 19, 1998.
17. Tobacco Resolution. Available at: http://www.tobaccoresolution.com/mainsite.html. Accessed August 19, 1998.
18. Strategy outline for Maryland Occupational Safety and Health regulations. April 1994. Bates no. 2023899204/7 or 2024105654/7. Philip Morris Incorporated document site. Available at: http://www.pmdocs.com. Accessed August 19, 1998.
19. Media plan for Maryland Citizens for Individual Rights. April 20, 1994. Bates no. 2024102370. Philip Morris Incorporated document site. Available at: http://www.pmdocs.com. Accessed March 12, 1999.
20. To: Tina Walls. From: Jim Lemperes. Subject: Smokefree regulation (proposal). Philip Morris, USA inter-office correspondence. November 8, 1993. Bates no. 2024198539/40. Philip Morris Incorporated document site. Available at: http://www.pmdocs.com. Accessed March 10, 1999.
21. To: Tina Walls. From: Jim Lemperes. Subject: MD—regulation banning workplace smoking. Philip Morris, USA inter-office correspondence. November 11, 1993. Bates no. 2024198537/8. Philip Morris Incorporated document site. Available at: http://www.pmdocs.com. Accessed March 10, 1999.
22. Political assessment of tobacco legislation and regulation: state of Maryland. February 7, 1994. Bates no. 2047897348/50. Philip Morris Incorporated document site. Available at: http://www.pmdocs.com. Accessed March 8, 1999.
23. Maryland/Washington OSHA regulations: strategy and budget. April 5, 1994. Bates no. 2044321567. Philip Morris Incorporated document site. Available at: http://www.pmdocs.com. Accessed March 15, 1999.
24. To: James R. Cherry, Mr Thomas C. Griscom, Mr John H. Hager, and Ms Ellen Merlo. From: Kurt L. Malmgren. RE: New York City, Maryland OSHA, and Washington labor and industry assessment. April 13, 1994. Bates no. 2024329149/51. Philip Morris Incorporated document site. Available at: http://www.pmdocs.com. Accessed March 10, 1999.
25. Campaign against state OSHA anti-smoking regulations. March 30, 1994. Bates no. 2023899055/9. Philip Morris Incorporated document site. Available at: http://www.pmdocs.com. Accessed March 15, 1999.
26. Maryland/Washington state budget; OSHA regulations. April 1994. Bates no. 2023899208. Philip Morris Incorporated document site. Available at: http://www.pmdocs.com. Accessed August 19, 1998.
27. Memo to: Kurt L. Malmgren. From: Pat Donoho. RE: Maryland OSHA grassroots funding. August 8, 1994. Bates no. 2024105518. Philip Morris Incorporated document site. Available at: http://www.pmdocs.com. Accessed March 12, 1999.
28. Dept of Licensing and Regulation, Division of Labor and Industry. 09.12.23 Prohibition on

smoking in an enclosed workplace, notice of proposed action. *Maryland Register*. 1994;21(8): 682–683.

29. Bero LA, Glantz SG. Tobacco industry response to a risk assessment of environmental tobacco smoke. *Tob Control*. 1993;2:103–113.
30. Gambrill ED. *Critical Thinking in Clinical Practice: Improving the Accuracy of Judgments and Decisions About Clients*. San Francisco, Calif: Jossey-Bass Publishers; 1990.
31. *H & G Restaurant Inc v Fogle* (Cir Ct Talbot Co 1994).
32. *Fogle v H & G Restaurant Inc* (Md Court of Appeals 1994).
33. Monardi F, Glantz SA. Are tobacco industry campaign contributions influencing state legislative behavior? *Am J Public Health*. 1998;88: 918–923.
34. Harris MS. Letter to Bruce Bereano from the executive vice president of the Restaurant Association of Maryland. February 17, 1993. Bates no. 2045919780. Philip Morris Incorporated document site. Available at: http://www.pmdocs.com. Accessed March 12, 1999.

Failure to Defend a Successful State Tobacco Control Program: Policy Lessons From Florida

Michael S. Givel, PhD, and Stanton A. Glantz, PhD

ABSTRACT

Objectives. This investigation sought to define policy and political factors related to the undermining of Florida's successful Tobacco Pilot Program in 1999.

Methods. Data were gathered from interviews with public health lobbyists, tobacco control advocates, and state officials; news reports; and public documents.

Results. As a result of a recent legal settlement with Florida, the tobacco industry agreed to fund a youth anti-smoking pilot program. The program combined community-based interventions and advertisements. In less than 1 year, the teen smoking prevalence rate dropped from 23.3% to 20.9%. The program also enjoyed high public visibility and strong public support. Nevertheless, in 1999, the state legislature cut the program's funding from $70.5 million to $38.7 million, and the Bush administration dismantled the program's administrative structure. Voluntary health agencies failed to publicly hold specific legislators and the governor responsible for the cuts.

Conclusions. The legislature and administration succeeded in dismantling this highly visible and successful tobacco control program because prohealth forces limited their activities to behind-the-scenes lobbying and were unwilling to confront the politicians who made these decisions in a public forum. (*Am J Public Health.* 2000;90:762–767)

On November 23, 1998, the attorneys general of 46 states signed a master settlement agreement with the tobacco industry that established a national tobacco control foundation and restricted certain industry advertising and other activities.[1] Payments to the states will total an estimated $206 billion through the first 25 years.[2] Before this settlement, the attorneys general of 4 states—Mississippi, Minnesota, Texas, and Florida—obtained separate monetary settlements and injunctive relief for various tobacco control efforts.[1]

Florida was the first state to enact legislation designed to make it easier to sue the tobacco industry for tobacco-caused illnesses. This enabling legislation began in the waning hours of the 1994 Florida legislative session, when Democratic Governor Lawton Chiles, working with trial lawyers and sympathetic politicians, quietly attached an amendment to a Senate Medicaid fraud bill to make it less difficult to sue the tobacco industry to recover Medicaid costs.[3] The amendment passed without public debate, and Chiles signed it on May 26, 1994.

During the 1995 legislative session, the tobacco industry and other powerful Florida business interests mounted a major campaign that convinced the legislature to repeal the law, but Chiles vetoed the repeal legislation. The campaign to repeal the legislation continued in the 1996 and 1997 legislative sessions, but Chiles defeated the repeal proposals.[3]

In February 1995, Florida sued the tobacco industry[4,5] to recoup costs for treating Florida Medicaid patients suffering from smoking-induced illnesses, to fund smoking cessation, to restrict tobacco marketing, and to fund an anti-tobacco education campaign.[6] On August 25, 1997, the tobacco industry settled with Florida[7,8] for $11.3 billion over 25 years, with additional comparable amounts paid in perpetuity; a total of $200 million was allocated to a 2-year program, the Tobacco Pilot Program, to reduce smoking among teens. The initial settlement agreement prohibited the Tobacco Pilot Program from attacking the tobacco industry, even though this message had proven effective in California.[9] After settlement of a similar case in Texas, on September 11, 1998,[10] Florida renegotiated its agreement to eliminate the 2-year time limit and prohibition against attacking the tobacco industry.

Under Chiles's leadership, Florida moved quickly to develop and implement an aggressive anti-tobacco education program, which was launched in March 1998. The Tobacco Pilot Program reduced the prevalence of smoking among Florida teenagers from 23.3% to 20.9% in less than a year.[11] Nevertheless, in the 1999 Florida legislative session, the Tobacco Pilot Program's funding was reduced from $70.5 million to $38.7 million for the 1999–2000 fiscal year, and the administration of new Republican Governor Jeb Bush initially announced that it was shifting the policy direction of the program away from the successful and aggressive counter-marketing anti-tobacco focus. The legislature and administration succeeded in dismantling this highly visible and successful tobacco control program, because prohealth forces limited their activities to behind-the-scenes lobbying and were unwilling to confront the politicians who made these decisions in a public forum.

This article chronicles the political events and key junctures in the decision-making process that led to this substantial weakening of the pilot program. It provides lessons for policymakers, public health advo-

The authors are with the Institute for Health Policy Studies, Department of Medicine, University of California, San Francisco.

Requests for reprints should be sent to Stanton A. Glantz, PhD, Box 0130, University of California, San Francisco, CA 94143 (e-mail: glantz@medicine.ucsf.edu).

This article was accepted November 5, 1999.

cates, and practitioners on what future political and public policy approaches may be taken to defend and maintain high-quality tobacco control programs.

Methods

Data were gathered from interviews with public health lobbyists (including Ralph Devitto, Brian Gilpin, and Brenda Olsen of the Tri-Agency Coalition on Smoking or Health), tobacco control advocates, and state officials; news reports; research reports; and government documents. Public health lobbyist interviewees were allowed to review and comment on a draft of our detailed report of these events.[3]

Results

Florida Tobacco Pilot Program

Because of the original settlement's requirement of completing a youth anti-smoking program within 2 years, efforts to establish the program occurred soon after Florida received its first tobacco settlement payment in February 1998. Many observers worried that the tobacco industry had insisted on the 2-year limit so as to not allow enough time for the program to be developed and implemented and measurable results to be achieved. Failure to obtain results could be used as a justification for eliminating the program. Chiles took this challenge seriously and quickly established the Tobacco Pilot Program to facilitate implementation.

The first high-profile step in developing the program occurred in March 1998, when 600 teenagers met at the Governor's Summit on Tobacco Education[12] to develop a tobacco control plan. Four program goals emerged[3,13]: changing youth attitudes regarding tobacco use, empowering youth to lead community involvement against tobacco, reducing the availability of tobacco products to youth, and reducing exposure to secondhand smoke. A new statewide organization called Students Working Against Tobacco was formed to coordinate this effort. On June 18 and 19, 1998, 67 local representatives of this organization and 4 at-large representatives met in St. Petersburg. At the meeting, the youth representatives elected a 10-member executive board and chairs and vice chairs for each of the 5 Tobacco Pilot Program components[3,13]: Marketing and Communications, Youth Programs and Community Partnerships, Education and Training, Enforcement, and Research and Evaluation.

The Truth Campaign

The most visible and popular component of the Tobacco Pilot Program was the large ($26 million over 12 months) anti-tobacco media "Truth Campaign," designed to discourage youth from using tobacco.[3,13] On the basis of guidance from the teens, the advertisements concentrated on discrediting tobacco use and the tobacco industry's allies in the advertising, publishing, and moviemaking businesses (and later, after the settlement had been renegotiated, the tobacco industry itself) rather than simply discussing the dangers of tobacco use. The major theme was "Their brand is lies. Our brand is Truth."

The campaign began in late April 1998. This first phase included tough, "in-your-face" print and broadcast advertisements throughout Florida. The second, ongoing phase of the campaign began in June 1998 with billboard advertisements in all major markets.[13] Finally, in late July 1998, a "truth train" filled with teenagers departed from Pensacola, Fla, on a 13-day, 1000-mile journey through the state to build awareness of the Truth Campaign, recruit new Students Working Against Tobacco members, and present a petition to Hollywood calling for the end of glamorization of tobacco in movies.[13]

An initial Florida State University study,[14] conducted for the Florida Department of Health and released in September 1998, indicated that teens were increasingly aware of the program. This study involved a pretest survey conducted in April 1998, before the media campaign started, and a posttest survey conducted in September 1998, after the media campaign had run for 5 months. About 28% of the youth indicated that they heard or saw 1 or more anti-tobacco advertisements daily. About 66% indicated that they heard or saw 1 or more anti-tobacco advertisements weekly. When all media sources were considered, 77% of the youth reported that they saw or heard 7 or more anti-tobacco advertisements weekly.

In just 5 months, knowledge of the Truth Campaign grew, with 57% of youth stating that they knew about the campaign and 87% reporting that they were aware of specific anti-tobacco messages. About 90% demonstrated confirmed awareness of the campaign or 1 or more of its components (e.g., anti-tobacco advertisements). Finally, 47% of the youth stated that tobacco companies were initiating deception in their advertisements—an increase of 6% from April 1998. There was also a 15% increase in young people who thought that tobacco companies were targeting youth to replace dying smokers. The program was successfully reaching its target audience.

Almost immediately, political opposition emerged to discount the evidence that the program was working. On November 11, 1998, Florida House Appropriations Chair Jim King (R, Jacksonville) questioned the initial results and called for the program to be substantially reduced.[15]

The 1999 Florida Legislative Session

On January 5, 1999, Republican Governor Jeb Bush took office. Despite some concerns that he would not support the Florida pilot project, Bush offered at least nominal support. On January 21, 1999, he urged that the anti-tobacco Truth Campaign be continued,[16] and on February 28, 1999, the Florida Department of Health asked the legislature for $61.5 million to continue the Tobacco Pilot Program.[17] Despite the fact that this proposal represented a $9 million cut from the $70.5 million funding in place at the time, no one in the health community protested.

The legislature proposed cutting the program even more. Early in the 1999 legislative session, an initial recommendation by Sen Ronald Silver (D, North Miami), chair of the Florida Senate Budget Subcommittee on Health and Human Services, called for a cut in the Tobacco Pilot Program by 30%.[18] Silver's justification for the cut was that he was not convinced that the program was working. Silver's subcommittee subsequently recommended funding the program at $50 million, a nearly 30% cut.[19] On March 18, 1999, the full Senate Budget Committee concurred.[20] Health community advocates did not hold specific politicians who supported this legislation publicly accountable for the budget cut.

In the House, the chair of the Budget Subcommittee on Health and Human Services Appropriations, Rep Debby Sanderson (R, Fort Lauderdale), called for eliminating the Tobacco Pilot Program[21] as early as January 1999, on the grounds that the program was not working.[20] With the encouragement of House Speaker John Thrasher (R, Orange Park) in mid-March, the full House Fiscal Responsibility Committee eliminated all funding for the program.[22] These actions by the Republican-dominated Senate and House placed them in nominal conflict with Republican Governor Bush. However, Bush did little to press the legislature to adopt his proposal to fund the Florida pilot program at $61.5 million.

The American Heart Association, American Lung Association, and American Cancer Society worked together as the Tri-Agency Coalition on Smoking or Health. Before these budget committee proposals were enacted in February and March 1999, the coalition approached newspaper editorial boards to obtain general editorial support for the Tobacco Pilot Program.[23] Several of these newspapers subsequently ran editorials during the 1999 legislative session urging the legislature not to cut its funding. Neither the coalition nor its constituent members, however, offered public criticism of any politician who was proposing to cut the program at any time during the debate.

Rather than protesting the $9 million cut that Bush proposed or fighting to maintain or expand program funding, the health groups decided that their best strategy would be to support Bush's proposal to cut the program to $61.5 million. In an early response to the proposed legislative budget cuts, the coalition ran political advertisements on March 8, 1999, in the *Fort Lauderdale Sun-Sentinel* and *Miami Herald* calling on voters to contact their elected South Florida representatives to support the governor's budget recommendation.[24] Significantly, the advertisements did not mention that some key South Florida legislators in the Florida Senate and House (particularly Senator Silver and Representative Sanderson) were actively working to drastically reduce or eliminate the Tobacco Pilot Program. In addition, when contacted by the media for comment on Sanderson's proposal to end the program, lobbyists for the coalition refused to criticize Sanderson or make any definitive comment.

In contrast to the coalition's refusal to confront specific politicians, about 40 teenage supporters of the Tobacco Pilot Program held a noisy demonstration at the state capitol on March 16, 1999.[25] Sanderson refused to meet with them.

The next day, March 17, the Florida Department of Health's Office of Tobacco Control issued a press release[26] announcing that, after less than a year of operation, the Tobacco Pilot Program was making significant progress. In a survey of more than 20000 Florida middle and high school students, the Florida Youth Tobacco Survey, 15.6% more middle and high school students than in the previous year said they definitely would not use tobacco in the future.[27] The percentage of teenagers who were current smokers (i.e., those who had smoked in the previous 30 days) dropped from 23.3% to 20.9% in the 9 months from April 1998 to February 1999, the most rapid decline in youth smoking ever produced in a large-scale tobacco control program. This change in prevalence represented 31000 teenagers in Florida who had decided not to smoke.

The department's press release explicitly credited the Truth Campaign's irreverent anti-industry campaign with this success: "A telephone survey of teens in September showed nine out of 10 teens were aware of the program's irreverent advertising campaign, dubbed 'Truth' by the teens who helped develop it. That September survey also showed teen attitudes about tobacco, especially those targeted by the advertising campaign, were changing in the right direction."[26]

TABLE 1—Budgetary Allocation for the Florida Tobacco Pilot Program: Fiscal Years 1998–1999 and 1999–2000 (Millions of Dollars)

Funding Category	1998–1999	1999–2000	Change, %
Marketing	26.0	12.0	−53.8
Education and training	15.0	7.0	−53.3
Youth and community partnerships	15.0	5.6	−62.7
Enforcement	8.5	5.1	−40.0
Minority programs	. . .	4.0	. . .
Evaluation	4.0	4.0	0
Administration	4.0	1.0	−75.0
Total	70.5	38.7	−45.1

Note. Data were derived from the Tri-Agency Coalition on Smoking or Health, the Florida Senate,[33] and Bush.[34]

Rather than rewarding the Tobacco Pilot Program management for this success, the same day the results were announced, Governor Bush and his secretary of health, Bob Brooks, forced the acting director of the Tobacco Pilot Program, Peter Mitchell, to resign.[25] In explaining why Mitchell was dismissed, Brooks said, "We have to head in a different direction with more education and cessation campaigns. His strength is marketing. We're headed in the other direction."[26]

The irony of firing Mitchell the same day that favorable results were announced attracted widespread media coverage as well as the interest of some of the Democrats in the legislature, who sought to use the controversy to engage the public in the battle over the program.[25] When contacted by the media regarding Mitchell's forced resignation, the health groups declined comment.

Despite the generally negative signals sent by the administration about the future funding, administrative, and policy direction of the Tobacco Pilot Program, a few days later, on March 23, 1999, representatives of the coalition joined Brooks in a news conference to laud the new findings of the Florida Youth Tobacco Survey.[28,29] None of the health groups raised obvious questions about the future direction or tone of the program, much less about Mitchell's firing.

On March 25, 1999, as a result of public awareness and the media pressure generated by Mitchell's firing,[30] the Florida Senate, with bipartisan sponsorship by Senate Minority Leader Buddy Dyer (D, Orlando) and Majority Leader Jack Latvala (R, Palm Harbor), increased the proposed funding of the program by $11 million to $61 million.[30] One day later, the Florida House increased its proposed budget from $0 to $30 million.[31]

On April 6, 1999, the coalition released the results of a poll conducted during March 1999 and commissioned by the Washington, DC-based Campaign for Tobacco Free Kids.[32] Poll results indicated that 81% of the voters thought that the Tobacco Pilot Program should be funded at least at the $61 million proposed by Governor Bush, with 57% preferring no cuts. The poll also indicated that 77% of the respondents were more likely to vote for a legislator who supported the program; only 14% reported that cutting the program in half would make them more likely to vote for a legislator. Despite these poll results, on April 30, 1999, the House and Senate adopted a compromise budget that substantially reduced spending for the Tobacco Pilot Program from the 1998–1999 budget of $70.5 million to a 1999–2000 budget of $45.2 million—a 36% reduction.[33]

At the same time that the legislature was considering the fate of the Tobacco Pilot Program, the American Heart Association was lobbying to create a $20 million youth program, the Youth Fitness Program. This comprehensive program, unrelated to tobacco control efforts, was to provide funding for schools to encourage children to exercise more and build healthier hearts (interview with Brian Gilpin, October 22, 1999). In the end, the legislature decided to appropriate up to $3 million for this program from Tobacco Pilot Program funds.[33] (The American Heart Association did not request that the Tobacco Pilot Program be used to fund its program.)

In its 1999 session, the legislature also agreed to allow, on a one-time basis, about $10 million in unspent carryover funds from the 1998–1999 budget to be used for the 1999–2000 budget. Allocation of these funds for specific programs such as the Truth Campaign or administrative support for Students Working Against Tobacco is discretionary, based on the administrative and policy prerogatives of the secretary of health and the governor.

On May 27, 1999, Governor Bush vetoed and also withheld funding of some elements of the anti-tobacco program (such as the American Heart Association's Youth Fitness Program) totaling $6.5 million.[34] This decision further reduced spending for the Tobacco Pilot Program to $38.7 million, a reduction of 45.1% from the preceding year[35] (Table 1). Among the line items that received the largest cuts were funding for administrative support of community-based Students Working Against Tobacco organizations, which now operate in all Florida counties (reduced by 62.7%); the Truth Campaign (53.8%); and administration (75%).

After the budget passed, the Bush administration acted quickly to dismantle the program. On June 2, 1999, a third of the Tobacco Pilot Program staff members were laid off or reassigned. Three high school students integral to the Students Working Against Tobacco effort, who were employed part-time at the program at $6 per hour, were also dismissed.[36] Furthermore, on July 1, 1999, the administration initiated a major reorganization, with the Youth Programs and Community Partnerships (which supports the student youth organizations) and Education and Training components, the Marketing and Communications component, and the Research and Evaluation component being moved to different sections of the Department of Health. The Enforcement component was transferred to the Florida Division of Business and Professional Regulation. This division into several administrative units made it more difficult for the program to function as a coordinated unit. The health groups did not protest these actions.

Discussion

Despite the unprecedented success of the Tobacco Pilot Program in reducing teen tobacco consumption in Florida, and despite broad public and editorial support, the program was severely weakened by legislative and administrative actions. This weakening is largely attributable to the unwillingness of the health community in Florida to sufficiently raise the political stakes to counter the pro-tobacco influences seeking to dismantle the program.

An early indicator that the health groups would not take strong action to defend the Tobacco Pilot Program was their failure to criticize proposals by Representative King (in November 1998) and by Representative Sanderson (in January 1999) to drastically reduce or eliminate its funding. This silence was reinforced when the health groups ran newspaper advertisements designed to rally public support for the program in March. Despite clear threats by King, Sanderson, and other politicians, the advertisements did not mention these individuals by name (which would have placed heightened public scrutiny and increased political pressure on them) or even indicate that cuts were imminent.

Instead, the advertisements simply urged readers to call various legislators to support Governor Bush's $61.5 million proposal for the program, even though Bush was proposing a substantial $9 million program cut. (The proposed amount, $61 million, which the coalition is also supporting for the 1999–2000 fiscal year, is less than the minimum funding level of $78.3 million for Florida recommended by the Centers for Disease Control and Prevention[37]; the maximum is $221.2 million.) In addition, by positioning themselves behind the governor, the health groups temporarily lost any chance to exert leverage on him during this crucial juncture in the policy-making process.

Moreover, in a news conference held jointly with the Bush administration, the coalition lauded the first-year results of the program. However, the coalition chose not to raise the issue of how the firing of the program director just days earlier signaled an administrative and policy shift by the Bush administration away from the program's aggressive and successful advertising campaign.

Late in the 1999 legislative session, as it became apparent that the Tobacco Pilot Program and the Truth Campaign were about to incur substantial budget cuts, the health groups continued to maintain their quiet insider approach of not publicly singling out specific legislators who were responsible for the cuts or urging the governor to vigorously campaign for full funding of the program. In addition, the American Heart Association's preoccupation with the Youth Fitness Program appears to have contributed to its reluctance to engage in such public actions of accountability. While the health groups did mobilize a private effort to lobby and pressure legislators, they did not go public with their actions.

Throughout the 1999 legislative session, the health groups engaged in policy-making as if they were powerful insiders with direct access to and influence over the decisions of public officials. Such insiders participate in an "iron triangle"[38-40] in which a small and informal but stable group of agency bureaucrats, legislative committee members, and interest groups are focused on the advancement of particular public policies and programs. In the iron triangle, interest groups lobby (including providing policy information) and provide electoral support (including campaign contributions) to legislative committee members. They also lobby bureaucrats. Bureaucrats administer the program with the policy support and input of the interest groups and provide constituent services for the legislative committee members. The legislative committee members provide favorable legislation for the interest groups and budget and program support for the bureaucrats. Of course, other legislators are needed to enact the program. However, they tend to defer to the policy preferences voiced by the groups of the iron triangle because they best understand the needs and intricacies of a program.

Some of these informal groupings of officials, lobbyists, and policy specialists have also been described as "issue networks" because they are looser than the iron triangle; that is, more policy experts are involved owing to the complexity and interconnectedness of modern policy problems. Nevertheless, the narrowly focused knowledge that influences the policies of legislative committees remains mostly the knowledge of those with a vested interest in the final policy. In theory, this insider power relationship under the iron triangle or issue network works to the advantage of each of its participants. Such an arrangement has existed for years in Florida with regard to tobacco, with pro-tobacco interests dominating the state legislature through a combination of campaign contributions and well-connected lobbyists.[3]

With the health groups, however, this was not the case. Although the health groups lobbied the key Florida legislative committees and subcommittees, the Department of Health, and the governor's office as if they were part of an iron triangle (without the assistance of a network of policy experts) to maintain the integrity of the Tobacco Pilot Program, neither the key legislative members nor the Department of Health acquiesced to their insider lobbying efforts. The health groups provided both the legislature and the administration with reasoned arguments, but they were not able to back up this insider effort with either significant campaign contributions or election support (both of which are provided with great abundance by the tobacco industry). At the same time, they were unwilling to deny the politicians popular support by publicly criticizing them for their pro-tobacco stands.

The health groups' power lies in outside lobbying, which brings pressure to bear on public officials in terms of accountability for their actions. This approach is particularly effective if the policy has wide public support, which existed in the case of the Tobacco Pilot Program, and if the advocate has high public credibility, which the health groups did. The primary outside lobbying tactics (used in tandem with the insider lobbying approaches) that could have been used during the legislative session were newspaper advertisements highlighting negative and positive actions of specific legislators and members of the administration, public demonstrations, and media interviews that would reach a large audience and hold specific public officials publicly accountable for their actions. The decision by the health groups to avoid these approaches contributed to their failure to defend the program.

This broad policy lesson has already been observed in other states. For instance, health groups in California[41] lost ground on the state's anti-tobacco program for years using insider tactics[42] to oppose actions by Republican Governor Pete Wilson and the Democratic legislature to cut funding for the program and weaken the successful anti-tobacco media campaign by watering down messages and politicizing the approval process for advertising. In a change in strategy, these health groups, led by the American Heart Association and Americans for Nonsmokers' Rights, used a high-profile series of paid advertisements and free media to pressure Wilson and the legislature to restore funding for the program and toughen the advertisements.[42,43]

In Massachusetts,[44,45] when Republican Governor William Weld proposed to divert anti-tobacco funds to other programs, the health groups compromised on an insider deal that allowed diversion of funds to non-tobacco activities. Later, when Weld attempted to cut the program even more drastically, the health groups, led by the American Cancer Society, took him on publicly and forced him to back down.[46] In Arizona,[47,48] health groups prevented diversion of anti-tobacco funds to other programs but failed to protest when the director of the program was removed because she was perceived as having an overly anti-tobacco stance. The result has been a weak program.

Another factor that may have contributed to this failure is the fact that health groups such as the American Cancer Society, the American Lung Association, and the American Heart Association have multiple goals, not just the reduction of tobacco use. Concern that strong action on tobacco could alienate political support in other areas has often led these groups to avoid the kinds of confrontational strategies that are necessary to prevail in battles over tobacco.[49] Indeed, during the battle over the Tobacco Pilot Program, the American Heart Association was giving passage of its Youth Fitness Program priority. This situation of conflicting goals and diffuse public interest[50,51] contrasts with the situation of the tobacco industry, a single-interest group with a direct financial stake in the outcome.

The situation in Florida provides important lessons for public health advocates everywhere. In 1998, all states participated in some sort of settlement of litigation with the tobacco industry, which produced more than $200 billion over 25 years.[7] A portion of this money could provide significant funding for anti-tobacco programming; as of this writing, however, few states have allocated funds for substantial anti-tobacco programs.

In the final analysis, the voluntary agencies in Florida were advocating for a popular, high-profile program that had achieved stunning results. If they had been willing to use outside lobbying tactics that have been used successfully by health groups in other parts of the country—or, for that matter, by most other interest groups—the likelihood of the Tobacco Pilot Program's not being weakened would have substantially increased. Voluntary health agencies need to make tobacco prevention their top priority and allocate the necessary financial and political resources. They must also be willing to take high-profile public positions in support of programs and to highlight those politicians advocating pro-tobacco positions. Otherwise, it is unlikely that they will succeed in defending these programs, even with their proven efficacy and popularity. If voluntary health agencies are to secure and defend high-quality tobacco control programs, they will have to learn this practical political lesson and change their behavior accordingly. □

Contributors

Both authors contributed to the design of the study, the analysis of the results, and the writing of the paper.

Acknowledgments

This work was supported by National Cancer Institute grant CA-61021, American Cancer Society grant CCG-294, and Tobacco-Related Disease Research Program grant 8FT-0095.

References

1. Daynard R, Enrich P, Parmet W, et al. *The Multistate Master Settlement Agreement and the Future of State and Local Tobacco Control: An Analysis of Selected Topics and Provisions of the Multistate Master Settlement Agreement of November 23, 1998.* Boston, Mass: Tobacco Control Resource Center, Northeastern University School of Law; 1999.
2. *Attorney General Announces Tobacco Settlement Proposal.* Olympia: Attorney General's Office of Washington; 1998.
3. Givel M, Glantz S. *Tobacco Industry Political Power and Influence in Florida From 1979 to 1999.* San Francisco: Institute for Health Policy Studies, University of California, San Francisco; 1999.
4. Woo J. Tobacco firms face greater health liability. *Wall Street Journal.* May 3, 1994:A1, A3.
5. Nickins T. With smoke and mirrors, he beat big tobacco. *Miami Herald.* March 14, 1995:1A, 5A.
6. *State of Florida, et al. v The American Tobacco Company, et al.*, Civil Action NP 95-1466-AH (Fla 1995).
7. Fox B, Lightwood J, Glantz S. *A Public Health Analysis of the Proposed Resolution of the United States Tobacco Litigation.* San Francisco: Institute for Health Policy Studies, University of California, San Francisco; 1998.
8. *Stipulation of Amendment to Settlement Agreement and for Entry of Consent Decree in Case of: State of Florida, et al. v The American Tobacco Company, et al.* Tallahassee: Florida Attorney General's Office; 1997.
9. Goldman L, Glantz S. Evaluation of antismoking advertising campaigns. *JAMA.* 1998;229:772–777.
10. *Participating Florida Counsel Agreement in Case of: State of Florida, et al. v The American Tobacco Company, et al.* Tallahassee: Florida Attorney General's Office; 1998.
11. *1999 Florida Youth Tobacco Survey.* Tallahassee, Fla: Florida Dept of Health; 1999.
12. *The Chiles/Mackay Years 1991–1998: This Time the People Won.* Tallahassee: Florida Governor's Office; 1998.
13. *Florida Tobacco Pilot Program Experts Meeting.* Tallahassee: Florida Tobacco Pilot Program; 1998.
14. *Florida Anti-Tobacco Media Evaluation: Report on September 1998 Survey Results.* Tallahassee: Florida State University; 1998.
15. McKinnon J. Lawmaker questions the effectiveness of antismoking ads. *Wall Street Journal.* November 11, 1998:F4.
16. Wallsten P. Bush proposes to honor Chiles [*St. Petersburg Times* Web site]. January 21, 1999. Available at: http://www.sptimes.com/News/12199/State/Bush_proposes_to_hono.html. Accessed March 4, 1999.
17. Florida's key legislative issues for 1999. *Tallahassee Democrat.* February 28, 1999:A9.
18. Klas M. House panel moves to end teen smoking effort. [*Palm Beach Post* Web site]. March 16, 1999. Available at: http://gopbi.com:80/news/1999/03/16/smoke.html. Accessed March 24, 1999.
19. Kennedy J. 'Truth' drive director is ousted. [*Orlando Sentinel* Web site]. March 18, 1999. Available at: http://www.orlandosentinel.com/news/legislature/s031899_smoke18_20.htm. Accessed March 25, 1999.
20. Clark L. State ads against teen smoking imperiled. *Miami Herald.* March 13, 1999:A1.
21. Kennedy J, Perez R. State house may pull plug on 'truth.' [*Orlando Sentinel* Web site]. March 12, 1999. Available at: http://www.orlandosentinel.com/news/legislature/s031299_smoke12.htm. Accessed March 24, 1999.
22. Kassab B. Students sense runaround, antismoking plea stalls at capitol. [*Florida Times-Union* Web site]. March 17, 1999. Available at: http://www.jacksonville.com/tu-online/stories/

031799/met_2b5stude.html. Accessed May 17, 1999.

23. *Tri-Agency Editorial Board Visits.* Tallahassee, Fla: Tri-Agency Coalition on Smoking or Health; 1999.
24. *Help Governor Bush Use Tobacco Dollars for Tobacco Prevention.* Tallahassee, Fla: Tri-Agency Coalition on Smoking or Health; 1999.
25. Clark L. Director of anti-smoking campaign says he was asked to quit. *Miami Herald.* March 17, 1999:B1.
26. *More Kids Are Saying No to Smoking* [press release]. Tallahassee: Florida Office of Tobacco Control, Marketing Office; 1999.
27. Pierce J, Choi WS, Gilpin EA, Farkas AJ, Merritt RK. Validation of susceptibility as a predictor of which adolescents take up smoking in the United States. *Health Psychol.* 1996;15:355–361.
28. Bauman C. *Public Health Advocates Release Tobacco Survey Results.* Tallahassee: Florida Tobacco Pilot Program; 1999.
29. Wallsten P. Cancer society joins democrats in tobacco fight: the charity's officials encounter partisan bickering they don't understand. [*St. Petersburg Times* Web site]. March 24, 1999. Available at: http://www.sptimes.com/News/32499/State/Cancer_society_joins_.html. Accessed March 24, 1999.
30. Clark L. Senate adds $11 million to anti-smoking fight. [*Miami Herald* Web site]. March 25, 1999. Available at: http://www.herald.com/search?NS-search-pa...erald&NS-docs-matched=20&NS-doc-number = 42. Accessed July 12, 1999.
31. Silva M. House yields to pressure, restores funding for anti-tobacco campaign. *Miami Herald.* March 27, 1999:B5.
32. Thorp J, Williams S. *Florida Voters Want the "Truth."* Tallahassee, Fla: Tri-Agency Coalition on Smoking or Health; 1999.
33. *Conference Report on Senate Bill 2500: General Appropriations for 1999–2000.* Tallahassee: Florida Senate; 1999.
34. Bush J. *Governor's Veto Message of May 27, 1999.* Tallahassee: Florida Governorís Office; 1999.
35. *Continuing the Fight: Florida Tobacco Pilot Program—Year 2.* Tallahassee: Florida Tobacco Pilot Program; 1999.
36. Clark L. Anti-tobacco ad staff reduced; activists alarmed. [*Miami Herald* Web site]. June 3, 1999. Available at: http://www.herald.com/content/today/news/florida/digdocs/035563.htm. Accessed June 3, 1999.
37. Centers for Disease Control and Prevention. *Best Practices for Comprehensive Tobacco Control Programs.* Atlanta, Ga: Office on Smoking and Health; 1999.
38. Freeman L. *The Political Process.* New York, NY: Random House; 1965.
39. Hamm K. Patterns of influence among committees, agencies, and interest groups. *Legislative Stud Q.* 1983;8:378–426.
40. Miroff B, Seidelman R, Swanstron T. *The Democratic Debate: An Introduction to American Politics.* New York, NY: Houghton Mifflin; 1998.
41. Balbach E, Glantz S. Tobacco control advocates must demand high-quality media campaigns: the California experience. *Tob Control.* 1998;7:397–408.
42. Glantz S, Balbach E. *Tobacco War: Inside the California Battles.* Berkeley: University of California Press; 2000.
43. Begay ME, Traynor M, Glantz SA. The tobacco industry, state politics, and tobacco education in California. *Am J Public Health.* 1993;83:1214–1221.
44. Begay M, Glantz S. Question 1 tobacco education expenditures in Massachusetts. *Tob Control.* 1997;6:213–218.
45. Heiser PF, Begay ME. The campaign to raise the tobacco tax in Massachusetts. *Am J Public Health.* 1997;87:968–973.
46. Phillips F. Weld maps $70M smoking fight, 18-month plan for funds from new cigarette tax. *Boston Globe.* February 22, 1993:1, 6.
47. Aguinaga S, Glantz S. *Tobacco Control in Arizona, 1973–1997.* San Francisco: University of California, San Francisco; 1997.
48. Bialous S, Glantz SA. Arizona's tobacco control initiative illustrates the need for continuing oversight by tobacco control advocates. *Tob Control.* In press.
49. Jacobson P. *Tobacco Control Laws: Implementation and Enforcement.* Santa Monica, Calif: Rand Corp; 1997.
50. Schattschneider E. *Semi Sovereign People: A Realist's View of Democracy in America.* New York, NY: Harcourt Brace Jovanovich; 1975.
51. Kingdon JW. *Agendas, Alternatives, and Public Policies.* New York, NY: HarperCollins College Publishers; 1995.

Tobacco Industry Allegations of "Illegal Lobbying" and State Tobacco Control

Stella Aguinaga Bialous, DrPH, MScN, Brion J. Fox, JD, and Stanton A. Glantz, PhD

ABSTRACT

Objectives. This study assessed the perceived effect of tobacco industry allegations of "illegal lobbying" by public health professionals on policy interventions for tobacco control.

Methods. Structured interviews were conducted with state health department project managers in all 17 National Cancer Institute–funded American Stop Smoking Intervention Study (ASSIST) states. Documentation and media records related to ASSIST from the National Cancer Institute, health advocates, and the tobacco industry were analyzed.

Results. The tobacco industry filed formal complaints of illegal lobbying activities against 4 ASSIST states. These complaints had a temporary chilling effect on tobacco control policy interventions in those states. ASSIST states not targeted by the tobacco industry developed an increased awareness of the industry's tactics and worked to prepare for such allegations to minimize disruption of their activities. Some self-reported self-censorship in policy activity occurred in 11 of the 17 states (65%).

Conclusions. Public health professionals need to educate themselves and the public about the laws that regulate lobbying activities and develop their strategies, including their policy activities, accordingly. (*Am J Public Health.* 2001;91:62–67)

In 1988, the Institute of Medicine[1] identified policy development as one of public health's core functions and emphasized the need for public health practitioners to be more politically involved in developing and implementing policy changes to improve the public's health. Public health professionals have shown the value of public policy interventions to reduce tobacco use, including clean indoor air laws[2–7] and tobacco tax increases.[8–13]

Policy interventions were at the center of 2 large-scale government tobacco control efforts: California's Proposition 99 Tobacco Control Program,[14] started in 1989, and the National Cancer Institute's (NCI's) American Stop Smoking Intervention Study (ASSIST), started in 1991. ASSIST was a 7-year, 17-state, federally funded comprehensive tobacco control project, in partnership with the American Cancer Society (ACS), state health departments, and public and private organizations, that emphasized the policy dimension in tobacco control.[15]

Both the California program and ASSIST required formation of tobacco control coalitions of health, business, and education groups. These coalitions work with, but are not part of, the health departments. Both programs significantly accelerated the decline in tobacco consumption. In the early years of the California program, the rate of decline in tobacco consumption tripled compared with historical rates,[8] and prevalence declined 1.9 times faster than in the rest of the United States.[16–18] Per capita cigarette consumption in ASSIST states was significantly lower than consumption in non-ASSIST states; by 1996, this difference reached 7%.[19]

The tobacco industry understood the potential effectiveness of these policy-based public health interventions and decided to take action against these programs.[20,21] A Philip Morris internal memorandum written around 1991, as ASSIST was starting, observed: "In California our biggest challenge has not been the anti-smoking advertising. . . . Rather it has been the creation of an anti-smoking infrastructure, right down to the local level. . . . ASSIST will hit us in our most vulnerable areas—in the localities and in the private workplace. It has the potential to peel away from the industry many of its historic allies."[22] By 1992, Philip Morris identified the strategy of claiming that federal funds were being used for "illegal lobbying" as a way to forestall the development and implementation of tobacco control policies. Philip Morris' "Counter Assist Plan" included

> 1) Congressional Investigation: . . . A more thorough investigation should be launched, particularly in terms of the NCI/ACS relationship and the use of federal funds for state and local lobbying purposes. With the current budget debate in Washington, this would be a good time to launch an investigation. Various tax and fiscally-responsible organizations could get involved. This should be coordinated with the Washington office.
> 2) Legal Challenges: Washington Legal Foundation/other groups could at the same time launch concurrent injunctive challenges in ASSIST states to stop dispersal of funds while the Congressional investigation is going on as well as to determine whether the program violates Federal or state ethics/Lobbying laws.[23]

Groups linked with the tobacco industry, such as the American Smokers Alliance, have been key to implementation of this strategy. Consistent with earlier industry strategies,[20] a 1995 American Smokers Alliance newsletter urged readers to use the Freedom of Information Act to collect information to make allegations of misuse of taxpayers' funds and provided guidelines for "concerned citizens" to

The authors are with the Institute for Health Policy Studies, Cardiovascular Research Institute, Department of Medicine, University of California, San Francisco.

Requests for reprints should be sent to Stanton A. Glantz, PhD, Cardiovascular Research Institute, University of California, San Francisco, San Francisco, CA 94143-0130 (e-mail: glantz@medicine.ucsf.edu).

This article was accepted July 18, 2000.

discover and stop "illegal lobbying activities" by tobacco control advocates.[24]

Lobbying with public funds is restricted in all states and the federal government; each has adopted a definition of lobbying that reflects different purposes and different federal, state, and local influences. (To describe all of the federal, state, and local laws addressing lobbying is beyond the scope of this paper.) These restrictions on lobbying do not mean that public health officials cannot do policy work but rather that rules exist for what they can do and how they can do it. Indeed, several laws regulating lobbying by public employees provide exceptions for public employees communicating with government officials and others in the conduct of their official duties.

To assess the perceived effect of tobacco industry claims of "illegal lobbying" on tobacco control activities, we examined the ASSIST states. (This study was meant not to assess the legitimacy of the claims or the value of the laws restricting lobbying behavior but merely to acquire a better understanding of public health officials' perceptions and responses to claims of "illegal lobbying.") We found that the tobacco industry's strategy of accusing public health professionals of "illegal lobbying" has had a self-reported chilling effect on some activities to implement tobacco control policies.

Methods

We identified the 4 ASSIST states—Colorado, Washington, Minnesota, and Maine—where formal complaints about the use of taxpayers' funds for allegedly illegal activities were filed. (New Jersey had a formal investigation by the inspector general against one of the ASSIST grantees, but we could not trace it to the tobacco industry. ASSIST was found innocent of any misuse of federal funds.) We collected documentation of these charges, formal responses, newspaper and other media reports, and information about these incidents from the NCI.

To test whether these 4 incidents had a broader effect on the ASSIST project, we conducted structured interviews with the state health department's project director or project manager in all 17 ASSIST states (Colorado, Indiana, Massachusetts, Maine, Michigan, Minnesota, Missouri, North Carolina, New Jersey, New Mexico, New York, Rhode Island, South Carolina, Virginia, Washington, Wisconsin, West Virginia), with assurances that individual responses would be kept confidential and anonymous. The interview contained 17 questions and an opportunity for interviewee comments. The interview questionnaire was designed to elicit the knowledge and perception of the interviewee without disclosing the underlying hypothesis of the research. The interview focused on 3 different themes: (1) the individual's knowledge of the laws restricting various lobbying activities; (2) the individual's assessment as to whether the laws themselves affect public health behavior; and (3) the individual's assessment as to whether third-party claims of illegal lobbying, either formal or informal, affected public health behavior. We also reviewed NCI written records related to ASSIST and conducted a limited review of the tobacco industry documents from the Minnesota Tobacco Document Depository and available on the Internet at Web sites maintained by the tobacco industry. This review was to confirm the hypothesis that the tobacco industry considered allegations of illegal lobbying as a strategy against tax-funded state and local tobacco control efforts.

Our results represent a view into the interaction between public health behavior and the lobbying laws in the area of tobacco control as self-reported by selected members of the ASSIST states. Results are based on self-report. Others who were involved in the process, including representatives of the tobacco industry, may have had a different perspective on these events.

Document data collection was limited to documents necessary to confirm or clarify a point made in the interviews and were mostly obtained from the NCI files. Many more documents relevant to ASSIST likely exist, but a complete search of these documents was beyond the scope of this paper.

Results

Colorado

In the early 1990s, 5 complaints were filed against tobacco control professionals and volunteers and the Colorado Department of Health, alleging the misuse of public funds and misconduct of government employees, allegedly for illegitimate political purposes. Although the cases did not all address the specific issue of illegal lobbying, claims of illegal lobbying were part of a campaign to disrupt public health activities. During this time, tobacco control advocates were attempting to develop and pass a $0.50 per pack tobacco tax increase initiative; some of the revenues would be used to fund antitobacco education programs. (The initiative was defeated in November 1994, 61% to 39%.[25]) The 5 complaints were as follows:

1. In March 1994, the Colorado Department of Health began to receive requests for public records based on Colorado's Open Records Law and the US Freedom of Information Act. These requests came from the Hays, Hays and Wilson, Inc, lobbying/law firm, which represented the Tobacco Institute, and included requests for records of the Coalition for a Tobacco Free Colorado, which were stored at the Colorado Department of Health. To protect the privacy of Coalition for a Tobacco Free Colorado records, a Coalition for a Tobacco Free Colorado officer removed them from the Colorado Department of Health after the request was filed.

A lawsuit was filed by the tobacco industry to obtain the Coalition for a Tobacco Free Colorado records after they had been removed from the Colorado Department of Health. Tobacco industry attorneys argued that because these records were at the Colorado Department of Health, they were public, and the Colorado District Court determined that because state employees had access to the records, they were public and had to be disclosed. The information obtained was used by the tobacco industry to discredit a pending media campaign in the press and to discourage potential bidders for the campaign (S.L. Temko, Covington & Burling, written communication to Edward Robbins, The Robert Wood Johnson Foundation, July 12, 1994; F.L. Hayes III, Hays, Hays & Wilson Inc, written communication, July 15, 1994). Nonetheless, the Colorado Department of Health received 2 bids and ran the media campaign (S. Young, MD, oral communication, February 1999).

2. The tobacco industry–funded group Citizens Against Tax Abuse and Government Waste filed a complaint with the secretary of state against ACS volunteers.[25–27] The complaint alleged that ACS volunteers were bribing voters to sign a petition for the 1994 tobacco tax initiative because they were collecting signatures at the same place where a Denver, Colo, radio station, KOA, was sponsoring a nonsmoking campaign. The ACS made the complaint public, and KOA publicized it. The plaintiff then dropped the complaint.[26,27]

3. The American Constitutional Law Foundation filed a complaint in July 1994 with the Colorado secretary of state that alleged that the Pueblo City and County Health Departments, Colorado Department of Health, and Snip Young, then director of the Colorado Department of Health Division of Prevention Programs, had helped to plan the tobacco tax initiative that was going to be on the November 1994 ballot.[28] (The American Constitutional Law Foundation received $60000 in 1995 from the Tobacco Institute.[29]) The secretary of state rejected most of the allegations, except for 3 violations.[30] One of the violations related to the publishing of factual information about the initiative in an ASSIST newsletter before the campaign had formally begun but after the initiative received a title, which was inappropriate.[31] The other 2 violations referred to Young's efforts to promote the initiative.

4. In September 1994, Citizens Against Tax Abuse filed a fourth complaint with the secretary of state against the Fair Share for Health Committee, the nonprofit organization that was created to pass the tobacco tax initiative, and its chairman, Arnold Levinson, alleging that the campaign had not disclosed 63 in-kind contributions that the Colorado Department of Health had made to the tax campaign.[26,32] On March 16, 1995, the secretary of state determined that 3 items should have been reported, and the Fair Share for Health Committee amended its campaign contribution reports as required.

5. The American Constitutional Law Foundation and Colorado Smokers' Alliance filed a federal civil suit with the Denver Federal District Court in September 1994 against the Colorado Department of Health and the Boulder County Health Department and specific staff, charging them with interfering with the petition process, using "government funds, resources and facilities to promote private and/or agency agendas," and violating several federal constitutional guarantees.[33] The suit was dismissed in February 14, 1995, because of lack of evidence; it was appealed and dimissed again on May 4, 1995, in response to the motion to dismiss.

Tobacco control advocates in Colorado contacted the media to denounce these allegations as a tobacco industry strategy to disrupt tobacco control activities and to create controversy around the tobacco tax initiative by questioning its propriety. However, most of the media reports focused on the accusations of illegal activities by government employees and questioned how much involvement in an initiative campaign was appropriate.[26,34]

The series of allegations made tobacco control advocates temporarily wary about conducting more aggressive policy work, but since then, activities have resumed as planned (S. Young, MD, oral communication, February 1999).[25]

Washington State

Between March and October 1995, the Washington State Health Department received 3 letters containing a total of 49 requests for -ASSIST-related documents under the state Freedom of Information Act.[35] The law firm Byrnes and Keller sent the letters on behalf of Stuart Cloud, owner of a chain of smoke shops (stores selling smoking paraphernalia) in Seattle, Wash.[36] Although the local smoke shop owner was the client and presented himself as a "concerned citizen," the Tobacco Institute paid the legal bills. (Washington Health Department staff discovered that the Tobacco Institute was paying the law firm when they noticed that the courier service slip that accompanied the request for documents listed the Tobacco Institute as the law firm's client.[35]) In the letters, requests were made not only for documents related to the activities of the Tobacco Free Washington Coalition, which is partly funded by ASSIST, but also for documents related to the activities and funding details of individual coalition members. After Cloud received the documents, he filed a 425-page complaint with the Washington Public Disclosure Commission in November 1995, charging Project ASSIST with illegally using taxpayer funds to conduct lobbying activities through the coalition.[37,38]

Members of the coalition and of the health department denied wrongdoing and developed a media plan to publicize the complaint, stressing that the complaint was financed by the Tobacco Institute. They successfully framed the issue as an attempt by the tobacco industry to harass and intimidate tobacco control professionals.[38,39] Nonetheless, even though coalition members understood that restrictions on using ASSIST funds for lobbying did not preclude them from using private funds to do so, some of them became reluctant to get involved in advocacy activities that used private funds or even to talk to public officials about tobacco control because of concern that their actions would be misinterpreted as illegal lobbying.[35] The issue was not the legal restrictions but the tobacco industry's often frivolous allegations, which, despite being frivolous, nevertheless must be addressed.

As reported in the Public Disclosure Commission Report of the Investigation on the claims of illegal lobbying, Washington ASSIST Project Manager Kim Dalthrop linked the decision to pursue a more cautious approach to public policy-making activities directly to the presence of tobacco industry complaints.[40]

In December 1999, the Washington Public Disclosure Commission issued a final order that implemented a stipulated agreement between the commission enforcement staff and the health department.[41] In this agreement, the department conceded that it unintentionally violated the state statute requiring the disclosure of lobbying expenses by failing to disclose the funding of 4 separate program activities. The penalty imposed on the department was a $2500 fine and the implementation of a departmental training program regarding compliance with the lobbying laws.[41]

Minnesota

Beginning in September 1993, a series of requests for documents were filed with Project ASSIST by tobacco industry allies, such as the Minnesota Grocers Association and the Minnesota Candy & Tobacco Association,[42,43] (also T. Briant, Minnesota Candy and Tobacco Association Inc, written communication to Alice O'Connor, The Tobacco Institute, February 20, 1991) which led to a complaint filed by the Minnesota Grocers Association with the Minnesota Ethical Practices Board and to a letter to the state auditor alleging unlawful use of federal taxpayer dollars in October 1995.[44] The complaint accused 16 groups that were ASSIST grantees of misusing ASSIST funds by encouraging stronger tobacco control laws and of violating the state's lobbying disclosure rules. Tobacco control professionals used the media to denounce these complaints as an attempt by the tobacco industry to intimidate them.[45]

The timing of the complaint coincided with the introduction of youth access legislation in the legislature. The youth access legislation was defeated. Tobacco control advocates in Minnesota believed that the complaints had a temporary chilling effect on tobacco control activities. Jeanne Weigum of the Association for Nonsmokers–Minnesota told the *Los Angeles Times*: "But the complaint still had an impact. They wanted people such as myself to be intimidated and fearful and confused—and at least to some extent they succeeded. Truly, we did almost nothing in the way of tobacco control for about three months."[45]

In January 1996, the State Ethical Practices Board fully exonerated 14 of the groups from any wrongdoing and cited the other 2 for minor violations. One group had failed to report $15 worth of staff time used in preparing an op-ed piece as a lobbying expense, and the other failed to report a $40 expense.[45]

Maine

In spring 1997, Maine was considering legislation to increase the tobacco excise tax. Jon Doyle, from the law firm Doyle & Nelson (which lobbied on behalf of the Tobacco Institute), distributed a notebook titled *Survey of DHS ASSIST Files* at the legislative hearing, which described how taxpayers' money had been wasted on tobacco control efforts in Maine. The information was presumably obtained through a large Freedom of Information Act request submitted to the Maine Department of Health in November 1996 by attorney Peter Dawson (with no known ties to the tobacco industry) (D. Mills, MD, personal communication, 1999).

This effort of derailing the tax effort failed, and the tax doubled from $0.37 to $0.74 per pack of cigarettes.

In April 1997, Jon Doyle sent a letter to the attorney general making 3 allegations of misuse of ASSIST money by the Maine Department of Health[46]: (1) use of money for lobbying activities, (2) failure to follow state bidding procedures, and (3) inappropriate use of monies and/or personnel to negatively influence clients of law firms representing the tobacco companies. The accusations that ASSIST money was used for illegal lobbying activities were very broad and insinuated that those activities occurred at both the state and the local level through contacts with local policymakers, efforts to pass state legislation to repeal existing laws that prevented communities from enacting tobacco control laws, and efforts to pass local tobacco control ordinances.

On May 19, 1997, the Maine attorney general wrote to Doyle & Nelson and refuted all allegations of illegal or inappropriate conduct by the Maine Department of Health staff or its grantees. For example, the attorney general stated that the director of public health for the city of Portland, Me, in her professional capacity, "had a right to discuss public health issues with a state representative."[47] He also concluded that there was no wrongdoing on the part of Coalition for a Tobacco Free Maine members, who had contact with state legislators either at their request or for educational purposes. More important, in this response, the attorney general referred to the laws governing the use of ASSIST funds, such as 42 USC §284-289 and 31 USC §1352, and expressly declined to provide Doyle & Nelson a state and federal definition of lobbying. He stated the following:

> I am using the term "lobbying" in the most generic, commonly-understood sense for purposes of making a point. If there appeared to be actual violations of state or federal law prohibiting "lobbying", it would then be necessary to apply the actual legal definition of lobbying under federal or state law. We have not done this, for as explained in this letter, there is not sufficient evidence to find that any "illegal" lobbying has taken place.[47]

The other 2 complaints also were dismissed because no evidence substantiated the charges of violating the bidding process or engaging in other inappropriate use of ASSIST monies. With the support from the attorney general and the knowledge of public health professionals, these accusations did not lead to a disruption of the work of tobacco control professionals in Maine, except for the labor involved in responding to the Freedom of Information Act request and to Doyle's letter.

Reaction to These Events in the 17 ASSIST States

All 17 interviewees believed that public health professionals in their state had a good understanding of the limitations imposed by lobbying laws restrictions, and 5 added that to maintain this level of understanding, ongoing education on the issue of lobbying is necessary. Three respondents thought that the lobbying restrictions limited the policy accomplishments of ASSIST; they used words such as "curtail," "timid," "chilling," and "hands-tied." However, at least 12 of the states overcame these limitations by working in close partnership with coalition members not affected by lobbying restrictions and focusing on local-level policy development. These states did not perceive the lobbying restrictions as having an effect on achieving ASSIST goals. Only 3 states responded that some groups involved with - ASSIST chose to focus on activities that did not involve policy changes.

Although formal complaints of improper use of taxpayer funds occurred in only 4 of the ASSIST states, tobacco control professionals in all 17 ASSIST states were aware of them. When asked if they were aware of informal complaints against ASSIST on the basis of using funds for illegal lobbying in their state, 11 of the 17 interviewees (65%) said "yes." Informal complaints were in the form of contacts with legislators, letters to the editors or articles in newspapers, and testimony at hearings or open meetings and were made by tobacco lobbyists, members of the press, members of trade associations, and individuals (often, but not always, linked to tobacco interests).

The effect of these informal complaints varied from no effect at all to strengthening the tobacco control professionals' determination. Five states felt so secure in their knowledge of the lobbying restrictions that such allegations had no effect. However, 4 states felt that the allegations created anxiety, even if unfounded, and led people to act more conservatively. The desire to avoid creating an impression of illegal lobbying often motivated states to avoid activities that were legal but that could be perceived by the public and the tobacco industry as illegal.

When asked if public health professionals were self-censoring their behavior because of fears that claims of illegal lobbying would be made against them (i.e., not doing things that they would otherwise do if there were no threat of allegations of illegal lobbying activities), 6 states said "yes," 5 states said "yes to a certain degree," and 6 states said "no." Thus, fear of allegations of illegal lobbying led public health professionals to report self-censoring their activities to some degree in 11 of the 17 states (65%). For example, the states that said "yes" or "yes to a certain degree" claimed that after allegations of illegal lobbying were made against ASSIST, people became more careful and more aware of the amount of scrutiny they were operating under, and when in doubt, they chose to err on the side of caution. They also believed that this caution was justified to avoid the administrative burden that accompanies those claims, which they feared could effectively shut down the program. In addition, not all ASSIST states felt that their attorney general would be supportive if a claim were made against them. States also said that they became more aware of the public perception of what can be viewed as lobbying activity, thus avoiding controversy.

The states that said that there was no self-censorship claimed that public health professionals were well aware of the limitations and felt comfortable developing activities within the restrictions imposed by law. They said that professionals had an increased awareness of the limitations, although that did not affect the development of their actions. Those states also claimed that having a strong communication network helped them keep within the boundaries and develop activities with other partners who were not restricted by lobbying laws.

Discussion

The tobacco industry has used various strategies in an attempt to disrupt tobacco control efforts by administratively burdening public health agencies and groups. For example, as has been discussed earlier in this paper, the tobacco industry routinely uses the Freedom of Information Act as a tool to slow the implementation of tobacco control programs[20,45] and has systematically requested ASSIST states to provide program-related documents. The tobacco industry, through different representatives (lawyers, front groups, local businesses), has requested many documents from state and local health departments. At first, health department employees were not prepared to respond to such demands, and, as a consequence, their work was disrupted. As employees became better versed in the requirements involved in responding to Freedom of Information Act requests, the industry demands became less disruptive.[20,45] Indeed, some public health professionals turned this strategy against the tobacco industry by focusing public attention on it.

Internal tobacco industry documents show that the industry considered a similar strategy to disrupt administrative actions by making claims that public health professionals were violating various lobbying laws.[23] Based on the paucity of formal complaints filed and their limited success in derailing tobacco control, one would not have thought that making claims of illegal lobbying and filing lawsuits would have been an effective strategy to protect the interests of the tobacco industry. Our interviews with the health department officials responsible for ASSIST in the 17 states, however, suggested that the industry achieved some success. Eleven of the 17 states (65%) reported an increase in the level of self-censorship as a result of concerns about accusations of illegal lobbying. Most often, this self-censorship was triggered by a desire to avoid the costs and administrative work that can be associated with refuting the tobacco industry's claims, which in many cases could lead to a complete halt of other program activities. These actions did not imply the cessation of policy work but rather the avoidance of activities that could be perceived as lobbying by the public, even if legal under lobbying restrictions.

Several states have sought the support of their department legal counsel or attorney general, but not all were successful in obtaining such support. In some states, the legal advice was to keep a lower profile on the lobbying issues because it was not worth the cost and the legal and administrative problems to deal with allegations, if any were made. Thus, the net effect of the industry strategy was an increase in the "cost of doing business" in tobacco control, to the level that some states may be more conservative than the law would warrant.

Understanding of the role of lobbying laws in restricting public policy activities is evolving. Historically, many of the laws prohibiting the use of public funds for lobbying purposes were enacted to prevent the government's power and resources from being used to promote private gain or to affect the outcome of an election. These first laws were not designed to restrict the involvement of government officials and programs in the public policy process.

Understanding the proper application of either the original laws or the more modern versions has been challenging. One problem is that reading the lobbying laws too broadly will render an interpretation that will inevitably come into conflict with the modern conception of public health. As noted by the Institute of Medicine,[1] participation of public health advocates in public policy–making is a crucial element of their activities. By its very nature, public health involves public policy–making. To accept an overly broad construction of what constitutes "illegal lobbying," such as that alleged in the complaints against tobacco control professionals in the 4 states in this study, would be to abandon one of public health's most effective tools for promoting health: public policy change.[48]

If public health professionals act too conservatively, assuming that the laws will be interpreted broadly, the result could compromise the ability of public agencies to promote public health. Such an interpretation could restrict communications with policymakers or the public during the times that public health policy is the subject of serious debate. As the Institute of Medicine report states:

> [P]ublic health agency leaders [should] develop relationships with and educate legislators and other public officials on community health needs, on public health issues, and on the rationale for strategies advocated and pursued by the health department. These relationships should be cultivated on an ongoing basis rather than being neglected until a crisis develops.[1(p154)]

Thus, to avoid problems with either violating the lobbying laws or becoming too conservative, public health practitioners must not wait for the solutions and guidance to come to them but must actively interpret the laws and policies they are presented with and conduct their activities accordingly. They must develop the political sophistication to understand how the laws are currently being interpreted and how they are likely to be changed. Public health practitioners should be proactive and should actively seek guidance from appropriate legal and political bodies while moving forward with their public health agenda. Furthermore, public health advocates should work to ensure that lobbying laws do not restrict the legitimate involvement of government workers in developing and implementing public policies to control tobacco and conduct other public health activities. □

Contributors

S. A. Bialous, B. J. Fox, and S. A. Glantz participated in the design of the study, the analysis of the data, and the preparation and revision of the paper. S. A. Bialous and B. J. Fox conducted the interviews.

Acknowledgments

This study was supported by National Cancer Institute grant CA-61021 and University of California Tobacco Related Diseases Research Program grant 6FT-0105.

This work was ruled "exempt" by the Committee on Human Research at the University of California, San Francisco. All interviewees knew that they were being interviewed for the purposes of this study and agreed to the interviews.

We thank the ASSIST project personnel, at both the state and the national level, for providing us with their time, information, and documentation and those who reviewed earlier versions of this paper.

References

1. Institute of Medicine. *The Future of Public Health.* Washington, DC: National Academy Press; 1988.
2. Glantz S. Back to basics: getting smoke free workplaces back on track [editorial]. *Tob Control.* 1997;6:164–166.
3. Stillman F, Becker D, Swank R, Glantz S. Ending smoking at The Johns Hopkins Medical Institutions: an evaluation of smoking prevalence and indoor air pollution. *JAMA.* 1990;264: 1565–1569.
4. Woodruff TJ, Rosbrook B, Pierce J, Glantz SA. Lower levels of cigarette consumption found in smoke-free workplaces in California. *Arch Intern Med.* 1993;153:1485–1493.
5. Patten C, Gilpin E, Cavin S, Pierce J. Workplace smoking policy and changes in smoking behavior in California: a suggested association. *Tob Control.* 1995;4:36–41.
6. Farrelly M, Evans W, Sfekas A. The impact of workplace smoking bans: results from a national survey. *Tob Control.* 1999;8:272–277.
7. Chapman S, Borland R, Scollo M, Brownson R, Domimello A, Woodward S. The impact of smoke-free workplaces on declining cigarette consumption in Australia and the United States. *Am J Public Health.* 1999;89:1018–1023.
8. Glantz S. Changes in cigarette consumption, prices, and tobacco industry revenues associated with California's Proposition 99. *Tob Control.* 1993;2:311–314.
9. Showalter M. The effect of cigarette taxes on cigarette consumption. *Am J Public Health.* 1998;88:1118–1119.
10. Lewit E, Hyland A, Kerrebrock N, Cummings KM. Price, public policy, and smoking in young people. *Tob Control.* 1997;6(suppl 2):S17–S24.
11. Grossman M, Chaloupka F. Cigarette taxes: the straw that broke the camel's back. *Public Health Rep.* 1997;112:290–297.
12. Centers for Disease Control and Prevention. Cigarette smoking before and after an excise tax increase and an anti-smoking campaign—Massachusetts, 1990–1996. *MMWR Morb Mortal Wkly Rep.* 1996;45:966–970.
13. Hu T, Bay J, Keeler T, Barnett P, Sung H. The impact of California Proposition 99, a major anti-smoking law, on cigarette consumption. *J Public Health Policy.* 1994;15:26–36.
14. Bal DG, Kizer KW, Felten PG, Mozar HN, Niemeyer D. Reducing tobacco consumption in California: development of a statewide anti-tobacco use campaign. *JAMA.* 1990;264: 1570–1574.
15. Manley M, Lynn W, Payne Epps R, Grande D, Glynn T, Shopland D. The American Stop Smoking Intervention Study for cancer prevention: an overview. *Tob Control.* 1997;6(suppl 2):S5–S11.
16. Pierce JP, Gilpin EA, Emery SL, et al. Has the California tobacco control program reduced smoking? *JAMA.* 1998;280:893–899.
17. Pierce J, Gilpin E, Emery S, et al. *Tobacco Control in California: Who's Winning the War? An Evaluation of the Tobacco Control Program.* La Jolla: University of California, San Diego; 1998.
18. Siegel M, Mowery P, Pechacek T, et al. Trends in adult cigarette smoking in California compared with the rest of the United States, 1978–1994. *Am J Public Health.* 2000;90:372–379.
19. Manley M, Pierce J, Gilpin E, Rosbrook B, Berry C, Wun L. Impact of the American Stop Smoking Intervention Study on cigarette consumption. *Tob Control.* 1997;6(suppl):S12–S16.
20. Aguinaga S, Glantz S. The use of public records acts to interfere with tobacco control. *Tob Control.* 1995;4:222–230.
21. Glantz S, Balbach E. *Tobacco War: Inside the California Battles.* Berkeley: University of California Press; 2000.
22. *Overview of State ASSIST Programs.* Philip Morris, undated. Report No. Bates 2021253353/57.
23. Joshua Slavitt. Counter Assist Plan. Memo to Jack Nelson, Todd Lattanzio, Tina Wells. Philip Morris. January 13, 1992. Report No. Bates 2023667193/7.
24. Scigliano E. Smoke screens. *Seattle Weekly.* November 15, 1995.
25. Monardi F, O'Neil A, Glantz S. *Tobacco Industry Political Activity in Colorado.* San Francisco: Institute for Health Policy Studies, University of California, San Francisco; May 1996.

26. Lipsher S. 4th complaint filed against tobacco tax. *Denver Post.* September 16, 1994.
27. Ross M. *Tobacco Tax Campaigns: A Case Study of Two States.* Washington, DC: The Advocacy Institute; 1996.
28. Colorado Secretary of State. Administrative Law Court With State Government Court Case No. 94-OS 94-02. Denver, Colo; 1994.
29. Adams W. Memorandum to Thomas Griscom, Denise Keane, Ernest Pepples, Arthur Stevens. Subject: 1996 Tobacco Institute Budget. Washington, DC: Philip Morris; 1995. Bates No. 2041212102.
30. Lipsher S. Buckley clears health agency. *Denver Post.* August 5, 1995.
31. Colorado Secretary of State. Final Agency Order, August 4, 1995. Case No. OS-02. Denver, Colo; 1995.
32. Colorado Secretary of State. Case No. OS 94-04. Denver, Colo; 1994.
33. Colorado USDCftDo. Civil Action File No. 94-2239. Denver, Colo; 1994.
34. Health officials must stay out of tobacco-tax campaign [editorial]. *Denver Post.* July 23, 1994.
35. Monardi F, Glantz S. *Tobacco Industry Political Activity and Tobacco Control Policy Making in Washington: 1983–1996.* San Francisco, Calif: Institute for Health Policy Studies; November 1996.
36. Paulson T. Cough up documents, agency told. *Seattle Post-Intelligencer.* October 24, 1995.
37. Mapes L. Smokers' rights advocate says foes aren't fighting fair. *The Spokesman Review.* November 10, 1995:A1, A8.
38. Murakami K. Tobacco Institute backs complaint against state anti-smoking programs. *Seattle Times.* November 10, 1995.
39. Paulson T. Smokers' rights advocate files complaint against state. *Seattle Post-Intelligencer.* November 10, 1995.D10.
40. *Report of Investigation, In re Compliance With RCW 42.17 by Washington State Department of Health.* Olympia, Wash: Washington Public Disclosure Commission; 1999:45. PDC Case No. 97-192.
41. *Final Order, December 21, 1999, In the Matter of Enforcement Action Against Washington State Department of Health.* Olympia, Wash: Washington Public Disclosure Commission; 1999. PDC Case No. 97-192.
42. Chilcote S. *Letter to Thomas Briant, Esq.* Washington, DC: The Tobacco Institute; December 14, 1990. Bates No. TIMN 218495. Available at: http://www.tobaccoinstitute.com. Accessed November 21, 2000.
43. Briant T. *Letter to Samuel Chilcote, President of the Tobacco Institute.* Minnesota Candy and Tobacco Association Inc; December 28, 1990. Bates No. TIMN 218493. Available at: http://www.tobaccoinstitute.com. Accessed November 21, 2000.
44. Baden P. Anti-tobacco organizations challenged. *Star Tribune.* November 9, 1995:B1.
45. Levin M. Legal weapon. *Los Angeles Times.* April 21, 1996;D1.
46. Doyle JR. Letter to Andrew Ketterer, Esq, Attorney General. Augusta, Me: Law Offices of Doyle & Nelson; 1997.
47. Ketterer A. *Letter to Jon R. Doyle, Esq.* Augusta: State of Maine Department of the Attorney General; 1997.
48. Mullan F. Don Quixote, Machiavelli, and Robin Hood: public health practice, past and present. *Am J Public Health.* 2000;90:702–706.

Implications for Tobacco Control of the Multistate Tobacco Settlement

Richard A. Daynard, JD, PhD, Wendy Parmet, JD, Graham Kelder, JD, and Patricia Davidson, JD

The 1998 master settlement agreement between major tobacco manufacturers and the US states will have a profound effect on many tobacco industry practices and will significantly influence future settlements with the tobacco industry. This article analyzes the settlement's key provisions pertaining to youth sales, advertising, marketing, and lobbying. It also examines the ways in which the settlement restricts industry practices as well as the many industry practices that remain unregulated. (*Am J Public Health.* 2001;91:1967-1971)

IN THE WAKE OF THE $145 billion in punitive damages awarded by a Florida jury in July 2000, Philip Morris launched a nationwide television campaign extolling the virtues of the "master settlement agreement" (MSA). Implicit in the advertising is the claim that the MSA fundamentally changed the way cigarettes are sold, obviating the need for further reform or punishment. This commentary examines that claim by reviewing the effects of the MSA on tobacco control efforts.

On November 23, 1998, the attorneys general of 46 states and the major tobacco manufacturers entered into the MSA, resolving outstanding state lawsuits against the tobacco companies.[1] Under this settlement and previous settlements with the other 4 states, the tobacco companies are obligated to pay the states an average of $10 billion per year for the indefinite future. In addition, the companies have agreed to significant restrictions on their advertising, marketing, and lobbying practices. The companies have not accepted responsibility for their past misdeeds, however. Nor have they agreed to cease many troubling practices.

BACKGROUND

The MSA arose out of efforts by 41 states to sue tobacco manufacturers for state health care costs attributable to tobacco-related illnesses. These suits represented a major threat to the industry, which had previously avoided all liability.[2]

Faced with potentially bankrupting liability, on June 20, 1997, the industry agreed with a group of state attorneys general and private attorneys to enter into a so-called "global settlement"[3] that would have resolved all of the tobacco industry's domestic liability concerns.[4] Because this global settlement would have affected the Food and Drug Administration's authority over tobacco, as well as closed the door to private litigation, legislation was required.

Various versions of the proposed global settlement were introduced in Congress. In March 1998, the Senate Commerce Committee endorsed one version, the McCain bill, that was less favorable to the tobacco industry than the original settlement. As a result, industry representatives withdrew their support[5] and successfully campaigned to defeat the bill.[6]

Industry representatives then met with attorneys general to discuss a less comprehensive settlement. By then, 4 states had reached individual agreements with the industry. In November 1998, the attorneys general of the remaining states and the participating manufacturers, including Brown & Williamson Tobacco Corp, Lorillard Tobacco Co, Philip Morris Inc, and RJ Reynolds Tobacco Co, agreed to the MSA.

Because the MSA had no direct impact on federal policies or private litigation, it did not require federal approval. Instead, it takes its effect from consent decrees approved by each relevant state court. The states that had not previously sued then did so solely to obtain such consent decrees. Enforcement is left primarily to the attorneys general, although the agreement calls for the National Association of Attorneys General to monitor the settlement and attempt to reconcile conflicting interpretations.

MONETARY TERMS

In their suits, the states sought billions of dollars for tobacco-related health care expenses. This amount might have been tripled if the states had prevailed on antitrust or racketeering grounds. In some states, punitive damages might also have been assessed. The MSA relieved the tobacco companies of these potentially crippling judgments.

In return, the industry agreed to pay each state each year an amount, set through a schedule and a series of adjustment formulas, designed as a reasonable estimate of each state's future tobacco-related health care costs. Including the 4 states that had settled previously, the industry will owe in total about $10 billion per year, adjusted for inflation, to be paid by the companies largely on the basis of their market shares.[7] The companies are expected to cover these costs by raising cigarette prices, with only modest adverse effects on their future profitability.[8]

The MSA provides each state, on average, a $200 million annual revenue enhancement. The settlement also relieved states of paying their outside counsel; the industry agreed to pay these lawyers through a complicated arrangement that reduced or eliminated the lawyers' claims on the states' receipts.[9]

From a public health perspective, however, the MSA's accomplishments are more modest. Perhaps the clearest benefit derives from the cigarette price increase imposed to cover the first year's payments. That increase has produced a decline of about 10% in cigarette sales.[10]

The settlement money could produce further public health benefits if it is spent on tobacco control. Experience with comprehensive programs in California and Massachusetts[11] indicates that such programs can yield significant declines in cigarette sales. The Centers for Disease Control and Prevention (CDC) therefore recommended a range of expenditures of MSA money for states to allocate to comprehensive tobacco control programs.[12] The MSA, however, did not require states to earmark their receipts for public health purposes.

Predictably, early results indicate that, contrary to widespread public opinion,[13] most states will spend little for public health, much less for tobacco control. As of August 4, 2000, for example, approximately 18 states had allocated $1 million or more of the settlement money for tobacco control, and of these states only 4 had allocated settlement funds for tobacco control in amounts that fell within the CDC's recommendations.[14]

The MSA also created an industry-funded foundation to run tobacco control programs and make grants to the states and their subdivisions.[15] The American Legacy Foundation is charged with supporting studies and programs designed to reduce use of tobacco products and substance abuse among young people and to prevent diseases associated with tobacco products (see www.americanlegacy.org).

The MSA describes more than 10 specific foundation activities, including a major national counteradvertising campaign. In addition, foundation grants will separately fund state and local advertising and educational programs to counter youth tobacco use and to educate consumers about tobacco-related diseases. However, the MSA imposes some significant limits on foundation funds. For example, the agreement prohibits use of foundation funds for personal attacks or vilification of any person, company, or government agency. This could censor hard-hitting advertising campaigns that put the spotlight on industry manipulation.

LIMITATIONS ON TOBACCO INDUSTRY PRACTICES

Youth Access Provisions

The MSA declares that tobacco manufacturers and settling states are "committed to reducing underage tobacco use by discouraging such use and by preventing Youth access to Tobacco Products."[16] The actual provisions, however, do little toward achieving that end.

Some reduction in youth access may be accomplished by the MSA's prohibition of gifts, credits, or coupons based on proof of purchase without documentation that the recipient is an adult.[17] However, a careful reading of how the MSA defines the critical terms *adult* and *underage* suggests that the restriction may apply only in states that have made the purchase or possession of tobacco products by minors illegal.

According to the MSA, an "underage" person is one who is "under the minimum age to purchase or possess (whichever minimum age is older) cigarettes applicable in the settling states."[18] Whereas all states prohibit the *sale* of tobacco products to minors, not all outlaw youth purchase or possession, and many public health advocates believe that "criminalizing" youth purchase and possession may be counterproductive.[19]

Another significant loophole permits redemption of proofs of purchase by mail. Although recipients must provide a copy of age identification, this requirement could be easily circumvented.

The MSA appears to restrict the distribution of free sample cigarettes. This provision also is more limited than initially evident, because manufacturers can distribute free samples at adult-only facilities.[20] Again, the definition of *adult-only facilities*[21] is tied to the problematic definition of *underage*. As a result, states that do not outlaw youth purchase or possession may not be able to enforce the ban. Manufacturers may also be able to continue to distribute free samples to college students in many venues.[22]

Another provision prohibits participating companies from

producing, selling, or distributing so-called kiddie packs, cigarette packs containing fewer than 20 cigarettes and packages of loose tobacco with fewer than 0.60 oz (16.80 g) of tobacco.[23] However, this prohibition expires in December 2001.

The MSA fails to include certain key tools for reducing youth access. For example, it does not limit self-service displays, vending machines, or point-of-sale advertising. And, unlike the proposed global settlement, the MSA does not establish any specific targets for reducing youth smoking. Nor does it impose any "look-back" financial penalties on tobacco manufacturers for failing to reduce youth smoking.

In short, the MSA advances only 3 very limited youth access measures. However, it does not expressly diminish the power of states and localities to adopt and enforce additional youth access laws.

Advertising Restrictions

The MSA's advertising restrictions[24] also involve many loopholes. They follow past industry concessions by allowing tobacco companies to shift advertising dollars to other media while restricting a carefully defined set of activities.[25] Indeed, in the first year of the MSA era, the industry increased tobacco advertising by 33% in magazines with high (15% or greater) youth readership.[26]

The MSA prohibits cartoon tobacco advertising,[27] but the definition of *cartoon* limits the ban's scope.[28] For example, although "Joe Camel" cartoons are banned, drawings of a camel are permitted unless they exaggerate or attribute human or superhuman qualities to the camel. Moreover, the "no cartoon" rule does not ban the use of the "Marlboro Man" or other human characters. The MSA also "grandfathers" existing cigarette logos.[28]

Under the MSA, tobacco product billboards, transit advertising, and certain other types of outdoor advertising (signs and placards in open-air or enclosed arenas, stadiums, shopping malls, and video game arcades) must be removed. However, tobacco retailers may continue to post any number of advertisements, each up to 14 sq ft (1.26 m^2) in size, on the windows of their establishments or anywhere else on their property.[29] Retailers are thus likely to remain an important venue for tobacco advertising.

The advertising restrictions are distinct from provisions applying to brand name sponsorships. These complex provisions ban 4 types of sponsorships: concerts, events at which "the intended audience" is composed of "a significant percentage of youth," events featuring paid youth contestants or participants, and "any athletic event between opposing teams in any football, basketball, baseball, soccer or hockey league."[30] Exceptions exist, however, for certain concerts, such as the Kool Jazz Festival.[31] And important questions remain as to how the ban will be interpreted. For example, it is unclear what percentage of an audience must consist of young people in order for the youth ban to apply.

The MSA also contains a complex series of restrictions on other types of brand name sponsorships, including a "one brand name sponsorship per year" rule.[32] These rules have many detailed exceptions that will permit tobacco companies to engage in a wide variety of brand name sponsorship activities and advertising.

Limitations on Endorsements and Other Marketing Restrictions

Under the MSA, tobacco manufacturers may not give anything of value to induce a person or entity to refer to, use, or display a tobacco product, package, or advertising "in any motion picture, television show, theatrical production or other live performance, live or recorded performance of music, commercial film or video, or video game."[33] However, media viewed in an adult-only facility, adult use of instructional media for nonconventional cigarettes, and media not intended for public distribution or display are excepted. In addition, the ban on endorsements and product placement does not apply to the permitted brand name sponsorships.[34]

The MSA also prohibits participating tobacco manufacturers from marketing, distributing, offering, selling, or licensing any merchandise or apparel bearing tobacco product brand names.[35] Once again, there are exceptions. For example, the ban does not apply to merchandise distributed in an adult-only facility.

Restrictions on Lobbying

Historically, tobacco industry lobbying, either directly or via proxy groups, has impeded the enactment of state and local tobacco control laws.[36] The MSA addresses this problem, but only to a limited extent. Rather than banning all industry efforts to derail tobacco control laws, the MSA prohibits lobbying against specific hypothetical state laws or regulations,[37] including laws limiting youth access to vending machines and laws enhancing preexisting prohibitions on youth tobacco sales. Participating manufacturers remain free to oppose other significant youth access restrictions such as limits on self-service displays.

The MSA makes clear as well that participating manufacturers may oppose all tobacco-related excise or income tax provisions.[37] The industry can also continue to oppose enforcement of existing legislation or rules. Given that enforcement is often key to the success of tobacco control measures, this limitation may undermine the efficacy of the lobbying restriction.

The status of industry lobbying in support of state laws that preempt local tobacco control initiatives is not entirely clear. Because such laws would forbid local legislation pertaining to the initiatives covered by the lobbying ban, tobacco control advocates may argue that preemption falls within the ban. However, manufacturers can counter that the MSA preserves their right to support statewide bills that are not explicitly included within the lobbying ban.

The MSA also restricts participating manufacturers from supporting any diversion of the settlement proceeds to any other than tobacco- or health-related uses. However, it leaves the industry free to seek the diversion of the funds to health-related uses other than those focusing on tobacco.

Finally, the MSA dissolves the Council for Tobacco Research—USA (CTR) and the Tobacco Institute, Inc, and includes the statement that the industry "may not reconstitute CTR or its function in any form."[38] Manufacturers may, however, create new tobacco-related trade associations.

EFFECT OF THE MSA ON OTHER TOBACCO LITIGATION

The MSA settled the states' claims for past, present, and future tobacco caused health care expenses. Because localities are subdivisions of states, their claims are also resolved. However, the states are not prevented from enforcing the MSA or from seeking court orders to enjoin tobacco industry misbehavior.

Nor does the MSA impede individual or class action cases brought by smokers, families of smokers, or afflicted nonsmokers. Indeed, the millions of pages of documents released in the course of the state litigation,[39] many of which will be made publicly available under the MSA,[40] have been crucial in fueling additional successful litigation. In 1999 alone, 2 large punitive damage verdicts were handed down in individual actions against Philip Morris,[41,42] along with a detailed and damning verdict against all of the major cigarette manufacturers in the first phase of a Florida class action.[43]

Other third-party payers, such as BlueCross BlueShield plans, may also seek tobacco-related health care costs. The most dramatic such case was the one filed by the Justice Department in 1999, seeking recovery of tobacco-caused health care expenses. The costs at issue in the case were estimated to total more than $20 billion per year. However, these claims were recently dismissed by the court.[44]

The federal action still raises claims under the Racketeer Influenced and Corrupt Organizations Act. That action seeks the disgorgement of the tobacco industry's profits from its decades-long pattern of fraudulent behavior, as well as the cessation of future misbehavior and the funding of public information projects. A successful conclusion to the case could contribute substantially to public health goals by increasing the price of cigarettes, thereby discouraging consumption, and by plugging many of the MSA's loopholes.

LESSONS LEARNED

The MSA and the 4 individual state settlements that preceded it represent a watershed in regard to tobacco control efforts. For the first time, the industry has assumed a significant share of the costs related to the illnesses it causes. And, for the first time, the industry has agreed to many restrictions on advertising, marketing, and lobbying.

Still, the MSA has not fundamentally changed the way cigarettes are sold. Nor has it punished the industry for its misdeeds. Even the ban on billboard advertising, arguably the most significant MSA restriction, has been circumvented through redirecting tobacco advertising to youth-oriented magazines.[24] Tobacco company profits actually increased subsequent to the MSA.[45]

Several lessons seem to follow. First, bargains struck without substantial public health input may be less meaningful than they initially appear. Second, federal, state, and local regulations are as needed as ever. Finally, tobacco litigation remains an important public health tool. Litigation brought the industry to the bargaining table in the first place. Even after the MSA, it may be a potent tool for exposing industry misbehavior and weakening the industry's power to resist effective controls. ■

About the Authors

Richard A. Daynard is with the Tobacco Control Resource Center, Northeastern University School of Law, Boston, Mass. Wendy Parmet is with the Northeastern University School of Law, Boston, Mass. Graham Kelder is with the Massachusetts Association of Health Boards, Cambridge. Patricia Davidson is with the Suffolk University Law School, Boston, Mass.

Requests for reprints should be sent to Wendy Parmet, JD, School of Law, Northeastern University, 400 Huntington Ave, Boston, MA 02115 (e-mail: w.parmet@neu.edu).

This commentary was accepted December 13, 2000.

Note. Any opinions, findings, and conclusions expressed in this article are those of the authors and do not necessarily reflect the views of the prime sponsor.

Contributors

The authors worked together to plan and structure the paper. R.A. Daynard took primary responsibility for sections pertaining to the monetary implications of the settlement. W. Parmet was primarily responsible for discussion of the settlement's background and editing the paper. G. Kelder was the primary author of the section on lobbying provisions. P. Davidson was primarily responsible for sections pertaining to the youth access provisions and advertising restrictions.

Acknowledgments

This article is based on work supported by a National Institutes of Health/National Cancer Institute award (grant 1 R01 CA67805-01).

References

1. Master settlement agreement. Available at: http://www.naag.org/cigmsa.rtf. Accessed October 1, 2001.
2. Kelder GE, Daynard RA. The role of litigation in the effective control of the sale and use of tobacco. *Stanford Law Policy Rev.* 1997;8:63–87.
3. Broder JM. The tobacco agreement: the overview: cigarette makers in a $368 billion accord to curb lawsuits and curtail marketing. *New York Times.* June 21, 1997:A1.
4. Proposed tobacco industry settlement, 12.3 TPLR 3.203–3.233 (1997).
5. Rosenbaum DE. Tobacco strategy, when no means yes and vice versa. *New York Times.* April 4, 1998:D5.
6. Mitchell A. The tobacco bill: news analysis. *New York Times.* June 18, 1998:A1.
7. Master settlement agreement: section IX. Available at: http://www.naag.org/cigmsa.rtf. Accessed October 1, 2001.
8. Associated Press. Philip Morris matches predictions with a 2% rise in earnings. *New York Times.* October 20, 1999:C11.
9. Master settlement agreement: section XVII. Available at: http://www.naag.org/cigmsa.rtf. Accessed October 1, 2001.
10. Hays CL. RJR Nabisco earnings slid by 54% in the first quarter. *New York Times.* April 23, 1999:C4.
11. Cigarette smoking before and after an excise tax increase and an antismoking campaign–Massachusetts, 1990–1996. *MMWR Morb Mortal Wkly Rep.* 1996;45:966–970.
12. *Best Practices for Comprehensive Tobacco Control Programs–August 1999.* Atlanta, Ga: Centers for Disease Control and Prevention; 1999.
13. Scherer R, Wood D. States plan for tobacco windfall. *Christian Science Monitor.* November 14, 1998:1.
14. National Center for Tobacco-Free Older Persons of the Center for Social Gerontology. Tobacco settlement funds: state updates. Available at: http://www.tcsg.org/tobacco/settlement/updates.htm. Accessed August 4, 2000.
15. Master settlement agreement: section VI. Available at: http://www.naag.org/cigmsa.rtf. Accessed October 1, 2001.
16. Master settlement agreement: section I. Available at: http://www.naag.org/cigmsa.rtf. Accessed October 1, 2001.
17. Master settlement agreement: section III(h). Available at: http://www.naag.org/cigmsa.rtf. Accessed October 1, 2001.
18. Master settlement agreement: section II(yy). Available at: http://www.naag.org/cigmsa.rtf. Accessed October 1, 2001.
19. Graham K. The perils, promises and pitfalls of criminalizing youth possession of tobacco. *Tob Control Update.* 1997;1:17–34.
20. Master settlement agreement: section III(g). Available at: http://www.naag.org/cigmsa.rtf. Accessed October 1, 2001.
21. Master settlement agreement: section II(c). Available at: http://www.naag.org/cigmsa.rtf. Accessed October 1, 2001.
22. Wechsler H, Rigotti NA, Glendhill-Hoyt J, Lee H. Increased levels of cigarette use–a cause for national concern. *JAMA.* 1998;280:1673–1678.
23. Master settlement agreement: section III(k). Available at: http://www.naag.org/cigmsa.rtf. Accessed October 1, 2001.

24. Master settlement agreement: section III. Available at: http://www.naag.org/cigmsa.rtf. Accessed October 1, 2001.

25. Kluger R. *Ashes to Ashes: America's Hundred-Year Cigarette War, the Public Health, and the Unabashed Triumph of Philip Morris.* New York, NY: Alfred A Knopf; 1996.

26. Turner-Bowker D, Hamilton WL. Cigarette advertising expenditures before and after the master settlement agreement: preliminary findings. Available at: http://www.tobacco.org/news. Accessed May 22, 2000.

27. Master settlement agreement: section III(b). Available at: http://www.naag.org/cigmsa.rtf. Accessed October 1, 2001.

28. Master settlement agreement: section II(l). Available at: http://www.naag.org/cigmsa.rtf. Accessed October 1, 2001.

29. Master settlement agreement: sections II(ii) and III(d). Available at: http://www.naag.org/cigmsa.rtf. Accessed October 1, 2001.

30. Master settlement agreement: section III(c)(1). Available at: http://www.naag.org/cigmsa.rtf. Accessed October 1, 2001.

31. Master settlement agreement: section III(c)(2)(B)(ii). Available at: http://www.naag.org/cigmsa.rtf. Accessed October 1, 2001.

32. Master settlement agreement: section III(c)(2). Available at: http://www.naag.org/cigmsa.rtf. Accessed October 1, 2001.

33. Master settlement agreement: section III(e). Available at: http://www.naag.org/cigmsa.rtf. Accessed October 1, 2001.

34. Master settlement agreement: section III(c)(3)(c). Available at: http://www.naag.org/cigmsa.rtf. Accessed October 1, 2001.

35. Master settlement agreement: section III(f). Available at: http://www.naag.org/cigmsa.rtf. Accessed October 1, 2001.

36. Jacobsen PD, Wasserman J. The implications and enforcement of tobacco control laws: policy implications for activists and the industry. *J Health Policy Polit Law.* 1999;24:567–598.

37. Master settlement agreement: section III(m). Available at: http://www.naag.org/cigmsa.rtf. Accessed October 1, 2001.

38. Master settlement agreement: section III(o)(5). Available at: http://www.naag.org/cigmsa.rtf. Accessed October 1, 2001.

39. About tobacco industry documents. Available at: http://www.cdc.gov/tobacco/industrydocs/about.htm. Accessed October 1, 2001.

40. Master settlement agreement: section IV. Available at: http://www.naag.org/cigmsa.rtf. Accessed October 1, 2001.

41. *Henley v Philip Morris,* 14.2 TPLR 2.27–2.33 (Super Ct Cal 1999).

42. *Williams v Philip Morris,* 14.2 TPLR 3.111–3.112 (Ore 1999).

43. *Engle v RJ Reynolds Tobacco Co,* 14.3 TPLR 2.101–2.107 (Cir Ct Fla 1999).

44. *US Dept of Justice v Philip Morris,* 116 F Supp 2d 131 (DDC 2000).

45. *Tobacco Industry Monthly Report.* New York, NY: Suisse First Boston; August 2000.

Simulated Effect of Tobacco Tax Variation on Population Health in California

Robert M. Kaplan, PhD, Christopher F. Ake, PhD, Sherry L. Emery, PhD, and Ana M. Navarro, PhD

ABSTRACT

Objectives. This study simulated the effects of tobacco excise tax increases on population health.

Methods. Five simulations were used to estimate health outcomes associated with tobacco tax policies: (1) the effects of price on smoking prevalence; (2) the effects of tobacco use on years of potential life lost; (3) the effect of tobacco use on quality of life (morbidity); (4) the integration of prevalence, mortality, and morbidity into a model of quality adjusted life years (QALYs); and (5) the development of confidence intervals around these estimates. Effects were estimated for 1 year after the tax's initiation and 75 years into the future.

Results. In California, a $0.50 tax increase and price elasticity of −0.40 would result in about 8389 QALYs (95% confidence interval [CI]=4629, 12113) saved the first year. Greater benefits would accrue each year until a steady state was reached after 75 years, when 52136 QALYs (95% CI=38297, 66262) would accrue each year. Higher taxes would produce even greater health benefits.

Conclusions. A tobacco excise tax may be among a few policy options that will enhance a population's health status while making revenues available to government. (*Am J Public Health.* 2001;91:239–244)

In January 1999, California enacted Proposition 10, an initiative to raise the state excise tax on cigarettes by $0.50 a pack. Several other states have also instated cigarette excise tax increases. Cigarette excise taxes are an attractive public policy tool for 2 reasons. First, they generate substantial revenue for the governmental unit levying the tax. Second, there is substantial evidence that a cigarette excise tax increase will reduce cigarette consumption by motivating some smokers to quit and many others to reduce their daily consumption.[1–9] These behavioral changes may ultimately manifest themselves in improved population health status.[10] In this report, we estimate the health status effects of increases of $0.50 and $1.00 per pack for California residents.

Most models of health outcome emphasize effects on mortality or on life expectancy.[11] However, such studies often underestimate the impact of smoking on public health. In addition to early death, tobacco consumption causes significant and prolonged loss in quality of life through illnesses such as chronic obstructive pulmonary disease.[11] Other models estimate the effect of smoking on specific diseases, such as lung cancer or heart disease, but often fail to account for all the diverse effects of tobacco consumption.[11] Smoking-related problems range from hearing loss to heart disease and a multitude of cancers.[12]

In this analysis, we use a combined index of morbidity and mortality known as the quality adjusted life year (QALY) to demonstrate changes in life expectancy with adjustments for quality of life. In cost–utility analysis, the relative value of medical care is often expressed as the cost per QALY. Typically, QALYs are produced at some cost in available resources. A tobacco excise tax may offer a unique situation in which QALYs are saved while resources are made available to government.

Methods

Overview

On the basis of current literature, we projected the expected changes in smoking prevalence that would result from a range of cigarette tax increases. These estimates were made for 2 points in time: 1 year after the tax was initiated and 75 years into the future, when the effects on the current cohort of smokers and potential smokers would be fully dissipated. Using the Smoking-Attributable Mortality, Morbidity, and Economic Costs (SAMMEC) program[13] and quality of life estimates from the National Health Interview Survey (NHIS), we then translated these changes in smoking prevalence into changes in population mortality and morbidity and then into QALYs for the California population.

Elasticity Estimates

Elasticity is a concept economists use to measure responsiveness to price changes. It is calculated as the percentage change in overall demand that results from a 1% change in a good's price. An elasticity estimate of −0.4 indicates that overall demand will decrease 4% in response to a 10% price increase.

An expert panel convened by the National Cancer Institute arrived at a consensus estimate of the adult overall price elasticity of demand for cigarettes of −0.4.[4] Generally accepted estimates[1–6,13–15] range from −0.2 to −0.6 (Table 1). Since the literature[2,9,15] also presents

The authors are with the Department of Family and Preventive Medicine, University of California, San Diego.

Requests for reprints should be sent to Robert M. Kaplan, PhD, Department of Family and Preventive Medicine, 0628, University of California, San Diego, La Jolla, CA 92093-0628.

This article was accepted August 17, 2000.

TABLE 1—Selected Econometric Estimates of the Price Elasticity of Demand For Cigarettes

Overall Adult Price Elasticity Estimate	
Adult studies	
Lewit and Coate[1]	−0.89
Becker et al.[2]	−0.40 (short run)
	−0.76 (long run)
Keeler et al.[3]	−0.20 to −0.36 (short run)
	−0.46 to −0.58 (long run)
NCI expert panel[4]	−0.3 to −0.5
Hu et al.[6]	−0.3 to −0.4 (short run)
	−0.5 to −0.6 (long run)
Farrelly and Bray[5]	−0.25
Overall Adolescent Price Elasticity Estimate	
Adolescent Studies	
Lewit et al.[7]	−1.44
Wasserman et al.[8]	0.86
Chaloupka and Grossman[9]	−1.31

Note. NCI = National Cancer Institute.

higher adult long-term estimates, in the range of −0.8, we used overall adult demand elasticity estimates of −0.2, −0.4, −0.6, and −0.8 in our models.

While a price increase may encourage current smokers (adults) to quit or cut back, it will also discourage potential future smokers (adolescents or young adults) from starting to smoke. The literature has consistently shown that price elasticity varies inversely with age: younger people appear more sensitive to the price of cigarettes than older people. As a result, estimates of adolescent elasticity of demand can be much higher than the adult estimates, varying from insignificant[8,16] to the more accepted range of −0.8 to −1.2.[7,9,12] (Although the studies that produced nonsignificant estimates of adolescent price elasticity introduced some controversy about the role of price in deterring adolescent smoking owing to limitations regarding their data, the higher estimates are given more weight in the literature.)

We know of no previous studies that have examined the impact of excise tax increases as large as $1.00. However, most studies have examined how price or excise tax differences across states influence patterns of smoking. Such cross-state cigarette price differences can approach $1.00 per pack. For example, in 1996, the average price of cigarettes in North Carolina was $1.52 per pack, while the average price in Massachusetts was $2.45 per pack. Therefore, it is appropriate to use elasticity estimates reported in this literature to simulate the impact of the $0.50- and $1.00-per-pack price increases in California in 1999.

For both adults and adolescents, a change in the price of cigarettes can influence consumption in 2 ways, both of which are captured in the estimate of overall elasticity of demand. First, a change in price can affect smoking prevalence: the number of individuals who decide to become smokers or to quit smoking. This is quantified as the elasticity of smoking participation. The literature generally agrees that the elasticity of smoking participation represents about half of overall elasticity of demand among adults and about 60% to 80% of overall elasticity among adolescents.[2,7,9] Thus, for instance, an overall estimate of adult elasticity of demand of −0.4 would imply an adult elasticity of participation of approximately −0.2. In our modeling, we assumed throughout that adult participation elasticity was 50% of overall adult elasticity of demand and that adolescent participation elasticity was 70% of overall adolescent elasticity of demand.

Second, a change in cigarette prices can influence the number of cigarettes consumed. This is the conditional demand elasticity (i.e., conditional on being a smoker). Because modeling changes in consumption is much more complicated than modeling changes in prevalence, the initial work we report here made the conservative assumption that consumption levels among those who continued to smoke did not change as a result of a price increase. In light of evidence showing that smokers facing higher taxes (prices) smoke cigarettes higher in tar and nicotine—thereby mitigating or removing altogether any beneficial health effects for continuing smokers from a tax increase[17]—we consider this assumption appropriate, since it produces the equivalent result of no health benefit increase for continuing smokers.

Model Cases and Assumptions

We calculated figures for 3 scenarios. Two of these scenarios use adult elasticities for overall demand and 1 uses adolescent elasticities. Using the adult estimates discussed above for overall elasticity of demand of −0.2, −0.4, −0.6, and −0.8, with a 50% portion attributed to elasticity of participation, we considered the effect of a tax increase (a) 1 year into the future and (b) 75 years into the future. Using the adolescent estimates for overall elasticity of demand of −0.8, −1.0, and −1.2, with a 70% share attributed to participation, we also considered the effect (c) 75 years hence. We selected the time point of 75 years into the future because it is reasonable to assume that by then everyone 85 or younger would have been subject to the increased tax during the years they initiated smoking.

For case a, we assumed that only some smokers will quit immediately (cessation) and that within each age group of adult smokers the same percentage will do so; we made no assumption of a change in initiation. For both our 75-year cases, we assumed that the effect of the 1999 tax increase manifests itself entirely in lessened initiation. Smoking initiation occurs almost exclusively among adolescents, and the prevalence among any age group whose adolescence occurred subsequent to the tax increase would reflect the reduced initiation that would result from higher prices and greater price sensitivity among teens. Thus, for our 75-year estimates, we compared the effect assuming adult elasticity estimates (case b) with that using adolescent elasticity estimates (case c).

For our adult elasticity cases (a and b), we examined 6 subcases: 3 with a tax increase of $0.50 and 3 with an increase of $1.00. For the $0.50 increase, we simulated results for overall elasticities of demand of −0.20, −0.40, and −0.60. For the $1.00 increase, we used −0.4, −0.6, and −0.8. The combination of a $0.50 increase and an overall elasticity demand of −0.8 was not used, since it yields the same results as a $1.00 increase with an overall elasticity of demand of −0.4. Similarly, the $1.00 increase with a −0.2 overall elasticity of demand was not used, because it is equivalent to the $0.50 increase with a −0.4 overall elasticity of demand. For these adult elasticity cases, we used the $0.50 increase with −0.4 overall elasticity of demand as our basis for comparison (our "base case").

For our adolescent elasticity case (case c), we looked at 6 subcases: the $0.50 and $1.00 tax increases each with an overall demand elasticity of −0.8, −1.0, and −1.2. Table 2 shows the expected changes in tobacco consumption based on the various assumptions of tax increase and elasticity. For the adolescent elasticity case, our base case was the $0.50 tax combined with a −1.0 overall elasticity of demand.

To derive our 75-year estimates in cases b and c, we assumed that the 1999 tax would be adjusted as necessary for inflation (or deflation) over time. Both cases also assume constant population size and composition over the

TABLE 2—Relation Between Tobacco Tax Increases and Estimated Changes in Tobacco Use, by Case

Simulation Run	Tax Increase, $	Increase/Price	Elasticity	Change in Overall Demand	Participation Elasticity[a]	Change in Use (a) or Initiation (b)[b]	Change in Participation Use[c]
Cases a and b: adult elasticities[d]							
1	0.50	0.20	–0.2	–0.04	–0.1	–0.02	
2	0.50	0.20	–0.4	–0.08	–0.2	–0.04	
3	0.50	0.20	–0.6	–0.12	–0.3	–0.06	
4	0.50	0.20	–0.8	–0.16	–0.4	–0.08	
2a	1.00	0.40	–0.2	–0.08	–0.1	–0.04	
4a	1.00	0.40	–0.4	–0.16	–0.2	–0.08	
5	1.00	0.40	–0.6	–0.24	–0.3	–0.12	
6	1.00	0.40	–0.8	–0.32	–0.4	–0.16	
Case c: adolescent elasticities							
1	0.50	0.20	–0.8	–0.16	–0.56		–0.112
2	0.50	0.20	–1.0	–0.20	–0.7		–0.14
3	0.50	0.20	–0.12	–0.24	–0.84		–0.168
4	1.00	0.40	–0.8	–0.32	–0.56		–0.224
5	1.00	0.40	–1.0	–0.40	–0.7		–0.28
6	1.00	0.40	–1.2	–0.48	–0.84		–0.336

[a]For case c, participation elasticity = 0.70 of total demand elasticity.
[b]In case a, change is in use, while in case b, change is in initiation.
[c]In case c, change in use rate in the future is a function of change in initiation rate.
[d]Subcase 2a is not distinct for purposes of analysis from subcase 2, since both result in the same percentage change in participation; this is also true for subcases 4a and 4.

75-year period. We recognize that population size will change, but we kept it constant so that the output could be interpreted in relation to current benchmarks. We also assumed that 75 years hence, the effect of a tax increase in 1999 would be to decrease the number of former smokers at that future time relative to what their number would have been without the tax increase by the same percentage as such a presently imposed tax increase would reduce the future number of current (i.e., 75 years hence) smokers relative to its nonintervention level.

For all cases, we used an average cigarette price per pack in California of $2.50. We also assumed that the tax increase would be completely passed on as a price increase. Thus, a $0.50 tax increase would represent a 20% price increase. With an assumed elasticity of –0.2, for example, the overall change in smoking demand would then be –4%.

Estimating Mortality Effects

The effects of changes of smoking prevalence on population mortality were estimated with SAMMEC software, available from the Centers for Disease Control and Prevention (CDC).[13] Version 3.0 can estimate 3 outcomes: smoking-attributable mortality, years of potential life lost (YPLL), and indirect mortality costs. Our model uses the YPLL component.

SAMMEC uses attributable risk formulas to estimate the number of deaths from neoplastic, cardiovascular, respiratory, and pediatric diseases, together with burn deaths, associated with cigarette smoking. SAMMEC requires 4 types of data as input: (1) mortality figures from the population of interest for a given year, broken down by sex, age, and *International Classification of Diseases, Ninth Revision* (*ICD-9*) classification, for which we used 1996 mortality data from California state vital records; (2) smoking prevalence figures by sex, smoking status (current vs former), and age (35–64 vs ≥65 years) and among pregnant women, which we derived from the 1996 California Tobacco Survey[18]; (3) population estimates by sex and 5-year age category, for which we also used 1996 California Tobacco Survey figures; and (4) YPLL due to smoking-related diseases, the calculation of which requires as input average years of life remaining, by sex, for each 5-year age category of the study population; for this, we used SAMMEC-supplied 1991 US figures.

Estimating Quality of Life Effects

To represent outcomes, we applied a comprehensive model of health-related quality of life.[19–23] With data from the 1994 NHIS, we estimated the morbidity consequences of smoking by using the Health and Limitations Index measure of years of healthy life. To estimate QALYs, we used the method of Erickson et al. that was developed by the National Center for Health Statistics, CDC.[24] The method requires 4 sources of information. The first source, life expectancy, is described above. Two other types of information, activity limitation and perceived health, come from the NHIS. Activity limitation describes performance of social role. In the NHIS, questions are contingent on a particular age group and are answered within this context for those who are working, homemaking, going to school, or retired. Each individual is classified into 1 of 6 categories on the basis of age and performance of major activity.

In addition to this classification by activity level, each respondent in the NHIS is asked to rate his or her perceived health status, in response to the question "Would you say your health, in general, is excellent, very good, good, fair, or poor?" The 5 levels of response to this question are factorially combined with the 6 levels of functional limitation to form a matrix with 30 cells. Each respondent in the NHIS is classified into 1 of these 30 categories.

The fourth source of information is used to assign a value to each of the 30 states on the continuum, ranging from death (0.0) to optimum functioning (1.0). The values are assigned by multiattribute utility scaling.[25] Each of the 30 states was matched to values corresponding to similar states as estimated by the Health Utilities Index.[26,27] Survival time for current, former, and never smokers was adjusted for quality of life as estimated by this index. The calculations were performed separately for men and women and adjusted by age.

To develop confidence intervals, Monte Carlo simulation was performed with the Crystal Ball 4.0 software program (Decisioneering Advanced Analytic Tools, Denver, Colo). For simulation purposes, we consider it highly plausible to assume that QALYs are normally distributed. Each simulation used 10000 trials.

Results

Under the base case of an 8% decline in overall demand for cigarettes, 2714 years (95% confidence interval [CI] = 2332, 3098) of potential life would be gained annually. Projecting 75 years forward (case b), the conservative estimate suggests that 5414 life years (95% CI = 4568, 6328) will be saved per year in the base case. Assuming that the tax increase works primarily to deter youth from smoking, and looking 75 years into the future (case c), the base model suggests that 18811 life years (95% CI = 15920, 21920) will be saved each year. Under case a, which considered changes in smoking demand of between 4% and 32%, the increase in life years ranged from 1136 to 11477 per year. Under case c, which considered a steady state and used a range of overall demand reduction of from 16% to 48%, the yield in life years ranged from 14828 to 47641 annually.

Using data from the NHIS, we also estimated the effect of a change in smoking status on health-related quality of life for individuals in age categories ranging from 18 to 19 years through 85 years and older. For women at each age, current smokers have lower scores on health-related quality of life than former or never smokers. After age 25, a similar pattern is seen for men. Beyond age 40, never smokers tend to have higher scores than former or current smokers.

Total QALYs were estimated by combining weighted YPLL (mortality) with quality of life (morbidity). The base case model suggests that in the first year the $0.50 tax would produce approximately 4321 QALYs per year for men and approximately 4067 QALYs per year for women in case a. For case b, 9254 QALYs per year would be produced for men and 5681 per year would accrue for women. Case c in the base scenario assumes an elasticity of demand of –1.0 and shows an outcome of 32158 QALYs per year for men and 19979 per year for women.

Figure 1 summarizes the yield in QALYs under different tax and adult elasticity assumptions. Reductions in tobacco consumption result from 2 sources, improved life expectancy and improved health-related quality of life. Our simulations suggest that about two thirds of the benefits reflect changes in quality of life and one third reflects changes in mortality. This is shown in Figure 1, which portrays the mortality and morbidity component of total annual QALYs saved given the various tax increase and elasticity settings under adult elasticity assumptions. The height of each column shows total QALYs gained, while the bottom section of each column shows the decrease in YPPL. Under the assumption of a $1.00 tax and a –0.60 elasticity, the model suggests that about 25380 QALYs (95% CI = 14279, 36334) would be produced in the first year. Under case b, the annual QALY yield would be about 44695 (95% CI = 32705, 56971), while under case c, if an adolescent elasticity of –1.0 is assumed, it would be about 105673 QALYs (95% CI = 76830, 134748), as shown in Figure 2. Since we are not comparing a present economic cost with a future anticipated benefit, discounting seems inappropriate, but for comparison purposes the latter 2 totals would become 4867 and 11508 per year, respectively, under the 3% rate recommended by Gold et al.[28] and 1153 and 2726 per year under a 5% discount. These totals would produce 10950 and 25880 QALYs saved annually per million present-day smokers in California, respectively.

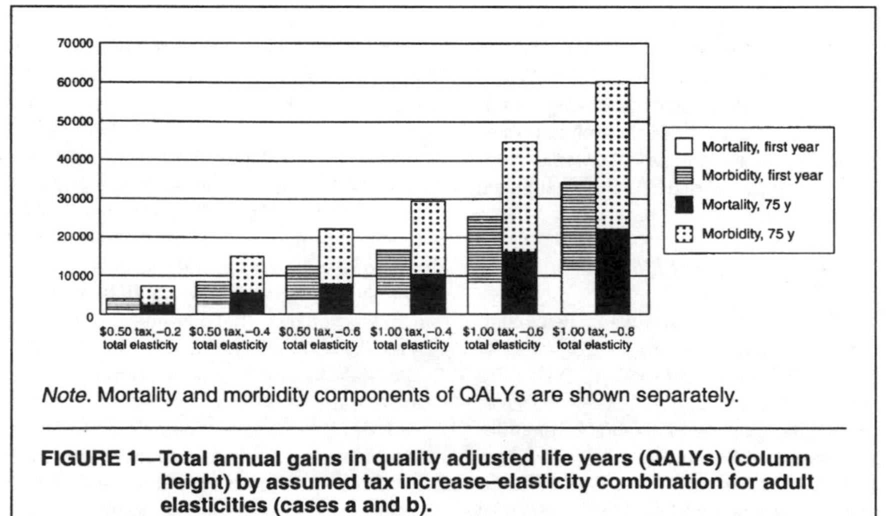

Note. Mortality and morbidity components of QALYs are shown separately.

FIGURE 1—Total annual gains in quality adjusted life years (QALYs) (column height) by assumed tax increase–elasticity combination for adult elasticities (cases a and b).

Discussion

In 1999, as a result of 2 separate $0.50-per-pack increases, smokers in California experienced an increase in the price of premium brand cigarettes amounting to at least $1.00 per pack. The first increase occurred with the implementation of the additional $0.50-per-pack tax on cigarettes, along with taxes on other tobacco products, which resulted from California voters' approval of Proposition 10. The second $0.50-per-pack increase resulted from the tobacco industry's response to the provisions of the Multistate Master Settlement Agreement. By the terms of this agreement, which California signed soon after Proposition 10 was passed, the tobacco industry will pay California and 45 other states $206 billion over the next 25 years. Unlike earlier settlement proposals, this one did not mandate any increases in the price of cigarettes or other tobacco products. However, by late November 1998, the 2 largest US cigarette manufacturers had announced their intention to raise the price of its premium brand cigarettes by $0.45 per pack to offset the settlement costs. (Owing to coupon redemption programs and carton price decreases, California smokers could potentially avoid the industry-driven price increases.) Distributors and retailers generally added an additional $0.05 to the wholesale price increase, so consumers realized a full $0.50-per-pack increase due to the settlement.[29,30] On top of the excise tax increase and the retail price increase driven by the agreement, the tobacco industry announced a further $0.22-per-pack increase in the price of cigarettes in late 1999. Therefore, even with new marketing approaches that use coupons and other incentives, California smokers faced an unprecedentedly large increase in cigarette prices in 1999.

Even in California, with one of the lowest smoking rates in the nation, the 1999 $0.50-per-pack tax increase is expected to generate about $700 million a year in revenues. In addition to these tax-generated revenues, the reductions in tobacco use that result from both the increased excise taxes and the industry-driven price increases will also produce an eventual savings by reducing the cost of providing health services for adults with tobacco-related chronic

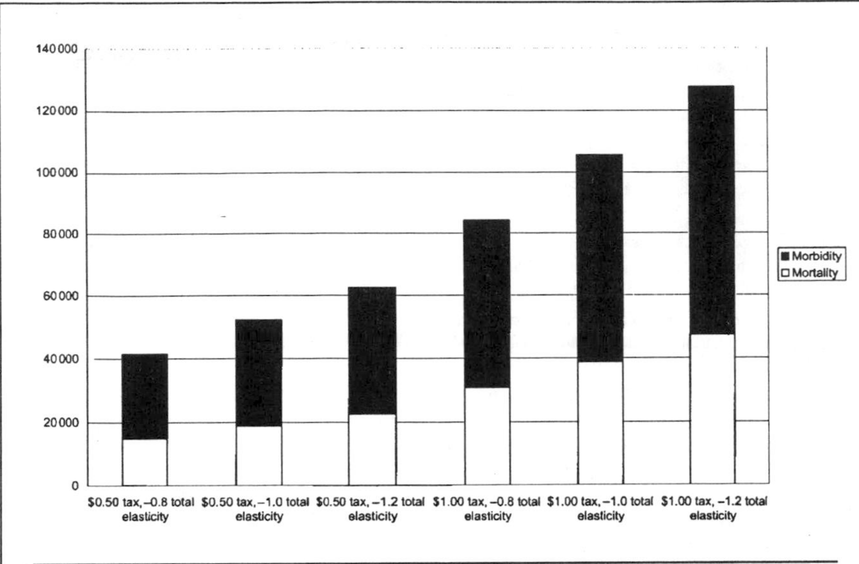

FIGURE 2—Total annual gains in quality adjusted life years (QALYs) by assumed tax increase–elasticity combination for adolescent elasticities (case c), showing mortality and morbidity components.

illnesses.[31,32] Despite decades of public health efforts and declining US smoking rates, the use of tobacco products remains a widespread problem. McGinnis and Foege estimated that tobacco was responsible for about 19% of approximately 2 150 000 deaths in the United States in 1990.[11] The World Health Organization projects that, worldwide, there will be 10 million tobacco-related deaths per year by 2030.[33]

Previous analyses may underestimate the impact of tobacco use by disregarding morbidity. The most widely cited analyses by Warner,[10] Manning et al.,[34] and Harris[35] all consider mortality, but not morbidity. Those studies that consider morbidity often estimate only the economic costs of smoking-related illnesses[31,36] or smoking-related health care use. Importantly, our results also probably underestimate the potential improvements in QALYs due to reduced smoking because we focus on participation (via initiation or cessation) and ignore benefits that might accrue to those who continue to smoke but reduce the number of cigarettes they consume. Doll and Peto estimated the incidence of lung cancer as a function of the number of cigarettes smoked[37]; to expand this analysis to include all smoking-related diseases is beyond the scope of this report. Nonetheless, the omission of the health impact of reduced cigarette consumption among smokers is likely to bias our results downward.

Another important finding from the present study was that the public health benefit of a tobacco tax increase grows for each of the first 75 years following its inception. This happens because a higher tax will significantly reduce initiation of the smoking habit among adolescents. Since smoking is rarely initiated among adults, the effect serves to reduce the pool of people who will later develop smoking-related diseases. A broad time perspective is needed to fully appreciate the benefits of the tax. It might be argued that many smokers over the age of 40 are confirmed, addicted users who are unlikely to change their habits in response to a tax. Cases b and c recognize this possibility by representing the effect of the tax to be on initiation rather than cessation. Further, some recent evidence suggests that the number of hard-core, addicted smokers is small.[38] This suggests that smokers throughout the life cycle may be responsive to quitting incentives. If this is true, our results are even more conservative.

Several other important limitations of our analyses must be considered. One potential problem is that we used national estimates of elasticity, even though our inferences apply to California. This was necessary because there has been only 1 study of the impact of the California tobacco tax.[3] However, this study offered elasticity estimates near the median for all studies. Thus, using elasticity estimates specific to California would not have substantially affected the results, and using national estimates may make our generalizations more robust.

Our analyses assumed that differences in self-reported health status between smokers and nonsmokers are attributable to smoking. It is possible that other health habits contribute to these differences. Unfortunately, the NHIS has few data on other health habits. In our data, adjustment for socioeconomic status, a crude proxy for health habits, did not eliminate the difference. Peto et al. have argued that all differences between smokers and nonsmokers are appropriately attributed to tobacco use.[33] However, we must recognize that our estimates may be inflated because smokers also tend to have other unhealthy health habits.

In summary, the motivation for health policy is to save lives and improve the health of the nation. It is often assumed that the best way to accomplish this goal is to invest in medical care. Tobacco tax programs may be unique in that they produce substantial public health benefits and at the same time produce revenues that might be used for other public health programs. Although the benefits we estimated appear small, compared with those of other preventive interventions, the tax increase clearly emerges as one of the best public health alternatives. Further, our findings suggest that the public health benefits of the California tobacco tax will grow stronger the longer the tax increase has been in effect. We believe that these estimates are conservative. Indeed, the elasticity values used in our base case were lower than those used in other recent analyses.[39] Near-term evaluations may misstate the full impact of the tobacco tax because elasticities are larger for those who are young and not using or not addicted to tobacco. Cases b and c in our models suggest that the impact of the tax will grow with the duration of time since the initiation of higher prices. The large future benefits suggested in case c are realistic given current data. □

Contributors

R. M. Kaplan designed the analysis, wrote the original grant proposal, and developed the conceptual model for the studies. C. F. Ake was the primary data analyst; he generated the computer runs, developed the mortality model, and computed the confidence intervals. S. L. Emery was also actively involved in the execution of the analysis and developed the economic components of the paper; she contributed the sections on elasticity and economic evaluation. A.M. Navarro worked on the estimates of QALYs by using the NHIS database. All authors contributed extensively to the writing and rewriting of the manuscript and systematically reviewed the analysis.

Acknowledgments

The research was supported by grant 6PT-2004 from the California Tobacco Related Disease Research Program (TRDRP).

References

1. Lewit EM, Coate D. The potential for using excise taxes to reduce smoking. *J Health Econ.* 1982;1:121–145.
2. Becker GS, Grossman M, Murphy KM. An empirical analysis of cigarette addiction. *Am Econ Rev.* 1994;84:396–418.

3. Keeler TE, Hu TW, Barnett PG, Manning WG. Taxation, regulation, and addiction—a demand function for cigarettes based on time-series evidence. *J Health Econ.* 1993;12:1–18.
4. *The Impact of Cigarette Excise Taxes on Smoking Among Children and Adults: Summary Report of a National Cancer Institute Expert Panel.* Bethesda, Md: National Cancer Institute; 1993.
5. Centers for Disease Control and Prevention. Response to increases in cigarette prices by race/ethnicity, income, and age groups—United States, 1976–1993. *MMWR Morb Mortal Wkly Rep.* 1998;47:605–609.
6. Hu TW, Sung HY, Keeler TE. Reducing cigarette consumption in California: tobacco taxes vs an anti-smoking media campaign. *Am J Public Health.* 1995;85:1218–1222.
7. Lewit E, Coate D, Grossman G. The effects of government regulations on teenage smoking. *J Law Econ.* 1981;24:545–569.
8. Wasserman J, Manning WG, Newhouse JP, Winkler JD. The effects of excise taxes and regulations on cigarette smoking. *J Health Econ.* 1991; 10:43–64.
9. Chaloupka F, Grossman M. *Price, Tobacco Control Policies and Youth Smoking.* Washington, DC: National Bureau of Economic Research; 1996.
10. Warner KE. Smoking and health implications of a change in the federal cigarette excise tax. *JAMA.* 1986;255:1028–1032.
11. McGinnis JM, Foege WH. Actual causes of death in the United States. *JAMA.* 1993;270: 2207–2212.
12. US Dept of Health and Human Services. *Reducing the Health Consequences of Smoking: 25 Years of Progress: A Report of the Surgeon General.* Washington, DC: Public Health Service, Office on Smoking and Health; 1989. DHHS publication CDC 89-8411.
13. Shultz JM, Novotny TE, Rice DP. Quantifying the disease impact of cigarette smoking with SAMMEC II software. *Public Health Rep.* 1991; 106:326–333.
14. Chaloupka F, Warner K. The economics of smoking. In: Newhouse J, Culyer A, eds. *The Handbook of Health Economics.* New York, NY: Elsevier Science; 2000:1540–1627.
15. Evans W, Ringel J, Stech D. Tobacco taxes and public policy to discourage smoking. In: Poterba J, ed. *Tax Policy and the Economy.* Vol. 13. Cambridge, Mass: National Bureau of Economic Research; 1999:1–55.
16. Douglas S, Hariharan G. The hazard of starting smoking: estimates from a split population duration model. *J Health Econ.* 1994;13: 213–230.
17. Evans WN, Farrelly MC. The compensating behavior of smokers: taxes, tar, and nicotine. *Rand J Econ.* 1998;29:578–595.
18. Pierce JP, Gilpin EA, Emery SL, et al. Has the California tobacco control program reduced smoking? *JAMA.* 1998;280:893–899.
19. Anderson JP, Kaplan RM, Coons SJ, Schneiderman LJ. Comparison of the Quality of Well-Being Scale and the SF-36 results among two samples of ill adults: AIDS and other illnesses. *J Clin Epidemiol.* 1998;51:755–762.
20. Kaplan RM. Decisions about prostate cancer screening in managed care [review]. *Curr Opin Oncol.* 1997;9:480–486.
21. Kaplan RM, Patterson TL, Kerner DN, Atkinson JH, Heaton RK, Grant I. The Quality of Well-Being Scale in asymptomatic HIV-infected patients. HNRC Group. HIV Neural Behavioral Research Center. *Med Decis Making.* 1997;6: 507–514.
22. Kaplan RM, Alcaraz JE, Anderson JP, Weisman M. Quality-adjusted life years lost to arthritis: effects of gender, race, and social class. *Arthritis Care Res.* 1996;9:473–482.
23. Kaplan R, Anderson J. The general health policy model: an integrated approach. In: Spilker B, ed. *Quality of Life and Pharmacoeconomics in Clinical Trials.* New York, NY: Raven; 1996: 309–322.
24. Erickson P, Wilson R, Shannon I. *Years of Healthy Life.* Washington, DC: National Center for Health Statistics; 1995.
25. Boyle MH, Torrance GW. Developing multiattribute health indexes. *Med Care.* 1984;22: 1045–1057.
26. Feeny D, Furlong W, Barr RD. Multiattribute approach to the assessment of health-related quality of life: Health Utilities Index. *Med Pediatr Oncol.* 1998;Suppl 1:54–59.
27. Torrance GW, Feeny DH, Furlong WJ, Barr RD, Zhang Y, Wang Q. Multiattribute utility function for a comprehensive health status classification system. Health Utilities Index Mark 2. *Med Care.* 1996;34:702–722.
28. Gold MR, Siegel JE, Russell LB, Weinstein MC. *Cost-Effectiveness in Health and Medicine.* New York, NY: Oxford University Press; 1996.
29. Meier B. Cigarette makers announce large price rise. *New York Times.* November 24, 1998:A20.
30. Broder J. Clinton wants big increase in federal tax on cigarettes. *New York Times.* January 15, 1999:A21.
31. Hodgson TA. Cigarette smoking and lifetime medical expenditures. *Milbank Q.* 1992;70: 81–125.
32. Burns DM, Shanks TG, Choi W, Thun MJ, Heath CW Jr, Garfinkel L. The American Cancer Society Cancer Prevention Study, I: 12 year follow-up of 1 million men and women. *NIH/NCI Smoking Tob Control Monogr.* 1997;8: 113–304.
33. Peto R, Lopez AD, Boreham J, Thun M, Heath C Jr. Mortality from tobacco in developed countries: indirect estimation from national vital statistics. *Lancet.* 1992;339:1268–1278.
34. Manning WG, Keeler EB, Newhouse JP, at al. *The Costs of Poor Health Habits.* Cambridge, Mass: Harvard University Press; 1991.
35. Harris J. The 1983 increase in the federal cigarette excise tax. In: Summers J, ed. *Tax Policy and the Economy.* Cambridge, Mass: MIT Press; 1994:87–111.
36. Barendregt JJ, Bonneux L, van der Maas PJ. The health care costs of smoking. *N Engl J Med.* 1997;337:1052–1057.
37. Doll R, Peto R. Cigarette smoking and bronchial carcinoma: dose and time relationships among regular smokers and lifelong non-smokers. *J Epidemiol Community Health.* 1978;32: 303–313.
38. Emery S, Gilpin EA, Ake C, Farkas AJ, Pierce JP. Characterizing and identifying "hard-core" smokers: implications for further reducing smoking prevalence. *Am J Public Health.* 2000; 90:387–394.
39. Evans WN, Ringel JS. Can higher cigarette taxes improve birth outcomes? *J Public Econ.* 1999; 72:135–154.

The New Battleground: California's Experience With Smoke-Free Bars

ABSTRACT

Objectives. This study examined the tobacco industry's tactics in the political, grassroots, and media arenas in attempting to subvert California's smoke-free bar law, and the efforts of health advocates to uphold and promote the law by using the same 3 channels.

Methods. Interviews with key informants involved in the development and implementation of the smoke-free bar law were conducted. Information was gathered from bill analyses, internal memoranda, tobacco industry documents, media articles, and press releases.

Results. The tobacco industry worked both inside the legislature and through a public relations campaign to attempt to delay implementation of the law and to encourage noncompliance once the law was in effect. Health groups were able to uphold the law by framing the law as a health and worker safety issue. The health groups were less successful in pressing the state to implement the law.

Conclusions. It is possible to enact and defend smoke-free bar laws, but doing so requires a substantial and sustained commitment by health advocates. The tobacco industry will fight this latest generation of clean indoor air laws even more aggressively than general workplace laws. (*Am J Public Health.* 2001;91:245–252)

Sheryl Magzamen, MPH, and Stanton A. Glantz, PhD

In 1994, the California Legislature enacted the California Smoke-Free Workplace Law (Assembly Bill [AB] 13), which required indoor workplaces in California to be smoke free.[1,2] AB 13 went into effect January 1, 1995, except for the provisions governing bars, taverns, and gaming rooms; these provisions, which aimed to give bar employees the same protections as other workers, took effect on January 1, 1998. The tobacco industry claimed that making bars smoke free would devastate business, deny adults the freedom to smoke, violate the rights of business owners, and be difficult to enforce[3] (also J. Miller, interview with authors, December 4, 1998).

The tobacco industry always opposes smoke-free workplace legislation.[4–6] Except for 1 unsuccessful attempt to undermine implementation of a local clean indoor air ordinance after it passed in 1987,[7] the industry generally retreats and accepts the law after it takes effect. However, the tobacco industry went to extraordinary lengths—9 repeal attempts, an unsuccessful $18 million initiative campaign,[4] and a statewide public relations campaign—to prevent the implementation of the Smoke-Free Workplace Law in California bars. Public health groups countered with surveys and community activities to demonstrate that the personal testimonials the tobacco industry solicited did not reflect the broader public sentiment, which favored smoke-free bars. Tobacco control groups upheld smoke-free bars by expending considerable resources to mobilize public support, working in the legislature, and remaining focused on smoke-free bars as a workplace safety measure.

Methods

We interviewed representatives from voluntary health organizations, legislative offices, advocacy groups, state agencies, state contractors, interest groups, trade groups, and media observers. We obtained information from news reports, internal tobacco industry memoranda, personal correspondence, public documents, and legislative meetings. We contacted tobacco industry agency Burson-Marsteller for an interview; it deferred questions to its client, the National Smokers' Alliance (NSA), which declined to participate.

Results

Delaying Initial Implementation of the Smoke-Free Bar Provisions of AB 13

On February 23, 1996, AB 3037 was introduced to extend the bar exemption in AB 13—originally scheduled to expire on January 1, 1997—to January 1, 2000, to give the state Occupational Safety and Health Standards Board or federal Environmental Protection Agency additional time to develop a ventilation standard.[8] Neither AB 13 nor the proposed AB 3037 placed an affirmative duty on either agency to produce ventilation standards. In the more than 2 years between the passage of AB 13 in 1994 and January 1, 1997, no representatives from bars, taverns, gaming clubs, or the tobacco industry petitioned either agency to create a standard (L. Aubry Jr, memorandum to Gov. Pete Wilson, September 12, 1996).

The senate reduced AB 3037 to a 1-year extension (to January 1, 1998), and the bill passed without controversy. The health groups did not oppose the 1-year extension. John Miller, chief of staff for the Senate Health and Human Services Committee, explained why:

The authors are with the Institute for Health Policy Studies, Department of Medicine, University of California, San Francisco.

Requests for reprints should be sent to Stanton A. Glantz, PhD, Professor of Medicine, Division of Cardiology, Box 0130, University of California, San Francisco, CA 94143 (e-mail: glantz@medicine.ucsf.edu).

This article was accepted January 3, 2000.

"When we imposed a statewide ban on restaurants and workplaces, it was the first [such state law] in the country. Nobody really knew if it would work or not. And we did not know what the effects would be. We never anticipated what the [tobacco industry] said they were. But you need to demonstrate that. And you need to win the sympathy of the press. It took a little time for the public to get used to that idea" (J. Miller, interview with authors, December 4, 1998).

1997–1999 Attempts to Repeal Smoke-Free Bar Law

After AB 3037 passed, 8 additional bills were introduced to overturn the smoke-free bar provisions of AB 13, both before and after the law took effect.[9] Rather than the tobacco industry or its known front groups, the organizations publicly supporting the repeal laws were Tavern Owners United for Fairness, Northern California Coalition Against Prohibition, Northern California Tavern and Restaurant Association, and California Licensed Beverage Association, as well as individual bars and bowling alleys. Groups on record as opposing the repeal included the American Cancer Society, the American Lung Association, the American Heart Association, Americans for Nonsmokers' Rights, the California Medical Association, California Labor Federation (American Federation of Labor and Congress of Industrial Organizations [AFL-CIO]), the California Nurses Association, and the League of California Cities.

Two bills illustrate the key legislative battles.

AB 297. AB 297 was introduced by Assemblyman Ed Vincent (D-Inglewood) in February 1997 to amend the law relating to gaming clubs. In May 1997, Vincent inserted amendments into AB 297 written by a lobbyist[10] for Philip Morris and Hollywood Park, a casino and racetrack in Vincent's district.[11] AB 297 would have extended the exemption for bars until January 1, 2001, and required that if the federal Occupational Safety and Health Administration adopted a standard for secondhand smoke exposure, bars would have 2 years to comply.

AB 297 passed the Assembly Labor Committee in July, too late to be enacted during the current legislative session,[12] so it could not delay implementation of the smoke-free bar provisions on January 1, 1998. The bill, however, would remain alive when the legislature returned on January 5, 1998, and would provide a vehicle for tobacco industry efforts to overturn the law after it was in effect.

Senate Bill 137. In August 1997, Vincent amended Senate Bill (SB) 137, a horse-racing bill authored by Senator Ken Maddy (R-Fresno), to extend smoking in bars until January 1, 2001. SB 137 had already passed in the senate and could still be enacted during the 1997 legislative session to prevent the smoke-free bar law from going into effect. Assembly Speaker Cruz Bustamante (D-Fresno) granted SB 137 rule waivers that suspended the normal filing and hearing deadlines.[13,14] The California Occupational Safety and Health Administration was to create standards for safe levels of smoke in the bars and casinos by January 1999 or smoking would be permitted until 2001.[12] Because of the cost of developing such standards, the bill would have been sent to the Assembly Appropriations Committee, where the committee chair, a strong public health advocate who refused tobacco industry campaign contributions, opposed it.[12] To avoid this hostile committee, Vincent and Maddy removed the requirement that the state Occupational Safety and Health Administration develop ventilation standards. Bustamante then referred SB 137 to the Assembly Governmental Organization Committee, which approved it 11–2. This parliamentary maneuvering illustrates how the tobacco industry is able to use insider strategies to operate quietly through legislative leaders who control the process.[15]

Between July and September, the media reported on Maddy and Vincent's intentions to use SB 137 to delay implementation of smoke-free bars.[12,14,16] To counter the industry's insider strategies, the health groups publicized its activities. On August 28, 1997, the day SB 137 was amended into a smoke-free bar repeal law, the American Heart Association and Americans for Nonsmokers' Rights took out a full-page advertisement in the *New York Times* Western Edition headlined "Don't all workers deserve smoke-free workplaces? The law says yes. Big tobacco says no."

On August 29, the assembly passed SB 137 by a vote of 44–28. Legislators voting yes on SB 137 (pro-tobacco) received a total of $433 700 in tobacco industry campaign contributions in the period 1997 to 1998 (mean, $9857 per vote)[9]; those voting no on SB 137 (pro-health) received $1000 in tobacco industry campaign contributions in the period 1997 to 1998 (mean, $36 per vote) ($P<.001$ by Mann-Whitney test). Previous research in California,[9,17,18] other states,[15] and the US Congress[19] has shown that tobacco industry campaign contributions both influence legislators' voting patterns on tobacco issues and serve as a reward for voting favorably for the tobacco industry.

The amended bill went back to the senate for concurrence. Senate President Pro Tem Bill Lockyer (D-Hayward), who had been a strong ally of the tobacco industry,[18,20] had come to view protection of bar employees from secondhand smoke as a "worker's rights issue."[21] He referred SB 137 to the Senate Judiciary Committee to kill it.

The week before SB 137 was to be heard in the Judiciary Committee, the American Cancer Society held a widely covered press conference and took out a full-page advertisement in the *Sacramento Bee*—headlined "Can Californians Afford the Best Legislature Money Can Buy?"—lambasting the assembly and exposing the industry's manipulation of the legislative process.

The day before SB 137 was heard in the Senate Judiciary Committee, the American Heart Association, American Lung Association, American Cancer Society, and California Medical Association took out a full-page advertisement in the *Sacramento Bee* headlined "Big Tobacco Is At It Again!" The advertisment highlighted the industry's unjustified claims that the law was hurting business and costing jobs and contested the industry's claim that ventilation standards could control secondhand smoke. The advertisement also listed phone numbers of the members of the Senate Judiciary Committee and urged constituents to call. The next day, September 9, 1997, the Judiciary Committee deferred a vote on SB 137, killing it.

During the last days of the 1997 legislative session, a tobacco industry lobbyist proposed a 5-cent tax increase on cigarettes to Lockyer in exchange for legislation allowing smoking to continue in bars.[22] Lockyer refused, and California became the first state to have smoke-free bars.

AB 297 revisited. AB 297 was alive when the legislature returned on January 5, 1998, just 4 days after the smoke-free bar provisions went into force. According to American Lung Association lobbyist Paul Knepprath, "As soon as the [smoke-free bar provisions] went into effect, it changed the legislative landscape completely. Now the onus was on the tobacco industry and [its] supporters and allies to undo and repeal a law that had gone into effect, which is much more difficult than stopping something from going into effect" (P. Knepprath, interview with authors, November 23, 1998). Nevertheless, on January 28, the assembly passed AB 297 by 42–26. Those voting yes received $412 800 in tobacco industry contributions in the period 1997 to 1998 (mean, $9829), and those voting no received $1000 (mean, $38) ($P<.001$).[9]

AB 297 then moved to the senate. Lockyer had stepped down as president pro tem, and Senator John Burton (D-San Francisco), who had a strong public health record, succeeded him. Recognizing the controversy the tobacco industry's public relations campaign generated, Burton was willing to consider the alleged negative economic impact of smoke-free bars.[23] Because he viewed the law as a "worker safety issue" and not a "customer-preference issue,"[24] Burton put the burden of proof on opponents to prove that the law was actually hurting business.[21,25,26]

Burton directed the bill to the Senate Health and Human Services Committee, chaired by anti-tobacco Senator Diane Watson (D-Los Angeles), who planned a public hearing.[21] Watson was concerned that the industry was "undermining the implementation of this public health law"[27] by urging noncompliance. Vincent wanted the hearing delayed until June, which would give the industry more time to build opposition, so he attempted to pull the bill off the voting calendar (J. Miller, interview with authors, December 4, 1998) and did not appear at the hearing in an effort to prevent a vote.[27] Watson kept AB 297 on the calendar and held the hearing.

The health advocates used the hearing as a focal point for their activities (M. Burgat, interview with authors, November 17, 1998). On March 12, 16, and 23, 1998, the health groups ran advertisements in the *Sacramento Bee*, *New York Times* Western Edition, and *La Opinion*, countering the tobacco industry's argument that AB 297 was about individual rights rather than employee protection from secondhand smoke.

On March 25, the day of the hearing, the American Cancer Society released the results of a poll conducted in February 1998 demonstrating public support for smoke-free bars[28]; 61% of voters surveyed supported the 2-month-old law. In another survey conducted for the California Department of Health Services, 61% reported that the new law had no effect on the likelihood of their visiting a bar, and 24% reported that they would be more likely to visit a smoke-free bar.[29] In addition, 75% of bar patrons who were smokers reported complying with the law when in a bar. This poll was consistent with other independent polls (Table 1) indicating public support for smoke-free bars and was used to counter widely accepted anecdotal claims of lost income and noncompliance in news reports orchestrated by the tobacco industry, mostly through the NSA, an organization created by the public relations firm Burson-Marsteller for Philip Morris.[36]

Americans for Nonsmokers' Rights linked groups such as the Northern California Bar and Tavern Association (created by the Dolphin Group, under contract with Philip Morris[37]) back to the tobacco industry or the NSA (C. Hallett, interview with authors, November 16, 1998). It also publicized Philip Morris documents disclosed during Minnesota's litigation against the tobacco industry that demonstrated that the NSA was a front group for the industry rather than an organization representing smokers.[38]

The hearing was a direct confrontation between the tobacco industry and the health groups. Bar owners, club owners, and bartenders opposing the law complained of lost business and infringement of their rights as business owners.[39] The health groups presented evidence that smoke-free workplaces were an integral part of the decline in smoking prevalence in California.[39] The president of the California Labor Federation (AFL-CIO) stated, "We believe disease and death should not be a condition of employment."[27] To put a human face on the issue, the health groups were also represented by individual bartenders, waitresses, and club owners who supported the law (M. Burgat, interview with authors, November 17, 1998; P. Knepprath, interview with authors, November 23, 1998).

AB 297 died in committee.

Putting the Economic Argument to Rest

In May 1998, the American Beverage Institute released a survey[3] of selected bar owners and managers in California that claimed a decline in business of 59.3% since January 1998, with stand-alone bars claiming a 81.3% drop.[3] Similar anecdotal claims of lost revenues have been used to fight smoke-free restaurant laws,[40–42] despite the fact that they have been repeatedly shown to be false in studies of actual restaurant[43–52] and bar[48] revenues.

Burton requested that the state Board of Equalization, California's sales tax collection agency, rapidly produce a preliminary analysis of taxable sales. On June 24, 1998, the board reported that the state's smallest 1161 establishments that serve alcohol (less than $50 000 in taxable sales per month) had a 1.06% increase in revenues in January 1998 compared with January 1997.[53] The board also found that the state's 131 smallest bars—those the industry claimed would be hurt most—showed the largest increase in business, 35% over the previous January.[53] Later, the board released data comparing January 1997 and 1998 sales for 1175 larger bars and restaurants with bars that showed a 1.07% increase in sales.[54] For the first quarter of 1998, there was a 6.0% increase in taxable sales for all eating and drinking establishments compared with 1997.[55] While the tobacco industry continued to press its economic claims in the media, the board reports ended the economic argument in the legislature.

State Efforts to Implement Smoke-Free Bars

As with other public health laws, the primary mode for implementing the Smoke-Free Workplace Law in 1995 was education, with formal enforcement actions (citations and fines) kept to a minimum. A public education campaign focusing on the dangers of secondhand smoke (the justification for the law) that started 6 months before the law took effect eased implementation and minimized the need for formal enforcement (R. Shimizu, California Department of Health Services (DHS), memo to J. Howard, D. Bal, and D. Lyman, May 27, 1997; C. Stevens, DHS, memo to M. Genest, September 30, 1997; C. Stevens, DHS, memo to L. Frost, May 23, 1997).

Refusal to use media campaign. Public health advocates were concerned that the tobacco industry would run a campaign to undercut compliance with the smoke-free bar provisions and felt it was important that the health message reach the public first. The Tobacco Control Section of the California Department of Health Services had 2 resources to undertake this task, a contract agency responsible for the implementation of the smoke-free bar provisions and a large statewide media campaign funded by the tobacco tax.[56,57] The Tobacco Education and Research Oversight Committee, the body with the legislative mandate to oversee the California Tobacco Control Program, recommended that an educational campaign begin as early as August 1997.[58]

The administration of Governor Pete Wilson (R) ignored this advice (M. Genest, memo to J. Howard and J. Stratton, May 28, 1997) and refused to implement an educational campaign on the grounds that promoting the new bar law would be considered "lobbying" against tobacco industry's efforts to overturn the law.[58,59] By October 1997, the American Heart Association and the American Cancer Society were complaining that bar patrons would be unprepared for the new provisions and that the tobacco industry would incite bar owners and patrons to violate the law.[60]

The Tobacco Education and Research Oversight Committee and public health advocates asked that, even if the administration would not allow advertisements while the legislature was in session, it at least develop and approve advertising that could air quickly after the legislature adjourned in September 1997. The administration refused (M. Genest, DHS, memo to J. Howard and J. Stratton, May 28, 1997), despite the fact that detailed advertising concepts had been presented by its advertising agency in April 1997 (A. Schafer, Asher/Gould Advertising, letter to C. Stevens, April 8, 1997). Only when legislative attempts to repeal the smoke-free bar law failed when the legislature adjourned did the administration begin working on an advertising campaign.[1] The first advertisement promoting smoke-free bars aired just 6 weeks before the law went into effect.

Supporting local agencies. By July 1996, when planning of the implementation of the smoke-free bar provisions began, 85% of California localities already had agencies designated to enforce the Smoke-Free Workplace Law because of the general workplace provisions implemented in 1995 (D. Kiser, interview with authors, November 11, 1998). In 1996, the Tobacco Control Section conducted

TABLE 1—Surveys of Popular Support of and Compliance With the California Smoke-Free Bar Law

Study Sponsor	Major Findings	Additional Findings
California Smokefree Cities[a] (March 1996)	64% agreed that bar employers had a responsibility to protect bar employees. 61% agreed that bar employers had a responsibility to protect bar patrons.	36% reported that they would be less likely to go to a bar that allowed smoking, as opposed to 11% who reported that they would be more likely to go to a bar that allowed smoking.
California Department of Health Services[b] (July 1997)	60% of bar patrons reported that they would prefer a smoke-free bar. 87% of bar patrons stated that it would make no difference *or* that they would be more likely to visit bars if they went smoke free.	75% of bar patrons reported that they did not smoke at all or did not smoke in bars. 64% of Californians had visited a bar in the past year; 11% reported being weekly bar patrons.
Los Angeles County Department of Health[c] (March 4, 1998)	85% of bar patrons were more likely to go to a smoke-free bar, or it made no difference. 70% of bar patrons reported that it was very or somewhat important to have smoke-free bars.	78% of frequent bar goers (1 or more times per week) reported that law increased or had an effect on their intent to visit bars. 61% of frequent bar goers strongly or somewhat approved of the smoking ban.
American Lung Association, Contra Costa–Solano[d] (March 11, 1998)	100% of bars in Jack London Square (Oakland) were smoke free. 96% of bars in Fisherman's Wharf (San Francisco) were smoke free.	The 2 areas are heavily patronized by tourists.
American Cancer Society, California Division[e] (March 25, 1998)	61% of voters supported the smoke-free bar law. 69% of voters were concerned about the effects of secondhand smoke on bar workers and patrons.	61% strongly agreed that the tobacco industry spent too much money on lobbying and advertising. 90% agreed that secondhand smoke is harmful to health. 75% favored a complete ban on smoking in all workplaces.
California Department of Health Services[f] (March 1998)	66% of bar patrons reported that having smoke-free bars was important. 61% reported that the law would have no effect on their likelihood of visiting a bar. 24% reported that they were more likely to visit a bar because of the new law.	33% of bar patrons reported that having smoke-free bars was not important. 14% reported that they were less likely to visit a bar because of the new law. 75% of smokers abided by the law the last time they were in a bar after January 1.
Los Angeles Times Poll[g] (May 27, 1998)	60% of respondents approved of the smoke-free bar law.	25% of smokers approved of the new law. 20% of respondents were smokers. 65% of Democrats, 57% of Republicans, and 59% of Independents supported the new law.
California Department of Health Services[h] (October 5, 1998)	65% of bar patrons approved of the smoke-free bar law. 68% reported that it was important to have a smoke-free environment inside bars.	87% went to bars more often, or did not change their behavior, after law was implemented. Since poll conducted in March, an increased number of smokers went outside to smoke (63% compared with 53% before March poll).
San Francisco Tobacco Free Project[i] (December 14, 1998)	Patrons were in compliance with AB 13 in 78.3% of San Francisco bars visited. 96.5% of restaurant bars visited in San Francisco were in compliance. 100% of hotel bars visited were in compliance.	50.6% of stand-alone bars visited were in compliance. 77.8% of nightclubs visited were in compliance. 57.9% of complying bars posted no-smoking signs. 76.5% of noncomplying bars posted no-smoking signs.

[a]Random-digit-dial telephone survey from February 7 to March 17, 1996, of 1283 adult members of California households. Sampling error is ±2.7%; sampling error with subsample of smokers (n=411) is ±4.8%. Survey was conducted by the Gallup Organization, Princeton, NJ.[30]

[b]Random-digit-dial telephone survey from July 11 to 17, 1997, of 1023 California adults 21 years or older, including 686 who were bar patrons. Sampling error is ±3.2%. Survey was conducted by the Field Research Corporation, San Francisco, Calif.[31]

[c]Random-digit-dial telephone survey in February 1998 of 455 Los Angeles County residents who had been inside a bar, nightclub, lounge, or bar attached to a restaurant after January 2, 1998, and who were 21 years or older. Sampling error is ±4.7%. Survey was conducted by Communication Sciences Group, San Francisco, Calif.[32]

[d]Site visits to 36 bars in Fisherman's Wharf, San Francisco, and 11 bars in Oakland by American Lung Association staff.[33]

[e]Random-digit-dial telephone survey in March 1998 of 600 California registered voters. Participants were 18 years or older. Sampling error is ±4.0%. Survey was conducted by Charlton Research Company, Walnut Creek, Calif.[28]

[f]Random-digit-dial telephone survey in February and March 1998 of 1001 California bar patrons, 21 years or older. A patron was defined as any adult 21 or older who reported visiting a bar, tavern, or nightclub, including one attached to a restaurant, hotel, or card club, in the last 12 months. Sampling error is ±3.2%. Survey was conducted by Field Research Corporation, San Francisco, Calif.[34]

[g]Random-digit-dial telephone survey in May 1998 of 1514 adults in California. Sampling error is ±3%. Survey was conducted by the *Los Angeles Times* Poll.

[h]Random-digit-dial telephone survey in August 1998 of 1020 bar patrons 21 years or older who in the last 12 months had visited a bar, tavern, or nightclub, including one attached to a restaurant, hotel, or card club. Sampling error is ±3%. Survey was conducted by Field Research Corporation, San Francisco, Calif.[35]

[i]Random sample of 225 bars in the city of San Francisco were generated. Each bar was initially contacted to confirm that a bar was in operation and to find out hours and location. A total of 217 bars were open and received compliance checks from 5 PM to 10 PM by consultants for the project for a 3-week period in November and December 1998.[29]

a Gallup poll to gauge public opinion on the Smoke-Free Workplace Law[28] and surveyed the county and city health departments (known as local lead agencies) to assess how to handle the transition to smoke-free bars.[61] The local lead agencies suggested various activities, including text for no-smoking signs informing people about the law, tip sheets for bar owners, bartenders, and wait staff, and enforcement suggestions.[61] In addition, by the end of 1996, 77 California communities had already implemented smoke-free bar ordinances, so the Tobacco Control Section could identify individuals who could advise state and local officials on implementation (T. Buffington, interview with authors, November 18, 1998). These efforts were less visible to political appointees within the Wilson administration and were easier for the Tobacco Control Section to complete than a media campaign.

To support the local implementation of the bar provisions, on March 1, 1997, the Tobacco Control Section awarded an American Lung Association affiliate a contract to assist the local lead agencies in implementing smoke-free bars. This project, named BREATH, allowed the Tobacco Control Section to support smoke-free bar implementation in a way that was more resistant to political interference.

In June 1997, information about the new law, answers to common questions, results from the Department of Health Services' 1997 poll showing public support for smoke-free bars (Table 1), and a letter from the department's director were sent to all 36000 bars in the state. BREATH followed with a poster mailing in late 1997 describing the new legal requirements regarding smoke-free bars, penalties for noncompliance, myths about ventilation and anticipated impacts, and public support. After the bar provisions went into effect, BREATH published 2 full-page advertisements in the *New York Times* Western Edition listing 140 well-known bars and restaurants with bars that supported the law to protect the health of their workers and customers.

The War of Perceptions

In 1994, well before implementation of the smoke-free bar provisions, Philip Morris contracted with a political public relations firm, the Dolphin Group, to develop a "California Action Plan" to "safeguard bars and taverns against the threat of a total smoking ban" and "protect and support point of sale retail/marketing strategies, visibility, and promotion."[37] Both Philip Morris and the NSA contacted bar owners and smokers through direct mail campaigns using Philip Morris's database of smokers[36,62–64] (also C. Hallett, interview with authors, November 16, 1998) to mobilize them against smoke-free bars.

Starting in February 1996, the NSA mounted a bar poster and coaster campaign, warning bar patrons, "You are being targeted," in more than 2000 bars[16] to enlist them in the campaign to postpone the phase-in of smoke-free bars (C. Hallett, interview with authors, November 16, 1998). The April 1996 NSA newsletter claimed that "California consumers now have a way to send a message to state lawmakers that they won't stand for an upcoming smoking ban that will force every bar in the state to quit serving their smoking customers."[65] Customers were asked to fill out the "action coasters" that were sent to state legislators. The NSA also took out a 4-page advertisement in the *Nation's Restaurant News* to promote the message that it wanted to help restaurateurs fight for their rights and that restaurants lose business when smoking ordinances go into effect.[38]

In December 1997 and January 1998, the NSA supplied 3000 bars with "action kits," which included a window sticker to register the bar's opinion of smoke-free bars, customer awareness posters to place in the bar, and customer action coasters that stated, "I'm a constituent, not a criminal," to be sent in NSA-provided envelopes to the bar owner's state legislator.[66] By March 1998, 4119 printed cards reached the Senate Health and Human Services Committee.[67]

The NSA, working through Burson-Marsteller, used print and electronic media to convey the impression that there were rampant public dissatisfaction with smoke-free bars and negative economic effects on small businesses (C. Hallett, interview with authors, November 16, 1998). Between January 1998 and June 1998, Burson-Marsteller issued more than 70 press releases claiming problems with the implementation of smoke-free bars.

The tobacco industry dominated early media coverage of the impact and popularity of smoke-free bars. Articles that were published the week before the smoke-free bar provisions went into effect, and until 3 months afterward, emphasized opposition to the law and claims of lost business, lost jobs, and problems with enforcement, as well as the probability that the law would be repealed[25,66,68–76] (also J. Miller, interview with authors, December 4, 1998). The Department of Health Services had tried to anticipate this argument by commissioning opinion polls in 1996 and 1997, which demonstrated that about two thirds of the population supported smoke-free bars (Table 1). These polls, however, did not have the same emotional appeal as the personal stories that the tobacco industry's media operation generated. Even so, support for smoke-free bars increased throughout 1998[34] (also C. Hallett, interview with authors, November 16, 1998).

Discussion

The tobacco industry's campaign to fight smoke-free bars in California was unprecedented in its duration and intensity and evolved over time.

The industry's initial arguments against the law centered on predictions of economic disaster and government interference with free choice. The economic argument lost steam after studies showed no effect of local smoke-free bar laws on bar revenues[48] and effectively ended after the Board of Equalization reported that bar business increased (D. Kiser, interview with authors, November 11, 1998; P. Hunting, interview with authors, December 18, 1998). The free-choice argument subsided as polling data from the state, voluntary health agencies, and the *Los Angeles Times* showed that most bar patrons supported smoke-free bars.[77] Research showing that bar workers' health improved 4 to 8 weeks after the law took effect[78] reinforced the concept of smoke-free bars as a workplace safety issue.

Throughout these battles, the industry tried to create a positive feedback loop in which smokers would be encouraged to ignore the law because it was going to be repealed, and the industry then used the noncompliance as an argument in the legislature for repeal. Although this strategy failed to get the law repealed; however, it did create compliance problems.

Although the health groups were outspent by the tobacco industry,[79] they were willing to make the implementation of smoke-free bars a priority and commit resources to defending the law (P. Knepprath, interview with authors, November 23, 1998). In addition to funds for polling and advertising, these groups used their credibility to garner public support for smoke-free bars and to counter the tobacco industry's activities, both outside and inside the legislature. Repeating the successful strategy used in other legislative battles,[1] the groups directly attacked the tobacco industry and state legislators willing to support the industry through a series of advertisements, which served as both a call to action for the public and a message to the legislature that the health groups were willing to use their public regard to hold the industry's political allies accountable. In addition, the health groups were able to attract critical support for smoke-free bars from entities outside the traditional public health community, including the California Labor Federation, the California League of Cities, and individual cities across the state (M. Burgat, interview with authors, November 17, 1998; P. Knepprath, interview with authors, November 23, 1998).

The public health groups also were aided by powerful legislators sympathetic to their cause. For years, Democrat Willie Brown, who received more tobacco industry campaign contributions than any other legislator in the country,[18,80] used his power as speaker of the assembly to protect the tobacco industry. After Brown left the legislature in 1996, anti-tobacco senators in the Democratic Caucus convinced President Pro Tem Lockyer that the Democrats were on the wrong side of the tobacco issue, particularly since the industry was favoring Republicans in its campaign contributions (D. Watson, T. Hayden, N. Petris; memorandum to Caucus Position on Tobacco Interests; April 24, 1996). As the bar law went into effect in 1998, new President Pro Tem Burton made it clear that the only reason the senate would reconsider the smoke-free bar law was if there was a substantial negative economic impact. After the Board of Equalization results were released, repeal of the smoke-free bar provisions was a dead issue in the senate.

The health groups were not as successful in getting the Wilson administration to ensure implementation of the smoke-free bar law. Despite the recommendations of the Department of Health Services' advertising agency, the Tobacco Education and Research Oversight Committee, and the health groups, the administration delayed using the statewide media campaign to educate the public. It also refused to use the licensing power of the Department of Alcoholic Beverage Control to see that bars did not participate in the tobacco industry's efforts to encourage people to ignore the law (M. Espinoza, letter to Assemblyman Brett Granlund, December 18, 1997). As elsewhere,[81,82] the health groups were not willing to be as public or aggressive in dealing with the administration as they were with the legislature, and they enjoyed less success there.

This situation left pro-health forces limited to lower-profile implementation efforts that would not attract the attention of high-level political figures in the administration. Fortunately, they could build on the infrastructure present in California, created by its large tobacco control program[57] and through the implementation of smoke-free workplaces and restaurants in 1995. Because approximately 90% of the state's bars are part of bar–restaurant combinations[83] (also D. Kiser, interview with authors, November 11, 1998), a large majority of bar owners and managers had already implemented the Smoke-Free Workplace Law in the restaurant sections of their establishments in 1995. As a result, compliance in bar–restaurant combinations was high from the beginning (88% of local lead agencies estimated that "most," "almost all," or "all" bar–restaurant combinations in their jurisdictions were complying with AB 13 by the end of January 1998[83]) and remained high (D. Kiser, interview with authors, November 11, 1998). Virtually all the controversy and problems centered on stand-alone bars.

Why Bars?

Why did the tobacco industry fight so hard against the smoke-free bar law, particularly since the number of cigarettes smoked in bars is much smaller than the number smoked in workplaces? Part of the answer may lie in the fact that bars have become viewed as the "last bastion"[84] of socially acceptable smoking, and smoke-free bars send a strong message that smoking is not socially desirable (A. Henderson, interview with authors, February 12, 1999).

A more direct reason may have to do with marketing tobacco products. In recent years, the tobacco industry's marketing efforts directed at young children have become a political liability. As a result, the industry may be shifting at least some of its marketing efforts to young adults, where the arguments that public health advocates have mounted about smoking and children do not apply. Smoking is increasing among college-age students (aged 18–24),[85,86] and young adults (aged 21–30) represent a substantial percentage of bar patrons.[87] The industry explicitly protected bars as promotional venues in the Master Settlement Agreement that settled lawsuits that the states brought against the tobacco industry.[88]

As early as 1996, Philip Morris and RJ Reynolds started marketing efforts in bars and clubs through the Camel Club and Marlboro Days campaigns.[89–96] The Camel Club program seeks to "create an alternative marketing campaign and cigarette distribution network that will not be affected by changing federal regulations or the scores of tobacco related lawsuits."[90] KBA Marketing, the Chicago firm that runs the Camel Club program, states in its marketing material that "[b]y operating in the nightlife scene, the objective is to directly reach the trend influencers, the people who start and maintain trends. Our association with trend influencers will have a lasting impact on club goers who will begin to associate Camel with what is 'cool.' "[97] In addition to reaching these young adults, this group serves as important role models for teens. Increasing smoking among young adults also promotes teen smoking.[98]

Although there is nothing in AB 13 that prohibits these promotional activities in bars, conducting them in a smoke-free bar presumably may reduce the effectiveness of these promotional campaigns: smoke-free bars send a strong social message that smoking is no longer socially acceptable.

Lessons Learned

Don't start with bars. The smoke-free bars were phased in 3 years after all other workplaces in California went smoke free. It was beneficial to implement the Smoke-Free Workplace Law incrementally to prepare for the tobacco industry responses to the law and to conduct educational efforts targeting bar owners and workers and the public.

Don't let the tobacco industry define the issue. The industry attempted to make the fight over smoke-free bars an economic debate, framing the small business owner as the victim of this law. Instead of using public appearances to respond to the tobacco industry's message, the health groups framed AB 13 as a health and worker safety issue.

Health groups must commit resources to upholding the law. The health groups spent an estimated $200 000 to promote and uphold the law. Polling, advertising, action alerts, and lobbying all take commitment and resources. The health groups were also willing to take on not only the tobacco industry but also tobacco's political allies in the legislature.

Once the law passes, the fight has just begun. The passing of AB 13 was only the beginning of the fight over smoke-free bars. The tobacco industry will continue to seek to undermine the law, even after it is passed. Although low-level officials in the Department of Health Services sought to implement the law, they did not receive high-level political support, and this reduced the effectiveness of their efforts. The private health groups did not apply effective pressure on the administration to secure optimal implementation. Long-term success requires that public health groups work to ensure not only passage but active implementation of clean indoor air laws. □

Contributors

Both authors contributed to the design of this study, the analysis of results, and the writing of the paper.

Acknowledgments

This work was supported by National Cancer Institute grant CA-61021.

This work was presented at the American Public Health Association Conference, November 7–11, 1999.

References

1. Glantz S, Balbach E. *Tobacco Wars: Inside the California Battles.* Berkeley: University of California Press; 2000.
2. Macdonald H, Glantz SA. Political realities of statewide smoking legislation: the passage of California's Assembly Bill 13. *Tob Control.* 1997;6:41–54.
3. American Beverage Institute. *American Beverage Institute Market Research Study.* Los Angeles, Calif: KPMG Peat Marwick; April 1998.
4. Macdonald H, Aguinaga S, Glantz SA. The defeat of Philip Morris' "California Uniform Tobacco Control Act." *Am J Public Health.* 1997; 87:1989–1996.

5. Samuels B, Glantz SA. The politics of local tobacco control. *JAMA*. 1991;266:2110–2117.
6. Traynor M, Begay ME, Glantz SA. New tobacco industry strategy to prevent local tobacco control. *JAMA*. 1993;270:479–486.
7. Samuels B, Begay ME, Hazan AR, Glantz SA. Philip Morris's failed experiment in Pittsburgh. *J Health Polit Policy Law.* 1992;17:329–351.
8. Regardie J. Tobacco Road: can smoking ban for bars possibly be good for health and business? *Downtown News.* September 9, 1996:12.
9. Magzamen S, Glantz S. *Turning the Tide: Tobacco Industry Political Influence and Tobacco Policy Making in California 1997–1999.* San Francisco: Institute for Health Policy Studies, School of Medicine, University of California, San Francisco; September 1999.
10. *AB 297 Bill Analysis.* Sacramento: Occupational Safety and Health Standards Board, California Dept of Industrial Relations; June 3, 1997.
11. Vanzi M. Smoking foe mounts offensive. *Los Angeles Times.* March 23, 1998:A3.
12. Morain D. Smoking ban is hazardous to capitol rules. *Los Angeles Times.* September 8, 1997.
13. California State Assembly. *Assembly Rule 77.2, Joint Rule 61.* Sacramento: California Legislature, 1997–98 Session; 1997.
14. Lucas G. Lobbyists try to delay smoking ban: state's bars, card clubs scheduled to be smoke-free. *San Francisco Chronicle.* July 17, 1997:A1.
15. Monardi F, Glantz S. Are tobacco industry campaign contributions influencing state legislative behavior? *Am J Public Health.* 1998;88: 918–923.
16. Vellinga M. Foes of bar smoking ban ready new tactic. *Sacramento Bee.* August 28, 1997:A20.
17. Glantz S, Begay M. Tobacco industry campaign contributions are affecting tobacco control policy making in California. *JAMA.* 1994;272: 1176–1182.
18. Balbach E, Monardi F, Fox B, Glantz S. *Holding Government Accountable: Tobacco Policy Making in California, 1995–1997.* San Francisco: Institute for Health Policy Studies, University of California, San Francisco; June 1997.
19. Moore S, Wolfe S, Lindes D, Douglas C. Epidemiology of failed tobacco control legislation. *JAMA.* 1994;272:1171–1175.
20. Glastris P. Frank Fat's napkin: how the trial lawyers (and the doctors!) sold out to the tobacco companies. *Washington Monthly.* December 1987:19–25.
21. Vanzi M. Bid to lift smoking ban comes before key opponent. *Los Angeles Times.* March 25, 1998:A18.
22. Ainsworth B. Smoking out the tobacco lobby's true intention. *San Diego Union-Tribune.* October 13, 1997:A3.
23. Vanzi M, Ingram C. Bid to lift smoking ban faces fight. *Los Angeles Times.* January 30, 1998:4.
24. Jordan H. Tax proposals taking aim at pockets of state smokers. *San Jose Mercury News.* February 13, 1998:A1.
25. Salladay R. Bar smoking ban still controversial. *San Francisco Examiner.* February 11, 1998.
26. Sweeney J. Smoking ban under review in the Senate. *San Diego Union-Tribune.* January 30, 1998:A3.
27. Vanzi M. Senate committee upholds ban on indoor smoking. *Los Angeles Times.* March 26, 1998.
28. American Cancer Society California Division. *Smoke-Free Workplace Law Public Opinion Poll.* Walnut Creek, Calif: Charlton Research Co; March 25, 1998.
29. San Francisco Tobacco Free Project. *San Francisco Smoke-Free Bar Compliance Survey Results.* San Francisco, Calif: San Francisco Tobacco Free Project; December 17, 1998.
30. California Department of Health Services. *A Survey on California's Law for a Smokefree Workplace (AB 13): Attitudes After the First Year of Implementation.* Lincoln, Neb: Gallup Organization; March 1996.
31. California Department of Health Services. *A Survey of California Adults Age 21 or Older About Smoking Policies and Smoke-Free Bars.* San Francisco, Calif: Field Research Corp; July 1997.
32. Los Angeles County Health Department. *Bar Patrons in LA County Overwhelmingly Support Smoke-Free Bars.* San Francisco, Calif: Communication Sciences Group; February 25, 1998.
33. Collins L, Gaynes M, Weitz A, Kleinschmidt K. Fisherman's Wharf and Jack London Square go for smoke-free bars [press release]. San Francisco, Calif: American Lung Association; 1998.
34. California Department of Health Services. *A Survey of California Bar Patrons About Smoking Policies and Smoke-Free Bars.* San Francisco, Calif: Field Research Corp; February 24–March 2, 1998.
35. California Department of Health Services. *Smoke-Free Bars Follow-Up Survey.* San Francisco, Calif: Field Research Corp; August 1998.
36. Stauber J, Rampton S. *Toxic Sludge Is Good for You.* Monroe, Me: Common Courage Press; 1995.
37. Philip Morris Companies Inc. California action plan, 1994. Available at: http://www.library.ucsf.edu/tobacco/calminnesota/html/3560/001. Accessed December 18, 2000.
38. Americans for Nonsmokers' Rights Foundation. *National Smokers Alliance: Exposed.* Berkeley, Calif: Americans for Nonsmokers' Rights; October 1998.
39. California State Senate Television Program. *Senate Health and Human Services Committee Hearing—March 25, 1998.* Sacramento: California State Senate Television Program; 1998.
40. San Diego Tavern and Restaurant Association. *Potential Economic Effects of a Smoking Ban in the City of San Diego.* San Diego, Calif: Price Waterhouse; October 1992.
41. Southern California Business Association. *Summary of Findings From LA Restaurant Owners/Managers Survey.* San Francisco, Calif: Charlton Research Co; December 1993–January 1994.
42. Southern California Business Association. *The Impact of the Current and Proposed Smoking Bans on Restaurants and Bars in California.* Los Angeles, Calif: KPMG Peat Marwick; February 1996.
43. Bartosch W, Pope G. *The Economic Impact of Brookline's Restaurant Smoking Ban.* Waltham, Mass: Health Economics Research; 1995.
44. Bartosch W, Pope G. The economic effect of smoke-free restaurant policies on restaurant business in Massachusetts. *J Public Health Manage Pract.* 1999;5:53–62.
45. Biener L, Siegel M. Behavior intentions of the public after bans on smoking in restaurants and bars. *Am J Public Health.* 1997;87:2042–2044.
46. Enz C, Corsun D, Young Y. To dine or not to dine: restaurant patrons' responses to the New York City smoke-free air act. *Cornell Hotel Restaurant Adm Q.* December 1996;37(6):8–12.
47. Glantz S, Smith LRA. The effect of ordinances requiring smoke-free restaurants on restaurant sales [published correction appears in *Am J Public Health.* 1997;87:1729–1730]. *Am J Public Health.* 1994;84:1081–1085.
48. Glantz S, Smith LRA. The effect of ordinances requiring smoke-free restaurants and bars on revenues: a follow-up [published correction appears in *Am J Public Health.* 1998;88:1122] *Am J Public Health.* 1997;87:1687–1693.
49. Goldstein A, Sobel R. Environmental tobacco smoke regulations have not hurt restaurant sales in North Carolina. *N C Med J.* 1998;59:284–288.
50. Huang P, Toblas S, Kohout S, et al. Assessment of the impact of a 100% smoke-free ordinance on restaurant sales—West Lake Hills, TX, 1992–1994. *MMWR Morb Mortal Wkly Rep.* 1995;44: 370–372.
51. Hyland A, Cummings K, Nauenberg E. Analysis of taxable sales receipts: was New York City's smoke-free air act bad for restaurant business? *J Public Health Manage Pract.* 1999;5:14–21.
52. Sciacca J, Ratliff M. Prohibiting smoking in restaurants: effects on restaurant sales. *Am J Health Promot.* 1998;12:176–184.
53. State Board of Equalization, Statistics Section. *Comparison of January 1997 and January 1998 Taxable Sales of Selected Eating and Drinking Places With General On-Sale Licenses.* Sacramento: Agency Planning and Research Division, California State Board of Equalization; June 24, 1998.
54. State Board of Equalization, Statistics Section. *Comparison of 1st Quarter 1997 and 1st Quarter 1998 Taxable Sales of Selected Eating and Drinking Places With General On-Sale Licenses.* Sacramento: State Board of Equalization, Agency Planning and Research Division; October 1, 1998.
55. Tobacco Control Section. *Final Taxable Sales Figures for Bars and Restaurants for the First Quarter of 1998.* Sacramento: California Dept of Health Services; December 22, 1998.
56. Bal D, Kizer KW, Felton PG, Mezar MN, Niemeyer D. Reducing tobacco consumption in California. Development of a statewide anti-tobacco use campaign. *JAMA.* 1990;264: 1570–1574.
57. Balbach E, Glantz SA. Tobacco control advocates must demand high-quality media campaigns: the California experience. *Tob Control.* 1998;7:397–408.
58. Hunting L. *TEROC Meeting Minutes.* Berkeley, Calif: Tobacco Education and Research Oversight Committee; September 30, 1997. Bates No. 7–12.
59. Russell S. Delay of smoking ads irks panel: campaign backs state law against lighting up in bars. *San Francisco Chronicle.* October 1, 1997.
60. Vellinga M. Wilson urged to publicize bar-smoking ban. *Sacramento Bee.* October 3, 1997:A3.
61. Tobacco Control Section. *AB 13 LLA Smoke-free Bar Survey Results.* Sacramento: California Dept of Health Services, Tobacco Control Section; July–September 1996.
62. Morain D. Behind fuming bar owners is savvy,

well-heeled group. *Los Angeles Times.* January 30, 1998.
63. Levin M. Smoker group's thick wallet raises questions. *Los Angeles Times.* March 29, 1998:A21.
64. Merlo E. Memo to D. McCloud re: National Smokers Alliance Membership. November 10, 1993. Minnesota Depository Bates No. 2023343150 (Philip Morris, Inc).
65. National Smokers' Alliance. California bar owners and smokers send message to lawmakers: "Lighten up!" *NSA Voice.* April 1996:1, 4.
66. Claiborne W. Unfiltered defiance: with tobacco industry's support, California taverns increasingly allow patrons to violate smoking bans. *Washington Post.* February 17, 1998:A3.
67. Miller J. *AB 297 Bill Analysis.* Sacramento, Calif: Senate Committee on Health and Human Services; March 25, 1998.
68. Weintraub D. Fight over smoking ban is likely to last a while. *Orange County Register.* January 30, 1998:1.
69. Gorman T. Bars still exhibit plenty of puffing—and huffing. *Los Angeles Times.* January 30, 1998.
70. Leeds J. Bar patrons still smoke despite ban. *Los Angeles Times.* January 15, 1998.
71. Lelyveld N. Where there's smoke—and ire; some tavern owners in California defy the new law that bans smoking. *Philadelphia Inquirer.* February 11, 1998:E1.
72. Howard J. Lifting of tavern smoking ban OK'd. *San Diego Union-Tribune.* January 29, 1998:A3.
73. Hubert C, Lindelof B. Enforcement of smoking ban is spotty: region's counties issue few citations despite complaints. *Sacramento Bee.* February 9, 1998:A1.
74. Romano B. Barkeeps fume over smoking ban: local tavern owners join statewide chorus saying new law is harming their business. *San Jose Mercury News.* February 27, 1998:B2.
75. Glionna J. Ban on bar smoking is target of protests stages in 5 cities. *Los Angeles Times.* February 27, 1998.
76. Nguyen D. Ban the ban bar owners say: effort launched to repeal smoking law. *San Diego Union-Tribune.* January 10, 1998.
77. Morain D. Bar smoking ban gets wide backing. *Los Angeles Times.* May 27, 1998:A3.
78. Eisner M, Smith AK, Blanc PD. Bartenders' respiratory health after establishment of smoke-free bars and taverns. *JAMA.* 1998;280: 1909–1914.
79. Jacobson P, Wasserman J, Raube K. *The Political Evolution of Anti-Smoking Legislation.* Santa Monica, Calif: Rand Corp; 1992.
80. Monardi F, Balbach E, Aguinaga S, Glantz S. *Shifting Allegiances: Tobacco Industry Political Expenditures in California, January 1995–March 1996.* San Francisco: Institute for Health Policy Studies, University of California, San Francisco; April 1996.
81. Aguinaga S. *The Politics of Tobacco Control: The Case of Arizona.* Berkeley: University of California, Berkeley; 1999.
82. Jacobson P, Wasserman J. The implementation and enforcement of tobacco control laws: policy implications for activists and the industry. *J Health Policy Polit Law.* 1999;24:567–598.
83. California Dept of Health Services. *January 1998 Assessment Survey.* Sacramento: California Dept of Health Services, Tobacco Control Section; January 27, 1998.
84. Morain D. Smoke set to clear in bars—but will it? *Los Angeles Times.* December 22, 1997:A1.
85. Emmons K, Wechsler H, Dowdall G, Abraham M. Predictors of smoking among US college students. *Am J Public Health.* 1998;88: 104–107.
86. Wechsler H, Rigotti N, Geldhill-Hoyt J, Lee H. Increased levels of cigarette use among college students. *JAMA.* 1998;280:1673–1678.
87. Clark W. Public drinking context: bars and taverns. In: Harford T, Gaines L, eds. *Social Drinking Context (NIAAA Research Monograph No. 7).* Washington, DC: Dept of Health and Human Services; 1981:8–33. Publication APM-81-1097.
88. National Association of Attorneys General. *Master Settlement Agreement.* Washington, DC: National Association of Attorneys General; 1998: 10, 12, 16, 19, 20, 109, 110.
89. Gellene D. Joining the clubs; tobacco firms find a venue in bars. *Los Angeles Times.* September 25, 1997:D1.
90. Naymik M. Night light: Camel kids push smokes at "cool clubs." *Winston-Salem Journal.* October 27, 1997.
91. Obermayer J. Marlboro fires up marketing campaign in Triangle bars. *News-Observer.* July 28, 1998.
92. Carreon C. Joe Camel turns up in Portland nightclubs. *Oregonian.* July 31, 1998.
93. Solomon C. Tobacco companies bankroll their own. *Seattle Times.* December 10, 1997:A1.
94. Danielson R. Camel promotion trots into clubs. *St Petersburg Times.* February 22, 1998:B3.
95. Davis H. Cigarette promotions target the college crowd: a party to die for? *Buffalo News.* July 27, 1998.
96. Cooper N. Warning: tobacco companies' advertising money may be addictive to Houston's club scene. *Houston Press.* October 1, 1998.
97. Romero D. The detectors are going off. *Los Angeles Times.* October 9, 1997.
98. Asher/Gould Advertising. *1998 Advertising Strategy Recommendations.* Los Angeles: California Dept of Health Services, Tobacco Control Section; December 10, 1997.

Constructing "Sound Science" and "Good Epidemiology": Tobacco, Lawyers, and Public Relations Firms

The tobacco industry has attacked "junk science" to discredit the evidence that secondhand smoke—among other environmental toxins—causes disease. Philip Morris used public relations firms and lawyers to develop a "sound science" program in the United States and Europe that involved recruiting other industries and issues to obscure the tobacco industry's role. The European "sound science" plans included a version of "good epidemiological practices" that would make it impossible to conclude that secondhand smoke—and thus other environmental toxins—caused diseases.

Public health professionals need to be aware that the "sound science" movement is not an indigenous effort from within the profession to improve the quality of scientific discourse, but reflects sophisticated public relations campaigns controlled by industry executives and lawyers whose aim is to manipulate the standards of scientific proof to serve the corporate interests of their clients. (*Am J Public Health.* 2001;91:1749-1757)

| Elisa K. Ong, MD, MS, and Stanton A. Glantz, PhD

THE TERMS "SOUND SCIENCE" and "junk science" have increasingly appeared in the media, medical literature,[1,2] and litigation.[3] Industries—those responsible for products ranging from silicone gel breast implants[4,5] to hormone-treated beef[6] to secondhand smoke[7]—claim to be victimized by lawsuits and regulations based on "junk science,"[2,8] while the scientific, public health, and regulatory communities claim their actions are based on "sound science."[9–12]

The tobacco industry has always contested the evidence that secondhand smoke endangers nonsmokers[13–17]; during the last decade the Philip Morris (PM) tobacco company appropriated the "sound science" concept to attack studies on secondhand smoke. To deal with the tobacco industry's lack of credibility, it developed "sound science" coalitions involving other industries opposed to regulation to support its position, similar to smokers' rights[18,19] and restaurant association[20,21] front groups. PM also mounted a sophisticated public relations campaign to promote "good epidemiology practices" (GEP) to shape the standards of scientific proof to make it impossible to "prove" that secondhand smoke—among many other environmental toxins—is dangerous.

We analyzed tobacco industry documents made public as a result of litigation in the United States and available on the Internet in an online repository to which documents are continually added as additional and unrelated legal cases are resolved. The documents cited in the reference list were originally accessed between January 2000 and May 2001. Search terms included "IARC," "TASSC," "sound science," "junk science," "GEP," and the names of key players. We did not use documents from a related depository covering British American Tobacco in Guildford, England, because of the depository's practical inaccessibility to researchers.[22] If we had used the Guildford documents, they probably would have contributed to a broader story.

PHILIP MORRIS'S "SOUND SCIENCE" ORGANIZATION IN THE UNITED STATES

PM began its "sound science" program in 1993 to stimulate criticism of the 1992 US Environmental Protection Agency (EPA) report,[23] which identified secondhand smoke as a Group A human carcinogen. Ellen Merlo (vice president, PM Corporate Affairs) wrote to William Campbell (chairman, PM USA):

> OBJECTIVES
> *Our overriding objective is to discredit the EPA report and to get the EPA to adopt a standard for risk assessment for all products.*
> Concurrently, it is our objective to prevent states and cities, as well as businesses from passing smoking bans.
> And finally, where possible we will proactively seek to pass accommodation legislation with preemption.
> STRATEGIES
> *To form local coalitions to help us educate the local media, legislators and the public at large about the dangers of "junk science" and to caution them from taking regulatory steps* before fully understanding the costs in both economic and human terms [emphasis added].[24]

In February 1993, PM and its public relations firm, APCO Associates, worked to launch a "sound science" coalition in the United States, with approximately $320 000 budgeted for the first 24 weeks.[24] Three months later, The Advancement for Sound Science Coalition (TASSC) had been formed.[25] TASSC described itself as "a not-for-profit coalition advocating the use of sound science in public policy decision making,"[26] even though APCO created it to help PM fight smoking restrictions.[27,28] TASSC's public positioning and media campaign were designed to minimize its connections with the tobacco industry[29,30]; TASSC's member survey mentioned only secondhand smoke among a list of other potential examples of "unsound, incomplete, or unsubstantiated science."[31]

A broad base of issues and members was necessary to provide credibility to the new organization. Charles Lister, a lawyer at the tobacco industry's Washington, DC, law firm, Covington & Burling, wrote, "No one would take seriously a meeting even partly sponsored by PM in which

EPA was more than one example among several. In any event, our points can be made more effectively and persuasively if EPA is discussed within a larger context."[32] Lister suggested that "foods, plastics, chemicals, and packaging would be natural candidates" in broadening the scope of TASSC's sponsors and issues beyond EPA and the tobacco industry.[32]

To develop TASSC into "a broad-based and diverse national coalition,"[33] more than 20000 recruitment letters were mailed, with 100 letters mailed to "key scientists,"[34] signed by TASSC's chairman Garrey Carruthers (former Republican governor of New Mexico). The leadership and members, which included prominent scientists and policymakers[35–37] plus representatives from corporations,[37,38] would be provided PM's secondhand smoke agenda suggestions through APCO but made to feel the agenda was their own.[39]

PM hid its role[40] so successfully that when longtime tobacco industry consultant Gary Huber, then a professor at the University of Texas Health Center, received the letter inviting him to join TASSC, he contacted Tony Andrade of the PM law firm Shook, Hardy & Bacon (SH&B) to inform him that the organization might be helpful to the tobacco industry.[41] Andrade, also unaware of PM's role with TASSC, forwarded the information to PM, which subsequently "filled him in on TASSC."[41]

TASSC's overall effectiveness in serving PM's initial goal of discrediting the EPA report may not have met PM's expectations; by April 1994, Merlo expressed concern that, despite its $880000 cost in 1994,[42,43] TASSC was not proving to be a "tool to affect legislative decisions"[28] to stem smoking restrictions.

Even so, by 1995, a TASSC Web site was being planned with PM to distribute scientific papers and polls to support PM's position.[44] TASSC and its Web site are now defunct, but its executive director Steve Milloy, an adjunct scholar at the Cato Institute (a libertarian think tank in Washington, DC, that has received funds from the tobacco industry[45]), now produces a "junk science" Web site.[46] Milloy's Web site continues TASSC's original work in criticizing and "debunking" the science behind public health and environmental issues, including secondhand smoke.[46]

THE EUROPEAN "SOUND SCIENCE" PROGRAM AND "GOOD EPIDEMIOLOGY PRACTICES"

PM also developed a "sound science" program in Europe to subvert[47] the effects of a large ongoing European epidemiologic study of passive smoking and lung cancer being conducted by the International Agency for Research on Cancer (IARC),[48] which the tobacco industry feared would stimulate smoking restrictions in Europe. PM sought to "develop a programme to generate support for 'junk science' and education on use and abuse of epidemiology, possibly through a coalition on bad science,"[49] which would prepare a skeptical environment for interpreting the study's results. PM used the public relations firms Burson-Marsteller and APCO[39,50–54] to address the need that "science must be managed according to clear, scientifically based criteria, e.g., good epidemiology,"[55] consistent with the industry's interests.

PM's interest in promoting "good epidemiology" developed after the Chemical Manufacturers Association (CMA) published its suggested "Good Epidemiology Practices" (GEP) in 1991 as a framework for "consumers of epidemiology" (policymakers and regulators) to determine the quality of a study and address poorly conducted studies.[56] The CMA's GEP promoted the "sound science" and "good epidemiology" concepts for each step in the conduct of an epidemiologic study.[57,58] Covington & Burling lawyer Charles Lister distributed the CMA's GEP to PM in February 1994:

> Their [CMA's] announced goals are essentially our own. The GEP Guidelines are intended to be analogous to Good Laboratory Practices (GLP) and Good Manufacturing Practices (GMP), both of which are expressly now endorsed and required by Community law.
>
> The GEP Guidelines themselves seem disappointingly vague to me.
>
> ...GEP is being pushed in Europe by a number of companies, including particularly Monsanto and ICI.
>
> ...I was informally told that DG V [European Union's Directorate General for Employment, Industrial Relations and Social Affairs] is quite interested in GEP, although reticent about proposing new legislation. Nonetheless, there seems to be a realistic prospect that they might be persuaded to issue a [European] Commission Communication or other policy document.[59]

PM saw the CMA's GEP as an opportunity to promote an official epidemiologic standard that would challenge the methodology of IARC's work.[60] Thomas Borelli (Director, PM Science and Environmental Policy), however, expressed concern that the CMA guidelines did not go far enough to meet the tobacco industry's needs because

> . . . it lacks teeth and as written it does not have enough meat to help us on ETS [environmental tobacco smoke, another term for secondhand smoke]. However setting up our own standards is a good project for us and our consultant's [sic] program. It would be good offensive strategy for our consultant's [sic] to be out there trying to fix epidemiology instead of being critical all the time.[61]

PM's scientific personnel agreed that PM could adapt GEP to include secondhand smoke studies and that PM's consultants, a network of scientists being financed by industry lawyers to contest the evidence that secondhand smoke caused disease,[47,62,63] should "fix" epidemiology proactively.[64,65] Mitch Ritter (PM Scientific Affairs) noted the obstacles, and appeal, of this approach: "It is difficult to imagine epidemiologists—or the health lobby in general—accepting this [CMA] initiative as it stands, though they will have to accept the principle of a set of good practices."[64,65] PM decided to appropriate the GEP movement by broadening its GEP support base to the scientific community, European government bodies, and other industries with similar concerns about low-level risks. PM's 1994 "Legislative Guidelines on GEP" included the following:

> Objective
> * Impede adverse legislation
>
> Strategy
> * Endorsement by scientific world
>   * International gathering of world's top epidemiologists (October)
>
> Tool: GEP guidelines
> * Expand debate to EU [European Union] political targets
>   * Political conference opportunities (DG V, STOA [EU Directorate General for Em-

ployment, Industrial Relations and Social Affairs; Science and Technology Office of Assessment])
* Legislative opportunities (EAC, Biomed, public health framework)

Tool: GEP resolution
* Motivate concerned industry sectors
  * GEP lobby

  Physical agents:
  - Mobile phones, electricity (EMF)
  - Computers (UV rays)

  Chemical agents:
  - Food (sugar, dairy, flavorings)
  - Chemicals
  - Metals
  * Sound science lobby

  Widen to
  - Packaging
  - Pharmaceutical
  - Forestry/paper[66]

PM wanted GEP guidelines to be endorsed by the scientific community, a GEP resolution to be passed through European legislation, and a GEP lobby with other industries facing regulation and a broad-based "sound science" lobby. As with the initial "sound science" efforts, the tobacco industry's role would be minimized. The industry sought broad support of numerous endorsers on a variety of issues to provide credibility for PM's GEP objective—to avert increased smoking restrictions.

With the help of its legal, public relations, and scientific resources, PM began drafting a GEP resolution that would be "authored" by a "sound science" coalition. In June 1994, APCO drafted a potential TASSC-sponsored list of "17 Guiding Scientific Principles,"[67] which PM found "too vague" and not supportive enough of its GEP plans.[68] SH&B drafted GEP guidelines to be sponsored by an "Executive Committee of the Sound Science Coalition" (Table 1).[54] SH&B's GEP resolution[54] promoted the tobacco industry's position, subsequently advocated publicly by SH&B,[69] that odds ratios of 2 or less are highly questionable and that a statistically significant association is not strong enough evidence for causation to warrant regulatory action. (This concentration on odds ratios was not in the original CMA proposal.)

PM consultant Roger Walk restructured the GEP resolution, relying "heavily on the content of the [SH&B] drafts" to "look more like a 'scientist's' version of guidelines."[70,71] With the relative risk for lung cancer due to passive smoking at about 1.2,[17,23,48,72–75] and the relative risk for heart disease about 1.3,[74–76] this standard would prevent action to protect the public from lung cancer and heart disease caused by secondhand smoke.

To obtain scientific endorsement of PM's GEP, PM needed scientists to promote it to government bodies.[77] In June 1994, PM sought scientists to participate in a GEP seminar in Germany[54] and planned for a subsequent long-term coalition that would help criticize the IARC study.[78] Burson-Marsteller identified scientists interested in "sound science" and "good epidemiology," but found that some scientists were concerned that corporate sponsorship—especially sponsorship by PM—would limit their scientific independence, even though Burson-Marsteller had not mentioned PM.[79,80] In August 1994, Covington & Burling created a list of potential epidemiologists who might be approached for the GEP seminar, excluding "influential epidemiologists known to have strongly antitobacco views."[81]

The plan to use prescreened epidemiologists may have changed just as PM was ready to introduce GEP to them.[82] An October 1994 memo from Joanna

TABLE 1— Shook, Hardy & Bacon's Draft GEP Resolution for a "Sound Science" Coalition[54]

THE EXECUTIVE COMMITTEE RECOMMENDS that the members of the Sound Science Coalition adopt and actively promote in the scientific community at large and within their individual disciplines, appropriate and specific professional standards for epidemiological research, to be carried out by accredited individuals and institutions, reflecting the following principles:

1. The study design should clearly define all objectives and hypotheses. Possible problems in design and data interpretation should be described and the intended method for addressing each fully set out. Every effort should be made to address possible confounders to avoid the need for subsequent adjustments.

2. In case-control studies, special attention should be given to how the control group will be selected and what matching procedures will be utilized. Also, case selection should be explained with emphasis on efforts to ensure a high participation rate. A pre-calculation of required sample size should be carried out to ensure that the sample is sufficient to produce meaningful results.

3. Statements of study design should contain a description of statistical techniques. This should include underlying assumptions for distribution, variance, correlation and regression procedures. The degree to which violation of these assumptions would invalidate the analysis should be specified whenever possible.

4. Adherence to the study protocol should be as close as possible. Any deviations (e.g., errors in randomization, low participation rate, suspected confounders, possible misclassification) should be documented.

5. Special care should be given to the training and monitoring of those administering questionnaires and surveys; blinded techniques are preferred.

6. After the study is conducted, the results should be analyzed as specified by the study protocol. Two-sided hypothesis tests are encouraged. If a one-sided test is employed, this should be noted and the rationale for using it provided. The presentation of confidence intervals for the estimate of risk gives more information than a single point value with an associated p value. Generally, 95% confidence intervals are preferred.

7. An adequate description of the raw data should precede and complement formal statistical analysis. If the data are not supportive of the stated hypotheses, no further analysis is necessary. Subsequent treatment of the data should only be for hypothesis generating purposes.

8. Odds ratios of 2 or less should be treated with caution, particularly when the confidence intervals are wide. There is a likelihood that the odds ratio is artefactual and the result of problems with case or control selection, confounders or bias.

9. Meta-analysis and pooling techniques are best used for homogenous data gathered under a uniform pool.

10. Observations that are inconsistent with the main body of the data should not be excluded from the analysis.

11. Journal articles and scientific conferences are the appropriate forum for the presentation of research results. Every effort should be made to publish and report on all completed research, regardless of outcome. Only by such efforts can the entire sample of conducted research be made available to the scientific community and publication bias minimized.

12. Generally, hypotheses tests not specified by the study protocol should not be reported. When many hypotheses tests are performed on data from a single study, a number of positive results can be expected to arise by chance alone, creating serious problems of interpretation.

13. Recognizing that a statistically significant association does not in itself provide direct evidence of causal relationship between the variables concerned and that causation can only be established on nonstatistical grounds, particular care should be taken when comparing two variables that have changed over time. Such comparisons often produce apparent associations.

14. Graphic display of results and figures that show individual observations are to be encouraged. For example, when appropriate, fixed regression lines should be presented together with a scatter diagram of the raw data. Any complex statistical methods should be communicated in a manner that is comprehensible to the reader.

15. Rigorous scientific objectivity should be the standard when reporting on epidemiological results. Defects in study design, conduct and analysis should be frankly admitted. It is helpful for abstracts accurately to reflect any study deficiencies. Advocacy and objectivity rarely comfortably coexist.

Sullivan (PM Corporate Services Brussels) announced, "the GEP project would be halted as previously discussed because the [PM IARC] Task Force agreed that it could be counterproductive."[83] PM's planned long-term "sound science" coalition is now likely to be the Cambridge-based European Science and Environment Forum, which sought funding from tobacco companies in addition to PM for its 1996 inception and has actively criticized the IARC study.[47]

PM still sought official European Union endorsement of GEP, which other industries were already seeking,[59] and PM hoped it would contain "the necessary language to catch the IARC study."[77] In July 1994, PM had a draft of a possible European Union GEP resolution,[54] and Covington & Burling lawyer John Rupp drafted a European Council resolution about GEP for PM's consideration.[84] In early 1995, PM was considering holding a GEP seminar in Germany and introducing PM's GEP at an October 1995 conference on the use of science in public health regulations to be funded by the European Union's Directorate General V (Employment, Industrial Relations and Social Affairs) and the nonferrous metal industry.[85]

In September 1995, Joanna Sullivan (PMCS Brussels) wrote to Richard Carchman (director, Scientific Affairs, PM USA) stating that the SH&B GEP guideline revision[71] "should be given to Professor [Ernst] Wynder for passing onto Dr [Henriette] Chamouillet of DGV of the European Commission."[86] Wynder, whose early work linked smoking and cancer, had developed a financial relationship with the tobacco industry.[87–99] PM described Wynder as "being in favor of the [GEP] project" and helping PM organize a GEP conference.[100]

It is unclear whether Wynder and Chamouillet did indeed meet, but by late 1995, the European Union Data Protection Directive was adopted, stating that "the Commission shall encourage the drawing-up of codes of conduct [for studies involving the processing of medical data]" and that "the Commission may ensure publicity for [approved] codes."[101,102] This European Union directive led to a new GEP proposal, drafted in 1995, with limited distribution in 1997, by a group of European and American epidemiologists from industry and academia, in hopes of international review and subsequent European Union Working Group approval.[101] Despite PM's efforts, no European Union resolution on GEP had been produced as of mid-2000.

WORLDWIDE SEMINARS ON GOOD EPIDEMIOLOGY PRACTICES

From 1994 to 2000, seemingly independent seminars on GEP have been conducted by several organizations in the United States, United Kingdom, European Union, and China. In fact, PM is connected to all these events.

Federal Focus, Inc, a nonprofit foundation based in Washington, DC, that engages in research and education pertaining to federal government policy issues, conducted 2 seminars[103] on epidemiology and risk assessment that appear to have been part of PM's GEP program. In 1994, Federal Focus convened a 19-member panel in the United States that advocated uniform epidemiology principles.[104] In October 1995, a second 18-member panel met in London, England, and drafted the "Principles for Evaluating Epidemiologic Data in Regulatory Risk Assessment," or "London Principles,"[105] which pose a series of questions to guide a risk assessor about the overall quality of the data and its potential weight for a risk assessment. The panel comprised scientific representatives from academia and industry, including some who had received tobacco industry funding or served as tobacco industry consultants.[47,105,106]

The London Principles do not criticize relative risks of less than 2, but the Federal Focus leaders have, while working under contract with PM. Federal Focus received at least $200 000 from PM in 1993.[107] Federal Focus' chairman, Jim Tozzi of Multinational Business Services, was under contract with PM for $40 000 a month in 1993 and up to $610 000 in 1994.[108,109] Thorne Auchter, director of Federal Focus' Institute for Regulatory Policy, has testified to the US Occupational Safety and Health Administration Public Meeting on Standards Planning Process that "a determination needs to be made regarding the reliability of relative risks in the "weak association (RR<2.0–3.0) range."[110] In 1993 and 1994, Tozzi was to work with PM "to develop materials designed to intensify the debate on the need for scientific standards on meta-analysis and epidemiology such as electromagnetic fields, chlorinated water, and radon in water," with the purpose of "supporting legislative mandates on epidemiological standards" and "increasing debate on ETS risk assessment within EPA."[108]

PM, Covington & Burling, and Tozzi collaborated on 8 "Criteria for Epidemiology" of which "all guidelines for conducting epidemiological studies should incorporate consideration," including "[d]oes the relative risk fall into the realm of 'weak association' (RR<2.0–3.0) relative to background?"[111] In July 1995, Tozzi sought PM to discuss the Federal Focus "EPI Principles" from the "first conference" with NATO and IARC officials, as "EPA, through IARC and NATO, continues to market its indoor air quality program overseas."[112]

The Weinberg Group, a consultancy run by Myron Weinberg that testifies for the tobacco industry on clean indoor-air issues,[63] worked with PM to conduct "Good Risk Management Practices" conferences in Europe and Asia. An October 1997 European conference, "The Challenges of Responsible Good Risk Management Practices," included PM as one of 11 corporate supporters with official sponsorship by the European Union Commission.[113] The speakers included tobacco industry consultant Ragnar Rylander[63] (who has consulted for PM about GEP's utility,[114,115] stated that relative risks of less than 2 have severe methodological problems,[116] and advocated GEP at a 1996 scientific conference[117]) and the European Science and Environment Forum's executive director, Roger Bates.[113] Government administrators were session moderators, which Weinberg described to PM as a "valuable concept" because they were "the target of the expert presentations."[113] PM wanted to repeat a similar Weinberg seminar in Asia in 1998, to be endorsed by the Association of South East Asian Nations,[113] which PM expected to establish guidelines for risk assessment.[118] PM planned to commit $220 000[113] for a conference in Kuala Lumpur or Bangkok by

November 1998 and hoped for published journal articles or conference proceedings.[118]

The tobacco industry's Center for Indoor Air Research cohosted a July 1997 "International Workshop on Risk Assessment and Good Epidemiological Practices" in China with the Guangzhou Institute for Chemical Carcinogens and the Chinese Epidemiological Association.[119] (The Center for Indoor Air Research financed projects "specially reviewed" by tobacco industry lawyers, as opposed to its peer-reviewed projects; the former are more likely to conclude that secondhand smoke does not cause disease.[120,121]) The China conference brought together 100 lung cancer specialists within China[122] with a few scientists from outside China, including scientists funded by the tobacco industry.[47,63,106,123] This China GEP workshop was part of the tobacco industry's "Asia-specific IARC preparation,"[124] and PM hoped to produce GEP resolutions by Chinese science organizations.[125] An organizer of the conference coauthored a paper on GEP and the etiology of lung cancer[126] with industry consultant Joseph Wu,[106] who had been paid $235 000 in 1995 and 1996 to organize and conduct "Chinese projects" through SH&B.[127] Wu authored an accompanying editorial[128] on risk assessment and GEP in the *Chinese Journal of Epidemiology* that states that relative risks of less than 2 may be artifactual for secondhand smoke studies, and that scientists need to examine other factors, such as pollution and diet, for lung cancer.[128]

Several European epidemiologic societies have developed GEP guidelines, including the International Epidemiological Association (IEA),[129] the Danish Society of Epidemiology,[129] and the Association des Epidémiologistes de Langue Française (ADELF, Association of French-Speaking Epidemiologists).[130] PM may have sought to participate in these processes; John Rupp, the lawyer from Covington & Burling who had drafted a European Council GEP resolution for PM,[84] lobbied ADELF on GEP, as well as in Italy and Germany.[131,132] The ADELF and IEA epidemiologists who headed the GEP efforts for their organizations state that they had no idea that PM had such subversive intentions. The GEP guidelines developed by the epidemiologic societies do not discuss relative risks of less than 2, and the IEA guidelines emphasize the ethical conduct of epidemiologic studies.

CHANGES IN PHILIP MORRIS'S GOOD PRACTICE PROGRAM

By April 1998, PM began to scale back its GEP program. Ted Sanders (PM Worldwide Scientific Affairs), who was to inherit the GEP program, expressed concern about the GEP program's value to Cathy Ellis (senior vice president of research and development, PM USA):

> . . . the concept of GEP's was discussed in considerable detail in PM. *Corporate Affairs thought it was a wonderful idea, because at first they . . . felt that part of a code for Good Epidemiological Practices would state that any relative risk of less than 2 would be ignored. This is of course not the case. No epidemiological organization would agree to this, and even Corporate Affairs realizes this now* [emphasis added].[131]

Sanders describes PM's initial objective as to discredit epidemiologic results with relative risks of less than 2, but the company realized that no epidemiological organization would agree to such a standard. Sanders' memo also suggests that if PM had succeeded in securing a GEP code as initially planned, there was a good chance PM would not be able to criticize future errors in epidemiologic studies, and a better alternative would be to continue developing GEP with other companies. PM seems to have followed Sanders' advice; by July 20, 1998, "no further work was to be done on GEP's" by Rupp, who had continued his activities in France.[131]

GEP has most recently been a focus for Toxicology Forum, a nonprofit organization that fosters interaction between scientists in academia, government, and industry.[133] The 1999 Brussels conference included "Epidemiology in a Policy and Regulatory Context: Considering a Code of Good Epidemiology Practice," and the May 2000 Brussels conference discussed "Determinants and Structure of Guidelines of Epidemiological Practice."[133] (Note: When the referenced Web site was accessed on September 24, 2001, the title of the May 2000 conference had been changed to "Comparison of the Principles and Practice of Risk Assessment Performed at the Global and European Level," and the list of pending participants had been removed.) The May 2000 session speaker list included tobacco industry consultants.[63,133–135] PM, R.J. Reynolds, and the Tobacco Institute contributed $35 000 through Covington & Burling for a 1992 Toxicology Forum meeting[136] that included the session "Weak Epidemiological Associations and the Limitations of Meta-Analysis."[137] The international discussion of GEP continues, although the tobacco industry's interest in the 1999 and 2000 GEP Toxicology Forum conference remains unclear.

DISCUSSION

PM appropriated the "sound science" concept to shape the standards of epidemiology and to prevent increased smoking restrictions. The "sound science" coalition was viewed by PM and its public relations firms as a launching point to introduce the tobacco industry version of "good epidemiological practices" that would be accepted by the scientific community. The "sound science" coalitions are similar to other tobacco industry front groups used as third-party spokesmen without disclosing the tobacco industry's involvement.[18–21] PM's GEP was constructed by their lawyers and internal scientific resources. To gain support for its GEP programs and perspectives, PM capitalized on the concerns of other industries facing regulation and the good intentions of the scientific community, which sought to improve the conduct of epidemiology.

PM has gone beyond "creating doubt"[63] and "controversy"[120,121] about the scientific evidence that demonstrates that active and passive smoking cause disease, to attempting to change the scientific standards of proof. PM's higher level of activity in Europe with GEP reflects the reason for this strategy shift. PM sought to establish a tactically advantageous scientific and policy-making environment before a scientific threat materialized in Europe, whereas in the United States, PM was reacting against an already damaging scientific government publication. The versions of GEP PM and its allies promoted discount relative risks below 2 and would set the standard in such a way that would make it impossible to conclude that secondhand smoke, as well as many other environmental toxins, is dangerous.

This approach ignores the fact that a comprehensive assessment of risk involves considering all the evidence related to a toxin, not just the epidemiology. This distinction was highlighted in the response to a news article in *Science*,[138] which represented several epidemiologists as concluding that there was a high threshold for a relative risk's being worth considering.[139] One of the epidemiologists quoted in the article responded that the news story

> ... writes that I have expressed the view that only a fourfold risk should be taken seriously. That is correct, *but only when the finding stands in a biological vacuum or has little or no biological credibility*. We all take seriously small relative risks when there is a credible hypothesis in the background. Nobody disputes that the prevalence of boys at birth is higher than that of girls (an excess of 3%), that men have a 30% higher death rate compared with women of the same age, or that fatality in a car accident is higher when the car is smaller [emphasis added].[140]

The risks mentioned are similar in magnitude to (or smaller than) the risks associated with secondhand smoke.

The industry's strategy for dealing with secondhand smoke may be shifting again. In 2000, PM released a Web site that acknowledges that many scientific studies report a small increased risk in disease with secondhand smoke exposure, but also claims that "exposure levels outside the home are lower than regulators have generally assumed."[141]

These claims of inconsequential exposures are based on tobacco industry–funded studies of dubious accuracy that were carried out within the same construct as the GEP efforts and other efforts to subvert the scientific process. Indeed, the pilot studies for these exposure studies have been demonstrated in government proceedings to be unreliable.[47]

As greater understanding of the tobacco industry's subversive operations accumulates, scientists and policymakers face the question of whether or not to include the tobacco industry in their discourses. Pros and cons of publishing any material funded by the tobacco industry have been debated, and some journals and organizations have rules to exclude those who are funded by the tobacco industry.[142]

The World Health Organization's tobacco control effort is the most prominent global case to observe in the near future, as the WHO deals with both the scientific and policy-making worlds and has been targeted by the tobacco industry. The WHO recently published a special inquiry on the tobacco documents, which concluded that the tobacco industry views the WHO as one of its leading enemies and strategized to "contain, neutralise, reorient" WHO's tobacco control initiatives.[143] The WHO is also conducting hearings, which include the tobacco industry, for its international Framework Convention on Tobacco Control. (Uncannily similar to projects of the TASSC and to Junkscience.com, a Web site for Guest Choice Networks, which claims to represent more than 30000 restaurant and tavern owners in promoting consumer choice, proclaims the WHO's Framework Convention as "Junk Science Goes Global."[144])

Publicly, the tobacco industry is now shifting to a campaign touting responsible corporate citizenship[145,146] and nominal efforts purportedly to discourage youth smoking prevention.[147] The industry's many past efforts—beginning with the "Frank Statement" advertisement and creation of the Tobacco Industry Research Committee in the United States in 1954[63(pp32–44)]—to publicly reinvent itself, while privately doing everything it can to protect itself from meaningful regulation and maximizing sales and profits, suggest that the WHO (and other government and scientific bodies) maintain an arm's-length relationship with the tobacco industry until it visibly reduces its aggressive efforts to promote tobacco use, whether to children or adults, worldwide.

Because the US Supreme Court is allowing judges more freedom to decide whether to admit or exclude scientific evidence,[148,149] the question of what work constitutes "junk science" or "sound science" comes to the forefront in discussions of the health effects of industry products and activities. Discussions of how to improve epidemiology should be ongoing, although there is continued debate as to the necessity for epidemiologic guidelines.[150,151] While every practicing scientist agrees that scientific work should be rigorously done, the scientific, public health, and regulatory communities need to be more aware that the "sound science" and "GEP" movement is not simply an effort from within the profession to improve the quality of scientific discourse. This movement reflects sophisticated public relations campaigns controlled by industry executives and lawyers to manipulate the scientific standards of proof for the corporate interests of their clients. ■

About the Authors

The authors are with the Institute for Health Policy Studies, University of California, San Francisco. Stanton A. Glantz is also with the Department of Medicine, Division of Cardiology.

Requests for reprints should be sent to Stanton A. Glantz, PhD, Department of Medicine, Division of Cardiology, Box 0130, University of California, San Francisco, CA 94143–0130 (e-mail: glantz@medicine.ucsf.edu).

This commentary was accepted April 6, 2001.

Contributors

E. K. Ong performed the document research. Both E. K. Ong and S. A. Glantz prepared and revised the manuscript.

Acknowledgments

This work was supported by National Cancer Institute grants CA-61021 and CA-87472 and the Richard and Rhoda Goldman Fund.

The authors would like to acknowledge Paolo Boffetta, Rodolfo Saracci, Marcus Goldberg, and Jorn Olsen for their helpful discussions, and Norbert Hirschhorn and Stella Aguinaga Bialous for providing several relevant references.

References

1. Hollingsworth P. The "junk science" dilemma. *Am Scientist.* 2000; 88:2–4.
2. Huber P. *Galileo's Revenge: Junk Science in the Courtroom.* New York, NY: Basic Books; 1991.
3. Schwartz J. Only good science to keep on debating "junk science." *Houston Chronicle.* March 28, 1999:5
4. Price J, Svitak L. It's time we took "junk science" out of the courtroom. *Star-Tribune* [Minneapolis]. June 20, 1999:5D.
5. Price J, Rosenberg E. The war against junk science: the use of expert panels in complex medical-legal scientific litigation. *Biomaterials.* 1998;19: 1425–1432.
6. McCullough L. Two views on Europe's ban of US beef: beef ban based in social issues, not sound science. *Wisconsin State Journal.* July 18, 1999:2B
7. Luik J. Toronto smoking debate fogged by junk science. *National Post* [Toronto]. July 8, 1999:C7
8. Crane M. Is "junk science" finally on the way out? *Med Econ.* 1996;73: 59–61, 65–66.

9. Pear R. Research web site idea fuels junk-science fears. *San Diego Union-Tribune.* June 16, 1999:E3

10. Fenske R. Pesticide limits based on sound science. *Seattle Times.* August 5, 1999:B4.

11. Coggon D, Cooper C. Fluoridation of water supplies: debate on the ethics must be informed by sound science. *BMJ.* 1999;319:269–270.

12. Kizer K, Warriner T, Book S. Sound science in the implementation of public policy: a case report on California's Proposition 65. *JAMA.* 1988;260: 951–955.

13. Reinken J. *Through the Smoke-screen—A Critique of Environmental Tobacco Smoke: A Review of the Literature by the Tobacco Institute of New Zealand.* Wellington: New Zealand Department of Health; 1990.

14. Bero L, Glantz S. Tobacco industry response to a risk assessment of environmental tobacco smoke. *Tob Control.* 1993;2:103–113.

15. Benitez JB, Idle JR, Krokan HE, et al., eds. *Environmental Tobacco Smoke and Lung Cancer: An Evaluation of the Risk.* Trondheim, Norway: European Working Group on Environmental Tobacco Smoke and Lung Cancer; 1996.

16. Davey Smith G, Phillips A. Passive smoking and health: should we believe Philip Morris's "experts"? *BMJ.* 1996; 313:929–933.

17. *The Health Effects of Passive Smoking.* Canberra, Australia: National Health and Medical Research Council; November 1997.

18. Samuels B, Glantz S. The politics of local tobacco control. *JAMA.* 1991; 266:2110–2117.

19. Americans for Nonsmokers' Rights Foundation. The National Smokers Alliance: exposed. Available at: http://www.no-smoke.org/nsa.html. Accessed August 27, 1999.

20. Traynor M, Begay M, Glantz S. New tobacco industry strategy to prevent local tobacco control. *JAMA.* 1993;270:479–486.

21. Dearlove J, Glantz S. 1999. Tobacco control policymaking in New York. Institute for Health Policy Studies, University of California San Francisco. February 1999. Available at: http://www.library.ucsf.edu/tobacco/ny. Accessed September 24, 2001.

22. Glantz SA. The truth about big tobacco in its own words. *BMJ.* 2000; 321:313–314.

23. *Respiratory Health Effects of Passive Smoking: Lung Cancer and Other Disorders.* Washington, DC: Office of Research and Development, US Environmental Protection Agency; 1992.

24. Merlo E. Memo to William Campbell [re: PM USA ETS actions]. February 17, 1993. Document no. 2021183916/3930. Available at: http://www.pmdocs.com. Accessed September 24, 2001.

25. Lattanzio T. ETS Task Force update. May 20, 1993. Document no. 2021178204. Available at: http://www.pmdocs.com. Accessed September 24, 2001.

26. The Advancement of Sound Science Coalition. [Information sheet describing TASSC.] 1993. Document no. 2046989061. Available at: http://www.pmdocs.com. Accessed September 24, 2001.

27. Kraus M. [Letter to PM Director of Communications re: TASSC]. September 23, 1993. Document no. 2024233677/3682. Available at: http://www.pmdocs.com. Accessed September 4, 2001.

28. PM USA. Corporate Affairs 1994 budget presentation. October 21, 1993. Document no. 2046847121. Available at: http://www.pmdocs.com. Accessed September 4, 2001.

29. Kraus M, Cohen N, Hockaday T. Revised 1993 TASSC launch program. October 15, 1993. Document no. 2045930491. Available at: http://www.pmdocs.com. Accessed September 4, 2001.

30. Kraus M. [Memo to Matt Winokur re: TASSC briefing.] October 26, 1993. Document no. 2025840783/0784. Available at: http://www.pmdocs.com. Accessed September 4, 2001.

31. TASSC. The Advancement of Sound Science Coalition Member Survey. 1993. Document no. 2024233662/3663. Available at: http://www.pmdocs.com. Accessed September 4, 2001.

32. Lister C. Memorandum to Dr. Reif Re: tolerance and junk science. February 2, 1993. Document no. 2028359740/9742. Available at: http://www.pmdocs.com. Accessed September 4, 2001.

33. Hockaday T. Update on the activities of The Advancement of Sound Science Coalition (TASSC). July 1, 1993. Document no. 2024233614. Available at: http://www.pmdocs.com. Accessed September 4, 2001.

34. The Advancement of Sound Science Coalition. Table of contents: TASSC—direct mail membership recruitment mailings. 1993. Document no. 2046989020. Available at: http://www.pmdocs.com. Accessed September 24, 2001.

35. National watchdog organization launched to fight unsound science used for public policy decisions. *US Newswire.* November 24, 1993.

36. Sound Science Coalition names former congressman Mickey Edwards to lead advisory committee. *PR Newswire.* August 16, 1995.

37. Science watchdog group celebrates third anniversary with renewed commitment to exposing use of junk science. *PR Newswire.* December 3, 1996.

38. Helvarg D. The big green spin machine: corporations and environmental PR (public relations). *Amicus Journal;* Summer 1996;18(2):13–21.

39. Kraus M. Sound science/lindheim meeting/next steps. April 26, 1994. Document no. 2025493192/3194. Available at: http://www.pmdocs.com. Accessed September 4, 2001.

40. Lenzi J. TASSC update. November 15, 1993. Document no. 2024233664. Available at: http://www.pmdocs.com. Accessed September 24, 2001.

41. Andrade A. The Advancement of Sound Science Coalition (TASSC). October 1, 1993. Document no. 2024233656. Available at: http://www.pmdocs.com. Accessed September 4, 2001.

42. Merlo E. TASSC. April 29, 1994. Document no. 2024233594. Available at: http://www.pmdocs.com. Accessed September 24, 2001.

43. Office of Victor Han. 1994 Communications plan. 1994. Document no. 2023918833/8852. Available at: http://www.pmdocs.com. Accessed September 24, 2001.

44. Office of David Cooper. Consumer issues program. October 1995. Document no. 2046039179/9194. Available at: http://www.pmdocs.com. Accessed September 24, 2001.

45. Levy R, Marimont R. Lies, damned lies, and 400,000 smoking-related deaths. *Regulation.* 1998;21:24–29.

46. Milloy S. JunkScience.com. Available at: http://www.junkscience.com. Accessed March 10, 2000.

47. Ong E, Glantz S. Tobacco industry efforts to subvert a secondhand smoke study by the International Agency for Research on Cancer. *Lancet.* 2000;355: 1253–1259.

48. Boffetta P, Agudo A, Ahrens W, et al. Multicenter case–control study of exposure to environmental tobacco smoke and lung cancer in Europe. *J Natl Cancer Inst.* 1998;90:1440–1450.

49. Sullivan J. IARC study. September 2, 1993. Document no. 2501117793/7797. Available at: http://www.pmdocs.com. Accessed September 24, 2001.

50. Winokur M. IARC situation overview and plan: presentation to PMCS. April 13, 1994. Document no. 2501355931/5944. Available at: http://www.pmdocs.com. Accessed September 24, 2001.

51. Hockaday T, Cohen N. Thoughts on TASSC Europe. March 25, 1994. Document no. 2024233595/5602. Available at: http://www.pmdocs.com. Accessed September 24, 2001.

52. Burson-Marsteller. Assessment project: Scientists for Sound Public Policy. March 1994. Document no. 2025493130/3138. Available at: http://www.pmdocs.com. Accessed September 4, 2001.

53. Lindheim J. Scientist group in Europe. April 18, 1994. Document no. 2025493128/3129. Available at: http://www.pmdocs.com. Accessed September 24, 2001.

54. Winokur M. IARC TF. July 5, 1994. Document no. 2028380422/0467. Available at: http://www.pmdocs.com. Accessed September 24, 2001.

55. Burson-Marsteller. Scientists for Sound Public Policy: assessment project and symposium. 1994. Document no. 2028363773/3791. Available at: http:// www.pmdocs.com. Accessed September 24, 2001.

56. Cook R. Overview of good epidemiologic practices. *J Occup Med.* 1991; 33:1216–1220.

57. Chemical Manufacturers Association. Guidelines for good epidemiology practices for occupational and environmental epidemiologic research. 1991. Document no. 2024005575/5604. Available at: http://www.pmdocs.com. Accessed September 4, 2001.

58. Chemical Manufacturers Association's Epidemiology Task Group. Guidelines for Good Epidemiology Practices for occupational and environmental epidemiologic research. *J Occup Med.* 1991;33:1221–1229.

59. Lister C. Memorandum to Messrs. Winokur and Bushong Re: epidemiological standards. February 24, 1994. Document no. 2026221042. Available at: http://www.pmdocs.com. Accessed September 24, 2001.

60. Walk R. Quality assurance in epidemiology: GEP. November 1996. Document no. 2063604594/5600. Available at: http://www.pmdocs.com. Accessed September 24, 2001.

61. Borrelli T. GEP review. March 15, 1994. Document no. 2028446631B. Available at: http://www.pmdocs.com. Accessed September 24, 2001.

62. Barnes D, Hanauer P, Slade J, Bero L, Glantz S. Environmental tobacco smoke. *JAMA.* 1995;274:248–253.

63. Glantz S, Slade J, Bero L, Hanauer P, Barnes D. *The Cigarette Papers.* Berkeley: University of California Press; 1996.

64. Ritter M. GEP proposal. March 17, 1994. Document no. 2028446632. Available at: http://www.pmdocs.com. Accessed September 24, 2001.

65. Reif H. GEP review. March 17, 1994. Document no. 2028446631. Available at: http://www.pmdocs.com. Accessed September 24, 2001.

66. Office of RA Walk. IARC tools. 1994. Document no. 2029059645. Available at: http://www.pmdocs.com. Accessed September 24, 2001.

67. Hockaday T. 17 Guiding Scientific Principles from The Advancement of Sound Science Coalition (TASSC). June 15, 1994. Document no. 2025492907/2909. Available at: http://www.pmdocs.com. Accessed September 4, 2001.

68. Winokur M. Sound science activities. June 16, 1994. Document no. 2025493118A/3119. Available at: http://www.pmdocs.com. Accessed September 24, 2001.

69. Sheehan T, Cameron C. Epidemiologic proof of causation. *For the Defense.* 1999:34–39.

70. Winokur M. [Roger Walk's revised GEP resolution.] July 26,1994. Document no. 2028381639. Available at: http://www.pmdocs.com. Accessed September 24, 2001.

71. Walk R. Proposed guidelines for Good Epidemiology Practices. July 25, 1994. Document no. 2029260524/0539. Available at: http://www.pmdocs.com. Accessed September 24, 2001.

72. *The Health Consequences of Involuntary Smoking.* Report of the Surgeon General. Washington, DC: Office of the Assistant Secretary of Health, Office of Smoking and Health; 1986. DHHS publication PHS 87-8398.

73. *Effects of Passive Smoking on Health.* Canberra, Australia: National Health and Medical Research Council; June 1986.

74. *Health Effects of Exposure to Environmental Tobacco Smoke.* Sacramento: California Environmental Protection Agency; 1997.

75. Report of the Scientific Committee on Tobacco and Health. March 1998. Available at: http://www.officialdocuments.co.uk/document/doh/tobacco/report.htm. Accessed September 24, 2001.

76. He J, Vupputuri S, Allen K, Prerost M, Hughes J, Whelton P. Passive smoking and the risk of coronary heart disease–a meta-analysis of epidemiologic studies. *N Engl J Med.* 1999;340:920–926.

77. Sullivan J. IARC next meeting. June 15, 1994. Document no. 2025493426/3427. Available at: http://www.pmdocs.com. Accessed September 24, 2001.

78. Lindheim J. Re: Scientist project. June 16, 1994. Document no. 2025493117. Available at: http://www.pmdocs.com. Accessed September 24, 2001.

79. Burson-Marsteller. Burson-Marsteller Milan Sound Science Project executive summary. June 17, 1994. Document no. 2025493074/3084. Available at: http://www.pmdocs.com. Accessed September 24, 2001.

80. Albinus S. Re: Sound Science Project and European Seminar in the autumn 1994. June 17, 1994. Document no. 2025493066/3069. Available at: http://www.pmdocs.com. Accessed September 4, 2001.

81. Lister C, Green J. Memorandum to Mr. Bushong re: Sound Science and GEP. August 14, 1994. Document no. 2028381627. Available at: http://www.pmdocs.com. Accessed September 4, 2001.

82. Walk R. IARC Task Force meeting. September 28,1994. Document no. 2028381446/1447. Available at: http://www.pmdocs.com. Accessed September 4, 2001.

83. Sullivan J. IARC Task Force meeting Brussels. October 4, 1994. Document no. 2028381444. Available at: http://www.pmdocs.com. Accessed September 4, 2001.

84. Winokur M. Draft EU Resolution on GEP. April 12,1995. Document no. 2050751334. Available at: http://www.pmdocs.com. Accessed September 24, 2001.

85. Walk R. EU GEP Conference. February 6, 1995. Document no. 2028381562. Available at: http://www.pmdocs.com. Accessed September 24, 2001.

86. Sullivan J. GEP. September 27, 1995. Document no. 2050761345. Available at: http://www.pmdocs.com. Accessed September 4, 2001.

87. Bowling J. American Health Foundation. May 22, 1973. Document no. 2015013864. Available at: http://www.pmdocs.com. Accessed September 24, 2001.

88. Wynder E. [Letter to PM USA president concurring animal research not necessarily relevant to smoking and human health.] May 30, 1974. Document no. 1003710586. Available at: http://www.pmdocs.com. Accessed September 24, 2001.

89. Wynder E. [Letter to PM research center head about collaborating in areas of mutual interest.] April 17, 1975. Document no. 1003710876/0877. Available at: http://www.pmdocs.com. Accessed September 24, 2001.

90. Warshaw S. Re: Report on luncheon meeting with Dr. Ernst Wynder of American Health Foundation. June 19, 1974. Document no. 2015013815. Available at: http://www.pmdocs.com. Accessed September 24, 2001.

91. Ruder W. [Letter to Wynder from Ruder & Finn suggesting R&F executive VP for American Health Foundation board and discussing PM as R&F client.] June 27, 1974. Document no. 2015013819/3820. Available at: http://www.pmdocs.com. Accessed September 24, 2001.

92. Ruder W. [Letter to PM stating American Health Foundation press kit by Ruder & Finn has no mention of smoking and health problem.] June 19, 1975. Document no. 2015013901. Available at: http://www.pmdocs.com. Accessed September 24, 2001.

93. Davies D. [Thank you letter to PM president for PM $20 000 for building fund.] November 4, 1974. Document no. 2015013916. Available at: http://www.pmdocs.com. Accessed September 24, 2001.

94. Osdene T. [Letter re: $25 000 for American Health Foundation.] October 14, 1986. Document no. 2021630516. Available at: http://www.pmdocs.com. Accessed September 4, 2001.

95. Osdene T. [Letter re: $25 000 for American Health Foundation.] October 13, 1987. Document no. 2021630797. Available at: http://www.pmdocs.com. Accessed September 4, 2001.

96. Osdene T. [Letter re: $25 000 for American Health Foundation.] April 18, 1988. Document no. 2021630850. Available at: http://www.pmdocs.com. Accessed September 4, 2001.

97. Osdene T. [Letter re $25 000 for American Health Foundation.] August 30, 1989. Document no. 2021630898. Available at: http://www.pmdocs.com. Accessed September 24, 2001.

98. Osdene T. [Letter re $25 000 for American Health Foundation.] October 10, 1990. Document no. 2021630953. Available at: http://www.pmdocs.com. Accessed September 24, 2001.

99. Bruckner E. Re Research project "Epidemiologic Study of Lung Cancer in Japan and the United States." April 10, 1995. Document no. 2050762685. Available at: http://www.pmdocs.com. Accessed September 24, 2001.

100. Monthly Activities HER, S&T, FTR/PM Neuchatel. November 29, 1994. Document no. 2028372914/2915. Available at: http://www.pmdocs.com. Accessed September 24, 2001.

101. Jackson J. Activity in 1998 in the development of standards of good epidemiological practice. *Int Arch Occup Environ Health.* 1999;72:M81–M85.

102. Bloemen L, Jackson J, Kightlinger M, Mundt K, Pastides H. A new proposal for a code of good epidemiological practice. Undated. Document no. 2063605907. Available at: http://www.pmdocs.com. Accessed September 4, 2001.

103. Federal Focus Inc. Available at: http://www.fedfocus.org. Accessed August 1999.

104. Graham JD. *The Role of Epidemiology in Regulatory Risk Assessment.* Amsterdam, the Netherlands: Elsevier Science; 1995.

105. *Principles for Evaluating Epidemiologic Data in Regulatory Risk Assessment: Developed by an Expert Panel at a Conference in London, England, October 1995.* Washington, DC: Federal Focus Inc; 1996.

106. Office of Thomas Osdene. ETS/IAQ scientific consultants. August 30, 1989. Document nos. 2023483171, 2023483161. Available at: http://www.pmdocs.com. Accessed September 24, 2001.

107. Auchter T. The need for Good Epidemiology Practices (GEPs) in studies used by regulatory agencies. November 21, 1994. Document no. 2050240421/0422. Available at: http://www. pmdocs.com. Accessed September 24, 2001.

108. Fuller C. [Letter to Jim Tozzi re: Federal Focus check.] July 13, 1993. Document no. 2046597569. Available at: http://www.pmdocs.com. Accessed September 24, 2001.

109. Borelli T. [Memo re monthly budget supplement re: ETS/OSHA federal activities.] March 16, 1993. Document no. 2046597148/7150. Available at: http://www.pmdocs.com. Accessed September 24, 2001.

110. Philip Morris Management Corporation. Re agreement dated January 1, 1994. August 8, 1994. Document no. 2029377061/7063. Available at: http://www.pmdocs.com. Accessed September 24, 2001.

111. Winokur M. Epi guidelines. August 25, 1994. Document no.

2028381624/1625. Available at: http://www.pmdocs.com. Accessed September 24, 2001.

112. Tozzi J. EPA. July 24, 1995. Document no. 2050761193. Available at: http://www.pmdocs.com. Accessed September 24, 2001.

113. Walk R. Proposed conference on "good risk management practices" in Asia 1998. August 1, 1997. Document no. 2063600682. Available at: http://www.pmdocs.com. Accessed September 24, 2001.

114. Dempsey R. Regarding: Good Epidemiological Practices. March 31, 1994. Document no. 2026221040. Available at: http://www.pmdocs.com. Accessed September 24, 2001.

115. vanHolt K. Re Good Epidemiological Practices. April 25, 1994. Document no. 2026221035. Available at: http://www.pmdocs.com. Accessed September 24, 2001.

116. Rylander R. Low risk epidemiology and good epidemiological practice. No date. Document no. 2050241534. Available at: http://www.pmdocs.com. Accessed September 24, 2001.

117. Etzel R, Windham G, Soskolne C. International Society for Environmental Epidemiology 8th Annual Conference. 1996. Available at: http://www.iseepi.org/NOFRAMES/96rep.htm. Accessed June 21, 2000.

118. Worldwide Scientific Affairs. Activities—project summaries. January 9, 1998. Document no. 2060565605/5617. Available at: http://www.pmdocs.com. Accessed September 24, 2001.

119. Zhang M. Press article in the *China Daily* on the CIAR's GEP workshop in Guangzhou. September 29, 1997. Document no. 2063608546. Available at: http://www.pmdocs.com. Accessed September 24, 2001.

120. Barnes D, Bero L. Industry-funded research and conflict of interest: an analysis of research sponsored by the tobacco industry through the Center for Indoor Air Research. *J Health Polit Policy Law.* 1996;21:515–542.

121. Barnes D, Bero L. Why review articles on the health effects of passive smoking reach different conclusions. *JAMA.* 1998;279:1566–1570.

122. Zhu B. Countries unite against cancer. *China Daily.* July 17, 1997. Document no. 2063608547. Available at: http://www.pmdocs.com. Accessed September 24, 2001.

123. Office of Richard Carchman. International Workshop on Risk Assessment and Good Epidemiological Practices. July 14–17, 1997. Document no. 2063608584/8602. Available at: http://www.pmdocs.com. Accessed September 24, 2001.

124. PM Scientific Affairs Hong Kong. Third Meeting of Asian Regional Tobacco Industry Science Team "ARTIST." May 26, 1997. Document no. 2063626181. Available at: http://www.pmdocs.com. Accessed September 24, 2001.

125. Walk R. Support of good science in Asia. October 4, 1996. Document no. 2060565640. Available at: http://www.pmdocs.com. Accessed September 24, 2001.

126. Du Y, Wu J. [Exploration of etiology of lung cancer and good epidemiological practices.] *Chung-Hua Liu Hsing Ping Hsueh Tsa Chih.* 1997;18:367–371.

127. Dreyer L. [Re Dr. Wu's expenses for Shook, Hardy & Bacon.] August 14, 1996. Document no. 2061683610/3620. Available at: http://www.pmdocs.com. Accessed September 24, 2001.

128. Du Y. [Risk assessment and good epidemiological practices.] *Chung-Hua Liu Hsing Ping Hsueh Tsa Chih.* 1997;18:323–324.

129. IEA/The European Epidemiology Group. Good Epidemiological Practice: proper conduct in epidemiologic research. October 1999. Available at: http://www.dundee.ac.uk/iea/euro_contents.htm. Accessed September 24, 2001.

130. Association des Epidémiologistes de Langue Française. *Recommendations: Professional Standards and Good Practices in Epidemiology.* Lyon, France: December 1998.

131. Sanders E. GEP's. July 20, 1998. Document no. 2060569954/9956. Available at: http://www.pmdocs.com. Accessed September 24, 2001.

132. Rupp J. [Re ADELF GEP September 1997 version.] October 2, 1997. Document no. 2063658334. Available at: http://www.pmdocs.com. Accessed September 24, 2001.

133. Toxicology Forum. March 10, 2000. Available at: http://www.toxforum.com/topics.htm. Accessed March 10, 2001.

134. Philip Morris Europe Science and Technology Neuchatel. ETS plan and budget for the years 1988, 1989, 1990, and 1991. April 19, 1988. Document no. 2028364436. Available at: http://www.pmdocs.com. Accessed September 24, 2001.

135. Covington & Burling. [Re invoice payments for consultants.] 1991. Document no. 2023856353/6357. Available at: http://www.pmdocs.com. Accessed September 24, 2001.

136. Buckley M. [Letter re Toxicology Forum invoice for tobacco industry.] August 7, 1992. Document no. 2024526242. Available at: http://www.pmdocs.com. Accessed September 24, 2001.

137. Toxicology Forum. 1992. Document no. 2028402242. Available at: http://www.pmdocs.com. Accessed September 24, 2001.

138. Taubes G. Epidemiology faces its limits. *Science.* 1995;269:164–169.

139. Willett W, Greeland S, MacMahon B, et al. The discipline of epidemiology [letter]. *Science.* 1995;269:1325–1326.

140. Trichopoulos D. The discipline of epidemiology [letter]. *Science.* 1995; 269:1326.

141. Philip Morris USA. Secondhand smoke: our actions to reduce unwanted ETS. 2000. Available at: http://www.philipmorrisusa.com/DisplayPageWithTopic.asp?ID=62. Accessed February 2001.

142. King J, Yamey G. Why journals should not publish articles funded by the tobacco industry. *BMJ.* 2000;321: 1074–1076.

143. Tobacco Free Initiative. An introduction to the WHO inquiry on tobacco industry influence. Available at: http://www.who.int/genevahearings/inquiry.html. Accessed February 2001.

144. Guest Choice Networks. WHO's fooling who? Junk science goes global. 2000. Available at: http://www.guestchoice.com/0420_junkscience.html. Accessed February 2001.

145. Philip Morris USA. 2000. Our mission and values. Available at: http://www.philipmorrisusa.com/DisplayPageWithTopic.asp?ID=63. Accessed February 2001.

146. Philip Morris International. Corporate reponsibility. 2000. Available at: http://www.pmintl.com/corp_resp/index.html. Accessed February 2001.

147. Brundtland G. Achieving worldwide tobacco control. *JAMA.* 2000; 284:750–751.

148. Marwick C. Court ruling on "junk science" gives judges more say about what expert witness testimony to allow [news]. *JAMA.* 1993;270:423.

149. Reichhardt T. Court affirms judges' right to reject "junk science" [news]. *Nature.* 1998;391:4.

150. Prineas RJ, Goodman K, Soskolne CL, et al. Findings from the American College of Epidemiology's survey on ethics guidelines. *Ann Epidemiol.* 1998; 8:482–489.

151. Rushton L. Reporting of occupational and environmental research: use and misuse of statistical and epidemiological methods. *Occup Environ Med.* 2000;57:1–9.

Strange Bedfellows: The History of Collaboration Between the Massachusetts Restaurant Association and the Tobacco Industry

ABSTRACT

Objectives. This article examines the historical relationship between the tobacco industry and the Massachusetts Restaurant Association, a nonprofit trade association aligned with the food and beverage industry.

Methods. The study analyzed data from Web-based tobacco industry documents, public relations materials, news articles, testimony from public hearings, requests for injunctions, court decisions, economic impact studies, handbooks, and private correspondence.

Results. Tobacco industry documents that became public after various state lawsuits reveal that a long history of collaboration exists between the Massachusetts Restaurant Association and the tobacco industry. For more than 20 years, their joint efforts have focused primarily on the battle to defeat state and local laws that would restrict smoking in public places, particularly in beverage and food service establishments. The resources of the tobacco industry, combined with the association's grassroots mobilization of its membership, have fueled their opposition to many state and local smoke-free restaurant, bar, and workplace laws in Massachusetts.

Conclusions. The universal opposition of the Massachusetts Restaurant Association to smoking bans in food and beverage establishments is a reflection of its historic relationship with the tobacco industry. (*Am J Public Health.* 2001;91:598–603)

Wendy A. Ritch, MA, MTS, and Michael E. Begay, PhD

The Massachusetts Restaurant Association ("the Association"), a nonprofit trade organization associated with the food and beverage industry in the Commonwealth of Massachusetts, was incorporated in February 1934.[1] According to its informational materials, the Association advocates for the interests of its members at the state and local levels, organizes annual trade shows, supports "food recycling" programs to supply edible food from restaurants and colleges to needy and homeless persons in participating communities, helps to sponsor "school-to-career" programs that provide interested high school students with paid internships and trained food service industry worksite mentors, and engages in various other activities that allow it to fulfill its mission, which is "to protect and improve the food and beverage industry."[2] The Association's membership exceeds 2000, and it represents "over 7000 restaurants and all phases of the food service industry" throughout Massachusetts.[2]

On the basis of information collected from archives of tobacco industry documents available as a result of various state class-action lawsuits, the Association is also an ally of the tobacco industry. Since the mid-1970s, the tobacco industry and the Association have worked together to defeat regulations to restrict smoking in public places, workplaces, restaurants, and bars. However, the Association has downplayed its relationship with "Big Tobacco." The *Boston Globe* published an article about the relationship between the Association and the tobacco industry on May 3, 1999, and a connection was admitted by Bruce Potter, the Association's director of membership services, but only insofar as the tobacco industry "might sponsor an event . . . that's all."[3] According to the *Boston Globe*, Potter also acknowledged that "Philip Morris and RJ Reynolds Tobacco," the nation's top 2 cigarette makers, "are dues-paying members, but . . . their role is entirely passive."[3] However, tobacco industry documents reveal that much more than a "passive" relationship exists between the Association and the tobacco industry.

In this article, we examine the history of collaboration between the Massachusetts Restaurant Association and the tobacco industry, and we discuss numerous documents that demonstrate the scope of this alliance. Contrary to public statements made by the Association that it is working independently of the interests of the tobacco industry, documentary evidence proves that the Association helps to mask the true extent of tobacco industry activity in Massachusetts. In addition, the documents show that the tobacco industry is engaged in similar relationships with restaurant associations in other American states. Therefore, state and local lawmakers, as well as local boards of health, must realize that when restaurant associations oppose anti-smoking legislation, they do so primarily because they are allies of the tobacco industry.

Methods

Data were collected from the following sources: tobacco industry documents released as a result of various state class-action lawsuits (http://www.tobaccoarchive.com), public relations materials, news articles, testimony from public hearings, requests for injunctions, court decisions, economic impact studies, handbooks, private correspondence, and additional public records.

The authors are with the Department of Community Health Studies, School of Public Health and Health Sciences, University of Massachusetts at Amherst.

Requests for reprints should be sent to Michael E. Begay, PhD, University of Massachusetts, School of Public Health and Health Sciences, Department of Community Health Studies, Arnold House, Amherst, MA 01003-9340 (e-mail: begay@schoolph.umass.edu).

This article was accepted July 18, 2000.

Results

1978: Ballot Question 8

The relationship between the Massachusetts Restaurant Association and the tobacco industry spans more than 20 years. In October 1978, the Association and the tobacco industry joined forces to oppose Question 8, a nonbinding ballot initiative that could have restricted smoking in public places to clearly marked, enclosed areas.[4] In a memorandum regarding Question 8, the Tobacco Institute, an industry political and public relations organization, indicated that low industry visibility had to be maintained and that "any public approach should be directed through locally based allies, such as the Massachusetts Restaurant Association, and not through either the Tobacco Institute or the member companies."[4] The Tobacco Institute estimated that it would cost less than \$50000 to mobilize groups to fight this initiative in communities throughout the state, and they used the Association to direct this opposition.[4]

The Tobacco Institute, with "concerned citizens of the Massachusetts Hotel and Restaurant industry," formed "a political committee," Independent Citizens for an Effective Government, to "fund the opposition to the referendum."[5] Dennis Dyer, the public affairs manager for the Tobacco Institute, was appointed the treasurer of the committee, while Stephen Elmont became the chairman.[5] Elmont was the president of the "Soups On" restaurant chain, a nonsmoker, and the incoming president of the Association.[5] Question 8, which would have required district representatives to vote for legislation to ban or restrict indoor smoking in public places, was defeated.

1984: Restaurant Restrictions in Boston

In March 1984, the State Activities Division of the Tobacco Institute compiled a report on a number of smoking restriction laws that were being proposed in the Massachusetts legislature, as well as those being considered by local governments and boards of health across the state.[6] For example, at the state level, bill S.1382, which called for the self-extinguishing of smoking materials in public places, was "killed in the Senate . . . on recommendation of [the] Joint Public Safety [Committee]."[6] It was also reported that there was "good news in Boston," where the city council "accepted the Government Operations Committee's unanimous 'ought not to pass' recommendation on [a] restaurant [smoking] restriction measure."[6]

According to the Tobacco Institute, "solid coalition building sunk [sic] Boston restaurant restriction ordinance . . . [the] Government Operations Committee hearing [was] attended by [the] Chamber of Commerce, [the] Massachusetts Restaurant Association, [the] Greater Boston Restaurant Association, [the] Massachusetts Hotel/Motel Association, two-thirds of the major Boston hotels as well as 30 of the City's major restaurants."[6] The defeat of the proposed restaurant smoking restrictions was aided by the testimony of the "President of Boston's oldest restaurant," who "experimented with voluntary 'no smoking' sections" and whose "two month test yielded only two 'no smoking' requests from 17000 customers."[6]

1985: Clean Indoor Air Acts

The Massachusetts legislature began to consider major clean indoor air legislation in the 1970s, and in 1975 it passed a law to regulate smoking in public elevators, supermarkets, museums, libraries, hospitals, and nursing homes and on trains, airplanes, single-car public transportation, and transportation provided by the Massachusetts Bay Transit Authority.[7] By February 1985, no further restrictions had been passed at the state level, but a \$0.05 tobacco tax increase was enacted in 1982.[7] Tobacco industry documents reveal that the industry was very successful in influencing the state legislative process during this period. In a 1985 memorandum, the Tobacco Action Network, an organization that furthers the political interests of the tobacco industry, stated that "historically, the industry has been successful by keeping tobacco issues off the floor. Legislative leadership changes effected in 1985 may limit our ability to keep legislation off the floor. A floor vote in either house would be, at best, a very narrow and difficult win for the industry."[7]

To help fight clean indoor air laws in the state legislature, the Tobacco Action Network created an elaborate plan of action that included direct lobbying, fostering legislative support, and creating alliances with businesses in Boston and throughout the state.[7] The Massachusetts Restaurant Association figured prominently in the tobacco industry's plan, as did hospitality associations, chambers of commerce, and organized labor. According to the Tobacco Action Network, "the education of their members and direct lobbying of legislators is the aid we seek from these groups," as well as contacting of subsidiaries, suppliers, and advertisers within Massachusetts to secure their early opposition to this legislation.[7] As an added boon, tobacco industry support in the form of materials or services would be almost impossible for the state to track because many of "the actions requested herein do not require the participants to register as legislative agents [or] lobbyists."[7]

1986–1989: Opposing Smoking Restrictions

The Association and the tobacco industry continued their joint opposition to state and local clean indoor air legislation, as well as to workplace and restaurant smoking restrictions, through the end of the 1980s.[8–10] One state-level smoking restriction bill, H.3697, that was in its third reading in the Senate in October 1987 was the target of pro-tobacco intervention; the "[Tobacco Institute] staff and legislative counsel continue[d] to work closely with the [Association] to defeat this bill."[9] The bill, which passed, required nonsmoking sections in restaurants, but it did not mandate the size of those sections.

Similar activities were mentioned in a Tobacco Institute report issued in September 1989 that discussed an Institute pilot program designed to reduce stringent smoking restrictions in 3 localities in eastern Massachusetts—Somerville, Malden, and Braintree—to the level of the state's statute requirements.[10] The Tobacco Institute, if successful in these efforts, planned to attempt to enact comparable restaurant restriction "rollbacks" in additional cities.[10] Even though the Tobacco Institute admitted that "in reality, most of these laws have been in place for a number of years" with "little impact [on restaurant businesses] and no legal ramifications," it was still determined to reverse these laws.[10]

Likewise, the Association knew that restaurants in these 3 cities experienced "little impact," yet it still led this rollback effort, with the support of local restaurant owners and managers.[10] However, "the function of the [Tobacco] Institute" was "limited to resources and organizational activities," because "direct tobacco contact with this effort would have a negative impact on its ultimate outcome."[10]

1990–1992: Economic Downturn

Although the Massachusetts economy was booming in the early and mid-1980s, an economic downturn began in 1988 that left the state with little option but to raise taxes. This fiscal reality was anticipated in a 1990 memorandum of the Tobacco Institute that foresaw an increase in tobacco taxes as inevitable for 2 reasons: first, because the industry had successfully defeated "proposed increases during the past eight years while all other taxes increased," and second, because a Democratic legislature would be "looking for minimal cost legislation that looks progressive," which could "prove to be a problem for the tobacco industry."[11]

To counter these "problems," the Tobacco Institute created a detailed plan of action for 1991 that ranged from the coordination of efforts with the legislature and Republican Governor William Weld's administration to the cultivation of alliances with organized labor, business associations, chambers of commerce, and other potentially interested parties.[11] The Tobacco Institute's plan of action contained a number of "Pro-Active Proposals" with section headings such as "State Tax Plan," "Hiring Discrimination," "Indoor Air Quality," "Minors," and "Restaurant Restriction Rollback."[11] Each proposal listed the coalition allies that needed to be developed or called upon, as well as the specific tobacco industry resources that had to be accessed or minimized to successfully implement the proposals.[11]

As "the primary sponsor" of these efforts, the Massachusetts Restaurant Association figured prominently in the tobacco industry's planned restaurant restriction rollbacks.[11] Once again, tobacco industry involvement was limited to "resources and organizational activities," such as providing the Association with smoker mailing lists, letters to local officials, and telephone scripts.[11] However, the Tobacco Institute also used its own public affairs organization to "assist the local business people and coordinate a media campaign."[11]

In 1990, Philip Morris launched the "It's the Law" campaign, which claimed to be aimed at curbing tobacco sales to minors.[12] Educational, training, and display materials were distributed to retailers in all 39 states where the minimum age to purchase cigarettes was 18 or 19 years. The Association was one of the 3 cosponsors of this program in Massachusetts.[12] In addition, the Association was listed as a general source of support for tobacco industry activities, specifically as a "state co-sponsor/participant" in 1991 and 1993, as indicated on in-house directories of Philip Morris allies.[13,14]

The Association also worked closely with the tobacco industry in 1992, when it provided witnesses and community attendees for a hearing in Marlborough. The Marlborough Board of Health considered a ban on couponing, self-service sales, and advertising on public transportation, as well as vending machine restrictions.[15] In the same year, the Tobacco Institute purchased "prime advertising space" in the Association membership directory, which was distributed to members and allied members constituting "75% of the buying power in the restaurant industry throughout the state."[16]

1993–1995: A Uniform Statewide Solution to the Smoking Issue

Many New England states, as well as localities within these states, considered adopting restaurant smoking bans in the early 1990s. In response to the US Environmental Protection Agency's report on the dangers of exposure to secondhand smoke, released in January 1993, some New England restaurant owners made their establishments smoke free to assuage liability concerns.[17] Other restaurateurs found support through Philip Morris' "Accommodation Program," a nonprofit program designed to address restaurant owners' concerns about tobacco smoke.[17] A free Accommodation Program packet that was sent to restaurateurs included signage to clearly demarcate smoking and nonsmoking sections, information on heating, ventilation, and air conditioning (HVAC) upgrades to provide cleaner air in these establishments, a toll-free hotline staffed by HVAC engineers, and other materials that would address these issues and would also discourage restaurateurs from making their establishments smoke free.[17]

In August 1993, Philip Morris stated that "restaurant owners know what their customers need and want, and they should be free to accommodate all of their customers as best they can. Feedback from restaurant owners that have been using the [Accommodation] program has been very positive."[17]

In December 1993, the Massachusetts Senate considered bill S.458, a "unified statewide smoking bill that allows restaurant owners the freedom to determine their own smoking policies that accommodate all of their customers and does not handicap some restaurants and give advantages to others."[18] The bill was supported by the Association for 2 reasons: it gave restaurateurs the power to decide how to handle the issue of smoking in their establishments, and it would have preempted all local restaurant smoking restrictions, which were generally much more stringent than S.458. Philip Morris, RJ Reynolds, and the Tobacco Institute issued a statement of support for S.458, stating that they "recognize the danger of government intervention and the competitive issues that [restaurants] are faced with" but that the bill was "common sense legislation that will simplify and unify state law while giving back policy making power to the private sector."[18]

The Association's executive summary on S.458 contained a question-and-answer section, so that its spokespeople would know how to address certain issues that would arise in interviews. One section of the executive summary directed spokespeople to avoid answering the question "Are you being used as a front group for the tobacco industry?" and instead to redirect the focus to S.458.[18] If asked, "Is your whole effort being bankrolled by the tobacco industry?" they were instructed to say, "No, but we certainly would encourage and appreciate any support the tobacco industry and anybody else for that matter can provide to help us get this legislation passed."[18] As for questions on statewide smoking bans and separate section restrictions, the spokespeople were to respond that the Association was "opposed to any kind of mandates."[18]

Statewide preemption bill S.458 did not pass, and communities throughout Massachusetts continued to consider and enact local restrictions and bans on restaurant smoking during 1994 and 1995. Consequently, the Association continued to oppose these smoking restrictions and bans and supported a statewide preemption bill so that the playing field would be level for all restaurants in the state.[19] In a March 1994 article in the *Boston Globe,* Cynthia Eid, a spokesperson for the Association, stated that restaurant owners would welcome "a national smoking ban, if only because it will be uniform from town to town, city to city, state to state."[20] However, once Peter Christie, the executive vice president of the Association, succeeded Eid as the organization's primary public voice, the Association no longer advocated for a national smoking ban.

Instead, Christie championed a statewide uniform legislative solution to the smoking issue that would allow restaurant owners to "reasonably accommodate" all of their patrons while establishing policy consistency throughout Massachusetts.[19,21] Christie and the Association endorsed Senate bill S.508 in 1995, a statewide bill that mandated that restaurant owners make at least 60% of their seating nonsmoking and no more than 40% of their seating smoking, with any restaurant owner allowed to go smoke free if he or she so chose.[21,22] S.508 would have preempted local legislative activity on the smoking issue and required that any changes to the statewide law be made only by city councils or township supervisors, "as opposed to local boards of health across the state."[22] This bill later died in the Committee on Senate Rules.

At this time, the legislature also considered bill S.514, which would have "preempt[ed] local decision-making authority by imposing a complete ban on smoking in restaurants" throughout Massachusetts.[22] S.514 failed to pass in the Senate. According to a news article written by Christie, "if we must have a law dealing with smoking in restaurants and bars, [the Association] prefers the uniform compromise. It is far more rational and accommodating than an outright ban, and most importantly, leaves the decision up to the restaurant owner[s] based on the needs of their customers."[22]

1996: An Economic Impact Study, a Congressional Report, and a Public Relations Campaign

In 1996, the Association and the tobacco industry jointly commissioned InContext, an "information company" based in Washington, DC, to conduct a study on the economic impact of smoking restrictions on restaurants in 23 cities and towns in Massachusetts.[23,24] The towns included in the study had passed smoking bans or restrictions between 1993 and 1995. InContext concluded that, with few exceptions, restaurant smoking bans were detrimental to business, and this was demonstrated by the study's finding that the highest losses of restaurant jobs typically were concentrated in those Massachusetts communities with the strictest restaurant smoking restrictions.[24]

InContext and the Association did not mention, in either the study's executive summary or in any of the publicity for the report, that restaurants in 5 "college towns" also participated in the study. College towns were defined as "those communities where the transient student population exceeds ten percent of the town's permanent population base."[24] When restaurant smoking bans in every college town positively correlated with a significant increase in restaurant jobs, from 20% to 70%, depending on the specific town, these results were excluded from the publicized study findings. According to InContext, "for college-town restaurants both the seasonal cycle and the non-local customer target base are derivative of the local higher education facility, not the local economy," so there was "no meaningful correlation" between smoking restrictions and restaurant job gains in college towns.[24]

The Association and InContext did not admit that any tobacco company or organization was involved in the financing, design, or production of the Massachusetts economic impact study, but several tobacco industry documents reveal that the Association, InContext, and the tobacco industry collaborated on this project. A Philip Morris memorandum dated March 1, 1996, stated that J. Dunham of Philip Morris "met with Bill Lilley," the chairman and cofounder of InContext, "to develop a methodology for determining the economic impact of restaurant smoking bans . . . [and] started work on [a] Massachusetts restaurant ban study."[25] A Philip Morris memorandum dated March 8, 1996, stated that Dunham "continued to work with Bill Lilley on [a] study showing [the] economic impact of restaurant smoking bans. Met with Bill Lilley and Matt Paluszek to discuss [a] similar study for Massachusetts . . . conference call scheduled for next Thursday with Matt Paluszek, Mass. Restaurant Assn, and Bill Lilley."[26]

In January 1996, the Association and the tobacco industry were joint proponents of study results released by the Congressional Research Service, a "non-partisan research component of the United States Congress" that "responds to inquiries from Congressional offices by providing statistical and historical research for the policy objectives of legislators."[27] The Congressional Research Service study, titled "Environmental Tobacco Smoke and Lung Cancer Risk," examined the same 30 studies that the Environmental Protection Agency analyzed in its 1993 report on the health risks associated with exposure to secondhand smoke.[28] According to an Association press release that was "sent to 175 newspapers and used for a radio talk show pitch," the study concluded that "the statistical evidence does not appear to support a conclusion that there are substantial health effects of passive smoking," and "it is clear that misclassification and recall bias plague [environmental tobacco smoke] epidemiology studies."[28]

However, Edward Sweda, the senior attorney for the Tobacco Products Liability Project in Boston, offered a different interpretation of the Congressional Research Service study in an article published in the *Middlesex News* on January 28, 1996. In this article, Sweda quoted passages from the study that contradicted the Association pro-tobacco interpretation of the report.[29] He also accused Christie and other "pro-tobacco apologists" of manipulating the study results in an attempt to "deflect public awareness away from the central issue: should nonsmokers . . . be forced . . . to breathe the poisons contained in secondhand tobacco smoke?"[29] In spite of arguments to the contrary, the Association used its interpretation of the study to urge town leaders to support the policy of accommodation for smokers instead of restricting or banning smoking at the local level.[28]

At the end of 1996, the Tobacco Institute mailed out materials for the "It's the Law" campaign, which was supposed to educate retailers about the illegality of tobacco sales to minors.[30] Flyers were distributed to retailers, for use by employees, that explained the law, how to ask for identification, and what to do if a customer refused to produce identification.[30] The "It's the Law" packets also included order forms for materials, such as point-of-purchase signs and buttons, that were specific to each retailer's state.[30] In Massachusetts, the Association was listed as one of the 4 "cooperating organizations" for the Tobacco Institute's "It's the Law" public relations campaign.[30]

1997–1999: A Mixture of Success and Failure

A July 1997 "issues update" report by RJ Reynolds discussed a number of smoking restrictions that were being considered by local boards of health throughout Massachusetts.[31] This report indicated that RJ Reynolds "met with [the Association] on July 8 to discuss alternatives to present to the [Wakefield] Board of Health," because restaurant owners wanted to change a 2-year-old smoking ban in this town.[31] An October 1997 issues update mentioned actions related to smoking bans and restrictions pending in 17 different localities throughout Massachusetts.[32] For example, Amherst, South Hadley, and Northampton conferred on the passage of a regional ban on smoking in bars to supplement the restaurant smoking restrictions that already existed in these towns.[32] Again, the restaurant industry figured prominently in the opposition to these ordinances.[32]

Local smoking bans and restrictions continued to occupy the attention of boards of health, the Massachusetts Restaurant Association, and the tobacco industry in 1998. An April 1998 internal memorandum between employees of RJ Reynolds indicated that "our partisans are prepared to challenge the [Falmouth] Board of Health with a series of questions and have speakers prepared to speak in opposition to the article [to ban smoking in restaurants], including restaurant owners, citizens, and the Chamber of Commerce."[33] The same week in April, RJ Reynolds also noted that they were "working with the [Association] to notify all partisans of [a] hearing [in Worcester on proposed new smoking restrictions] and [we] have a meeting on 4/21 at Tweed's Restaurant to prepare for the hearing."[33] The 1998 president of the Massachusetts Restaurant Association, Jim Donoghue, who joined the Association in 1982 and had been a member of its board since 1989, owned Tweed's Restaurant.[34]

In July 1998, the Association challenged the Boston Public Health Commission's ban on smoking in restaurants.[35] These restrictions had been adopted on March 19 and were scheduled to go into effect on September 30, 1998 (Lori Fresina, American Cancer Society [lfresina@cancer.org], e-mail, September 25, 1998). The Association filed a preliminary injunction against the new smoking regulations in Boston, claiming that (1) the regulations were not "reasonable" under Massachusetts general law 111 s.31, (2) the health commission considered economics in making the decision when it had only the authority to consider health, and (3) the regulations were "unconstitutionally vague" (Lori Fresina, American Cancer Society [lfresina@cancer.org], e-mail, August 31, 1998). On September 25, 1998, Judge Mitchell J. Sikora Jr of the Suffolk Superior Court ruled against the Association, denying its application for an injunction against the health commission's smoking regulations (Lori Fresina, American Cancer Society [lfresina@cancer.org], e-mail, September 30, 1998). In spite of the efforts of the Association and the tobacco industry to block the Boston smoking restrictions, they went into effect as scheduled. The health commission's smoking regulations made more than 1400 restaurants in Boston smoke free and restricted smoking to the bar areas of an additional 200 restaurants (Lori Fresina, American Cancer Society [lfresina@cancer.org], e-mail, September 30, 1998).

In 1999, many communities throughout Massachusetts, such as Northampton, considered the passage of smoking restrictions and bans, while others, such as Amherst, faced tremendous opposition to bans that had already been enacted.[36] The Association was an active participant in the opposition to the Northampton workplace smoking ban because bars were included in the scope of the ban. At the July 20, 1999, public hearing before the Northampton Board of Health, Andrea Bolton, the Association's legislative coordinator, referred to the proposed ban as "ludicrous." Bolton stated that "this kind of ban will wreak havoc. It will negatively affect these bars."

However, during her commentary, Bolton failed to address the earlier testimony of W. A. R., a tobacco policy researcher at the University of Massachusetts, who discussed the results of the 1996 Massachusetts Restaurant Association/Philip Morris/InContext economic impact study as they related to Northampton. The researcher speculated that because a restaurant smoking ban in Northampton had resulted in a 20% increase in restaurant jobs in 1996, a bar smoking ban in Northampton might have a similarly positive economic impact on the city's bar business. One year after this public hearing, Northampton had not yet adopted a workplace smoking ban.

Conclusions

The Massachusetts Restaurant Association and the tobacco industry have been allies in the battle against state and local smoking restrictions in Massachusetts for several decades. Multitudes of tobacco industry documents testify to the lengthy history of collaboration between the 2 parties. The Association and the tobacco industry have joined forces to sponsor and oppose tobacco-related bills in the Massachusetts legislature and in localities across the state and have collaborated on local restaurant restriction rollbacks.

The close political association between the Association and the tobacco industry has been mutually beneficial. The Association has helped to conceal the tobacco industry's state and local political activity in exchange for a variety of industry resources. Public documents also reveal that the tobacco industry has cultivated similar relationships with restaurant associations in states other than Massachusetts.[25,26] However, using information contained in tobacco industry archives, health advocates and tobacco control activists across the country now have the power to oppose state and local pro-tobacco policy initiatives by publicly exposing the alliance that exists between the tobacco industry and state restaurant associations. □

Contributors

W. A. Ritch and M. E. Begay designed the study, collected the data, and wrote the paper.

Acknowledgments

This research was supported by a grant from the American Cancer Society (RPG-97-033-01-PBR) and by a grant from the National Institutes of Health (1 R01 CA86314-01).

References

1. Massachusetts Restaurant Association. How it all started. Available at: http://www.marestaurantassoc.org/history.shtml. Accessed July 7, 1999.
2. Massachusetts Restaurant Association. MRA hospitality institute launches school-to-career program in nine Bay State schools; program expected to double next year [press release]. May 18, 1999. Available at: http://www.marestaurantassoc.org/school2career.shtml. Accessed July 28, 1999.
3. Restaurant group tied to Big Tobacco. *Boston Globe* [newspaper online]. May 3, 1999. Available at: http://www.boston.com. Accessed May 3, 1999.
4. Tobacco Institute. Memorandum from Dennis M. Dyer, public affairs manager, to Jack Kelly, senior vice president. October 2, 1978. Available at: http://www.rjrtdocs.com. Document no. 5000653393 -3398. Accessed May 10, 1999.
5. Tobacco Institute. Memorandum to Jack Kelly from Mike Kerrigan: report on Massachusetts Campaign/Independent Citizens for an Effective Government. October 21, 1978. Available at: http://www.pmdocs.com. Document no. 1005115395-5397. Accessed May 5, 1999.
6. Tobacco Institute, State Activities Division. Stateline report. March 29, 1984. Available at: http://www.tobaccoinstitute.com. Document no. TIMS0020109-0110. Accessed May 28, 1999.
7. Tobacco Action Network. Memorandum from Roger L. Mozingo, Tobacco Action Network, to State Activities Policy Committee re Massachusetts action request. February 27, 1985. Available at: http://www.rjrtdocs.com. Document no. 504984001 -4005. Accessed May 10, 1999.
8. Tobacco Institute. Memorandum to Peter Sparber from Susan Stuntz: corporate contacts re workplace smoking. January 16, 1986. Available at: http://www.pmdocs.com. Document no. 2025853944-3975. Accessed May 5, 1999.
9. Tobacco Institute. Executive summary. October 23, 1987. Available at: http://www.rjrtdocs.com. Document no. 506772572 -2573. Accessed May 10, 1999.
10. Tobacco Institute. Proactive legislative targets 1990, proactive proposal, Massachusetts local restaurant restriction rollback. October 2, 1989. Available at: http://www.rjrtdocs.com. Document no. 5076160656 -6064. Accessed May 10, 1999.
11. Tobacco Institute. Revised report of the State Activities Division of the Tobacco Institute—1991 preliminary state legislative forecast for consideration of major tobacco issues. October 1990. Available at: http://www.rjrtdocs.com. Document no. 512564768 -5124. Accessed May 10, 1999.
12. Philip Morris. Question and answers on "It's the Law" campaign. December 1990. Available at: http://www.pmdocs.com. Document no. 2054322723-2726. Accessed May 5, 1999.
13. Philip Morris. State co-sponsors/participants as of 10/1/91. October 1, 1991. Available at: http://www.pmdocs.com. Document no. 2025727042-7044. Accessed May 5, 1999.
14. Philip Morris. State co-sponsors/participants as of 9/23/93. September 23, 1990. Available at: http://www.pmdocs.com. Document no. 2023389716-9720. Accessed May 5, 1999.
15. RJ Reynolds. Local plan for board of health hearing—city of Marlborough, Massachusetts. January 8, 1991. Available at: http://www.rjrtdocs.com. Document no. 515198794 -8796. Accessed May 10, 1999.
16. Tobacco Institute. Memorandum to Don D'Errico from Kathy Getz, account manager, re Massachusetts Restaurant Membership Directory 1993. June 18, 1992. Available at: http://www.tobaccoinstitute.com. Document no. TIMN0206573. Accessed May 28, 1999.
17. Restauranteurs confront the smoking issue with Philip Morris' accommodation program. August 1993. Available at: http://www.pmdocs.com. Document no. 2021204015. Accessed May 5, 1999.
18. Massachusetts Restaurant Association. Executive summary: S.458. December 1993. Available at: http://www.pmdocs.com. Document no. 2046114219-4222. Accessed May 5, 1999.
19. Christie P. Restaurant group backs uniform legislative solution for nonsmoking and smoking clientele. *West Bridgewater Times* [newspaper online]. June 28, 1995. Available at: http://www.pmdocs.com. Document no. 2061878483. Accessed June 28, 1995.
20. Smoke ring tightens, eateries, bars, hotels hardest hit. *Boston Globe* [newspaper online]. March 26, 1994. Available at: http://www.pmdocs.com. Document no. TIMN0055880. Accessed May 28, 1999.
21. Massachusetts Restaurant Association. Christie P. Restaurant backs uniform legislative solution for nonsmoking and smoking clientele [general opinion piece]. 1997. Available at: http://www.pmdocs.com. Document no. 2061878381. Accessed May 5, 1999.
22. Smoking in restaurants: a compromise. *Middlesex News* [newspaper online]. June 29, 1995. Available at: http://www.pmdocs.com. Document no. 2061878482. Accessed May 5, 1999.
23. Massachusetts Restaurant Association. New study shows restaurant smoking bans cost jobs in Massachusetts communities [press release]. 1996. Available at: http://www.pmdocs.com. Document no. 2061878376-8379. Accessed May 5, 1999.
24. *Economic Impact Study Correlating Smoking Ban Severity With Restaurant Job Gains/Losses.* Westborough, Mass: Massachusetts Restaurant Association, InContext Inc; 1996.
25. Philip Morris. Weekly direct report to Lance Pressl from Josh Slavitt. Available at: http://www.pmdocs.com. Document no. 2045458609-8611. Accessed May 5, 1999.
26. Philip Morris. Weekly direct report to Howard Liebengood from Press/Issues Team. March 1, 1996. Available at: http://www.pmdocs.com. Document no. 2046946028-6030. Accessed May 5, 1999.
27. US Senate. Letter from Roger Fiske, staff assistant, to Bruce Potter, Massachusetts Restaurant Association. June 20, 1996. Available

at: http://www.pmdocs.com. Document no. 2061878462. Accessed May 5, 1999.

28. Massachusetts Restaurant Association. Congressional Research Service study casts doubt on local board of health smoking bans. 1996. Available at: http://www.pmdocs.com. Document no. 2061878456. Accessed May 5, 1999.
29. Is EPA exaggerating dangers of second-hand smoke? *Middlesex News* [newspaper online]. January 28, 1996. Available at: http://www.pmdocs.com. Document no. 2061878459. Accessed May 5, 1999.
30. Tobacco Institute. It's the law, we do not sell tobacco products to persons under 18 [brochure]. Available at: http://www.tobaccoinstitute.com. Document no. TIMN0384729-4730. Accessed May 28, 1999.
31. RJ Reynolds. Issues update, July 1997, legislation/regulation. July 1997. Available at: http://www.rjrtdocs.com. Document no. 517996439 -6444. Accessed May 10, 1999.
32. RJ Reynolds. Issues update, October 1997, legislation/regulation. October 1997. Available at: http://www.rjrtdocs.com. Document no. 517976643 -6648. Accessed May 10, 1999.
33. RJ Reynolds. Memorandum from Robert J. Stone to David M. Powers re Connecticut, Massachusetts, and Rhode Island. April 15, 1998. Available at: http://www.rjrtdocs.com. Document no. 518477870 -7871. Accessed May 10, 1999.
34. Massachusetts Restaurant Association. MRA names new president [press release]. July 9, 1998. Available at: http://www.marestaurantassoc.org/donoghue_rls.shtml. Accessed July 7, 1999.
35. RJ Reynolds. Issues update, July 1998, legislation/regulation. July 1998. Available at: http://www.rjrtdocs.com. Document no. 5169246607 -4611. Accessed May 10, 1999.
36. Blanchard E, Begay M. *Local Tobacco Control Policymaking and the Amherst Massachusetts Bar Smoking Ban.* Amherst, Mass: School of Public Health and Health Sciences, University of Massachusetts; 1999. Monograph Series.

Louisiana Tobacco Control: Creating Momentum With Limited Funds

| Sarah Moody Thomas, PhD, Elissa B. Schuler-Adair, PhD, Stacey Cunningham, MS, Michael Celestin, BA, and Charles Brown, MD

The influx of tobacco settlement money has generated unprecedented potential to address the public health problem of tobacco use.[1] In states such as California, Massachusetts, and Florida, where resources have been allocated to tobacco control efforts, much has been achieved.[2] Yet a recent survey of state legislatures found that less than 10% of settlement funds are designated for smoking prevention.[3] With this level of funding, existing blueprints for comprehensive tobacco control, such as the Centers for Disease Control and Prevention's (CDC's) "best practices," are beyond the reach of most states.[4]

The CDC, through the Louisiana Office of Public Health, funds the Louisiana Tobacco Control Program's Research and Evaluation Center (LTCP-REC). LTCP-REC's purpose is to provide resources to the general public, health care providers, educators, and state-funded tobacco initiatives; identify and distribute educational materials; offer technical assistance in design, implementation, and evaluation of community-based tobacco control programs; provide tobacco use prevention and cessation information and referrals via telephone and community outreach; assist with media campaigns; and provide information on model policies and state legislation.

LTCP-REC's operating budget for 1998–1999 was approximately $42 000 in direct costs, not including personnel. When resources are scarce and objectives are broad, opportunities are created through partnerships. For example, LTCP-REC initiated a pilot program in New Orleans public schools using the American Lung Association's "Teens Against Tobacco Use," a school-based smoking prevention program led by teenagers. Twenty-one youths were trained to deliver 4 presentations to elementary school children assigned to in-school suspension for disciplinary reasons.[5] This program was expanded, with American Lung Association sponsorship, in spring 2001. After a review of publications revealed a need for prevention materials for young adult African Americans, LTCP-REC conducted focus groups in collaboration with the Center for Substance Abuse Prevention to identify and develop anti-tobacco messages for African Americans aged 18 to 24 years.[6]

Strategic planning provides maximum flexibility and responsiveness. LTCP-REC began providing tobacco control education *before* all the resources were in place:

- The first educational presentation was held on August 29, 1998; 72 presentations had been made by July 2000. The experience provided immediate feedback about priorities, needs, and current challenges.
- LTCP-REC's newsletter, first published in May 1999, has grown from an initial distribution of 400 to 1277 (1000 posted, 277 e-mailed) by July 2000. It includes sections on local initiatives, national news, legislative updates, and statistical information.
- Surveys and focus groups of providers and smokers were conducted to assess cessation services in Louisiana.[7] Expansion was achieved by implementing small projects on multiple fronts.

Development of a tobacco control resource center requires networking, identification of communication channels, and management of educational materials (Table 1). Early progress indicators for LTCP-REC show positive feedback from clients, partners, and mailing list recipients; increasing recognition of LTCP-REC; growth in the number and extent of outreach and evaluation activities; and wider distribution of materials. ■

About the Authors

The authors are with the Stanley S. Scott Cancer Center, Louisiana State University Health Sciences Center, New Orleans, La.

TABLE 1—Strategies to Develop a Tobacco Control Resource Center

Activity	Description	Example
Networking	Sharing information, facilitating service provision, and working collaboratively with strategically positioned individuals, institutions, and organizations (state and national)	Hosted a conference covering the rationale for and barriers to tobacco control, implementation of control strategies, and treatment of nicotine addiction, attended by 58 individuals from a variety of disciplines and institutions; proceedings from the conference were summarized and distributed to participants, policymakers, and service agencies
Use of communication channels	Disseminating educational messages and materials (oral, written, electronic, and audiovisual) to groups of people and receiving their input and feedback	Allowed direct access for interested residents and enhanced customer responsiveness via a toll-free number (1-877-KICK-NIC) and Web site (http://www.lsuhsc.edu/centers/cancer/tobacco)
Management of educational materials	Evaluating suitability of materials and monitoring their use; stocking, purchasing, distributing, lending, and compiling materials into packets	Used a database to monitor available materials and their acquisition and distribution; standardized content analysis of tobacco control materials has informed purchasing and distribution decisions.[8]

Requests for reprints should be sent to Sarah Moody Thomas, PhD, Department of Public Health and Preventive Medicine, 1600 Canal Street, Suite 800, New Orleans, LA 70112 (e-mail: sthoma@lsuhsc.edu).

This brief was accepted May 30, 2001.

Contributors

All authors contributed to the conceptualization of the project, the compilation of lessons learned, and revision of the article. The team was led by S.M. Thomas. E.B. Schuler-Adair coordinated the project. S. Cunningham, M. Celestin, and C. Brown identified activities and extracted data.

Acknowledgments

Funding is provided by the Centers for Disease Control through the Louisiana Office of Public Health.

The authors would like to acknowledge the following individuals who have contributed to the development and implementation of the LTCP-REC activities described in this article: Diane Hargrove-Roberson, Josie White, Shawn Williams, and Betty Jo Lovell.

References

1. Green LW, Eriksen MP, Bailey L, Husten C. Achieving the implausible in the next decade's tobacco control objectives. *Am J Public Health.* 2000; 90:337–339.

2. National Cancer Policy Board, Institute of Medicine, National Research Council. *State Programs Can Reduce Tobacco Use.* Washington, DC: National Academy of Sciences Press; 2000. Available on-line at: http://www.nap.edu/catalog/9762.html. Accessed April 2, 2002.

3. *State Allocation of Tobacco Settlement Funds: FY2000 and FY2001.* Washington, DC: Health Policy Tracking Service, National Conference of State Legislatures; August 1, 2000.

4. *Best Practices for Comprehensive Tobacco Control Programs–August 1999.* Atlanta, Ga: National Center for Chronic Disease Prevention and Health Promotion, Office on Smoking and Health; August 1999.

5. Celestin M. Delivering school-based tobacco control programming through partnerships: a New Orleans pilot for Teens Against Tobacco Use (YIP-TATU). Paper presented at: Annual School Health Conference of the American School Health Association; October 25–29, 2000; New Orleans, La.

6. Hairston BK, Stewart T. *Louisiana Anti-Tobacco Focus Groups Among African-American Young Adults, Final Report.* Baltimore, Md: Marketing Resources; 2000.

7. Schuler-Adair E, Thomas SM, Cunningham S, Celestin M, Jarrett D, Jones-Lange K. Availability of smoking cessation services in Louisiana. Paper presented at: World Conference on Tobacco OR Health; August 6–11, 2000; Chicago, Ill.

8. Cunningham S, Schuler-Adair E, Celestin M, Quintal L, Lovell BJ, Thomas SM. A content analysis of tobacco prevention and cessation print materials. Paper presented at: meeting of the American Association for Cancer Education and the European Association for Cancer Education; November 2–5, 2000; Washington, DC.

Local Enactment of Tobacco Control Policies in Massachusetts

| William J. Bartosch, MPA, MA, and Gregory C. Pope, MS

In recent years, communities have turned to policymaking as a strategy to control both youths' access to tobacco products and the general population's exposure to environmental tobacco smoke. The number of local tobacco policies has grown—beginning in the 1970s and intensifying in the mid-1980s—with the emergence of research showing the health risks associated with environmental tobacco smoke.[1,2] At the forefront of this movement have been many Massachusetts cities and towns, which wield substantial regulatory authority in areas of public health and have aggressively pursued local tobacco control policies. This has been particularly evident since the implementation of the Massachusetts Tobacco Control Program (MTCP) in 1993.[3,4]

MTCP, one of the most prominent state tobacco control initiatives in the United States, is supported by the state's tobacco excise tax. The program funds various activities, including a media campaign; school health services; statewide and regional initiatives; smoking intervention programs; and research, demonstration, and evaluation projects.[5] It provides funds to local boards of health to raise public awareness of the need for tobacco control policies and supports their passage and enforcement.

We examined the effect of MTCP funding of local boards of health on the enactment of tobacco control policies by the 351 cities and towns in Massachusetts. To identify local policy status, we used data from multiple sources, including the MTCP Ordinance Update Database, a Massachusetts Association of Health Boards survey, data collected by Americans for Nonsmokers' Rights, and our own review of local policy documents. Table 1 shows the local enactment status of tobacco control policies in March 1999.

We created a local tobacco policy index to measure the extent of policy adoption. We began by identifying the range of policies that a community could enact, excluding policies that might apply to only a small number of large towns or cities (e.g., smoking bans in sports arenas). Then, as shown in Table 1, we assigned points to each policy. The maximum score for a town was 100 points, if it enacted all policies identified. Fifty points were assigned to each of 2 domains: environmental tobacco smoke policies and youth access policies. Within each domain, points were assigned to each policy according to the authors' assessment of the restrictiveness and significance of the policy and its difficulty of enactment. Index scoring was informed by interviews the authors conducted with local tobacco control officials. Additional analyses (not shown) indicate that our results are not very sensitive to the precise weights chosen for the policy index.[3]

Since tobacco policy enactment may be influenced by a number of factors, we conducted multiple regression analysis to identify the relationship between community characteristics and policy enactment as measured by our tobacco policy index. Total policy score was explained by MTCP funding and town characteristics. Since MTCP funding is based on a formula that is largely driven by town population, we created a binary variable indicating whether or not a town received funding or was part of a coalition of communities receiving funding. Explanatory variables also included demographics, political orientation, and town governance.

Results from the regression analysis are shown in Table 2. Our model explained 47% of the variation in policy enactment across communities. We found that MTCP funding was strongly related to enactment, with funded communities (76% of towns), on average, scoring 27 points higher than nonfunded communities, other factors being constant.

We also found that town size was an important factor related to tobacco control policy adoption. Very small towns were much less likely than larger towns to adopt tobacco control policies. Communities with populations between 25 000 and 40 000 had total local tobacco policy scores 40 points higher than communities with 2500 or fewer residents, other factors being equal. Interviews with local tobacco control officials suggested that very small towns have few retail establishments or restaurants and therefore do not

TABLE 1—Local Tobacco Control Policies in Effect: Massachusetts, March 1999

	No. of Communities With Policy[a]	Proportion of State Population, %	Weight in Tobacco Policy Index[b]
Environmental tobacco smoke policies (maximum score = 50)			
Any restaurant policy (maximum score = 20)	153	65.7	...
Highly restrictive[c]	75	32.3	20
Other	78	33.3	10
Municipal buildings	127	48.9	15
Private worksites	87	39.9	15
Nursing homes	80	31.0	NA
Hospitals	68	28.0	NA
Sports arenas	71	27.7	NA
Hotels/motels	63	24.1	NA
Malls	54	23.7	NA
Private secondary schools	37	16.7	NA
Private colleges/universities	27	12.2	NA
Outdoor stadiums	12	4.0	NA
Youth access policies (maximum score = 50)			
Any vending machine policy (maximum score = 10)	152	77.3	...
Ban on vending machines	85	22.0	10
Lock-out devices required, limited to adult-only establishments	24	22.4	8
Lock-out devices required	43	24.2	4
Limited to adult-only establishments	31	8.7	4
Licensing of tobacco retailers required	182	76.8	20
Limit on free-standing displays	169	69.6	3
Ban on distribution of free samples	157	67.9	3
Fines for selling to minors	157	66.7	8
Ban on sale of individual cigarettes	135	51.6	3
Ban on tobacco coupon redemption	41	12.0	3
Ban on public transit advertising of tobacco	20	7.6	NA
Ban on taxi advertising of tobacco	18	7.2	NA
Ban on tobacco billboards	5	2.0	NA

Note. NA = not applicable; these policies were relevant only to a small minority of towns.
Source. Data were taken from the Massachusetts Tobacco Control Program Ordinance Update Database; data collected by Americans for Nonsmokers' Rights and by the Massachusetts Association of Health Boards; the authors' review of local policy documents; and the 1990 US census.
[a]There are 351 cities and towns in Massachusetts.
[b]The tobacco policy index measures the extent of policy enactment by communities. Weights were assigned by the authors.
[c]The authors defined highly restrictive restaurant smoking policies as policies that completely prohibit smoking in restaurants or that allow smoking in physically segregated or separately ventilated areas.

perceive regulating tobacco sales or public smoking as a high priority. In addition, these officials reported that small towns, even those receiving MTCP funding, lack sufficient resources (particularly staff) to pursue tobacco policy enactment.

No factors other than MTCP funding and town population had a strong relationship to tobacco control policy enactment in our regression model.

Our analysis shows a clear correlation between MTCP funding of local boards of public health and local policy enactment. MTCP funding may be a function of unmeasured characteristics, such as the presence of local tobacco control advocates, that predispose towns both to apply for state support and to enact policies; however, our interviews with local tobacco officials support the interpretation that MTCP funding is an independent causal factor influencing policy enactment. Local public health staffs consistently reported that MTCP funding was critical to their success. They noted that MTCP funding allowed them to focus specifically on tobacco control policies, thus taking advantage of the considerable discretion that they are granted under state law.

Our study shows that state funding of local boards of health serves as a catalyst for local policy enactment. This is particularly important because although statewide tobacco control policies can have far-reaching impact, they can be difficult to enact. Research has shown that the tobacco lobby has operated more effectively at the federal and state levels than at the local level.[6–8] State laws that do get enacted may be less protective of public health than tobacco control advocates would like, and they may preempt passage of more stringent local policies.[9–14]

The Massachusetts experience shows that with state funding, tobacco control policies are adopted where local communities exercise a high degree of control over public health regulation. However, tobacco control in very small towns is limited. Very small towns may require additional state resources or innovative approaches, such as collaborative initiatives involving several localities, to stimulate policy action. ■

About the Authors

The authors are with the Center for Health Economics Research, Waltham, Mass.

Requests for reprints should be sent to William J. Bartosch, MPA, MA, Center for Health Economics Research, 411 Waverley Oaks Rd, Suite 330, Waltham, MA 02452 (e-mail: bbartosch@her-cher.org).

This article was accepted December 4, 2001.

***Note.** The statements contained in this article are solely those of the authors and do not necessarily reflect the views or policies of the Massachusetts Department of Public Health or the Robert Wood Johnson Foundation.*

Contributors

Both authors were involved in the study's conception, design, and analysis, as well as in drafting the manuscript and carrying out the final revision.

Acknowledgments

Support for this research was provided by the Massachusetts Department of Public Health, Tobacco Control Program (contract SCDPH290788HCHER) and the Robert Wood Johnson Foundation's Substance Abuse Policy Research Program (grant 028803).

The authors are grateful to Jerry Cromwell of the Center for Health Economics Research for his technical assistance.

TABLE 2—Factors Influencing Tobacco Policy Enactment in Massachusetts Cities and Towns (n=351)

Independent Variable	Coefficient (SE)
Constant	7.5 (40.64)
Local board of health received MTCP funding[a]	26.92 (3.56)***
Population (omitted: 0-1250)	
1251-2500	2.56 (6.24)
2501-5000	16.14 (6.76)**
5001-7500	21.17 (7.03)***
7501-10 000	30.15 (7.73)***
10 001-15 000	25.58 (7.54)***
15 001-25 000	31.06 (8.25)***
25 001-40 000	39.90 (10.19)***
>40 000	34.18 (11.43)***
Education (omitted: lowest quartile)[b]	
Low (second quartile)	3.50 (4.84)
Moderate (third quartile)	0.32 (5.59)
High (fourth quartile)	6.73 (8.04)
Income (omitted: lowest quartile)[c]	
Low (second quartile)	0.82 (4.45)
Moderate (third quartile)	-3.07 (5.25)
High (fourth quartile)	1.55 (6.91)
Percentage of White residents	-21.80 (29.80)
Percentage of residents < 18 y	-6.86 (49.12)
Percentage of blue-collar workers	-40.29 (35.59)
Percentage of Democrats	17.37 (18.38)
Percentage of registered voters	26.69 (14.01)*
Percentage who voted for tobacco excise tax	-14.54 (27.26)
Town governance (omitted: representative town meeting)	
Open town meeting	-5.38 (5.88)
City council	-2.53 (6.86)
Community has a town manager	2.45 (3.51)
Number of restaurants	1.21 (0.64)*
Percentage border towns with highly restrictive restaurant policy	-6.94 (3.87)*
Adjusted R^2 = 0.47	

Note. The dependent variable was the local tobacco policy index score (range = 0-100, mean = 37.70). MTCP = Massachusetts Tobacco Control Program.
Sources. Policy enactment status was determined from multiple sources of data, including the MTCP Ordinance Update Database, data collected by the Massachusetts Association of Health Boards, data collected by Americans for Nonsmokers' Rights, and the authors' analysis of policy documents. Sociodemographic variables were based on the 1990 US census. Voting records (1994) were provided by the Massachusetts Secretary of State's Office. Number of restaurants was based on meals tax data provided by the Massachusetts Department of Revenue. Town governance variables came from the Massachusetts Municipal Association.
[a]Funded boards of health included local boards of health that received MTCP funding or were part of a coalition of boards receiving MTCP funding between 1994 and 1998.
[b]Education quartiles were based on the percentage of college graduates aged 25 years and older.
[c]Income quartiles were based on town-level median household income.
*P<.1; **P<.05; ***P<.01.

References

1. *Monograph 3: Major Local Tobacco Control Ordinances in the United States.* Bethesda, Md: National Cancer Institute; 1993. NIH publication 93-3532.

2. Rigotti NA, Pashos CL. No-smoking laws in the United States. An analysis of state and city actions to limit smoking in public places and workplaces. *JAMA.* 1991;266:3162–3167.

3. Bartosch WJ, Pope GC. *Analysis of the Adoption of Local Tobacco Control Policies in Massachusetts, Final Report.* Waltham, Mass: Center for Health Economics Research; 2000.

4. Bartosch WJ, Pope GC. Local restaurant smoking policy enactment in Massachusetts. *J Public Health Manage Pract.* 1999;5:53–62.

5. Hamilton WL, Norton GD. *Independent Evaluation of the Massachusetts Tobacco Control Program, Fifth Annual Report, January 1994 to June 1998.* Cambridge, Mass: Abt Associates; 1999.

6. Samuels B, Glantz SA. The politics of local tobacco control. *JAMA.* 1991;266:2110–2117.

7. Glantz SA. Achieving a smoke-free society. *Circulation.* 1987;76:746–752.

8. Begay ME, Traynor M, Glantz SA. The tobacco industry, state politics, and tobacco education in California. *Am J Public Health.* 1993;83:1214–1221.

9. Magzamen S, Glantz SA. The new battleground: California's experience with smoke-free bars. *Am J Public Health.* 2001;91:245–252.

10. Conlisk E, Siegel M, Lengerich E, MacKenzie W, Malek S, Eriksen M. The status of local smoking regulations in North Carolina following a state preemption bill. *JAMA.* 1995;10:805–807.

11. Jacobson PD, Wasserman J, Raube K. The politics of antismoking legislation. *J Health Polit Policy Law.* 1994;18:787–819.

12. Ellis GA, Hobart RL, Reed DF. Overcoming a powerful tobacco lobby in enacting local smoking ordinances: the Contra Costa County experience. *J Public Health Policy.* 1996;17:28–46.

13. Macdonald H, Aguinaga S, Glantz SA. The defeat of Philip Morris' 'California Uniform Tobacco Control Act.' *Am J Public Health.* 1997;87:1989–1996.

14. Siegel M, Carol J, Jordan J, et al. Preemption in tobacco control. Review of an emerging public health problem. *JAMA.* 1997;278:858–863.

The Institute of Medicine Report on Smoking: A Blueprint for a Renewed Public Health Policy

| Gio Batta Gori, ScD, MPH

This past September, the Institute of Medicine (IOM) published the report *Clearing the Smoke: Assessing the Science Base for Tobacco Harm Reduction.*[1] The report's leading conclusion is that tobacco products of reduced risk, and especially less hazardous cigarettes, are within technical reach and should be officially endorsed and regulated. The report speaks of unparalleled public health opportunities in tobacco harm reduction and in the abatement of the awesome morbidity and premature mortality of more than 1 billion smokers worldwide.[1(p23)]

Since a preview draft was released in early 2001, the report has hardly been noticed by the public health community, because it implies a policy shift that many would find uncomfortable. Indeed, especially the endorsement of less hazardous cigarettes would be at odds with long-standing policies aimed exclusively at the elimination of tobacco use, policies whose effectiveness the proposed shift also may appear to question.

In reality, the IOM report continues to insist on reinforcing traditional tobacco control efforts to discourage users and would-be users while asserting that "[f]or many diseases attributable to tobacco use, reducing risk of disease by reducing exposure to tobacco toxicants is feasible."[1(p5)] The report covers the entire spectrum, from snuff to cigars, with potentially less hazardous cigarettes receiving prominent attention. The authors of the report find the technology of such cigarettes to be within short-term reach, given resolute official prodding of an industry that has to date resisted them on a variety of pretexts.

In a crucial departure from current tenets, the report affirms that there is "misinformation regarding the safety of nicotine,"[1(p110)] which it finds relatively safe: "Many studies of nicotine suggest that nicotine is unlikely to be a cancer-causing agent in humans,"[1(p167)] "high doses of nicotine do not seem to cause acute adverse events even among smokers who have experienced cardiovascular disease,"[1(p115)] and long-term nicotine replacement therapy has been "without an apparent cardiovascular hazard, not only in the general population . . . but also in patients with established cardiovascular disease."[1(p252)] The report also notes how the Food and Drug Administration has affirmed the safety of nicotine for more than 15 years, by approving over-the-counter sales of patches and gums that contain more nicotine than a pack of cigarettes.

The massive epidemiological evidence that risk relates to dose is found by the report to allow estimates of "a dose–response relationship between exposure to whole tobacco smoke and major diseases."[1(p9)] Building on these findings, the report considers a general strategy for cigarette harm reduction as "[r]etaining nicotine at pleasurable or addictive levels while reducing the more toxic components of tobacco."[1(p29)]

It continues by recommending that "Congress enact legislation enabling a suitable agency to regulate tobacco-related products that purport to reduce one or more tobacco toxicants or to reduce the risk of disease"[1(p205)] so that "[p]romotion, advertising and labeling of these products are firmly regulated to prevent false or misleading claims" and "[m]anufacturers have the necessary incentive to develop and market products that reduce exposure to tobacco toxicants and that have a reasonable prospect of reducing the risk of tobacco-related disease."[1(p7)] The report backs up such deeply heterodox but testable conclusions and prescriptions with an impressive review of the scientific evidence.

Coming full circle, the IOM's message reconnects with virtually the same science and public health recommendations advanced more than 20 years ago by the Smoking and Health Program of the National Cancer Institute and the National Heart, Lung, and Blood Institute[2]—recommendations that were suppressed with the adoption of "smoke-free America" policies from the late 1970s and onward. Although the IOM report does not broach the issue, the report is apt to raise disturbing regrets in the minds of those who for more than 20 years have contributed to delaying the life-saving benefits of less hazardous cigarettes. Such regrets, and the opposition they might engender, could be a significant hindrance to progress but should yield to determined action, because the evidence revisited by the report brings forth an unavoidable moral obligation to learn and act now.

Time is of the essence, because people are dying or at risk as we read these words, and the IOM report shows that there can be a remedy while also implying that, ethically speaking, the plight of smokers is no less deserving than that of people with other afflictions. Despite all warnings, close to a billion people will continue to smoke for decades to come, making a compelling case for a radically fresh approach in the prevention of tobacco-related diseases. The report makes it clear that action cannot be expected from a tobacco industry mired in controversy and of nonexistent credibility and aims its message directly toward Congress and the government, academic, and private institutions and charities that embody the public health community.

Aside from generally upbeat conclusions about the feasibility of less hazardous cigarettes, the IOM report leaves the operational detail largely unanswered and bristles with caveats and questions that need teasing out. Technical approaches to reduction of dose and risk ought to be sifted; methods and markers for toxicological evaluation need to be discussed and standardized; risk models and regulatory measures should be sensibly reconciled to avoid disabling complexities; ways for monitoring and surveillance should be devised; legislative issues have to be worked on. These and other questions must be aired and resolved in a broader dialogue that should begin immediately, in the pages of this venerable journal that strives to be the voice of our conscience. ■

About the Author

The author is with The Health Policy Center, Bethesda, Md. Requests for reprints should be sent to Gio Batta Gori, ScD, MPH, The Health Policy Center, 6704 Barr Rd, Bethesda, MD 20816 (e-mail: gorigb@msn.com).

This brief was accepted January 10, 2002.

References

1. Institute of Medicine. *Clearing the Smoke: Assessing the Science Base for Tobacco Harm Reduction.* Washington, DC: National Academy Press; 2001.

2. *A Safe Cigarette?* Gori GB, Bock FG, eds. Cold Spring Harbor, NY: Cold Spring Harbor Laboratory Press; 1980. Bambury report 3.

Tobacco Industry Surveillance of Public Health Groups: The Case of STAT and INFACT

| Ruth E. Malone, RN, PhD

Objectives. The goal of this study was to describe how the tobacco industry collects information about public health groups.

Methods. Publicly available internal tobacco industry documents were reviewed and analyzed using a chronological case study approach.

Results. The industry engaged in aggressive intelligence gathering, used intermediaries to obtain materials under false pretenses, sent public relations spies to the organizations' meetings, and covertly taped strategy sessions. Other industry strategies included publicly minimizing the effects of boycotts, painting health advocates as "extreme," identifying and exploiting disagreements, and planning to "redirect the funding" of tobacco control organizations to other purposes.

Conclusions. Public health advocates often make light of tobacco industry observers, but industry surveillance may be real, intense, and covert and may obstruct public health initiatives. (*Am J Public Health.* 2002;92:955–960)

Public health advocates increasingly focus attention on the tobacco industry's role as "the vector of the tobacco epidemic"[1(p206)] and highlight industry behaviors that undermine public health and raise ethical concerns.[2] Industry-focused campaigns are effective in changing views of tobacco use,[3–7] but the study described in this article shows that such a strategy may also invite aggressively conducted industry surveillance.

Many businesses use "competitive intelligence" to learn about their competitors.[8,9] For example, it is common for companies to request competitors' publicly filed business reports, to attempt to learn about sales, or to conduct analyses of competitors' products. However, tobacco industry intelligence gathering extends beyond other cigarette companies to include tobacco control organizations, which the industry calls "the antis." Although such groups are not cigarette "competitors," they do compete with the industry for public opinion and the ear of policymakers, and thus they are perceived as a threat. In this article, evidence from internal tobacco industry documents is used to describe how the industry responded to 2 such groups, STAT (Stop Teenage Addiction to Tobacco) and INFACT (formerly the Infant Formula Action Coalition), both of which were active during the 1990s in drawing public and media attention to industry behaviors.

METHODS

Data were collected from tobacco industry internal documents released as a result of the Minnesota Tobacco Settlement and other legal cases. Tobacco Institute (http://www.tobaccoinstitute.com), R.J. Reynolds (http://www.rjrtdocs.com), and Philip Morris (http://www.pmdocs.com) document Web sites were searched for combined text fields such as "anti," "intelligence," and public health group names, including STAT, INFACT, DOC (Doctors Ought to Care), and others. Searches of the Minnesota Tobacco Documents Depository were also conducted. Searches took place between January 1, 2001, and January 19, 2002, and involved systematic "snowball" searching techniques, as described elsewhere.[10,11] Data used included internal letters, memorandums, reports, and other documents. Findings were assembled chronologically into a narrative case study.

RESULTS

1985: STAT Is Formed

STAT, founded in 1985 by Stanford MBA and activist Joe Tye, was almost immediately perceived as a threat by the industry. A grassroots group focused on the industry's targeting of children, STAT was well organized and media savvy. The first issue of *STAT-News* reported that STAT was "beginning a major project to analyze, catalog and index the documentation that is being generated as a result of tobacco products litigation," threatening further public exposure of potentially embarrassing industry documents.[12]

The industry responded quickly. At the Tobacco Institute, the industry's public relations organization, A.H. (Anne) Duffin, vice president and director of publications, sent a terse message, apparently to her assistant: "Please start a file on this STAT group. And please run a complete search on it and Joe B. Tye."[13] Duffin advised colleagues that STAT had "implications for the industry in both legislative and litigative areas," describing its plans for a study with DOC on cigarette purchasing by minors and noting that the organization was selling copies of an anti–tobacco industry book, *Sixty Years of Deception.*[14]

This intelligence gathering had several purposes. In 1988, a Tobacco Institute public affairs division operational plan proposed "keep[ing] the Institute in the driver's seat" through "knowledge of anti-smoking announcements before the fact."[15] Betsy Annese of R.J. Reynolds public affairs attached a list of industry critics to a memorandum sent to Herb Osmon in 1987,[16] and Osmon presented several talks focusing entirely on tobacco control "zealots," apparently accompanied by slides with photographs of tobacco control activists and researchers.[17–19] Intelligence could be used to "discredit" public health groups, as recommended in a 1989 INFOTAB (the industry's international intelligence and research agency) report, *A Guide for Dealing With Anti-Tobacco Pressure Groups,* which advised executives to *"discredit* the often imported activists of the [tobacco control] coalition—ideally through third parties [emphasis in original]."[20]

1990: STAT Growth, Boycott of RJR–Nabisco

The industry used intermediaries to obtain STAT materials under the pretense of being interested members.[21] According to a STAT newsletter (found with numerous other STAT-generated materials among Philip Morris's internal documents), STAT had more than 5000 members by 1990 and was calling for a boycott of RJR–Nabisco products.[22] In August 1990, STAT held its first annual activists' conference in Boston. Cosponsored by DOC, it attracted participants from many organizations, including the Tobacco Institute. At least 1 industry spy "attended as an interested public relations specialist" and provided the Tobacco Institute with a detailed report on the conference.[23] "While the goal may be reduced tobacco use by minors, the actions encouraged are to harass two specific tobacco companies, Philip Morris and R.J. Reynolds Tobacco," the spy reported.[23]

Apparently, the spy was someone accepted and perhaps known by the "antis" but also recognizable within the industry: when conference attendees adjourned to picket at Fenway Park to protest tobacco advertisements, the spy left early, possibly fearing detection. "Because of my double status at the conference and because of likely media coverage, after consultation with [Tobacco Institute] personnel I departed," the spy reported.[23] The Tobacco Institute even received the summary of conference participant evaluations.[24]

Although R.J. Reynolds attempted publicly to minimize STAT's boycott, preparing a press release stating that "historically...boycotts have not been particularly successful,"[25] the extent of internal activity suggests concern. The Fleishman Hillard public relations agency sent regular intelligence reports to R.J. Reynolds, including copies of STAT's *Tobacco and Youth Reporter*. In addition, at least 1 R.J. Reynolds consultant, Susan Heenan Piscitelli, made a membership contribution to STAT as early as February 1991 and forwarded STAT mailings.[26] STAT was at that point writing letters about the industry's product placement in movies,[27] causing some consternation.

A letter from assistant general counsel Deborah Christie to Brennan Dawson, vice president for public affairs at the Tobacco Institute, sought advice on what the Liggett Tobacco Company should do: "Should we ignore the [STAT] letter? Can the Tobacco Institute respond on behalf of its industry members?"[28] In addition to the intelligence and public relations efforts of INFOTAB and the Tobacco Institute on behalf of their tobacco company funders, the individual companies sometimes shared intelligence about opponents. In a 1991 memo, R.J. Reynolds's Tom Ogburn Jr noted that Philip Morris "has agreed to share with us their 'no mail' list . . . the list of people they have compiled whom they know should not be on our mailing lists. We will share similar information with them."[29]

1991: Major Intelligence Report for R. J. Reynolds

In March 1991, Joe Rodota of the Benchmark Research Group described to R.J. Reynolds's Osmon the preparation of intelligence research on antismoking groups, including "a review of potential allies opposed to one or more aspects of these organizations' agendas." This research also included field visits to DOC, STAT, the Tobacco Divestment Project, and other organizations "to see if these groups share offices with other organizations; retrieve pamphlets or other materials from local libraries; and confirm through city or county business filings the ownership or size of the organization."[30]

Later in 1991, Rodota proposed selecting "certain documents concerning the antismoking movement" that would be kept in binders for use by "selected company officials."[31] Rodota noted that the documents assembled "undoubtedly comprise the nation's largest collection of materials on anti-smoking groups, apart from materials maintained by the groups themselves."[31] The study reported on 21 organizations and included more than 30 000 pages.

Yet even as this massive intelligence report was being prepared, some in the company wondered about the implications of such efforts. "Your comment that we don't want to be in a position of developing a Richard Nixonesque 'enemies' list is a point well-taken," wrote R.J. Reynolds's Rob Meyne in April 1991 to his public affairs colleague Tim Hyde. "The existence of such a list could, in and of itself, be a negative P.R. story . . . my bottom line recommendation . . . would be that we encourage the Field Coordinators to collect the names of known antis as they come across them, and delete from our database those who prove to be a problem." A handwritten response at the bottom, signed "T" (probably Tim Hyde), concurs: "Exactly! For now, at least, we should simply put these names on our 'grief' file, along with underages and those demanding to be taken off the list, and the known dead."[32]

Industry spies attended the 1991 STAT conference. Judy Provosty of Fleishman Hillard duly reported to R.J. Reynolds that tobacco control advocates ridiculed industry intelligence: "During the middle of his lecture, [tobacco control activist Michael] Pertschuk ripped off his STAT name tag and admitted to being a tobacco industry mole. He donned a tie and jacket and introduced himself as Walker Merryman [a well-known Tobacco Institute spokesman]."[33] R.J. Reynolds was particularly upset at press coverage STAT received about its assertions that Joe Camel used phallic imagery and appealed to children. "This is perverted and deviant," a draft R.J. Reynolds letter to the editor spluttered.[34] The planned response was to "position Joe Tye as too extreme in his tactics and condemn his involving children in cigarette advertising," according to an R.J. Reynolds public relations strategy document.[35]

1992: Illegal Audiotaping of STAT Sessions

Beth Lancaster of Fleishman Hillard and R.J. Reynolds consultant Susan Heenan attended STAT's 1992 meeting, according to the STAT participants list found among other Tobacco Institute documents.[36–38] Lancaster (and possibly others) secretly tape-recorded the sessions, despite careful and explicitly announced security measures by the conference organizers.[39] In a report prepared for the industry, a spy describes the STAT strategy session on shareholders' resolutions aimed at tobacco companies:

> This workshop was the strangest by far. Each participant was more or less searched and name badges were cross checked with the master list . . . (The tape sound quality is poor since the recorder had to be well hidden and once on, not adjusted. Several times you will hear random searches of belongings for security reasons). At one point . . . Mr. Garfield Ma-

> hood (NRA [Nonsmokers' Rights Association]–Toronto) challenged the meetings [sic] security by saying "do we know everybody in this room?" [A]t that time it was suggested that chairs be circled with individual introductions around the room. Chaos followed as chairs were moved and several people headed out the door. ([A]ll names were rechecked and those who left were so noted on the list). A light visual sweep was made for cameras or recorders. The tension was great and the group was giddy for awhile . . . The workshop ran 15 minutes over time and people were starting to filter out–in order to conceal the recorder the last 50 seconds were not recorded. It is impossible to accurately summerize [sic] this meeting. The paranoia alone was just unbelieveable [sic]. Needless to say you must hear it to believe it![40]

This industry report suggests that there may have been several other industry spies in attendance who left the room to avoid detection, leaving Lancaster, who was apparently convincing in her self-presentation. A tape recording of this session was apparently used by someone to try to discredit STAT, according to industry reports about the following year's STAT conference. A Philip Morris document regarding the 1993 STAT conference reports that "audio or video recordings of the sessions were not permitted this year since a 'tobacco spy' was in the audience last year and had attempted to discredit and harm the reputation of a Canadian researcher."[41] An R.J. Reynolds report on the same conference indicated that "security [was] intense–due to illegal recording obtained at 1992 conference that caused serious federal problems for STAT."[42] This spy also reported: "Have made connection with the Advocacy Institute–the Scarcnet [tobacco control advocacy network] people."[42]

A 1992 DOC internal organizational memo from Eric Solberg to the DOC executive committee, found on the R.J. Reynolds documents Web site, seems to indicate that industry surveillance reached the inner circles of some tobacco control groups. Written by Solberg shortly after the STAT conference, the confidential document expressed concern that DOC had not capitalized on its "Joe Camel" research and was marginalized. The copy on the R.J. Reynolds documents site shows that it was faxed from the Baylor Family Practice Center, where the organization's leaders practiced, suggesting that either someone at the clinic or a member of DOC's executive committee who received the fax provided it to the industry.[43]

1993–1998: INFACT Campaign

In 1993, STAT engaged a powerful ally in its tobacco industry campaign: INFACT. INFACT was a veteran of anticorporate boycott battles in public health, having spearheaded extended boycotts of Nestle and General Electric, both of which ended in industry concessions.[44] This caused new industry concern. At Philip Morris, covert intelligence gathering began with the Burson-Marsteller public relations firm, as described in a memo to Craig Fuller from Barry Holt: "The basic research with INFACT would be done without any mention of the [tobacco industry] client."[45] Burson-Marsteller, according to Holt, had "third-party contacts that can access information (anonymously) on the organization and its activities."[46] A 5-page report concluded with plans for a third-party meeting with INFACT leadership "to assess level and degree of resources and commitment to the campaign."[47] The material was probably prepared by Sheila Raviv of Burson-Marsteller.[48]

Burson-Marsteller recommended a wait-and-see response. However, by September 1993, the Interfaith Center on Corporate Responsibility (ICCR) had joined INFACT's campaign. According to the intelligence sources, "this is the type of action we feared . . . recommend that we expand our intensive information-finding to ICCR and step up our information-gathering of INFACT."[49] ICCR, a respected coalition of groups including several religious orders, would be more difficult for the industry to discredit as "extreme."

In early 1994, Philip Morris discussions of the INFACT/STAT/ICCR campaign began to refer to "the critic" rather than using the organizations' names, perhaps reflecting an increasingly sensitive internal climate. A presentation by Raviv in March emphasized that the "landscape of anti-tobacco activists is changing; new critics bring new tactics . . . [such as] corporate accountability, boycotting companies . . . mobilizing broader constituencies . . . e.g., human rights groups, children's and youth groups, religious groups *and even smokers* [emphasis in original]."[50,51] Burson-Marsteller's recommendation was as follows: "Responding to it legitimizes INFACT and gives the group credibility . . . but put in place mechanisms to counter expected offshoots of campaign. Continue critic monitoring . . . determine which groups have been solicited by INFACT to join campaign."[51] To date, no documents have been located that describe what these "mechanisms" were or whether they were used.

On April 11, 1994, Raviv notified Holt that the INFACT boycott media announcement was imminent.[52] She suggested "intensifying our efforts to identify the depth of support for the critics' efforts and to determine whether any organizations disapprove of the critics' tactics . . . identify and develop unofficial lines of communication with groups and individuals who may privately oppose these tactics."[53] As the boycott was launched, memos reflect Philip Morris's efforts to stay apprised of the situation on a moment-to-moment basis. "We are continuing to monitor the situation throughout the country, particularly keeping a close watch for any activities during this evening's rush hour," wrote Darienne Dennis, manager of external communications at Philip Morris. "We will update you on any new developments as we become aware of them."[54]

The INFACT/STAT/ICCR campaign was apparently very effective in generating a public response. As of May 10, 1994, Philip Morris reported receiving almost 15 000 postcards and letters.[55] A memo to Holt from Pat Ford and Eileen Burke of Burson-Marsteller noted that "we have also learned that the critic is reportedly receiving 200 inquiries a month on the boycott, several of which are international requests. . . . By capitalizing on its strong ties with [ICCR], the critic could easily increase the scope and size of its coalition. . . . This tactic could swiftly increase the number of boycotters and provide numerous vehicles for communicating the critic's message."[56] A meeting was scheduled for June 2 at Burson-Marsteller's Washington, DC, office to "coordinate a comprehensive strategy."[57] The agenda for this meeting included "techniques for dealing with critics," and the agenda packet included detailed descriptions of both STAT and INFACT.[58]

R.J. Reynolds was also a target of the campaign. Yancey Ford, executive vice president for sales, wrote to customers and retailers, suggesting that INFACT "is really interested in censorship" and asserting: "If our company believed that Camel advertising was causing children to start smoking, we would pull the campaign without having to be asked."[59,60] Ford requested customers to act as intelligence agents for the industry: "If you are contacted, please call . . . immediately and let us know."[60]

In August 1994, Pat Ford of Philip Morris warned colleagues again that INFACT's allies were "not typical 'anti' groups" but, rather, "established, respected religious organizations with a long history of corporate pressure."[61] An attached draft presentation also cautioned that the "risk always exists that [the] group will use innovative tactic[s], e.g., producing documentaries, that could involve and activate a larger segment of the population—particularly outside the United States, and especially in Europe." A major worry was that INFACT might produce a film and distribute it through nontraditional outlets, such as MTV.[61]

The next draft of the critic boycott plan encouraged use of the Philip Morris "sales force as [an] intelligence network to monitor local critic activities."[62] It included warnings for retailers who seemed sympathetic toward the boycott: "If you become one who is known to succumb to activist pressures, you will invite other extremist groups to threaten action against you in the future."[62] As the boycott continued into autumn 1994, Philip Morris began a training program for senior management officials at affiliated companies whose products were being boycotted. Training included "critic tactics and boycott history, guidelines for managing activists, media, customers, minimal 'paper trail.' "[63]

By the following spring, INFACT was reportedly in need of funding to continue its work, according to an April 4, 1995, memo to Barry Holt from Pat Ford and Eileen Burke. A handwritten note at the bottom of the confidential memo describing a fundraising letter and INFACT's "Face the Faces" campaign (a visual display of photographs of those killed by tobacco) added: "they aren't getting the funds but they still plan something."[64] It is unclear how the industry knew that INFACT was not "getting the funds."

In a 1992 speech, Steve Parrish of Philip Morris corporate affairs had expressed concern about the prospects of "antis with media *and* money" and product boycotts. The plan was to continue efforts to "redirect funding of antis to pressing social needs" instead of tobacco control efforts.[65] The speech did not identify which "antis" were being discussed, and to date no further documents addressing INFACT issues have been located. However, there is evidence the industry used this strategy to undermine state-funded tobacco control programs.[4] According to STAT activists, that organization was likewise in financial straits. Large funders were no longer supporting STAT, and other tobacco control groups, including the new, well-funded Center for Tobacco Free Kids, were competitors (B. Godshall, former STAT board director, oral communication, August 2001; J. Sopenski, former STAT executive director, oral communication, July 2001).

Despite INFACT's apparently weakening financial situation, Philip Morris executives worried about the coalition's plan to submit a shareholder proposal for the 1995 Philip Morris stockholder's meeting, especially if accompanied by protests. Darienne Dennis reassured several colleagues: "this is a 'dog bites man story,' in that there is not much news value to the fact that people do not like tobacco companies."[66] Four proposals from tobacco control advocates were presented. An industry public relations–advertising firm reported later: "All shareholder proposals were defeated despite the usual anti-activists having their four minutes of fame (Alan Blum, Father Crosby, INFACTS [sic] and Anne Morrow Donnelly/GASP)."[67]

Activists also were expected at the R.J. Reynolds annual meeting. Maura Ellis of R.J. Reynolds sent a note to Jim Johnston, the company's chairman and CEO, and Tom Griscom, vice president of external relations, on April 10 noting "known 'antis' who will be present at the annual meeting. . . . Attached is detailed background information Herb Osmon has collected on some of the people."[68] R.J. Reynolds apparently continued to receive information on tobacco control groups from third parties, as evidenced by the presence in the R.J. Reynolds documents of a signed letter sent in 1997 to Working Assets, a progressive telephone company that donates funding to public health and environmental groups. The letter, nominating INFACT for the Member Contribution Ballot, was copied to Kathy Mulvey, INFACT's executive director, whose name is circled.[69]

Postscript: STAT and INFACT Today

According to INFACT's Web site,[70] the Kraft Foods/Philip Morris boycott and campaign against the tobacco industry continue, with endorsements by groups in the United States and other countries. INFACT has become a major international tobacco control presence, now recognized in "official relations" with the World Health Organization. As a founding member of Accountability of the Tobacco Transnationals, a coalition of 65 organizations from 40 countries working to build support for strong corporate accountability measures in the International Framework Convention on Tobacco Control, INFACT has been able to expand its work despite the industry's efforts to thwart it. STAT's Web site is still operating, but the organization closed its doors in 2001 as a result of lack of funds.[71]

DISCUSSION

Although it may not be surprising that the tobacco industry would be interested in its opponents, the covertness and intensity of the surveillance described here are remarkable. For example, the covert taping of the 1992 STAT strategy meeting, in addition to violating social norms and meeting rules, also violated Massachusetts state law and the code of ethics for business intelligence professionals. Massachusetts Statute 272 §99 (amended 1968) calls for penalties of up to 5 years in prison and $10 000 for such "interception" of communication. The Society of Corporate Intelligence Professionals code of ethics requires compliance "with all applicable laws, domestic and international," and accurate disclosure of "all relevant information, including one's identity and organization, before all interviews."[9] The taping constitutes a clear violation of both and was apparently used by someone to attempt to discredit STAT.

Campaigns that focus on industry activities represent a special problem for the tobacco industry, because "negative statements in the media put the company on the defensive . . . causing greater scrutiny of our actions and activities by general public, shareholders, employees and plant communities."[72] The recent, well-publicized Philip Morris campaign to remake the company's image (even renaming the entire Philip Morris parent corporation "Altria" in an attempt to shed its tobacco associations) demonstrates the importance of public relations and public opinion to corporate legitimacy and, in turn, the importance of legitimacy to the tobacco industry's survival and growth.[73] As international tobacco control leaders have argued, the tobacco industry needs "respectability" to buttress its political power and avoid regulatory attention.[1] Industry-focused public health campaigns disrupt the industry's carefully constructed images and promote public discourse on the ethical aspects of tobacco promotion.

This study shows that tobacco industry surveillance extends beyond attendance at public meetings. The industry response in the case described above included aggressive intelligence gathering,[13,14] use of intermediaries to obtain organizations' printed materials under false pretenses,[21,45,46] use of public relations specialists as spies,[23] and covert audiotaping.[39,40] In addition, the documents show that cigarette companies coordinated among themselves to share information[29] and maintained detailed lists of industry critics.[16,74]

Other strategies the industry used or contemplated using against STAT/INFACT included publicly minimizing the effects of a boycott,[25] attempting to portray the organizations' leaders as too "extreme,"[35] attempting to exploit potential areas of disagreement with the organizations' allies,[51] and "redirecting" funding for "anti" organizations to other causes.[65] The tobacco industry finds campaigns that focus on its corporate activities particularly threatening, and it especially fears the effects of anti-industry documentaries aimed at a youth–young adult audience.

This study has several limitations. Because of the sheer volume of documents contained in the repositories and the inadequate indexing, it was not possible to ensure that all relevant documents were retrieved. For example, no documents describing how the industry may have attempted to derail funding for STAT/INFACT have been located, so it is not possible to say whether this strategy was implemented or merely contemplated. Further studies should compare the industry's response to STAT/INFACT with its response to other public health groups. Despite its limitations, this study shows that tobacco industry spying is real. Public health groups must anticipate industry surveillance, take steps to address it, and consider whether third parties may be involved in obstructing their activities. ■

About the Author

The author is with the Department of Social and Behavioral Sciences, School of Nursing, and Institute for Health Policy Studies, University of California, San Francisco.

Requests for reprints should be sent to Ruth E. Malone, RN, PhD, Institute for Health Policy Studies, Box 0936, Laurel Heights Campus, University of California, San Francisco, CA 94143-0936 (e-mail: rmalone@itsa.ucsf.edu).

This article was accepted February 11, 2002.

Acknowledgments

Work on this article was supported by grant 9RT-0095 from the California Tobacco-Related Disease Research Program and grants 1 R01 CA87472-01 and 1 R01 CA90789-01 from the National Cancer Institute. Legal assistance was provided by Brion Fox, JD, Center for Tobacco Control Research and Education, University of Wisconsin, and Christopher Banthin, JD, Tobacco Control Resource Center, Northeastern University.

References

1. Yach D, Bettcher D. Globalisation of tobacco industry influence and new global responses. *Tob Control.* 2000;9:206–216.

2. Hicks JJ. The strategy behind Florida's "truth" campaign. *Tob Control.* 2001;10:3–5.

3. Healton C. Who's afraid of the truth? *Am J Public Health.* 2001;91:554–558.

4. Balbach E, Glantz S. Tobacco control advocates must demand high quality media campaigns: the California experience. *Tob Control.* 1998;7:397–408.

5. British Columbia Ministry of Health and Ministry Responsible for Seniors. British Columbia's 'Tobacco industry's poster child': one part of a bigger picture. *Tob Control.* 1999;8:128–131.

6. Zucker D, Hopkins R, Sly D, Urich J, Kershaw J, Solari S. Florida's "truth" campaign: a counter-marketing, anti-tobacco media campaign. *J Public Health Manage Pract.* 2000;6(3):1–6.

7. Sly DF, Hopkins RS, Trapido E, Ray S. Influence of a counteradvertising media campaign on initiation of smoking: the Florida "truth" campaign. *Am J Public Health.* 2001;91:233–238.

8. Attaway MS. A review of issues related to gathering and assessing competitive intelligence. *Am Business Rev.* 1998;16:25–35.

9. Society of Competitive Intelligence Professionals. SCIP code of ethics for CI professionals. Available at: http://www.scip.org/ci/ethics.html. Accessed May 5, 2001.

10. Malone RE, Balbach ED. Tobacco industry documents: treasure trove or quagmire? *Tob Control.* 2000; 9:334–338.

11. Muggli ME, Forster JL, Hurt RD, Repace JL. The smoke you don't see: uncovering tobacco industry scientific strategies aimed against environmental tobacco smoke policies. *Am J Public Health.* 2001;91: 1419–1423.

12. Stop Teenage Addiction to Tobacco. *STAT-News.* Bates No. TIMN0331957/1962. Available at: http://www.tobaccoinstitute.com. Accessed June 21, 2001.

13. Duffin AH. Note to Laura, Tobacco Institute, August 20, 1986. Bates No. TIMN0319107. Available at: http://www.tobaccoinstitute.com. Accessed June 21, 2001.

14. Duffin AH. Memo to William Kloepfe, Jr, Fred Panzer, John Rupp, Peter Sparber, Tobacco Institute, December 14, 1986. Bates No. TIMN0331968/1969. Available at: http://www.tobaccoinstitute.com. Accessed June 20, 2001.

15. Tobacco Institute. Public affairs division proposed 1988 operation plans and budget. Bates No. 506644419 -4579. Available at: http://www.rjrtdocs.com. Accessed August 14, 2001.

16. Annese B. List of tobacco critics, November 11, 1987. Bates No. 506131600 -1602. Available at: http://www.rjrtdocs.com. Accessed April 20, 2001.

17. Osmon HE. Anti-smoking zealots: speech, January 17, 1991. Bates No. 507651081 -1108. Available at: http://www.rjrtdocs.com. Accessed April 20, 2001.

18. Osmon HE. Anti-smoking zealots. Bates No. 512014614 -4641. Available at: http://www.rjrtdocs.com. Accessed April 22, 2001.

19. Osmon HE. Letter to TC Harris and others: attached is the updated overview of anti-smoking organizations. October 26, 1990. Bates No. 507625356 -5412. Available at: http://www.rjrtdocs.com. Accessed April 21, 2001.

20. INFOTAB. A guide for dealing with anti-tobacco pressure groups, 1989. Bates No. 2504063806–3817. Available at: http://www.pmdocs.com. Accessed August 11, 2001.

21. Newman FS. Memo to Donald Fried and others: attached FYI materials from Joe Tye's group, June 27, 1990. Bates No. 2022972734. Available at: http://www.pmdocs.com. Accessed April 27, 2001.

22. Stop Teenage Addiction to Tobacco. *STAT-News,* March, 1990. Bates No. 2025685564/5567. Available at: http://www.pmdocs.com. Accessed July 7, 2001.

23. Anonymous. Report to Barclay Jackson, regional director, the Tobacco Institute, on the First Annual STAT Conference, August 28, 1990. Bates No. TIMN0378533/8543. Available at: http://www.tobaccoinstitute.com. Accessed April 20, 2001.

24. Stop Teenage Addiction to Tobacco. The 1990 STAT community organizers conference summary of participant evaluations, 1990. Bates No. TIMN0378545/8546. Available at: http://www.tobaccoinstitute.com. Accessed July 7, 2001.

25. Payne M. Proposed statement in response to query re: STAT boycott, August 30, 1990. Bates No. 507718775 -8775. Available at: http://www.rjrtdocs.com. Accessed April 20, 2001.

26. Stop Teenage Addiction to Tobacco. Letter to

Susan Heenan Piscitelli, thanking her for recent contribution to STAT, February 1, 1991. Bates No. 512003766 -3766. Available at: http://www.rjrtdocs.com. Accessed April 20, 2001.

27. Tye J. Letter to Samuel Chilcote, president, Tobacco Institute re: product placement in movies, February 14, 1991. Bates No. TIMN0373250. Available at: http://www.tobaccoinstitute.com. Accessed April 20, 2001.

28. Christie D. Letter to Brennan Dawson, vice president for public affairs, Tobacco Institute, March 6, 1991. Bates No. TIMN0373247. Available at: http://www.tobaccoinstitute.com. Accessed April 20, 2001.

29. Ogburn T Jr. Letter to Tom Griscom re: Tobacco Institute/PM meeting, March 7, 1991. Bates No. 507665665 -5669. Available at: http://www.rjrtdocs.com. Accessed April 20, 2001.

30. Rodota J. Status report on external environment: to Herb Osmon, March 19, 1991 Bates No. 507787073 -7076. Available at: http://www.rjrtdocs.com. Accessed April 20, 2001.

31. Rodota JD. Proposal for R.J. Reynolds Tobacco Company, July 15, 1991. Bates No. 507789428 -9430. Available at: http://www.rjrtdocs.com. Accessed August 13, 2001.

32. Meyne R. Anti-smokers database, April 2, 1991. Bates No. 507699824 -9824. Available at: http://www.rjrtdocs.com. Accessed April 20, 2001.

33. Provosty J. Memo to Sheila Consaul forwarded to other RJR personnel re: 1991 STAT conference, Fleishman Hillard, 1991. Bates No. 507783691 -3698. Available at: http://www.rjrtdocs.com. Accessed April 20, 2001.

34. Anonymous. Draft letter to the editor with marginalia. Bates No. 507721147 -1147. Available at: http://www.rjrtdocs.com. Accessed April 20, 2001.

35. Anonymous. Camel STAT response—public relations strategies, 1991. Bates No. 507721156 -1156. Available at: http://www.rjrtdocs.com. Accessed April 20, 2001.

36. Sutherland J. Note to Carol Hrycaj, Tobacco Institute, Fleishman Hillard, September 21, 1992. Bates No. TIMN0378708. Available at: http://www.tobaccoinstitute.com. Accessed April 27, 2001.

37. Carter P. Memo to Tom Griscom, Maura Payne, and others at RJR re: STAT, American Public Health and HHS/CDC meetings, November 13, 1992. Bates No. 512005259 -5260. Available at: http://www.rjrtdocs.com. Accessed April 27, 2001.

38. Stop Teenage Addiction to Tobacco. STAT-92 conference participant list. Bates No. TIMN0179253/9288. Available at: http://www.tobaccoinstitute.com. Accessed April 27, 2001.

39. Lancaster B. Memo to Carol Hrycaj, Tobacco Institute. Fleishman Hillard, December 2, 1992. Bates No. TIMN0179106/9107. Available at: http://www.tobaccoinstitute.com. Accessed April 27, 2001.

40. Sasso LA. Attached summary of lectures and workshops from STAT conference, December 17, 1992. Bates No. 519857020 -7046. Available at: http://www.rjrtdocs.com. Accessed April 27, 2001.

41. Poole J. Memorandum—4th annual STAT conference, November 15, 1993. Bates No. 2025381569/1587. Available at: http://www.pmdocs.com. Accessed April 27, 2001.

42. Anonymous. Overview: equally as productive as last year, October 3, 1993. Bates No. 512029252–9274. Available at: http://www.rjrtdocs.com. Accessed January 19, 2002.

43. Solberg E. STAT (Stop Teenage Addiction to Tobacco) conference, November 23, 1992. Bates No. 515847170 -7171. Available at: http://www.rjrtdocs.com. Accessed August 14, 2001.

44. INFACT. Infact: challenging corporate abuse, building grassroots power. Available at: http://www.infact.org. Accessed January 24, 2002.

45. Holt B. INFACT initial research: memo to Craig Fuller, June 29, 1993. Bates No. 2047904454. Available at: http://www.pmdocs.com. Accessed July 6, 2001.

46. Holt B. INFACT update to Craig Fuller, August 5, 1993. Bates No. 2047904452/4453. Available at: http://www.pmdocs.com. Accessed July 7, 2001.

47. Anonymous. INFACT—issues analysis, 1993. Bates No. 2047904455/4460. Available at: http://www.pmdocs.com. Accessed July 6, 2001.

48. Fuller C. Memo to distribution list, June 29, 1993. Bates No. 2047904502. Available at: http://www.pmdocs.com. Accessed July 2, 2001.

49. Anonymous. Unsigned intelligence report, September 1993. Bates No. 2047904440. Available at: http://www.pmdocs.com. Accessed July 7, 2001.

50. Holt B. Memo to Ellen Merlo and others re: Raviv presentation, March 1, 1994. Bates No. 2023437082. Available at: http://www.pmdocs.com. Accessed July 2, 2001.

51. Anonymous. Overview, 1994. Bates No. 2047904381/4399. Available at: http://www.pmdocs.com. Accessed July 2, 2001.

52. Raviv S, Perkins R. Memo to Barry Holt, April 11, 1994. Bates No. 2047904377/4377. Available at: http://www.pmdocs.com. Accessed August 2, 2001.

53. Raviv S, Perkins R. Memo to Barry Holt, April 12, 1994. Bates No. 2045994611/4612. Available at: http://www.pmdocs.com. Accessed July 2, 2001.

54. Dennis D. Annual meeting: update on INFACT activities, April 19, 1994. Bates No. 2046007917. Available at: http://www.pmdocs.com. Accessed July 2, 2001.

55. Dennis D. INFACT update, May 10, 1994. Bates No. 2047790195. Available at: http://www.pmdocs.com. Accessed July 2, 2001.

56. Ford P, Burke E. Critic to broaden boycott internationally, July 5, 1994. Bates No. 2046019692–9693. Available at: http://www.pmdocs.com. Accessed July 2, 2001.

57. Dennis D. INFACT planning meeting June 2, May 10, 1994. Bates No. 2023437010/7010. Available at: http://www.pmdocs.com. Accessed July 2, 2001.

58. Anonymous. Background briefing—consumer boycott, June 2, 1994. Bates No. 2046007849/7887. Available at: http://www.pmdocs.com. Accessed January 22, 2002.

59. Ford Y Jr. To our customers, April 28, 1994. Bates No. 513196537–6538. Available at: http://www.rjrtdocs.com. Accessed July 7, 2001.

60. Ford Y Jr. To our retail customers, May 2, 1994. Bates No. 513196516 -6517. Available at: http://www.rjrtdocs.com. Accessed July 7, 2001.

61. Ford P. Memo to Barry Holt and Darienne Dennis re: boycott presentation, August 4, 1994. Bates No. 2046019733/9755. Available at: http://www.pmdocs.com. Accessed July 2, 2001.

62. Philip Morris. Critic boycott: history and strategic recommendations, August 18, 1994. Bates No. 2046021034/1061. Available at: http://www.pmdocs.com. Accessed July 2, 2001.

63. Philip Morris. Discussion paper critic boycott: scenarios and proactive program, November 30, 1994. Bates No. 2045994659/4671. Available at: http://www.pmdocs.com. Accessed July 2, 2001.

64. Ford P, Burke E. Memo to Barry Holt re: critic unveils additional details of April events; seeks funds, April 4, 1995. Bates No. 2048240338. Available at: http://www.pmdocs.com. Accessed July 2, 2001.

65. Parrish S. Speech: goals for 2000, February 4, 1992. Bates No. 2024705949/5981. Available at: http://www.pmdocs.com. Accessed April 27, 2001.

66. Dennis D. Memo re: the critic, April 24, 1995. Bates No. 2054406112/6113. Available at: http://www.pmdocs.com. Accessed July 2, 2001.

67. Mulvihill M. To David Laufer, monthly report, Earl Palmer Brown, April 27, 1995. Bates No. 2044270323. Available at: http://www.pmdocs.com. Accessed July 2, 2001.

68. Ellis M. To Jim Johnston and Tom Griscom re: annual meeting attendees, April 10, 1995. Bates No. 520800981 -0981. Available at: http://www.rjrtdocs.com. Accessed July 2, 2001.

69. VanderBent T. Letter to Clarice Corell, donations manager, Working Assets, May 28, 1997. Bates No. 516930667 -0667. Available at: http://www.rjrtdocs.com. Accessed July 7, 2001.

70. INFACT. INFACT's tobacco industry campaign, 2001. Available at: http://www.infact.org/helpstop.html. Accessed August 25, 2001.

71. Stop Teenage Addiction to Tobacco. STAT Web page. Available at: http://www.stat.org. Accessed September 10, 2001.

72. Philip Morris Corporate Affairs Department. Corporate affairs 1994 budget presentation, October 21, 1993. Bates No. 2046847121/7137. Available at: http://www.pmdocs.com. Accessed April 27, 2001.

73. Meyer CR. Coverup: Philip Morris tries to polish its image. *Minn Med*. 2000;83(3):6.

74. R.J. Reynolds Tobacco Co. Anti-smoker database, October 17, 1990. Bates No. 507789259 -9284. Available at: http://www.rjrtdocs.com. Accessed April 20, 2001.

Independent Evaluation of the California Tobacco Control Program: Relationships Between Program Exposure and Outcomes, 1996–1998

Louise Ann Rohrbach, PhD, MPH, Beth Howard-Pitney, PhD, Jennifer B. Unger, PhD, Clyde W. Dent, PhD, Kim Ammann Howard, PhD, Tess Boley Cruz, PhD, MPH, Kurt M. Ribisl, PhD, Gregory J. Norman, PhD, Howard Fishbein, DrPH, and C. Anderson Johnson, PhD

Objectives. This study sought to determine the effects of the California Tobacco Control Program on tobacco-related attitudes and behaviors.

Methods. In 1996 and 1998, a telephone survey was conducted among adults in randomly selected households in 18 California counties. Tenth-grade youths in 84 randomly selected high schools completed a written survey. In analyses conducted at the county level, differences in outcomes were regressed on an index of program exposure.

Results. Among adults, program exposure was associated with decreased smoking prevalence rates, increased no-smoking policies in homes, and decreased violations of workplace no-smoking policies. Among youths, there was no effect of program exposure on outcomes.

Conclusions. These results suggest that the California Tobacco Control Program may have reduced adult smoking prevalence rates and exposure to environmental tobacco smoke. (*Am J Public Health.* 2002;92:975–983)

The California Tobacco Control Program (CTCP) was established in 1989, after the passage of a statewide referendum (Proposition 99) that increased the tax on tobacco products and earmarked the new revenues for tobacco control, medical care, and research activities. The program was the first of its kind in the United States, and it has stimulated other states to increase cigarette excise taxes[1–3] as well as serving as a model for those states that are developing programs funded by recent legal settlements with the tobacco industry.[4]

Annual funding for the CTCP has varied considerably over its 11-year history. With the exception of the 1990–1991 fiscal year, the California legislature underfunded the program from 1989 to 1996 by between 14% and 51% of the voters' funding mandate.[5] In 1997–1998, after civil lawsuits that challenged the state's redirection of funds for other purposes, the legislature restored program funding to its original level. However, total program funding declined again in the 1998–1999 and 1999–2000 fiscal years. Since its inception, per capita spending for the CTCP has ranged from $2.08 to $3.35, considerably below the $5.12 to $13.71 per capita range recommended by the Centers for Disease Control and Prevention for an effective statewide tobacco control program.[6]

The CTCP is a comprehensive program involving multiple, coordinated tobacco control strategies that aim to reduce tobacco use at the population level. Consistent with national trends in tobacco control,[7,8] the CTCP has evolved over time into a program approach focused on changing community norms regarding the acceptability of tobacco use.[9] The goal of the program is to alter the social–political environment in which tobacco initiation and cessation occur, and one of the primary mechanisms used to attain this goal is the passage and enforcement of local and statewide policies.

The specific strategies of the CTCP may be grouped into 3 program components. One component is the statewide media campaign, which disseminates anti-tobacco messages through television, radio, print media, and outdoor advertising. This program component is perhaps best known to public health professionals nationwide because of its hard-hitting ads designed to expose tobacco industry marketing tactics.[10,11] The second program component consists of local tobacco control initiatives, policy development, and public education programs implemented by county health departments and community-based organizations. The third component comprises school-based tobacco prevention programs, activities, and policies.

Since the inception of the CTCP, statewide surveillance of tobacco-related attitudes and behaviors among adults and adolescents has been used to evaluate program effectiveness.[12,13] The state has also sponsored 2 "independent evaluations" of the CTCP.[14–17] The first focused on process evaluation and assessed program inputs, such as the structure and staffing of programs, numbers and types of tobacco control activities, and characteristics of program participants, from 1990 to 1994.[15] The second independent evaluation, which we began in 1996, aims to determine the effectiveness of the CTCP by examining relationships between program inputs and exposure and program outcomes.[16,17]

Our evaluation differs from previous studies of the CTCP in 3 important respects. First, it has the capacity to link program implementation directly to changes in outcomes through the use of a repeated cross-sectional design in a sample of counties. Second, multiple, integrated data collection methods (e.g., surveys of in-school youths, adult residents, community program directors, school program personnel, enforcement agency staff, community opinion leaders) are used to measure program inputs, program exposure, and individual- and county-level outcomes. Third, the evaluation measures both intermediate outcomes—such as personal behaviors; public support for tobacco control strategies; and passage of restrictions on smoking, youth access, and tobacco industry promotions—and ultimate outcomes—such as smoking prevalence and exposure to environmental tobacco smoke.

Surveillance studies have indicated that the CTCP has been responsible for reductions in smoking prevalence and consumption beyond what would have been expected from a price increase alone.[12,13,18,19] During the early phase of the CTCP, smoking prevalence rates among adults decreased more rapidly than before the program began and more rapidly than for the United States overall. From 1993 to 1996, when funding allocations for the CTCP began to decrease, the rates of decline in adult smoking prevalence slowed. Among adolescents, the prevalence of 30-day smoking (i.e., having smoked on at least 1 day in the past 30 days) did not change in the early phase of the program; however, from 1993 to 1996, adolescent smoking prevalence rates increased.[13]

A comparison of smoking among youths in California relative to the rest of the United States, based on data from the Monitoring the Future study, suggested that the rate of increase in 30-day smoking from 1993 to 1996 was less dramatic in California.[16] Several econometric studies have shown the CTCP to be associated with a significant decline in per capita cigarette consumption, and the declines are attributable to both the cigarette tax increase and the tobacco control program.[18,19] Recently, the CTCP has been linked with declines in lung cancer incidence (during the period 1988 to 1997[20]) and heart disease mortality (during the period 1989 to 1997[21]).

To allow a more complete understanding of the effectiveness of comprehensive tobacco control programs, surveillance and econometric studies need to be supplemented by program evaluation studies that focus on measuring program implementation and strength, receipt of the program by the target population, intermediate outcome indicators, and tobacco industry efforts to counter program efforts.[22,23] The current study investigated the effectiveness of the CTCP by examining changes in program outcomes as a function of program exposure. In a representative sample of California counties, we assessed relationships between exposure to the media, community, or school tobacco control program components and changes in intermediate and ultimate outcomes among adults and youths from 1996 to 1998. On the basis of research suggesting that multicomponent prevention interventions (e.g., school-based programs supported by a media campaign) are more effective in reducing adolescent tobacco use than are single-component interventions (e.g., a school program alone),[24,25] we hypothesized that counties in which increased proportions of residents were exposed to multiple CTCP components would show enhanced program outcomes.

METHODS

Tobacco Control Program Intervention

The 3 primary CTCP components are designed to address the overall program objectives, which include (1) reducing exposure to environmental tobacco smoke, (2) countering pro-tobacco influences, (3) reducing youth access to tobacco products, and (4) promoting tobacco use cessation.[9] From January 1997 to June 1998, the media component included 40 media campaign spots that targeted the state's population overall (20 on television, 12 on radio, and 8 in outdoor locations). Of the total campaign expenditures during this period, 44% were allocated to spots that focused on reducing environmental tobacco smoke, 34% focused on countering pro-tobacco influences, 20% addressed smoking cessation, and 2% focused on reducing youth access.[26] Although the state also had media spots targeting ethnic-specific audiences, these spots were not the focus of our evaluation.

The community program component of the CTCP consists of a broad range of activities, implemented by county health departments and community-based organizations, that are designed to change community norms regarding tobacco use. From 1996 to 1998, efforts to counter pro-tobacco influences included activities such as mobilizing community support for policies designed to decrease tobacco advertising and sponsorship and conducting educational campaigns about the tobacco industry's manipulation of young people.

Efforts to reduce exposure to environmental tobacco smoke included activities such as expanding workplace policies to increase smoking restrictions and conducting campaigns to increase the number of families with personal policies restricting smoking in their homes and vehicles.[27,28] Efforts to reduce youth access to tobacco included activities such as creating local support for enforcement of laws to reduce illegal tobacco sales, educating tobacco retailers about youth access laws, and conducting educational campaigns to address social (i.e., nonretail) sources of tobacco. To facilitate tobacco use cessation, local programs provided cessation services and publicized the statewide cessation telephone counseling program.[29]

The school-based program component consists of school policies prohibiting tobacco use, classroom instruction focused on tobacco use prevention, schoolwide tobacco prevention events, and direct cessation services for smokers. During the 1996–1997 school year, the majority of high schools that received competitive tobacco use prevention grant funds provided tobacco use prevention lessons (84%) and on-site tobacco cessation services (92%). About half of these schools also implemented schoolwide activities such as Great American Smoke-Out events, tobacco prevention contests, and tobacco-specific assemblies. In 97% of school districts statewide, prevention activities were supported by policies prohibiting tobacco use by students, staff, and visitors.[30]

Study Design and Sample

This study focused on 2 waves of cross-sectional data from adult residents and 10th-grade youths in a sample of California counties.[16,17] Baseline measurement took place in October 1996 to February 1997, and the 18-month follow-up took place between March and July 1998. The conceptual framework for the evaluation measures has been described elsewhere.[16]

Counties. We chose counties as the primary sampling units for the study because the majority of funds for local tobacco control programs are awarded to county health departments. A cluster approach was used to select 18 counties that would be representative of the 58 counties in California. Because the statewide media campaign was one of the 3 program components to be evaluated, the 5 counties that overlap with the 5 largest media markets in the state were preselected. The cluster analysis was applied to the remaining 53 counties.

The analysis was designed to yield 3 strata based on county population density and rural area percentage. Thirteen counties were randomly selected from the 3 strata. The final sample included these 13 counties along with the 5 media market counties. Overall, these

18 counties represented approximately 75% of the population of California.

Adults. During each wave of data collection, approximately 388 adults in randomly selected households within each county were administered 20-minute computer-assisted telephone interviews. In the first wave, a randomly selected sample of 24 101 residential telephone numbers was contacted, and screening interviews were completed with 11 958 adults in those households (50% screening rate). As a means of achieving a random sample within the household, 1 of the screening questions identified the adult with the most recent birthday. Of those who completed screening interviews, 7127 were eligible to participate in the survey (60% eligibility rate). Eligibility was restricted to residents of the 18 counties who spoke English or Spanish, were 18 years or older, and had lived in the county for at least 6 months. Of the respondents who were eligible, 6985 completed the survey (98% completion rate).

In the second wave, in addition to the approximately 384 adults per county sampled, an oversample of 1218 Hispanic and African American households was included. A total of 26 682 randomly selected telephone numbers were contacted, and 15 573 screening interviews were conducted (58% screening rate). Of those screened, 8572 were eligible to complete the survey (55% eligible rate), and 8122 actually completed it (95% completion rate).

Youths. Within the 18 counties, a sample of high schools that had an enrollment of at least 100 students in grade 10 was randomly selected for participation in the study. Schools were sampled in 2 strata: (1) schools that had received a competitive Tobacco Use Prevention Education grant from the California Department of Education and (2) all other eligible high schools in the target counties. Of the schools selected for participation in either wave of data collection, 35% declined participation and were replaced. A total of 65 and 79 high schools, respectively, participated in the first and second waves, with 60 of these schools participating in both waves.

Within each school, approximately 5 classes of 10th-grade students enrolled in a required discipline, such as English or social studies, were randomly selected to participate in the survey. All students in the selected classes were eligible to participate. An implied parental consent procedure was used in which students were assumed to have parental consent if their parents did not return a signed form declining the youth's permission to participate. Students were free to decline participation if they so chose. In the first and second waves, only 1% and 3% of parents declined participation, respectively. In both waves, 99% of students whose parents provided consent chose to participate. The mean rate of absentees in both waves was 13.7%. The final samples included 6911 and 8186 grade 10 youths in the first and second waves, respectively.

Adult data collectors trained by the research staff administered the anonymous, 50-minute surveys during regular classroom periods. In each of the 2 waves, 95% of students completed the survey within the allotted period of time.

Measures

We addressed 2 ultimate program outcomes and a subset of intermediate outcomes that were selected a priori to represent the primary objectives of the program. Because most of the CTCP strategies target cigarette use, the outcome measures focused on cigarette smoking rather than other forms of tobacco use. Most of the survey items were based on previous surveillance studies.[5,31] Items with continuous scales that had nonnormal distributions were recoded into dichotomous variables.

Ultimate outcomes. Among adults, *cigarette smoking prevalence* was defined as the proportion of adults within the county who had smoked at least 100 cigarettes in their lifetimes and who now reported smoking "every day" or "some days"; among 10th-grade youths, it was defined as the proportion who had smoked on at least 1 day during the past 30 days. *Exposure to environmental tobacco smoke* was measured with 2 items. For adults, the items assessed the number of days in the previous week that respondents had been exposed to tobacco smoke in their homes and, if applicable, at work. Because the consent procedure for the study precluded asking any questions about the home environment, the items for youths assessed exposure to tobacco smoke in an indoor area and a car. All responses were recoded into 2 categories: 0 days vs 1 or more days.

Intermediate outcomes. Intermediate outcomes assessed included *reductions in environmental tobacco smoke exposure, countering of pro-tobacco influences,* and *reductions in youth access to tobacco.* In regard to reducing exposure to environmental tobacco smoke, perceived violations of workplace smoking policies were examined by asking adults how many smokers in their workplace break the no-smoking rules (0=none, 5=all). This item was recoded as having seen no smokers vs any smokers break the rules. Also, adult respondents were asked about personal policies regarding smoking in their home ("Can family and visitors smoke wherever they want or in certain rooms only or not smoke anywhere in your home?") and their family cars ("Is smoking never allowed in any car or allowed sometimes in some cars or there are no rules about smoking in your car?"). These items were recoded as total ban vs any smoking allowed.

In the countering pro-tobacco influences category, adults were asked how many items with a tobacco company brand name or logo they owned (0=none, 1=at least 1). Adults' support for advertising bans was assessed with a composite index that averaged responses to 3 items regarding whether tobacco advertising should be banned in stores, on billboards, and on buses and whether tobacco company sponsorship of sport and community events should be disallowed (1=strongly disagree, 4=strongly agree; Cronbach α=0.85). Youths' negative attitudes toward the tobacco industry were measured with a composite index that averaged 3 items regarding whether tobacco companies try to get people addicted to cigarettes, try to get young people to start smoking by using advertisements that are attractive to youths, and would keep selling cigarettes even if they knew for sure that smoking is harmful (1=strongly disagree, 4=strongly agree; Cronbach α=0.51).

Youths' perceptions of access to tobacco were measured with a single item asking how easy or difficult it would be for them to obtain cigarettes if they really wanted some (recoded as very or somewhat easy vs very or somewhat hard). In regard to other intermediate outcomes among youths, youths were classified as susceptible to smoking if they gave a response other than "definitely not" to one or both of the following questions: "If one of your best friends were to offer you a cigarette, would you smoke it?" and "At any time during the next year, do you think you will smoke a cigarette?" Also, youths' estimates of smoking prevalence among peers were measured with a single item: "Out of 100 students your age, about how many smoke cigarettes once a month or more?" (0=none, 10=about 100). Responses were multiplied by 100 to obtain a percentage estimate.

To assess the reliability of our outcome measures, we reinterviewed 7% of the second-wave adult telephone interview respondents (n=600) 2 to 4 weeks after they had completed the initial interview. The mean κ coefficient for the dichotomous outcome variables was 0.71; the mean intraclass correlation for the continuous variables was 0.63.

Program exposure. Adult and youth respondents were asked a series of questions about their awareness of and exposure to the media and community components of the CTCP; youths were also asked about their exposure to the school component. The question format was based on previous studies of exposure to pro- and anti-tobacco media campaigns.[32–39] Adults were asked whether they recalled seeing or hearing 6 of the CTCP media spots (e.g., "Have you seen the television commercial in which a woman named Debi is smoking through a hole in her throat?") and were aware of 12 community-based tobacco control activities during the year before the 1998 survey (e.g., "Have you heard of local efforts to reduce tobacco company sponsorship of community and sporting events?").

Youths were asked similar questions about 7 media spots and 12 community-based activities, as well as whether they had participated in 4 school-based tobacco prevention activities (e.g., lessons, special events). Recall of media spots was prompted by brief descriptions of the spots and validated with an additional question about their meaning. Among adults, the mean test–retest κ coefficient for the media and community program exposure items was 0.46.

A composite program exposure index was created as follows. For each program component (media, community, and schools), respondents received a score of 0 if they recalled none of the specific activities or spots and a score of 1 if they recalled at least 1 activity, media spot, or local initiative. Scores for the program components were summed, resulting in scores ranging from 0 to 2 for adults and 0 to 3 for youths. Next, these individual scores were aggregated to create county means. The county-level multicomponent exposure score represented the proportion of respondents who were exposed to the CTCP through 2 or more different program components.

Data Analysis

Adult survey data were first weighted to account for the number of adults and telephone lines in a given household. In the second step, weights were applied to match the target population parameters obtained from Claritas, an online database of current census estimates.[40] Within each of 12 regions of the state, distributions were weighted according to ethnicity, sex, and age.

TABLE 1—Independent Evaluation of the California Tobacco Control Program: Demographic Characteristics of Adult and Youth Samples, 1996 and 1998

	1996		1998	
	No.	Weighted %	No.	Weighted %
Adult sample				
Sex				
Female	4054	50.4	4509	50.7
Male	2931	49.6	3613	49.3
Race/ethnicity				
White non-Hispanic	5065	61.3	4866	55.8
Hispanic	1071	25.0	1770	28.4
African American	294	5.5	667	5.5
Asian/Pacific Islander	308	5.9	441	7.7
Native American	127	1.7	106	0.8
Other	60	0.6	174	1.8
Education				
Less than 12th grade	639	12.1	779	11.5
High school	1727	23.9	1898	23.6
Some college	2050	27.3	2508	29.8
College or more	2535	36.7	2883	35.0
Age, y				
18–24	783	13.2	968	13.8
25–34	1503	21.5	1702	20.0
35–44	1672	23.4	1925	22.2
45–54	1260	16.2	1498	18.0
55–64	771	12.7	856	12.5
≥65	905	13.0	1068	13.4
Youth sample				
Sex				
Female	3406	46.9	4016	47.4
Male	3505	53.0	4170	52.6
Race/ethnicity				
White non-Hispanic	2676	27.2	3406	32.6
Hispanic	1533	31.4	1800	27.7
African American	339	12.4	477	13.4
Asian/Pacific Islander	1110	13.5	1234	12.5
Multiethnic	863	12.3	975	12.4
Other	317	3.2	134	1.4

Note. Sample sizes are for raw data. Percentages represent weighted population estimates.

Weights for the youth data were based on school enrollment data obtained from the California Department of Education.[41] Each student was given a school weight based on the total number of 10th-grade students enrolled at that school. To create a final weight, we aggregated school weights to the enrollment counts. All final youth survey weights were divided by the average weight of the data set to obtain relative weights equating the weighted sample sizes to the actual sample sizes.

Each cross section of adult and youth data was weighted on the basis of population estimates from the same year the data were collected. Table 1 presents unweighted sample sizes and weighted percentages of demographic characteristics for the adult and youth samples in 1996 and 1998. We used SUDAAN, a software package that accounted for the complex sampling design and weighting factors in the data sets, to calculate the standard errors of the prevalence estimates.[42]

Analyses of relationships between program exposure and changes in outcomes were conducted at the county level, because the data were longitudinal at that level (i.e., the 2 waves of data collection consisted of 2 different random samples of individuals in the same 18 counties). This county-level analysis strategy also eliminated the effects of intraclass correlation on the standard errors of the regression coefficients. All weighted variables were aggregated to the county level through computation of weighted means for adult and youth respondents in each county. To assess changes in the outcome variables, each county's baseline mean was subtracted from its follow-up mean to create a difference score. These outcome difference scores then were regressed on the program exposure variable via SAS PROC GLM.[43]

The regression models, which we ran separately for adult and youth respondents, included no covariates. In some models, 1 of the counties was found to be an outlier. To eliminate the influence of this outlier, the county was represented as an additional dummy variable and allowed to enter the regression model through a forward selection process after the program exposure variable had been forced into the model. If the dummy variable for the county was significantly associated with the outcome variable at $P<.05$, we partialed out its effect before evaluating the regression coefficient for program exposure.[44]

RESULTS

In 1998, most Californians reported that they had been exposed to tobacco control messages during the previous year through at least 2 different program components (Table 2). Among adults, 80% were exposed to both media and community programs. Among 10th-grade youths, 55% were exposed to all 3 components (community, media, and schools), and 31% were exposed to 2 of the components.

Among adults, none of the 1996 to 1998 changes in outcome variables was significant (Table 3). Among 10th graders, there were significant decreases in prevalence rates of 30-day cigarette smoking and indoor environmental tobacco smoke exposure ($Ps<.05$).

Linear regression models at the county level showed that multicomponent exposure

TABLE 2—California Tobacco Control Program Exposure Among Adults and 10th-Grade Youths, 1998

Type of Program Component	Adults (n = 8122), %	Youths (n = 8186), %
None	2	4
Community only	16	2
Media only	2	6
School only	. . .	2
Community and media	80	22
Media and school	. . .	6
Community and school	. . .	3
School, community, and media	. . .	55

TABLE 3—California Tobacco Control Program Outcomes Among Adults and 10th-Grade Youths, 1996 and 1998

Outcome	1996 Estimate	1996 95% CI	1998 Estimate	1998 95% CI
Adults[a]				
Ultimate				
Cigarette smoking, %	17.7	16.1, 19.3	19.3	17.8, 20.8
ETS exposure, home, %	23.8	21.4, 26.6	22.5	20.0, 24.0
ETS exposure, work, %	28.4	25.4, 30.6	26.5	24.0, 28.0
Intermediate				
Have home smoking ban, %	75.7	73.8, 78.1	78.5	76.6, 79.7
Have car smoking ban, %	65.5	63.9, 68.1	66.9	65.2, 68.6
Have seen workers break no-smoking rule, %	26.3	23.3, 28.7	24.2	21.8, 26.2
Own tobacco promotional item, %	19.1	17.3, 20.7	19.5	17.1, 21.9
Support for advertising ban, mean[b]	2.76	2.73, 2.79	2.79	2.76, 2.82
Youths[c]				
Ultimate				
30-day cigarette smoking, %	27.4	23.6, 31.2	21.8	20.3, 23.3*
ETS exposure, indoors, %	65.9	62.3, 69.5	58.2	55.6, 60.8*
ETS exposure, car, %	44.5	40.5, 48.5	38.7	36.1, 41.3
Intermediate				
Susceptibility to smoking, %	59.0	55.1, 62.9	54.2	52.0, 56.4
Easy perceived access to cigarettes, %	89.1	86.4, 91.8	87.0	85.6, 88.4
Perceived peer smoking prevalence, %	50.6	48.5, 52.6	49.5	48.2, 50.8
Negative attitudes toward tobacco industry, mean[b]	3.37	3.28, 3.45	3.50	3.46, 3.54

Note. CI = confidence interval; ETS = environmental tobacco smoke.
[a]1996, n = 6985; 1998, n = 8122.
[b]On a 4-point scale.
[c]1996, n = 6911; 1998, n = 8186.
*$P<.05$

TABLE 4—Independent Evaluation of the California Tobacco Control Program: County-Level Analysis of Effects of Multicomponent Program Exposure on Changes in Outcomes Among Adults and 10th-Grade Youths, 1996 to 1998

	Standard β	P
Adults		
Ultimate outcomes		
Cigarette smoking	-0.634	.03
ETS exposure, home	-0.537	.13
ETS exposure, work	-0.165	.51
Intermediate outcomes		
Have home smoking ban	0.678	.04
Have car smoking ban	0.415	.25
Have seen workers break no-smoking rule	-0.703	.04
Own tobacco promotional item	-0.155	.62
Support for tobacco advertising ban	0.124	.63
Youths		
Ultimate outcomes		
Cigarette smoking	-0.024	.93
ETS exposure, indoors	-0.222	.44
ETS exposure, car	-0.355	.20
Intermediate outcomes		
Susceptibility to smoking	-0.141	.53
Easy perceived access to cigarettes	0.109	.67
Perceived peer smoking prevalence	-0.312	.21
Negative attitudes toward tobacco industry	0.218	.41

Note. ETS = environmental tocacco smoke.

was significantly associated with reductions in the prevalence of adult cigarette smoking, increases in home smoking bans, and reductions in perceived violations of workplace no-smoking rules (*P*s<.05; Table 4). Figure 1 demonstrates these effects graphically, dividing the sample of counties into tertiles based on levels of multicomponent exposure. Counties with the highest multicomponent exposure rates had the greatest reductions in adult smoking prevalence, the largest increases in home smoking bans, and the greatest reductions in workplace no-smoking policy violations. None of the changes in outcomes among youths was associated with multicomponent exposure (Table 4).

DISCUSSION

The results of this study indicate that exposure to the CTCP was associated with reductions in adult cigarette smoking prevalence rates from 1996 to 1998. These findings are consistent with those of previous studies that have shown correlations between trends in adult smoking prevalence and per capita cigarette consumption and fluctuations in CTCP funding, providing rough approximations of program impact.[5,12,13,18,19] Program evaluation studies conducted in Massachusetts and Oregon have also shown an association between implementation of a statewide tobacco control program and declines in adult smoking prevalence rates.[3,45–47]

We also found a significant relationship between program exposure and increases in the prevalence of no-smoking policies in homes, as well as a moderate, nonsignificant relationship between program exposure and decreased environmental tobacco smoke exposure in homes. Counties with higher levels of program exposure showed fewer perceived no-smoking policy violations in workplaces than did counties with less program exposure. These results suggest that the strongest effects of the CTCP may be related to the program objective of reducing the public's exposure to environmental tobacco smoke. California has been a leader in enacting strong, comprehensive state laws designed to reduce residents' exposure to environmental tobacco smoke in a variety of settings. Statewide and locally, efforts to reduce exposure, including promoting and enforcing state laws and encouraging voluntary adoption of smoke-free home and car policies, have been sustained over a longer period than have efforts related to the other CTCP objectives.

We found no evidence of an effect of program exposure on tobacco control outcomes among youths. Although there were significant decreases in prevalence rates of 30-day smoking and environmental tobacco smoke exposure among 10th-grade youths from 1996 to 1998, these changes were not associated with program exposure. These findings are consistent with results of surveillance studies in California, which have suggested that the tobacco control program has not brought about reductions in smoking prevalence rates among adolescents.[13]

In their review of the literature on comprehensive tobacco control programs, Wakefield and Chaloupka[23] suggested that the range of coordinated program strategies used in California, including school-based programs, a mass media campaign, enforcement of policies that restrict smoking in public places and youth access to tobacco, enactment and enforcement of policies restricting tobacco promotion and sponsorship, and price increases, ultimately will lead to reductions in teenage smoking. However, they speculated that a program approach such as California's, which focuses on environmental change through policy enactment, support, and enforcement, may require more time to affect adolescent smoking rates than to affect adult rates. These approaches aim to change social norms about smoking; as such, they affect youths more indirectly than directly. Thus, we may see reductions in smoking among California youths in the future, as the environmental approaches slowly bring about changes in social norms. On the other hand, reductions in adolescent smoking may be unlikely as long as tobacco industry advertising and promotional campaigns in the state continue to be strong.[13,48]

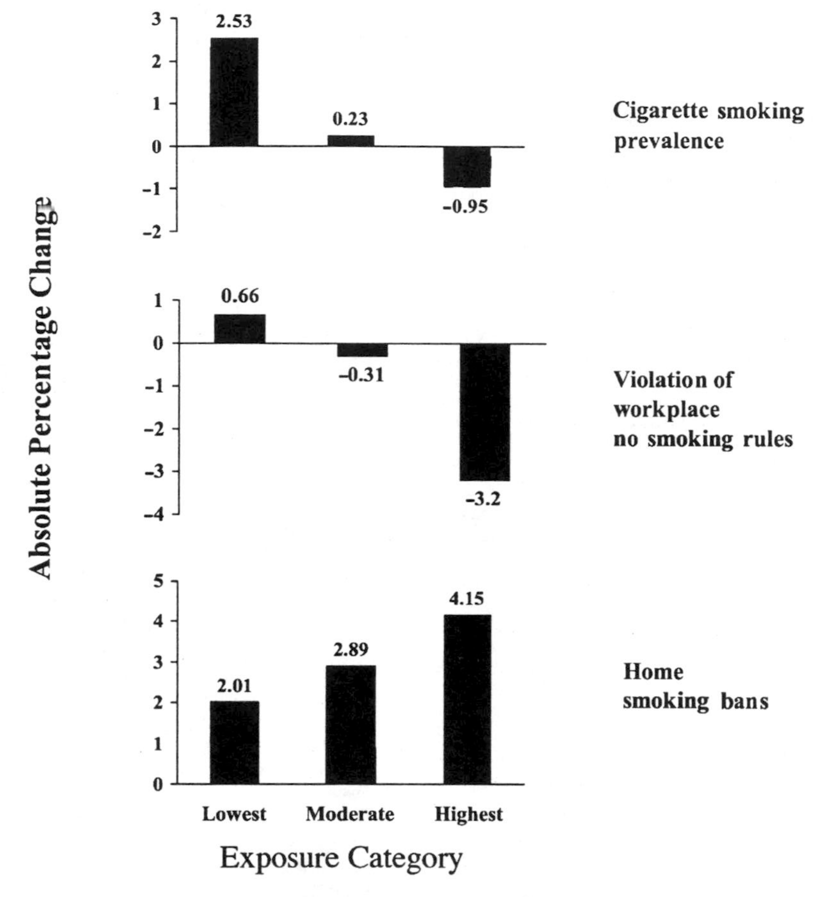

FIGURE 1—Changes in adult outcomes, by county-level multicomponent program exposure: California Tobacco Control Program, 1996–1998.

The conventional wisdom in the field of tobacco control is that comprehensive programs, involving a range of coordinated and complementary tobacco control strategies, are most effective in reducing tobacco use.[7,49,50] In our study, we investigated whether exposure to multiple tobacco control program components had a larger impact on outcomes than did exposure to only 1 component or to no components. In regard to tobacco control outcomes among adults, we found stronger effects in counties in which higher proportions of adults were exposed to multiple program components. These results provide support for a multifaceted approach to tobacco control such as that implemented in California.

The primary strengths of our study were its use of a repeated cross-sectional design in which changes in outcomes were examined in a representative sample of California counties and its ability to link program exposure to changes in outcomes for both adults and youths in these counties. Although the magnitude of the changes we were able to link with program exposure was small, these changes may have considerable significance for public health. For example, a decline of 1% in adult smoking prevalence in the counties with the highest program exposure represents about 70000 fewer smokers in the state.

Several limitations of the study should be noted. First, because we did not conduct a randomized controlled trial, the study was limited in the extent to which changes in program outcomes could be attributed to programmatic efforts. Examining changes as a function of exposure is an approach to investigating tobacco control program effectiveness that should be used cautiously, in conjunction with examination of time-series data and comparisons of outcomes with those of other states.[51] Second, although the field has great interest in determining the components of a comprehensive tobacco control program that are most effective, our evaluation was designed to determine whether exposure to a combination of tobacco control program components was more effective than exposure to a single component rather than to determine, for example, whether the media campaign was more effective than community or school programs.

Third, our program exposure measure assessed recall, not actual exposure to program activities. Although previous studies have shown dramatic increases in recall of anti-tobacco messages after mass media campaigns,[38,39] there is a need for more research on the validity of self-reported exposure to anti-tobacco campaigns. An alternative approach might be to measure program inputs and to relate the degree of program implementation to changes in outcomes. We used measures of program recall because they were available for all program components, whereas county-level program input measures were not. Fourth, using counties as the units of analysis for relationships between program exposure and outcomes provided only modest statistical power to detect small program effects. However, our calculations showed, for example, that with 18 counties and statistical power of .80%, the minimal detectable effects in outcomes among youths ranged from 0.66 to 2.78 prevalence points for every 1% change in the program exposure measure.

A fifth limitation of our study is that we tested multiple nonindependent hypotheses regarding associations between program exposure and outcomes without adjusting significance values. However, these hypotheses were developed a priori for both youths and adults, and they were conceptually related to one another. Finally, this evaluation was not funded until 8 years after initiation of the CTCP. Ideally, the evaluation would have been designed, and the baseline data collected, before program implementation. Surveillance data have shown that the most rapid changes in outcomes occurred in the early years of the program.[5] It is difficult to observe significant changes in outcomes in the middle of a program's history. The baseline for this evaluation assessed CTCP activities that occurred during 1995–1996, the lowest point in funding allocations for the program since its inception. Because this period was followed by a doubling in budget allocations for the program (by fiscal year 1997–1998), we might expect to observe greater changes in outcomes in future evaluations of the program.

CONCLUSIONS

This evaluation represents the first study of the CTCP to quantitatively link program exposure to changes in outcomes. We found significant associations between exposure to multiple program components and reductions in adult smoking prevalence rates, decreases in violations of workplace no-smoking rules, and increases in presence of personal policies prohibiting smoking in family homes. Although no effects of program exposure on youth outcomes were observed, the results suggest that the CTCP may be changing social norms about the acceptability of tobacco use and exposure to environmental tobacco smoke. Future research should examine the consistency between these findings and trends in state and national surveillance data. ■

About the Authors

Louise Ann Rohrbach, Jennifer B. Unger, Clyde W. Dent, Tess Boley Cruz, and C. Anderson Johnson are with the Institute for Health Promotion and Disease Prevention Research, Department of Preventive Medicine, University of Southern California, Los Angeles. Beth Howard-Pitney and Kim Ammann Howard are with the Stanford Center for Research in Disease Prevention, Stanford University School of Medicine, Stanford, Calif. Kurt M. Ribisl is with the School of Public Health, University of North Carolina at Chapel Hill. Gregory J. Norman is with the San Diego State University Foundation, San Diego, Calif. Howard Fishbein is with the Gallup Organization, Washington, DC.

Requests for reprints should be sent to Louise Ann Rohrbach, PhD, MPH, Institute for Health Promotion and Disease Prevention Research, University of Southern California, 1000 S Fremont Ave, Unit #8, Alhambra, CA 91803 (e-mail: rohrbac@hsc.usc.edu).

This article was accepted December 23, 2001.

Note. The analyses, interpretations, and conclusions presented in this article are those of the authors, not of the California Department of Health Services.

Contributors

L.A. Rohrbach was the scientific director of the study. L.A. Rohrbach, B. Howard-Pitney, C. Dent, K.A. Howard, T.B. Cruz, H. Fishbein, and C.A. Johnson designed the study. L.A. Rohrbach, B. Howard-Pitney, and H. Fishbein supervised the data collection. L.A. Rohrbach, B. Howard-Pitney, J.B. Unger, C.W. Dent, K.A. Howard, T.B. Cruz, K.M. Ribisl, and G.J. Norman contributed to the data analytic strategy and interpretation of the data. J.B. Unger and G.J. Norman conducted the data analyses. L.A. Rohrbach wrote the article, with contributions from B. Howard-Pitney, J.B. Unger, K.A. Howard, T.B. Cruz, and K.M. Ribisl.

Acknowledgments

This study was conducted by the Independent Evaluation Consortium, which consists of a team of investigators from the Gallup Organization, Stanford University, and the University of Southern California. The study was made possible by funds received from the Tobacco Tax Health Protection Act of 1988, under contract 97-105546 with the California Department of Health Services, Tobacco Control Section, and the California Tobacco-Related Disease Research Program (grant 9RT-0107).

We wish to thank June Flora, PhD, and Todd Rogers, PhD, for their contributions to the study design.

References

1. Connolly G, Robbins H. Designing an effective statewide tobacco control program—Massachusetts. *Cancer.* 1998;83(suppl 12):2722–2727.

2. Meister JS. Designing an effective statewide tobacco control program—Arizona. *Cancer.* 1998; 83(suppl 12):2728–2732.

3. Pizacani B, Mosbaek C, Hedberg K, et al. Decline in cigarette consumption following implementation of a comprehensive tobacco prevention and education program—Oregon, 1996–1998. *MMWR Morb Mortal Wkly Rep.* 1999;48:140–143.

4. Bauer U, Johnson T, Pallentino J, Hopkins R., Brooks RG. Tobacco use among middle and high school students—Florida, 1998 and 1999. *MMWR Morb Mortal Wkly Rep.* 1999;48:248–253.

5. Pierce JP, Gilpin EA, Emery SL, White MM, Rosbrook B, Berry CC. Has the California Tobacco Control Program reduced smoking? *JAMA.* 1998;280: 893–899.

6. *Best Practices for Comprehensive Tobacco Control Programs—August 1999.* Atlanta, Ga: Centers for Disease Control and Prevention; 1999.

7. Shopland DR. Smoking control in the 1990s: a National Cancer Institute model for change. *Am J Public Health.* 1993;83:1208–1210.

8. Manley M, Lynn W, Epps R, Grande D, Glynn T, Shopland D. The American Stop Smoking Intervention Study for cancer prevention: an overview. *Tob Control.* 1997;6(suppl 2):S5–S11.

9. Bal DG. Designing an effective statewide tobacco control program—California. *Cancer.* 1998;83(suppl 12): 2717–2721.

10. Stevens C. Designing an effective counteradvertising campaign—California. *Cancer.* 1998;83(suppl 12): 2736–2741.

11. Balbach ED, Glantz SA. Tobacco control advocates must demand high-quality media campaigns: the California experience. *Tob Control.* 1998;7:397–408.

12. Pierce JP, Evans N, Farkas AJ, et al. *Tobacco Use in California: An Evaluation of the Tobacco Control Program, 1989–1993.* La Jolla, Calif: University of California, San Diego; 1994.

13. Pierce JP, Gilpin EA, Emory SL, et al. *Tobacco Control in California: Who's Winning the War? An Evaluation of the Tobacco Control Program, 1989–1996.* La Jolla, Calif: University of California, San Diego; 1998.

14. Russell CM. Evaluation: methods and strategy for evaluation—California. *Cancer.* 1998;83(suppl 12): 2755–2759.

15. Elder JP, Edwards CC, Conway TL, Kenney E, Johnson CA, Bennett ED. Independent evaluation of the California Tobacco Education Program. *Public Health Rep.* 1996;111:353–358.

16. Independent Evaluation Consortium. *Final Report of the Independent Evaluation of the California Tobacco Prevention and Education Program: Wave I Data, 1996–1997.* Rockville, Md: Gallup Organization; 1998.

17. Independent Evaluation Consortium. *Interim Report. Independent Evaluation of the California Tobacco Prevention and Education Program: Wave 2 Data, 1998; Wave 1 and Wave 2 Data Comparisons, 1996–1998.* Rockville, Md: Gallup Organization; 2001.

18. Hu TW, Sung H, Keeler TE. Reducing cigarette consumption in California: tobacco taxes vs an anti-smoking media campaign. *Am J Public Health.* 1995; 85:1218–1222.

19. Hu TW, Sung H, Keeler TE. The state anti-smoking campaign and the industry response: the effects of advertising on cigarette consumption in California. *Am Econ Assoc Papers Proc.* 1995;85:85–90.

20. Centers for Disease Control and Prevention. Declines in lung cancer rates—California, 1988–1997. *MMWR Morb Mortal Wkly Rep.* 2000;49:1066–1069.

21. Fichtenberg CM, Glantz SA. Association of the California Tobacco Control Program with declines in cigarette consumption and mortality from heart disease. *N Engl J Med.* 2000;343:1772–1777.

22. Stillman F, Hartman A, Graubard B, et al. The American Stop Smoking Intervention Study: conceptual framework and evaluation design. *Eval Rev.* 1999;23: 259–280.

23. Wakefield M, Chaloupka F. Effectiveness of comprehensive tobacco control programmes in reducing teenage smoking in the USA. *Tob Control.* 2000;9: 177–186.

24. Tobler NS, Stratton HH. Effectiveness of school-based drug prevention programs: a meta-analysis of the research. *J Primary Prev.* 1997;18:71–127.

25. Worden JK, Flynn BS, Solomon LJ, Secker-Walker RH, Badger GJ, Carpenter JH. Using mass media to prevent cigarette smoking among adolescent girls. *Health Educ Q.* 1996;23:453–468.

26. Cruz TB, Flora J, Unger J, et al. The statewide media campaign. In: Independent Evaluation Consortium. *Interim Report. Independent Evaluation of the California Tobacco Prevention and Education Program: Wave 2 Data, 1998; Wave 1 and Wave 2 Data Comparisons, 1996–1998.* Rockville, Md: Gallup Organization; 2001:83–97.

27. Norman GJ, Ribisl KM, Howard-Pitney B, Howard

KA, Unger JB. The relationship between home smoking bans and exposure to state tobacco control programs and smoking behaviors. *Am J Health Promotion.* 2000;15:81–88.

28. Norman GJ, Ribisl KM, Howard-Pitney B, Howard KA. Smoking bans in the home and car: do those who really need them, have them? *Prev Med.* 1999;29:581–589.

29. Howard-Pitney B, Howard KA, Ribisl KM, Norman GJ. Local tobacco control programs. In: Independent Evaluation Consortium. *Interim Report. Independent Evaluation of the California Tobacco Prevention and Education Program: Wave 2 Data, 1998; Wave 1 and Wave 2 Data Comparisons, 1996–1998.* Rockville, Md: Gallup Organization; 2001:47–82.

30. Rohrbach LA, Skara S, Unger J, Dent C. School-based tobacco use prevention program. In: Independent Evaluation Consortium. *Interim Report. Independent Evaluation of the California Tobacco Prevention and Education Program: Wave 2 Data, 1998; Wave 1 and Wave 2 Data Comparisons, 1996–1998.* Rockville, Md: Gallup Organization; 2001:98–112.

31. Centers for Disease Control and Prevention. Youth risk behavior surveillance—United States, 1999. *MMWR Morb Mortal Wkly Rep.* 2000;49(SS-5):1–95.

32. Botvin GH, Goldberg CH, Botvin EM, Dusenbury L. Smoking behavior of adolescents exposed to cigarette advertising. *Public Health Rep.* 1993;108:217–224.

33. Schooler C, Feighery E, Flora J. Seventh graders' self-reported exposure to cigarette marketing and its relationship to their smoking behavior. *Am J Public Health.* 1996;86:1216–1221.

34. Sargent JD, Dalton M, Beach M. Exposure to cigarette promotions and smoking uptake in adolescents: evidence of a dose-response relation. *Tob Control.* 2000;9:163–168.

35. Biener L, Siegel M. Tobacco marketing and adolescent smoking: more support for a causal inference. *Am J Public Health.* 2000;90:407–411.

36. Pierce JP, Choi WS, Gilpin EA, Farkas AJ, Berry CC. Tobacco industry promotion of cigarettes and adolescent smoking. *JAMA.* 1998;279:511–515.

37. Aitken PP, Leathar DS, O'Hagan FJ, Squaire SI. Children's awareness of advertisements for cigarettes and brand imagery. *Br J Addict.* 1987;82:15–22.

38. Murray DM, Perry CL, Griffin G, et al. Results from a statewide approach to adolescent tobacco use prevention. *Prev Med.* 1992;21:449–472.

39. Murray DM, Prokhorov AV, Harty KC. Effects of a statewide antismoking campaign on mass media messages and smoking beliefs. *Prev Med.* 1994;23:54–60.

40. Claritas. Claritas update, 1998. Available at: http://www.claritas.com. Accessed September 30, 1998.

41. California Department of Education. California Board of Education data set, 1998. Available at: http://www.cde.ca.gov/demographics/files. Accessed September 16, 1998.

42. Shah BV, Barnwell BG, Bieler GS. *SUDAAN User's Manual, Release 7.5.* Research Triangle Park, NC: Research Triangle Institute; 1997.

43. *SAS/STAT User's Guide, Version 6, 4th ed.* Cary, NC: SAS Institute Inc; 1992.

44. Fox J. *Applied Regression Analysis, Linear Models, and Related Methods.* Beverly Hills, Calif: Sage Publications; 1997.

45. Siegel M, Biener L. The impact of an antismoking media campaign on progression to established smoking: results of a longitudinal youth study. *Am J Public Health.* 2000;90:380–386.

46. Harris JE, Connolly GN, Brooks D, Davis B. Cigarette smoking before and after an excise tax increase and an anti-smoking campaign—Massachusetts, 1990–1996. *MMWR Morb Mortal Wkly Rep.* 1996;45:966–970.

47. Rohde K, Pizacani B, Stark M, et al. Effectiveness of school-based programs as a component of a statewide tobacco control initiative—Oregon, 1999–2000. *MMWR Morb Mortal Wkly Rep.* 2001;50:663–666.

48. Cruz TB, Feighery E, Unger J, et al. The tobacco marketing environment in California. In: Independent Evaluation Consortium. *Interim Report. Independent Evaluation of the California Tobacco Prevention and Education Program: Wave 2 Data, 1998; Wave 1 and Wave 2 Data Comparisons, 1996–1998.* Rockville, Md: Gallup Organization; 2001:23–46.

49. Institute of Medicine. *State Programs Can Reduce Tobacco Use.* Washington, DC: National Cancer Policy Board, National Academy of Sciences; 2000.

50. Glynn TJ. Comprehensive approaches to tobacco use control. *Br J Addict.* 1991;86:631–635.

51. Siegel M, Biener L. Evaluating the impact of statewide anti-tobacco campaigns: the Massachusetts and California tobacco control programs. *J Soc Issues.* 1997;53:147–168.

Evaluating the Tobacco Settlement Damage Awards: Too Much or Not Enough?

Maribeth Coller, PhD, Glenn W. Harrison, PhD, and Melayne Morgan McInnes, PhD

Objectives. This study compared the present economic value of the 1998 tobacco settlement with the present economic value of the damages attributable to tobacco.

Methods. The 1987 National Medical Expenditure Survey was used to estimate the smoking attributable fraction (SAF) of medical expenditures. SAFs were then applied to Medicaid and other expenditures.

Results. Settlement payments covered only 40% of Medicaid treatment costs already incurred and only 30% of past and projected future Medicaid costs. Excess medical expenditures for all other payment sources were roughly comparable to those incurred by Medicaid.

Conclusions. Although the settlement may reduce future smoking prevalence rates by limiting the ability of tobacco companies to promote smoking and by raising cigarette prices, euphoria over the huge settlement funds should be balanced by a sober comparison with the even larger damage amounts. (*Am J Public Health.* 2002;92:984–989)

The recent wave of litigation brought by state attorneys general against tobacco companies resulted in a landmark settlement agreement in late 1998 for excess expenditures under Medicaid and other state and local health plans. The Master Settlement Agreement represents the largest financial recovery in the nation's history and is potentially one of the most significant public health interventions in decades. It includes graduated annual payments made in perpetuity, totaling $196 billion through the year 2025. These payments are guaranteed in that the terms of the agreement are legally enforceable. If any settling company undergoes bankruptcy, the remaining companies will be responsible for the bankrupt company's share of the payments.

These settlement amounts exclude $10 billion of other payments made by tobacco companies, as well as roughly $40 billion to be paid to Mississippi, Florida, Texas, and Minnesota. Attorneys' fees, not included in these amounts, will easily run into the tens of billions. Thus, the sum of the payments exceeds $250 billion.

This seems like a huge amount, and it is. But before one declares victory in this battle of the tobacco war, perspective is urgently needed. We consider 3 dimensions of the settlement from the perspective of plaintiff damages experts involved in individual state cases. (Glenn W. Harrison served as an expert and calculated damages for the cases brought by 13 states, while Maribeth Coller used these calculations to determine damages in terms of current dollars for the cases brought by 5 states. Harrison also serves as a damages expert in the case brought by 22 BlueCross BlueShield plans in federal court in New York, and both serve as damages experts for 2 HMOs in Minnesota.)

First, we illustrate the computation of the damages that the settlement is intended to compensate. Second, we compare the settlement amounts with these damages. Finally, we show that comparable damages have been incurred in terms of medical expenditures by private citizens, private insurance companies, worker's compensation, and Medicare. The legalities of collecting damages in each of these cases are complex, and many cases have been summarily dismissed by the courts. Without forming any judgment on the legal issues, we calculate the damages attributable to smoking in all of these cases.

The analysis involved 3 significant features. First, consistent with recent studies,[1–5] damages were not restricted to diseases known to be caused by smoking. Our estimates allowed for the possibility that smoking may cause the treatment costs to be higher for any given medical condition, even if smoking did not cause the condition that led to the medical intervention. Second, we took into account the effects of passive smoking by considering the current smoking status of all members of each dwelling unit.

Finally, we estimated a separate model for children that also measured the effects of the biological parents' smoking. Children constitute a substantial fraction of all Medicaid expenditures, and there are well-known clinical links between the smoking history of mothers and fathers and illness in their children. The only other damages calculation in the Medicaid litigation to include excess health expenditures for children was provided by Jeffrey Harris in the Florida case, and it was restricted to damages from specific respiratory conditions.[6]

METHODS

The discussion to follow illustrates the computation of excess Medicaid expenditures. Excess expenditures for other payer sources were determined in a similar manner. The objective was to determine how much more Medicaid spends on smokers than on nonsmokers after taking into account other differences in these populations. First, we used the National Medical Expenditure Survey (NMES) to estimate a model that allowed us to determine the effects of tobacco use on Medicaid expenditures.

Second, the smoking attributable fraction (SAF) of expenditures was calculated for each individual as follows: SAF=(EXPS−EXPNS)/EXPS, where EXPS is the predicted level of Medicaid expenditures for an individual, given his or her actual smoking history, and EXPNS is the predicted level of Medicaid expenditures if smoking were nonexistent. By equation construction, the SAF for a nonsmoker is zero. Finally, SAFs were applied to annual Medicaid expenditures to obtain the dollar amount of these expenditures attributable to smoking. Such "excess" expenditures constituted the damages that were the focus of the litigation.

We estimated the SAF with data from the NMES undertaken by the US Department of Health and Human Services in 1987, the most recent version of this survey for which complete results were available at the time damages reports were prepared for litigation. The Medical Expenditure Panel Survey of 1996 is now available, but the 1987 NMES represented a better choice for our purpose because it was completed in the middle of the period under consideration (1965–2008).

One advantage of our econometric approach, which is now widely used in the public health literature,[1–3,5,7] is that it directly estimates the SAF for medical expenditures rather than inferring it from an SAF for mortality or an SAF for utilization. Another advantage is that it makes no a priori judgments as to which medical conditions involve expenditures that are attributable to smoking, effectively "letting the data speak." Earlier traditions, such as the mortality risk approach, relied entirely on the best available clinical and epidemiological evidence that linked smoking causally to specific medical conditions, such as cancers and respiratory problems. More recent evidence points to a much broader medical impact of smoking.[8]

The expected levels of expenditures used to calculate the SAF represented the product of 2 terms: the probability that an expenditure will occur and the level of expenditure if it does occur. Decomposing the expected levels of expenditures into these 2 components allows for the possibility that various characteristics have different effects on the probability of incurring an expenditure than they do on the level of expenditure once it occurs. Similar 2-equation "hurdle" specifications[9–11] are common in the health economics literature.

In our specification, the first component is determined via a regression equation relating the probability of positive Medicaid expenditures to various individual characteristics. All Medicaid-eligible individuals in the NMES are included in the estimation of this equation, after deletion of some observations owing to missing values. The second component is determined via a regression equation relating the dollar amount of expenditures to individual characteristics, conditional on the individual's incurring positive Medicaid expenditures in 1987. Details of the estimation procedure, data set, and regression results are provided in an appendix available at http://dmsweb.moore.sc.edu/glenn/tobacco/ajph.htm.

Measures of Smoking Intensity

Eight measures of smoking were included among the individual characteristics used in the regressions. Smokers were identified as those who reported having smoked 100 or more cigarettes in their lives, and the model included number of years smoked, past smoking intensity, whether the individual currently smoked, and current smoking intensity. Smoking intensity was measured via typical number of cigarettes smoked per day. In the case of all variables in the regressions that were not dichotomous, we included squared values to capture possible nonlinear effects.

Other Explanatory Variables

We also included variables adjusting for factors other than smoking that might cause the health expenditures of smokers and nonsmokers to differ. Measures of income, education, risk attitude, and health status were included to control for differences in health care use not due to smoking. Measures of health status and risk attitude included body mass index and indicator variables for the following: medical treatment for drug use, medical treatment for alcohol use, pregnancy, regular exercise, regular seat belt use, and consideration of oneself as above average in terms of risk taking. Other variables included age, sex, race, census region, and indicators of whether the individual was married, employed, a veteran, a homeowner, a resident of an inner city, a resident of a suburb, or an English speaker. Measures of income and education were also included.

Passive Smoking

A notable feature of the NMES is that it provides information on all members of each family covered, as well as information on all members of each dwelling unit. Hence, we were able to identify the current smoking activities of everyone in the dwelling unit and thus to attribute some of the expenditures of other individuals living in that dwelling unit to the "passive" effects of smoking.

Children and Teenagers

Separate equations were estimated for adults 18 years or older and for children and teenagers up to the age of 13 years. For the latter, current and past smoking intensity of the biological father and mother were included in addition to the measures of passive smoking just described. Because the NMES contains no information on the smoking behavior of individuals younger than 18 years, we were unable to capture the possible effects of these individuals' smoking on Medicaid expenditures. The SAF for youths aged 14 to 17 years was assumed to be zero. This assumption created a conservative bias in estimated SAF values for children and teenagers. To allow for the possible confounding effect of alcohol abuse among mothers, we included a binary indicator for mothers who were receiving treatment associated with alcohol abuse. Because of smaller sample sizes, we used all medical expenditures rather than simply Medicaid expenditures when estimating the model for children.

Simulating the Absence of Smoking

Given the estimates from the 2 terms described earlier, one involving the probability that an expenditure will occur and the other involving the level of the expenditure if it occurs, we estimated the SAF for each individual in the NMES. To estimate EXPS, the expected level of Medicaid expenditures given the observed smoking history of the individual and all other individuals whose smoking affects expenditures, we used the estimated regression coefficients and the observed smoking history of everyone in the sample. To estimate EXPNS, the expected level of Medicaid expenditures in the absence of smoking, we assumed that all individuals had never smoked and did not currently smoke. By setting all smoking variables to zero, we were able to predict the probability of an expenditure's being incurred as well as the expected expenditure (conditional on expenditures being positive) for each individual had there been no history of smoking.

Disease-Specific Calculations

Earlier studies estimating smoking-attributable expenditures often restricted attention to specific diseases or conditions.[12]

Our broader approach, examining all expenditures viewed as being attributable to smoking, was made possible by the availability of the NMES database. Inclusion of these expenditures was appropriate, because smokers may have higher treatment costs for conditions not caused by smoking. For example, if smoking generates a degree of heightened surgical risk owing to the increased probability of anesthesia complications, then any smoker who undergoes surgery could have higher costs as a result of smoking.

It is possible to determine which damages arise from the disease-specific pathway (smoking causes the disease, which causes the medical intervention, which in turn causes the extra medical cost) and which damages arise from other pathways (smoking causes greater medical care use or cost, even if it did not cause the original medical intervention). We illustrate this breakdown, which played an important role in the litigation by explicitly linking the medical testimony on causality and liability to the testimony on economic damages.

Because the NMES includes codes from the *International Classification of Diseases, Ninth Revision (ICD-9)*, it was possible to identify expenditures by disease code. We were then able to modify the damages calculation to estimate a *smoking-disease-specific SAF* by including only those expenditures for diseases that could be viewed as directly attributable to smoking, relying on the best epidemiological and clinical evidence. We chose these categories of diseases and *ICD-9* codes on the basis of the advice of medical experts who were to testify in the trial taking place in Hawaii. Among adults, these diseases included certain cancers, cardiovascular and cerebrovascular disease, certain respiratory conditions, ulcers, and pregnancy complications; among children and teenagers, the diseases included were limited to asthma, ear infections, and respiratory infections.

RESULTS

Applying the SAF

The SAF was calculated for each Medicaid recipient in the NMES database. The weighted average adult SAF was then calculated for the sample, and the expected levels of Medicaid expenditures given the observed smoking history of the individual were the weights. Similarly, the SAF for children and teenagers was the weighted average of the individual SAFs for all children and teenagers in the sample.

Finally, we obtained a weighted SAF for Medicaid by averaging the SAF for adults with the SAF for children and teenagers and then weighting the result by their respective expenditure shares in the NMES. The adult SAF for Medicaid was 16.3%, and the SAF for children and teenagers was 1.7%. Because the adult share of Medicaid expenditures was 85%, the resulting overall weighted SAF for Medicaid was 14.1%. To estimate annual smoking-attributable Medicaid expenditures in dollars, we then multiplied the SAF by total annual Medicaid expenditures reported by the Health Care Financing Authority.

To illustrate the magnitude of disease-specific expenditures relative to general medical expenditures, we turn to 1 particular state for which these more detailed computations were finalized before the Master Settlement Agreement. The smoking-disease-specific SAF in Hawaii for those patients whose claims were paid by Medicaid was estimated to be 27%, higher than the overall SAF for Hawaii. This result was expected, given that we restricted attention to disease codes for which we had strong a priori beliefs that smoking was a causal factor.

When we applied the smoking-disease-specific SAF to the Medicaid expenditures of Hawaii associated with the identified *ICD-9* codes, we found that disease-specific damages constituted 65% of overall smoking-attributable Medicaid expenditures.[13] Thus, approximately one third of the overall smoking-attributable Medicaid expenditures in Hawaii can be viewed as due to increased treatment costs of conditions not caused by smoking.

Table 1 shows annual smoking-attributable expenditures by Medicaid and by other state and local plans that were covered in the settlement agreement. In terms of historical dollars, the total damages ranged from a low of $0.7 billion in 1965 to a high of $34.8 billion in 1998.

Our results can be compared with those of 2 published studies. Miller et al.[3] provided state-level estimates for Medicaid. Although they used the same NMES database used here, their statistical model was different in many respects. For example, it contained more "structural" detail on the processes that lead an individual to seek Medicaid medical care. Also, the model of Miller et al. estimated the effects of smoking on expenditures, controlling for self-reported health status but taking into account the fact that poor health status may be due to smoking, by using a 4-equation specification. This structural approach provided a useful counterpart to the "reduced form" approaches employed in most other studies, including ours. For the year 1993, Miller et al. calculated a national Medicaid SAF of 14.4% for adults, a value close to the 16.3% we calculated.

Cutler et al.[4] used the National Health Interview Survey, and a different methodology, to estimate a Medicaid SAF of 5.6% for Massachusetts. They used a 2-stage regression model for adult utilization and employed nonregression methods to ascertain extra utilization due to low-birthweight babies and nursing home admissions. Their statistical analysis focused on the calculation of a utilization SAF estimating the additional inpatient days, but not the additional treatment costs per day, attributable to smoking. This utilization SAF was then used as a proxy for an expenditure SAF. With the exception of the increased utilization associated with low-birthweight infants, they did not include children in their analyses. They also used a disease-specific approach in their analysis of nursing home utilization.

Aggregate Damages

To evaluate whether the settlement amounts were adequate, we converted all calculated damage amounts to 1998 dollars. We compounded historical damages by using the opportunity cost of the funds to the responsible party.[14,15] This rate is the weighted average borrowing rate on corporate bonds of the firms named in the settlement. The final column of Table 1 shows the effects of compounding at the rates applicable to each year.

In addition to past damages, the states also relinquished their right to sue in the future for damages associated with tobacco products. To evaluate the settlement in terms of

TABLE 1—Past Damages in Historical and Current Dollars (Billions)

Year	State and Federal Medicaid (Historical $)	Other State and Local Plans (Historical $)	Damages Covered in Suits: All Medicaid and State–Local	
			Historical $	1998 $
1965	0.0	0.7	0.7	9.5
1966	0.2	0.7	0.9	11.7
1967	0.4	0.7	1.1	13.8
1968	0.5	0.8	1.3	14.6
1969	0.6	0.8	1.4	16.2
1970	0.8	1.0	1.7	17.5
1971	1.0	1.0	2.0	18.5
1972	1.2	1.1	2.2	21.9
1973	1.3	1.2	2.6	21.5
1974	1.6	1.4	3.0	27.1
1975	1.9	1.6	3.5	25.4
1976	2.2	1.7	3.8	23.6
1977	2.5	1.9	4.4	22.4
1978	2.8	2.2	4.9	25.3
1979	3.2	2.5	5.7	30.0
1980	3.7	2.8	6.5	36.3
1981	4.3	3.2	7.5	54.1
1982	4.5	3.5	8.1	58.5
1983	5.0	3.7	8.7	38.6
1984	5.4	3.9	9.3	45.3
1985	5.8	4.3	10.2	34.4
1986	6.4	5.0	11.5	29.2
1987	7.1	5.6	12.8	31.9
1988	7.8	6.1	13.9	33.4
1989	8.8	6.8	15.6	35.5
1990	10.7	7.5	18.1	38.9
1991	13.3	7.9	21.1	39.3
1992	15.0	8.4	23.5	37.8
1993	17.2	8.7	25.9	38.8
1994	19.0	9.2	28.2	39.2
1995	20.7	9.3	29.9	37.3
1996	21.8	9.5	31.3	36.4
1997	22.6	10.1	32.7	35.2
1998	24.1	10.7	34.8	34.8
Total	243	146	389	1033

the damages, it is thus necessary to consider future medical costs. In fact, the damages calculations prepared for the trials in virtually all states included an allowance for future excess health expenditures to be incurred to treat smoking-related illnesses due to past smoking behavior.

Admittedly, quantification of future costs is relatively difficult, because future smoking prevalence is unknown. However, if we assume a continuation of historical trends in smoking and medical expenditures for 10 years into the future (with excess costs set to zero after 10 years), which was the assumption used in much of the litigation, we can estimate future costs with enough precision to evaluate the terms of the Master Settlement Agreement. Because the payments for the settlement of these future costs are guaranteed, we used the US Treasury bill rate in converting values to 1998 dollars.

Once we converted past damages (over the 1965–1998 period) to 1998 dollars and converted future damages (over the 1999–2008 period) to 1998 dollars, we summed these amounts to determine aggregate damages. This calculation yielded past damages of $1033 billion and future damages of $371 billion. Total estimated damages, in terms of 1998 dollars, were $1404 billion.

Comparison of Damages With the Settlement

Before comparing the terms of the settlement with the damages, we take into account 2 adjustment factors that will affect the stream of future payments. The settlement payments will be adjusted upward to reflect inflation but will be adjusted downward if cigarette sales fall. Beginning with payments made in 2000, the Master Settlement Agreement stipulated that all future payments would be adjusted upward annually to reflect inflation. This adjustment will be determined via the change in the consumer price index relative to the January 1999 level. If this change is less than 3% in any year, 3% will be used as the adjustment factor.

The Master Settlement Agreement also includes a provision for future payments to be adjusted to reflect the aggregate number of cigarettes shipped in the United States, with volume changes measured relative to 1997 levels. This provision specifies that payments will increase by 1% for each percentage point increase in volume and decrease by 0.98% for each percentage point decline in volume. Given the new marketing and advertising restrictions placed on the industry, as well as the increase in antismoking campaigns and recent increases in cigarette prices, it is likely that the volume adjustments will result in decreased future payments.

To estimate the present value of the settlement, we made 3 conservative assumptions. First, we assumed that the volume of cigarette sales would remain constant, so that there would be no downward adjustment in payments. Second, we assumed that inflation would be, on average, 3% and adjusted each year's payment upward by 3%. Finally, we used a low real discount rate of 2%. This brought the present value of all payments (including the "up front" payments due in 1998 and in 2000 through 2003, along with the annual payments beginning on April 15, 2000) to $417 billion.

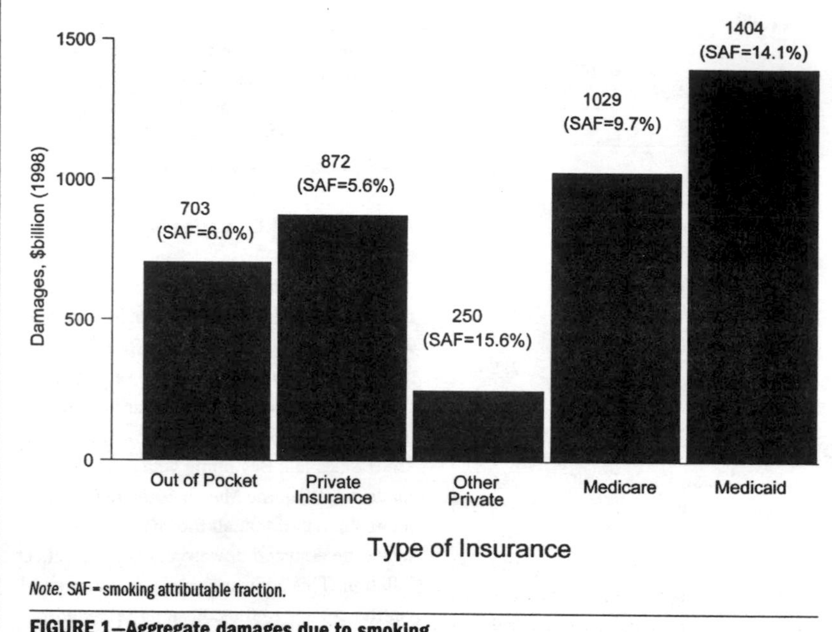

Note. SAF = smoking attributable fraction.

FIGURE 1—Aggregate damages due to smoking.

Although the dollar amount of the settlement appears staggering, one should bear in mind that it represents only 40% of past damages and 30% of total damages. Moreover, if the prevalence of smoking continues to decline, the percentage of total damages recovered will be even lower. For example, if we assume that smoking declines, such that the volume of cigarettes shipped is 5% less in 2000 than in 1997, and then further decreases by 1% for each of the next 20 years, the present value of the settlement, with a 2% real discount rate, is reduced to $332 billion, or just 24% of total damages.

Damages Beyond Medicaid

The same statistical methodology can be applied to calculate an SAF applicable to non-Medicaid medical expenditures. Figure 1 shows the SAFs and aggregate damages for each category of expenditure in billions of 1998 dollars. The Medicare SAF is 9.7%, close to the SAF of 9.4% estimated by Zhang et al.[16] for Medicare expenditures in 1993. It is apparent that although Medicaid accounts for about one half of total damages, the other categories are substantial. None have been settled as yet; indeed, there is much debate over the liability of tobacco manufacturers for these costs.

Economic theory suggests that the damages should include only the external costs of smoking: the costs that are imposed on others involuntarily. Some have argued that smokers should be assumed to have understood and accepted all of the health risks of smoking and are therefore responsible for any private health care costs they incur. Under this theory, Medicaid and Medicare damages are recoverable, but some or all of the excess expenditures of private individuals and private insurers may not be. Whether smokers tacitly understood and accepted the risk is something we cannot determine here. Rather, we present damage estimates with the recognition that determination of liability remains an open issue of fact and law.

Overall, we found that 8.3% of total US expenditures on medical care are attributable to smoking. In a review of the literature, Warner et al.[17] concluded that the estimates of 6.5% and 14.4% provided by Miller et al.[1,2] are plausible lower and upper bounds for the national SAF. If we consider only adult expenditures, our national SAF estimate of 9.0% falls in the middle of this range. Moreover, even though we used a lower SAF than did Miller et al.,[2] we included expenditures for nonadults, and thus our estimate of total US medical expenditures attributable to smoking in 1993 is very close to theirs ($74.5 billion vs $71.8 billion).

DISCUSSION

We developed our estimates of the excess medical expenditures due to smoking by using the most comprehensive data available. We included expenditures for diseases caused directly by smoking as well as other differences in treatment expenditures that are increased as a result of smoking. Furthermore, we included the effects of passive smoking and conducted separate analyses for adults and nonadults. We therefore view these estimates as reflecting good medical science as well as good statistical methods. Our methods yielded a final damage estimate of $1404 billion in 1998 dollars. When one compares this estimate with the present value of the settlement payments, it is apparent that the settlement did not achieve reimbursement for these expenditures.

Several other costs and benefits not calculated here should also be noted. First, 2 offsets are often mentioned: excise taxes on cigarettes and the so-called "death benefit" (cost savings that accrue to Medicaid, and especially Medicare, for smokers who die young).[18,19] In the case of Medicaid, it has been argued that savings on nursing home expenditures may offset some of the increased health costs of smokers. The death benefit offset was considered by many of the judges in the state Medicaid cases; most of those judges had decided that it could not be presented at trial. Hence, including this offset would not be appropriate when evaluating settlement amounts in proportion to the damage amounts that the defendants could claim in court.

Furthermore, damage calculations undertaken for litigation purposes need not necessarily include all factors that might be included in cost–benefit analyses undertaken for policymaking purposes. Although excise taxes and possible death benefits may be relevant to determining the overall effects tobacco has on society, the lawsuits were brought not by "society as a whole" but by specified legal entities. For example, it could be argued that the death benefit primarily saves federal expenditures under Medicare and pension payments.[19] For this reason, these savings should not be considered to offset the damages incurred by other entities.

Second, no attempt has been made to factor in the devastating psychosocial costs of reduced life spans and increased morbidity borne by smokers and their families, although such costs would probably dwarf the damages reported here. The question of whether smokers knowingly assumed risk continues to be a key point of contention in this litigation. The costs just described are appropriately considered in punitive damage awards, along with a factual determination of whether the plaintiff class assumed some share of the risk.

Although the settlement represents only a partial recovery of the damages from past smoking, it is a landmark victory against the tobacco industry and regarded by many as a favorable settlement in light of the risk and expense inherent in litigating separate suits in each state. It is also important to note that the Master Settlement Agreement includes significant restrictions on the marketing and advertising efforts of the tobacco companies. Such restrictions, including prohibitions on marketing aimed at youth smokers, use of cartoon characters in advertising, and payments by tobacco companies to have products placed in movies or television shows, would probably not have been implemented had the courts ruled on these cases, because they would violate the tobacco industry's rights to free (commercial) speech.

In addition, outdoor advertising and brand sponsorship of events have been severely restricted. The various restrictions carried differing phase-in dates, but all were effective on or before July 1, 1999. Although these elements of the Master Settlement Agreement do nothing to compensate the states for the costs they have already incurred in treating smoking-related illnesses, they should help to reduce smoking prevalence rates and thus medical expenditures due to smoking in the future. To the extent that future damages are reduced as a result of these restrictions, the settlement may be viewed as more favorable than indicated by our evaluation based on payments relative to damages.

However, the possibility of reduced smoking prevalence rates is a double-edged sword in terms of the settlement. The reduction in smoking is good news from a public health standpoint, but it further reduces the extent to which the states will be compensated for the medical costs they have incurred (and will incur) as a result of past smoking. Because of the volume adjustments included in the settlement, as cigarette sales fall, so will the dollars received in the future.

In complex litigation, it is common for settlements to represent "cents on the dollar." Is the tobacco settlement, which we calculate to be 30 cents on the dollar, a good settlement? The answer to this question depends on how we proceed from this point. The extent of future damages is, in large measure, in the hands of public heath officials, who can use settlement funds to attempt to reduce prevalence rates and hence future damages. States are free to impose excise taxes of their own that seek to cover future costs. For that matter, they could also use excise taxes on future smoking to cover some of the uncompensated costs of past excess Medicaid expenditures.

The main conclusion from our analysis is that the medical and public health communities need to understand what the tobacco settlement represents before victory is declared in the Medicaid settlement. We need to realize that the past costs of tobacco have not yet been reimbursed in the United States, that future costs are not reimbursed at all, and that huge settlement sums or excise taxes must be viewed in relation to the even larger damages to be correctly evaluated. We must be diligent in pressing for such an understanding as future lawsuits arise and settlements are agreed upon. ■

About the Authors

The authors are with the Moore School of Business, University of South Carolina, Columbia.

Requests for reprints should be sent to Glenn W. Harrison, PhD, Department of Economics, Moore School of Business, University of South Carolina, Columbia, SC 29208 (e-mail: harrison@moore.badm.sc.edu).

This article was accepted June 7, 2001.

Contributors

M. Coller conducted the present value analyses of the damages and the settlement. G.W. Harrison conducted the damages analyses on which the article was based. M.M. McInnes integrated the various aspects of the analysis. All of the authors contributed to the writing of the article.

References

1. Miller VP, James CR, Ernst C, Collin F. Smoking-attributable medical care costs: models and results. Available at: http://dmsweb.moore.sc.edu/tobacco/vmiller.pdf. Accessed April 1, 2002.

2. Miller LS, Zhang X, Rice DP, Max W. State estimates of total medical expenditures attributable to cigarette smoking, 1993. *Public Health Rep.* 1998;113:140–151.

3. Miller LS, Zhang X, Novotny T, Rice DP, Max W. State estimates of Medicaid expenditures attributable to cigarette smoking, fiscal year 1993. *Public Health Rep.* 1998;113:447–458.

4. Cutler DM, Epstein AM, Frank RG, et al. *How Good a Deal Was the Tobacco Settlement? Assessing Payments to Massachusetts.* Cambridge, Mass: National Bureau of Economic Research; 2000. Working paper 7747.

5. Miller VP, Ernst C, Collin F. Smoking-attributable medical care costs in the USA. *Soc Sci Med.* 1999;48:375–391.

6. Harris JE. Estimates of smoking-attributable Medicaid expenditures in Florida. Available at: http://dmsweb.moore.sc.edu/tobacco/FloridaEstimates.pdf. Accessed August 17, 1997.

7. Bartlett JC, Miller LS, Rice DP, Max W. Medical care expenditures attributable to cigarette smoking: United States, 1993. *MMWR Morb Mortal Wkly Rep.* 1994;43:469–472.

8. American Council on Science and Health. *Cigarettes: What the Warning Label Doesn't Tell You.* Amherst, NY: Prometheus Books; 1997.

9. Greene WH. *Econometric Analysis.* 3rd ed. Upper Saddle River, NJ: Prentice Hall; 1997.

10. Cragg J. Some statistical models for limited dependent variables with application to the demand for durable goods. *Econometrica.* 1971;39:829–844.

11. Melenberg D, van Soest A. Parametric and semiparametric modeling of vacation expenditures. *J Appl Econometrics.* 1996;11:59–76.

12. Centers for Disease Control and Prevention. Medical-care expenditures attributable to cigarette smoking during pregnancy—United States, 1995. *JAMA.* 1997;278:2058–2059.

13. Harrison GW. Tobacco damages to the state of Hawaii. Available at: http://dmsweb.moore.sc.edu/tobacco/hireport.pdf. Accessed April 1, 2002.

14. Coller M, Harrison GW. Time value and the expert witness: guidance from the tobacco litigation. *J Forensic Accounting.* 2001;2:145–160.

15. Pattel JM, Weill RL, Wolfson MA. Accumulating damages in litigation: the roles of uncertainty and interest rates. *J Legal Studies.* June 1982:341–364.

16. Zhang X, Miller L, Max W, Rice DP. Cost of smoking to the Medicare program, 1993. *Health Care Financ Rev.* 1999;20:179–196.

17. Warner KE, Hodgson TA, Carroll CE. Medical costs of smoking in the United States: estimates, their validity, and their implications. *Tob Control.* 1999;9:290–300.

18. Viscusi WK. The government composition of the insurance cost of smoking. *J Law Economics.* 1999;62:575–609.

19. Manning WG, Keeler EB, Newhouse JP, Sloss EM, Wasserman J. The taxes of sin: do smokers and drinkers pay their way? *JAMA.* 1989;261:1604–1609.

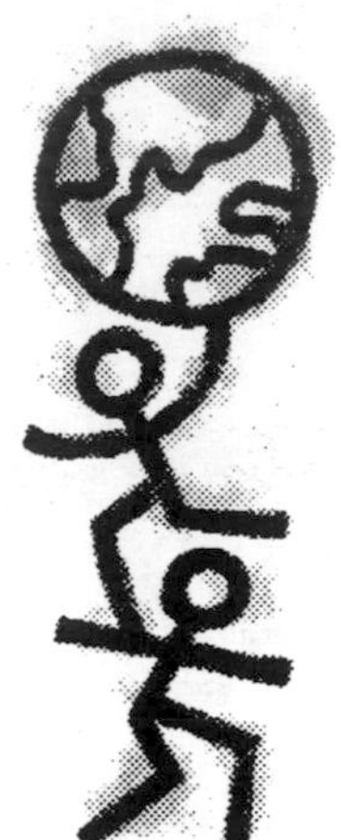

Tobacco: The Limits of Child Protection

Is Smoking Delayed Smoking Averted?

| Sherry Glied, PhD

Antismoking efforts often target teenagers in the hope of producing a new generation of never smokers. Teenagers are more responsive to tobacco taxes than are adults.

The author summarizes recent evidence suggesting that delaying smoking initiation among teenagers through higher taxes does not generate proportionate reductions in prevalence rates through adulthood. In consequence, the impact of taxes on smoking among youths overstates the potential long-term public health effects of this tobacco control strategy. (*Am J Public Health.* 2003;93:412–416)

CONTEMPORARY TOBACCO control policy has concentrated its fire on reducing smoking initiation among teenagers. According to Donna Shalala, former secretary of health and human services, the rhetoric used to justify measures designed to control adolescent smoking emphasizes that, "among children living in America today, 5 million will die an early preventable death because of a decision made as a child."[1] This focus is operationalized in the terms of the 1998 master settlement agreement between the state attorneys general and the tobacco industry; many of the agreement's clauses concern restrictions on tobacco advertising, promotion, and sales to young people. The focus is similarly reflected in the close attention tobacco use analysts pay to changes in annual data on patterns of cigarette smoking among youths.

Educating young people and helping them to make rational decisions in regard to smoking is sound and appropriate public policy. Yet, from a public health perspective, the harms of cigarette smoking are—with the important exception of the effects of smoking during pregnancy on fetal health[2]—only distantly connected to the smoking behavior of teens. Most of the health effects of smoking occur later in life, after years of exposure. Quitting can reverse many of the ill health consequences of earlier smoking.[3] Thus, the main purpose of programs designed to reduce smoking among teens is instrumental: to reduce smoking among adults.

The public health logic of concern over youth smoking is primarily that reducing youth smoking is the best way to reduce smoking overall. The principal conclusion of the 1994 surgeon general's report on smoking was that "[n]early all first use of tobacco occurs before high school graduation; this finding suggests that if adolescents can be kept tobacco free, most will never start using tobacco."[4(p543)]

While quitting smoking is very difficult, focusing on teens may, as Elders et al.[4] have suggested, produce a new generation of never smokers. Antismoking efforts focused on teenagers may be not only more politically saleable, but also more effective, than broader efforts. Teenagers are more susceptible than are adults to a range of inducements toward curbing smoking. For example, they respond more strongly to tobacco taxes. The price elasticity of demand for smoking—the standard measure of responsiveness to taxation—is 2 to 3 times as high among teenagers as it is among adults.[5,6]

Similarly, marketing analysts believe that teens are more responsive to advertising because their tastes have not yet been fully formed. As David Verklin, CEO of Cara International (a media buyer), stated recently in a National Public Radio report, younger buyers "haven't made all their brand choices . . . and if you could reach them and get them to be users of your brand at an early age, you'll have them for a lifetime." For this reason, a 30-second commercial on *The Late Show with David Letterman* produces 38% more revenue than a similar commercial on *Nightline*, although the *Nightline* audience is only 4 years older, and about 10% larger, than Letterman's audience. The literature on responsiveness thus suggests that targeting teen smokers will generate a larger reduction in smoking for a given cost than targeting adults.

Reducing smoking among teens is a necessary condition for a program aimed at young people to have an effect on adult smoking rates. But it may not be a sufficient condition. The smoking rate among adults in the United States is lower than the corresponding rate among youths.[7,8] Many factors intervene between youth and adulthood in terms of the decision to smoke. A complete evaluation of the effects of antismoking efforts cannot assume that delaying smoking initiation among teenagers will generate persistent reductions in prevalence through adulthood.

The effects of programs designed to reduce smoking among

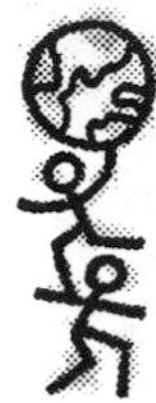

youths may remain constant, intensify, or diminish over time. Programs that discourage smoking may educate even those who do begin smoking. As these smokers grow older, such programs may increase later quit rates. Or it may be that tobacco control programs are most effective among those who are most susceptible to long-term addiction.

If late initiators find quitting easier (as some evidence suggests), programs that delay smoking may also increase quitting behavior.[9] In these cases, the program's effects intensify over time. Alternatively, adults who were discouraged from smoking by a program may change their minds as their incomes increase or they join new peer communities. In such cases, the program's effects diminish over time.

LONG-TERM EFFECTS OF CIGARETTE TAXES

Evaluations of programs designed to reduce smoking among teens generally examine effects on teenage smoking rates. To examine the long-term consequences of teen smoking reduction programs, however, analysts need to follow people over time. Two recent studies involved this type of design, assessing the long-term effects of cigarette taxes experienced during youth on adult smoking rates. Both focused on tobacco taxation, because taxes appear to be the best method of reducing smoking among teens.[5]

One study, that of Gruber and Zinman,[10] related the smoking behavior of pregnant women to the cigarette taxes in force in their youth. Gruber and Zinman matched Vital Statistics Natality File data on smoking during pregnancy among women 24 years or older to information on cigarette taxes in the women's state of birth when they were aged 14 to 17 years. They found that the price elasticity of smoking consumption (including both whether women smoked and how much they smoked) with respect to cigarette taxes when the women were 14 years of age was about 30% as high as the estimated effect of these taxes on adolescents. The corresponding effect on adult smoking participation (i.e., whether women smoked or did not smoke) was only 25% as great.

In a recent paper, I used data from the National Longitudinal Survey of Youth (NLSY), involving a panel of young people followed from 1979 (when they were aged 14–24 years) through 1994 (when they were 29–39 years old), to examine the same question.[11] The NLSY asked about current smoking and smoking initiation in its 1984 and 1992 surveys and about current smoking in its 1994 survey. Also, in addition to retrospective information on respondents' residence at the age of 14 years, information was collected on state of residency in each of the study years. These data can be matched to tax information, and thus a full cigarette tax history can be constructed for each member of the panel. The fact that the NLSY followed a single cohort eliminated problems involving changes in the information available to smokers over time.

My estimates of the effects of contemporaneous cigarette taxes on smoking are in line with the existing literature: they suggest that a 10% increase in cigarette taxes leads to about a 1% decline in adult smoking participation. However, my estimates of the effects of taxes at the age of 14 years on later smoking suggest that these effects attenuate considerably over time. I repeated the analyses for different subsamples of the population (men, women, and those who were members of low-income families when they were 14 years of age) and found attenuation effects in all of these subsamples, with the greatest effects exhibited among low-income people and women.

The overall results of my study and that of Gruber and Zinman are summarized in Figure 1, which shows the effect of a 10% increase in tobacco taxes faced at the age of 14 years on smoking participation at subsequent ages. It can be seen that, among pregnant women, the effect on smoking participation of a 10% increase in tobacco taxes at the age of 14 years is below 1%. Among women in the NLSY, the estimated effect of taxes had disappeared entirely by the time they were 39 years old. Among men, the effects persisted but were much smaller when the respondents were 39 years of age than when they were 14 years of age.

In themselves, the implications of these studies are limited and should be viewed as provisional. They are based on special populations (Gruber and Zinman) or small samples (Glied). Yet, they do raise the possibility that controlling smoking among teens may not, in itself, yield substantial reductions in adult smoking rates. These studies imply that measuring the impact of tax policies on smoking among youths is likely to overstate potential public health effects. Similarly, short-term changes in youth smoking rates may matter less than media attention might suggest. Fine-tuning policy to address fluctuations in youth smoking rates may be unwarranted.

These 2 studies also raise some doubt regarding the conventional wisdom that taxes are the best way to control youth smoking.[5] The studies examined only the effects of tobacco taxation; they did not assess the effects of other forms of tobacco control. It may well be that approaches aimed at changing adolescents' attitudes toward smoking, which are less effective than taxes in the short run, yield larger long-term benefits than approaches that target teen wallets. All in all, researchers need to take a longer term look at the effects of tobacco control policies.

TARGETING YOUTHS

The statistical fact that most people begin smoking when they are teens is simply not enough to draw the inference that reducing smoking among teenagers will, in itself, generate substantial reductions in this behavior among adults. This is confirmed by studies of other behaviors that typically begin in youth. For exam-

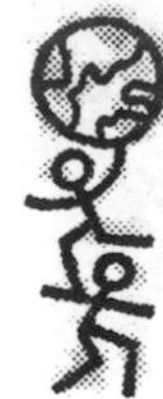

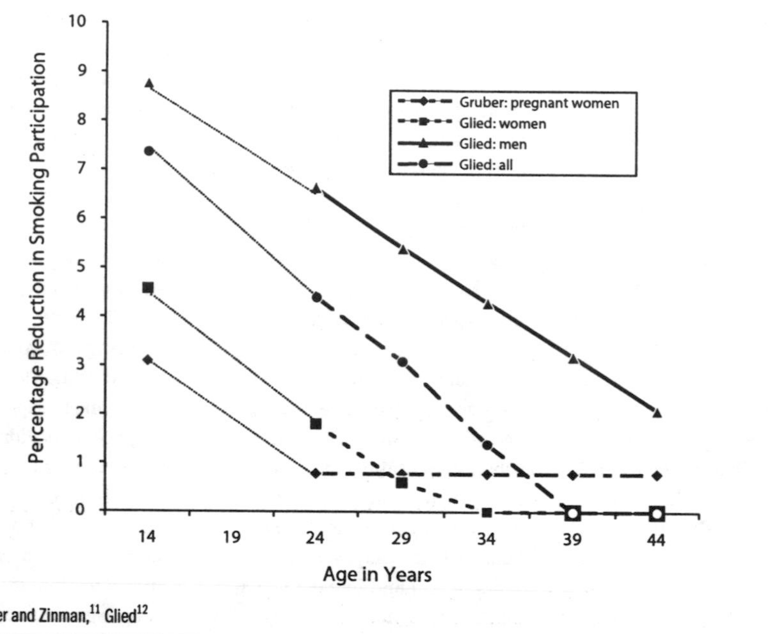

Sources: Gruber and Zinman,[11] Glied[12]

FIGURE 1—Long-term reductions in smoking participation produced by a 10% cigarette tax increase.

ple, Cook and Moore[12] found that raising the drinking age had no discernible effect on the probability that a youth would drink as an adult, although it might slightly lower his or her propensity toward later binge drinking (they found no persistent effects of beer taxes on either drinking or bingeing). Moreover, it has been shown that delaying initiation of childbearing beyond the teenage years has little, if any, effect on cumulative achieved parity among women who go on to have children.[13–15] Teen mothers have their babies earlier, but White and Black teen mothers appear to have correspondingly fewer children in young adulthood than do those who postpone childbearing. (Ribar[13] found that Hispanic teen mothers had higher parities than those who postponed childbearing.)

The evidence on average age of smoking initiation similarly suggests that there is no particular susceptibility to smoking associated with being a teenager that might imply that delaying smoking beyond the adolescent years would lead to overall reductions in smoking rates. Figure 2 shows median and 75th percentile ages of smoking initiation among different cohorts of men and women 25 years or older; data were derived from the 1997 National Health Interview Survey. If teenage irrationality leads to increased susceptibility, average age of initiation should have fallen after publication of the surgeon general's 1965 report, which led to large declines in initiation rates and increases in cessation rates. Yet, as can be seen in Figure 2, among cohorts born both before and after 1948, approximately 25% of men who had ever smoked initiated smoking after the age of 18 years.

Declines in age of initiation have occurred steadily among women. Women's smoking behavior has become more and more similar to that of men over time. The median age of smoking initiation among women who were born after 1968 and had ever smoked was 16 years (assuming that the women in this cohort are no longer initiating smoking). Among earlier generations of women, however, smoking initiation generally occurred in young adulthood. Among women born between 1948 and 1957, the median age of smoking initiation was 18 years, and among women born before 1928 who had ever smoked, the median age of initiation was 20 years. More than one fourth of the women older than 40 years who had ever smoked began smoking after 22 years of age. These data suggest that being a teenager is not a necessary prerequisite to initiating smoking.

CONCLUSIONS

Targeting young smokers is a politically appealing way to address the public health problem of tobacco use. In a recent poll, 77% of respondents agreed that "[t]he government should take steps to reduce teen-aged smoking. However, adults who want to smoke should be free to make their own decision."[16] Some economists have found evidence suggesting that adult smokers may behave rationally, weighing the costs and benefits of their decisions.[17] Such evidence lends weight to arguments that policies designed to discourage adult smoking are paternalistic and encroach on individual freedom.[18] By contrast, teenagers may not have the capacity to make rational decisions about substances that cause damage in the distant future.[19,20] Our concerns about teenage knowledge and rationality are implicit in rules that limit to adults the right to vote and to serve on a jury. In this light, preventing young people—or, as former secretary Shalala put it, children—from making decisions with long-term negative consequences is politically acceptable.

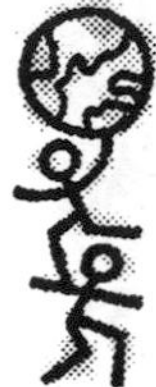

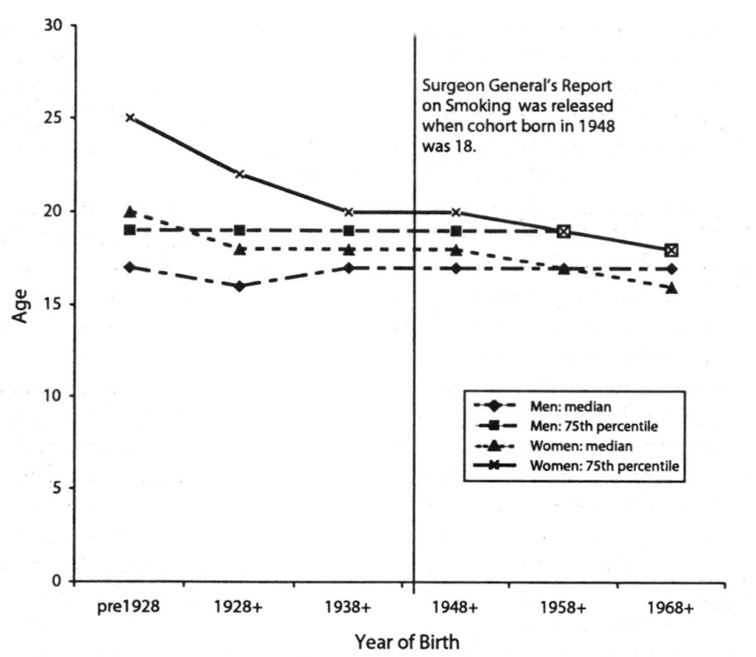

FIGURE 2—Age at smoking initiation, by sex and year of birth, median and 75th percentile: National Health Interview Survey, 1997.

If they are to have long-term effects, however, efforts to reduce smoking among teens need to be sustained into adulthood and should encompass changes in adult behavior rather than simply focusing on adolescent initiation. Indeed, the greatest long-term health benefit of raising taxes to prevent youth smoking is that it inevitably raises taxes for adults at the same time. In the study described earlier, Gruber and Zinman[10] found that the tobacco taxes pregnant women face as adults are 6 times as effective in reducing their current smoking participation as the taxes they faced in youth.

Focusing attention on adults is also consistent with the fact that more than 80% of current smokers want to quit[21] and about two thirds have made at least one serious attempt to do so.[22] Although quitting smoking is very difficult, the number of adult Americans who are former smokers is nearly as high as the number who are current smokers (44.8 million vs 47.2 million in 1998). Among those older than 45 years, among all Whites, and among all men, former smokers outnumber current smokers.[23] (Former smokers also considerably outnumber current smokers in the population older than 65 years, but this difference may be substantially attributable to differential mortality rates.) The continuing high rates of quitting suggest that encouraging adult cessation, while difficult, may be at least as effective a long-term policy strategy as reducing teenage initiation.

There is ample reason for public policy to help smokers engage in actions that promote public health and that smokers themselves wish to undertake. A growing literature in the area of behavioral economics highlights the efforts people make to develop self-control.[24,25] This literature has recently been applied to considering the time inconsistency of preferences surrounding smoking.[26] Recent empirical estimates based on these models suggest that, by promoting self-control, the raising of tobacco taxes might even result in adult smokers being subjectively better off in that their smoking rates may be reduced.[27] Consistent with these estimates, a surprisingly large minority of adult smokers (more than 25%) favor at least some smoking bans.[21]

Public opinion and public policy have long favored control of youth smoking. If delaying smoking among young people does not, in itself, lead to persistent reductions in smoking over the long term, as the 2 recent studies described here suggest it may not, we need to rethink this approach. Those responsible for public policy need to consider approaches that sustain delayed initiation into adulthood. In the long run, helping adults achieve their own goals may be as effective a tobacco control strategy as changing teenage minds. ■

About the Author

The author is with the Department of Health Policy and Management, Mailman School of Public Health, Columbia University, New York, NY.

Requests for reprints should be sent to Sherry Glied, PhD, Department of Health Policy and Management, Mailman School of Public Health, Columbia University, 600 West 168th, 6th Floor, New York, NY 10032 (e-mail: sag1@columbia.edu).

This article was accepted September 27, 2002.

References

1. *Hearings Before the Senate Labor and Human Resources Committee,* 105th Cong, 1st Sess (1997) (testimony of Donna Shalala).

2. Cliver SP, Goldenberg RL, Cutter GR, Hoffman HD, Davis RO, Nelson KG. The effect of cigarette smoking on neonatal anthropometric measurements. *Obstet Gynecol.* 1995; 85:625–630.

3. *Smoking Among U.S. Adults: Fact Sheet.* Atlanta, Ga: Centers for Disease Control and Prevention, Office of Smoking and Health; 1997.

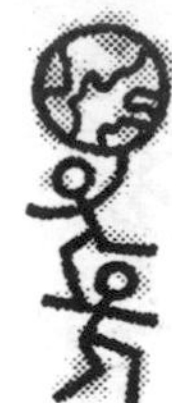

4. Elders MJ, Perry CL, Eriksen MP, Giovino GA. The report of the surgeon general: preventing tobacco use among young people. *Am J Public Health*. 1994; 84:543–547.

5. Chaloupka FJ, Warner K. The economics of smoking. In: Culyer A, Newhouse J, eds. *Handbook of Health Economics*. Vol. 1. Amsterdam, the Netherlands: Elsevier; 2000: 1539–1627.

6. Evans WN, Ringel JS, Stech D. Tobacco taxes and public policy to discourage smoking. In: Poterba J, ed. *Tax Policy and the Economy*. Vol. 13. Cambridge, Mass: National Bureau of Economic Research; 1999:1–55.

7. Centers for Disease Control and Prevention. Cigarette smoking among adults–United States, 1999. *MMWR Morb Mortal Wkly Rep*. 2001;50: 869–873.

8. Centers for Disease Control and Prevention. Trends in cigarette smoking among high school students–United States, 1991–2001. *MMWR Morb Mortal Wkly Rep*. 2002;51:409–412.

9. Breslau N, Peterson EL. Smoking cessation in young adults: age at initiation of cigarette smoking and other suspected influences. *Am J Public Health*. 1996;86:214–220.

10. Gruber J, Zinman J. Youth smoking in the U.S.: evidence and implications." In: Gruber J, ed. *Risky Behaviors Among Youths*. Chicago, Ill: University of Chicago Press; 2001:69–120.

11. Glied S. Youth tobacco control: reconciling theory and empirical evidence. *J Health Economics*. 2002;21:117–135.

12. Cook PJ, Moore MJ. Environment and persistence in youthful drinking patterns. In: Gruber J, ed. *Risky Behaviors Among Youths*. Chicago, Ill: University of Chicago Press; 2001:375–437.

13. Ribar DC. The effect of teenage fertility on young adult childbearing. *J Popul Economics*. 1996;9:197–218.

14. Heckman JJ, Walker JR. Economic models of fertility dynamics: a study of Swedish fertility. In: *Research in Population Economics*. Vol. 7. Greenwich, Conn: JAI Press; 1991:3–91.

15. Heckman JJ, Hotz VJ, Walker JR. The influence of early fertility on subsequent births and the importance of controlling for unobserved heterogeneity. *Bull Int Stat Inst*. 1985;51:1–15.

16. Portrait of America. *The Government Should Take Steps to Reduce Teen-Aged Smoking*. Mathews, NC: Rasmussen Research; 2000.

17. Becker GS, Grossman M, Murphy KM. An empirical analysis of cigarette addiction. *Am Econ Rev*. 1994; 84:396–418.

18. Schaler JA, Schaler ME. The smoking controversy: a right to protect versus a right to smoke. In Schaler JA, Schaler ME, eds. *Smoking: Who Has the Right?* New York, NY: Prometheus Books; 1998:9–20.

19. Orphanides A, Zervos D. Rational addiction with learning and regret. *J Political Economy*. 1995;103:739–758.

20. Suranovic SM, Goldfarb RS, Leonard TC. An economic theory of cigarette addiction. *J Health Economics*. 1998;18:1–29.

21. *The Gallup Poll: Public Opinion 2000*. Wilmington, Del: Scholarly Resources Inc; 2000.

22. *The Gallup Poll: Public Opinion 1999*. Wilmington, Del: Scholarly Resources Inc; 1999.

23. Centers for Disease Control and Prevention. Number (in millions) of adults 18 years and older who were current, former, or never smokers, overall and by sex, race, Hispanic origin, age, and education, National Health Interview Surveys, selected years–United States, 1965–1995. Available at: http://www.cdc.gov/tobacco/research_data/adults_prev/tab_3.htm. Accessed June 21, 2002.

24. Schelling TC. Self-command in practice, in policy, and in a theory of rational choice. *Am Econ Rev*. 1984;74: 1–11.

25. Thaler R, Shefrin HM. An economic theory of self-control. *J Political Economy*. 1981;89:392–406.

26. Gruber J, Koszegi. 2001. Is addiction 'rational'? Theory and evidence. *Q J Economics*. 2001;116:1261–1303.

27. Gruber J, Mullainathan S. *Do Cigarette Taxes Make Smokers Happier?* Cambridge, Mass: National Bureau of Economic Research; 2002.

A Balanced Tobacco Control Policy

| Stephen D. Sugarman, JD

By raising the price of cigarettes through tobacco taxes, policymakers might only be delaying some smokers' initiation of smoking rather than permanently preventing them from smoking. This is one of several reasons for adopting a balanced tobacco control policy that relies only in part on cigarette taxation. (*Am J Public Health*. 2003;93: 416–418)

IN RECENT YEARS, MUCH attention has been given to reducing the number of people who start smoking. Since historically a very high proportion of smokers have taken up the habit during the teenage years (or even younger), policy has concentrated on youths. In an accompanying article, Sherry Glied suggests that this focus may be unwise.[1]

Other tobacco control advocates have worried that, although it might be politically easier in the short run to enact measures with a "child protection" feel to them, most smokers are adults. Moreover, it seems highly unlikely for now that any youth-oriented policy (or combination of policies) would be fully effective. Hence, those who continue to start smoking in their teens are going to remain a public health concern in the future when they become adults. Furthermore, some fear that if public policy implies that smoking is bad for kids but all right for adults, it might make experimenting with smoking even more attractive to some youths.

DO TOBACCO TAXES ONLY DELAY INITIATION?

Glied suggests a possible additional unease about the youth focus of tobacco control policy. Suppose that smoking policy aimed at children merely delays initiation. At the extreme, imagine a hypothetical program that appeared at first blush to be astoundingly successful because, as a result of this intervention, no teenager in America smoked anymore. And yet, suppose further that, by the time they were 30 years old, as many in the cohort group were smoking as before the seemingly wondrous youth-oriented smoking program went into effect. That is, suppose this program merely pushed up

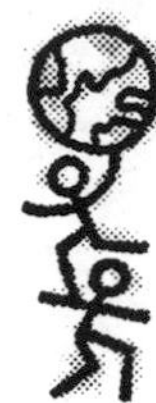

the start of smoking until people are aged 21 or so.

Such a result, of course, would be altogether contrary to assumptions that seem now widely held in the tobacco control community, where most believe that if people don't start smoking by age 20, they are unlikely ever to start. After all, a rather small share of smokers who are alive today began as adults. Explanations for this behavioral pattern seem to be that after the teen years, people will more rationally reject smoking because of the dangers to their health; or they will be less susceptible to tobacco company promotion campaigns or to the peer pressure of friends who smoke; or perhaps they will have found some other "vice" to engage in as teens that substitutes for smoking and precludes the need or wish ever to smoke. But what if this assumption about initiation is incorrect? What if policies that cause a dramatic reduction in teen smoking simply lead to an offsetting increase in initiation by those in their 20s?

That could plausibly happen if the effect of the youth smoking control policy somehow wears off over time. For example, those teens who are merely priced out of the tobacco market by higher taxes may well be able to afford to enter it later on. Or perhaps in response to an effective youth-oriented tobacco control policy, tobacco companies develop new and effective tobacco marketing campaigns aimed at 18- to 24-year-olds.

The basic point is that if delayed initiation were its real impact, then an apparently large public health success could actually be dramatically less than assumed. Because the main harms from smoking generally come much later in life, merely delaying when one begins to smoke is probably much less beneficial from the public health perspective than is delaying many other dangerous activities. For example, if teens did not drink or did not have children, specific dangers associated with youths engaging in such conduct would be avoided. Moreover, when these youths later take up those very same behaviors as adults, the negative consequences to others could well be much reduced. With smoking, by contrast, the benefits of merely delaying initiation may not be the same.

To be sure, if delayed initiation into smoking also meant that one were more likely to quit later on, or more likely not to relapse after quitting later on, it might be almost as beneficial as is assumed today, even if the benefit arises in a somewhat different form. In addition, if most long-term smokers started at age 25 instead of age 15, their encounters with tobacco-related diseases would probably, on average, come later in life and at a somewhat reduced incidence. Moreover, from the "free choice" perspective, it is much more attractive that new initiates are adults who presumably are able to make more reasoned choices about their own best interests than are children.

Glied's study, details of which have previously been reported,[2] as well as a report that she describes by Gruber and Zinman[3] suggest that today's policies, especially tobacco tax increases that appear to reduce youth smoking, primarily delay initiation. I believe, however, that it is uncertain whether this is so. Simplifying a lot, we are talking about a pattern roughly as follows. Suppose that in a cohort of 100 youths, 25 18-year-olds smoked before the intervention and 25 were smokers at age 30 (although this would include some new starters who had replaced some quitters). Now suppose a tax increase reduces the number of 18-year-old smokers to 20 of 100 (which would be initially viewed as a substantial public health gain) but that at age 30, 25 are smokers. Such a result, other things being equal, suggests that the tax merely put off initiation. But, of course, other things are by no means equal. And with so many other policy changes in play and so much else happening that might be influencing smoking behavior over time, one should be highly cautious about drawing a firm conclusion from these initial investigations, regardless of their statistical sophistication—especially when we are talking about changed conduct of 5% or less of the population.

REASONS NOT TO RELY ONLY ON TOBACCO TAXES

It must also be emphasized that tobacco tax increases are very different, for example, from public policies that impose high automobile insurance rates on teen drivers. The latter, which are meant to delay initiation into driving by some teens, are a highly targeted form of intervention. Tobacco taxes are not, and realistically cannot be, restricted to youths. Indeed, a huge share of tobacco taxes is borne by adults. Although adult demand for cigarettes may not be as price sensitive as is that of teens, the weight of scholarly opinion is that tobacco tax increases have an immediate impact on adults as well—giving some just the right financial nudge to quit or not to relapse, as well as discouraging others who would otherwise begin to smoke. Nor does Glied suggest the contrary.

Of course, tobacco tax increases may lose their potency over time simply because they are no longer the tax they once were. Unlike typical sales taxes, for example, that are imposed as a percentage of the price of some good or service, cigarette taxes are primarily levied as so many cents per pack of 20. If, because of inflation, for example, the price of the pack rises from $2.50 at time 1 to $3.50 at time 2, and a new tax of 50 cents a pack that was introduced at time 1 (and included in the $2.50 price) remains at 50 cents at time 2, then one would expect the impact of that tax to decline. That is why some have argued that tobacco taxes should be set by formula in relation to price.

NEED FOR BALANCE

Whether or not Glied's fears about the impact of tobacco taxes on youths are correct, there

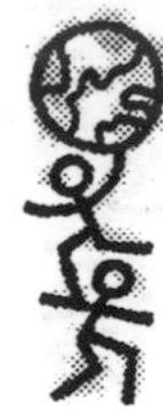

are other reasons not to make tobacco taxes almost the entire focus of tobacco control policy, whether we are talking about youth smoking or adult smoking. These taxes, in the end, burden adult smokers, who increasingly come from the ranks of the working class and the poor, most of whom are addicted. And while it is true that lower-income people are disproportionately influenced by cigarette price increases, I believe that most people would nonetheless consider the net tax consequence as regressive rather than progressive. In any event, as nonsmokers become an increasing majority of the voting public, the ease with which they can push more of the regular costs of government onto smokers is worrying as a matter of fairness. In turn, that makes public spending dependent on continued substantial rates of smoking. Higher tobacco taxes also can bring with them increased tobacco smuggling and the possible involvement of organized crime or other dangerous criminal elements. These points are not meant to be an argument against moderate or even substantial tobacco taxes. But they are meant as a caution against excessive reliance on this one policy instrument.

Of course, in a state like California that has been successful in reducing smoking rates, tobacco control policy is by no means restricted to tobacco tax increases. The other most effective policies seem to be very tough controls on indoor smoking at both work and leisure venues and a very aggressive antismoking advertising program (even if some of the advertisements strike me as unseemly propagandistic). A supposedly conservative US Supreme Court has recently given an extraordinarily liberal interpretation of the First Amendment and an extraordinarily anti–states' rights interpretation of the federal law on cigarette warnings. These rulings have precluded California and other states from strongly curbing tobacco industry advertising and promotional campaigns.

Yet, even in California, considerably more could be done to promote the free or inexpensive availability of effective smoking cessation (or smoking reduction) products and programs. Indeed, the ready availability of such programs and products may be thought a precondition for the fair imposition of high tobacco taxes on addicted smokers. After all, the strongest ethical justification for public health intervention to reduce smoking (putting aside the consequences of secondhand smoke) is that children are duped into starting to smoke and become hooked before they realize what they are getting into. But then to impose pain in the form of higher taxes on those very victims seems harsh, especially if those most burdened by tobacco taxes also find cessation programs and products financially daunting. ■

About the Author

Stephen D. Sugarman is with the School of Law, University of California, Berkeley.

Requests for reprints should be sent to Stephen D. Sugarman, JD, 327 Boalt Hall, University of California, Berkeley, CA 94720-7200 (e-mail: sugarman@law.berkeley.edu).

This article was accepted October 4, 2002.

References

1. Glied S. Is smoking delayed smoking averted? *Am J Public Health.* 2003; 93:412–416.

2. Glied S. Youth tobacco control: reconciling theory and empirical evidence. *J Health Econ.* 2002;21:117–135.

3. Gruber J, Zinman J. Youth smoking in the US: evidence and implications. In: Gruber J, ed. *Risky Behavior Among Youths.* Chicago, Ill: University of Chicago Press; 2001:69–120.

| SECTION II |

Tobacco Advertising & Marketing

Influence of a Counteradvertising Media Campaign on Initiation of Smoking: The Florida "truth" Campaign

David F. Sly, PhD, Richard S. Hopkins, MD, MSPH, Edward Trapido, ScD, and Sarah Ray, MA

ABSTRACT

Objectives. The purpose of this study was to assess the short-term effects of television advertisements from the Florida "truth" campaign on rates of smoking initiation.

Methods. A follow-up survey of young people aged 12 to 17 years (n=1820) interviewed during the first 6 months of the advertising campaign was conducted. Logistic regression analyses were used to estimate the independent effects of the campaign on smoking initiation while other factors were controlled for.

Results. Youths scoring at intermediate and high levels on a media effect index were less likely to initiate smoking than youths who could not confirm awareness of television advertisements. Adjusted odds ratios between the media index and measures of initiation were similar within categories of age, sex, susceptibility, and whether a parent smoked.

Conclusions. Exposure to the "truth" media campaign lowered the risk of youth smoking initiation. However, the analysis did not demonstrate that all such media programs will be effective. (*Am J Public Health.* 2001;91:233–238)

Media campaigns are being advocated to combat many public health problems.[1–4] Counteradvertising is salient in anti-tobacco campaigns.[5–8] Anti-tobacco counteradvertising campaigns are under way in 7 states, and the American Legacy Foundation has initiated a national campaign. As tobacco settlement funds become available, the Centers for Disease Control and Prevention (CDC) expects 27 more states to initiate campaigns by 2002. Media campaigns are costly, and it is important to document evidence linking advertisements to reductions in the prevalence of tobacco use and to determine what ad strategies work best.[9]

Early evaluations of anti-tobacco media campaigns yielded mixed results.[10–12] More recently, 2 evaluations of statewide media campaigns reported positive results.[13,14] Although both studies involved a longitudinal design, both also involved a dependent variable that did not directly measure behavior at 2 points in time. The researchers used a measure (having smoked 100 or more cigarettes in one's lifetime) difficult to interpret in conventional epidemiologic terms. This problem is compounded because in neither study was the measure used at both points in time, and no effects were reported for timing of cigarette use. The implications of having smoked 99 cigarettes the month before a second interview are different from the implications of having smoked the same number of cigarettes in the month after the first interview and having not smoked since. This difference is compounded when the period between interviews spans several years.

Our objective was to test the hypothesis that a counteradvertising campaign can lower the probability of smoking initiation. We used a longitudinal, multivariate design to examine an intense, statewide, industry manipulation counteradvertising campaign. Two levels of smoking behavior were measured at 2 points in time. Results showed that a measure of advertising effectiveness that rigorously assessed advertisement exposure, advertisement-specific content, and cognitive awareness of the campaign message was related to maintenance or change in cigarette use.

Background

In August 1997, Florida reached a settlement with the tobacco industry,[15] and the state embarked on an anti-tobacco campaign targeting young people aged 12 to 17 years starting in early 1998. An important and highly visible component of the initial effort was an intense counteradvertising campaign (the "truth" campaign). The strategy has been outlined in detail.[16] The campaign was intended to empower young people with the feeling that they could take on the tobacco industry and its executives and be part of a tobacco-free generation. The "industry manipulation strategy" used in the campaign attacked the industry and portrayed its executives as predatory, profit hungry, and manipulative. It argued that the tobacco industry has targeted young people, lied to and hid the truth from them, and used them to its own ends, knowing that tobacco use is detrimental to young people's health.

David F. Sly is with the Center for the Study of Population, College of Social Sciences, Florida State University, Tallahassee, and the Office of Smoking and Health, Centers for Disease Control and Prevention, Atlanta, Ga. Richard S. Hopkins is with the Florida Department of Health, Tallahassee. Edward Trapido is with the Department of Epidemiology and the Tobacco Research and Evaluation Coordinating Center, Sylvester Comprehensive Cancer Center, University of Miami School of Medicine, Miami, Fla. Sarah Ray is with the Center for the Study of Population, College of Social Sciences, Florida State University.

Requests for reprints should be sent to David F. Sly, PhD, Center for the Study of Population, College of Social Sciences, Florida State University, Tallahassee, FL 32306 (e-mail: dsly@coss.fsu.edu).

This article was accepted October 6, 2000.

Twelve advertisements were run statewide during the first 10 months of the campaign. The total media budget for the first year was approximately $26.5 million. The first flight, or "buy," included 2 ads, and successive flights generally included 3. Gross rating points per quarter (theoretical ad exposures per 1000 expected viewers) averaged 1606 over the year, with a somewhat higher point total (1900) in the first 2 quarters.

We believe that this program has been one of the most thorough and rigorously evaluated anti-tobacco counteradvertising campaigns in the United States. The evaluation included a quasi-experimental design involving 4 cross-sectional surveys (a baseline survey and a 1-year survey of the Florida target population and a national comparison group not exposed to the campaign) and 2 intermediate tracking surveys.[17,18] These surveys showed that at the end of 1 year (May 1999), there was a 91.5% confirmed awareness of the campaign and an 88.6% confirmed awareness of "truth" advertisements. There were significant increases in anti-tobacco attitudes and decreases in tobacco use prevalence in Florida but not in the national comparison group.

Ten months into the campaign, results from the Florida Youth Tobacco Survey showed an 11% decrease in smoking prevalence rates.[18,19] All results from the various cross-sectional surveys suggested that the campaign was having its desired effects, but there was no way to relate individual behavior change to the media campaign via these cross-sectional sources.

A longitudinal study was designed to observe change and maintenance in smoking behaviors at the individual level and to allow investigation of the campaign's effects on smoking behaviors.[18,20] The campaign was designed primarily with a prevention objective. Data from the longitudinal component were used to assess whether this objective was reached.

Methods

Follow-Up Sample

By the ninth month of the campaign, 4935 youths had been interviewed in one of the Florida Anti-Tobacco Media Evaluation (April, June, or September 1998) surveys; this was the sampling frame for the follow-up conducted in February 1999.[18,20] Names were arranged alphabetically and assigned a random number that determined calling order. We called 3712 numbers and completed 1820 interviews. Refusal rates were 4.9% for parents and 3.7% for children. Telephone numbers for 436 (11.7%) individuals were reported to be no longer in service. For 638 of the remaining 1100 numbers called, no contact was made after 5 callbacks; for 462 numbers, contact was made with the household, but not with a parent or the child, after 5 callbacks.

Interviews

Details on interviewer training and the telephone protocol have been reported elsewhere.[17,18] Interviewers asked for a parent or guardian of the child, using the child's name. Parents were informed of the purpose of the call and the content of the survey. If a parent gave permission, informed consent was obtained from the child, who had the opportunity to not participate. Interviews were conducted in English or Spanish. Average completion time was just over 28 minutes. Respondents received an incentive of $12.50.

Measures

To identify smokers, the CDC recommends a question that asks whether a person has smoked at all (even a puff or two) in the month before an interview. Some have rejected this criterion on the grounds that many youths smoke irregularly and cannot provide accurate information in regard to the 30-day referent. Researchers taking this position advocate a question asking whether a person has smoked 100 cigarettes in his or her lifetime.[14] We use the CDC criterion for 2 reasons. First, the length of recall and use criteria are much simpler than a lifetime, specific number of cigarettes. It makes little sense to argue that one can recall a lifetime of experience better than the events of the previous 30 days. Second, in comparison with an adolescent aged 11 years, a youth aged 17 years has 2190 more days to have smoked 100 cigarettes, a youth aged 16 years has 1825 more days to have smoked that number of cigarettes, and so on. A single lifetime criterion applied at each age does not measure progression, because it reveals nothing about when an individual started or stopped smoking the 100 cigarettes.

To measure progression to dependence, we used the CDC criterion and included 2 additional items: number of days in which respondents smoked in the previous month and number of cigarettes respondents smoked on days on which they smoked. For respondents who had smoked in the previous 30 days, number of days smoked and cigarettes smoked per day were cross tabulated to form a matrix. Across surveys, consistent patterns and clustering have been found. Detailed epidemiologic analyses of the follow-up data show that 3 clusters—identified as situational, occasional, and dependent—are highly predictive of future cigarette use.[20]

We used 2 measures of smoking. The first was the CDC-recommended question. Using this item, we determined whether each time-1 nonsmoker remained a nonsmoker (coded 1) or became a smoker at time 2 (coded 0). The second measure of change in smoking status was derived from the classification based on the matrix. In effect, we classified situational smokers as nonsmokers. Persons falling in the situational classification smoked on fewer than 6 days in the 30 days before the survey, and none reported smoking more than 5 cigarettes on days on which they smoked. More than 78% of "situational smokers" actually reported smoking no more than 1 cigarette on days on which they smoked. According to this definition, "smokers" are persons reporting smoking on 6 or more days in the previous 30 days and smoking 5 or more cigarettes on days on which they smoked. We refer to these individuals as "established" smokers.

Our measure of media effectiveness was designed to capture confirmed awareness of specific "truth" advertisements, their receptivity among target audiences, and the cognitive or perceived influence of the campaign as opposed to individual ads. If an ad is to be effective, its message needs to provoke a cognitive reaction. Also, campaigns are designed to present similar messages in different ads to communicate a general theme. If a campaign is to be effective, ad-specific messages must blend around a theme that becomes a salient feature of the decision-making matrix that influences targeted behaviors. Many advertising campaign assessments are based only on the former criterion, but ad campaigns are usually designed to communicate general messages that cut across and link various specific ads that are part of the campaign.

To tap the first dimension, we used an unaided as opposed to an aided approach. When an "aided" approach is used, respondents are provided with a description of the advertisement (in varying detail) and then are asked whether they can recall it. If they respond "yes," they are asked 1 or 2 additional questions. If a minimum of detail is provided in the description, respondents are asked for greater detail about the advertisement. The second item asks respondents to describe the major message of the specific advertisement. This item, referred to as a measure of confirmed awareness, is acknowledged to have shortcomings related to the detail of the ad's description provided, which can assist recall and even result in "coaching" for desired replies.

The more rigorous technique used in this study of measuring awareness involved asking a question that provides no advertisement-specific description but affords respondents the opportunity to offer such a description. We asked respondents whether they recalled having seen antismoking advertisements since the previous spring (i.e., since the start of the "truth" campaign). If respondents answered "yes" or "maybe," they were asked to (1) describe the ad they most liked and (2) relate to the interviewer the major theme or message of the ad. This sequence was repeated for the advertisement rated as second most liked.

For each set of items, respondents were given a score ranging from 0 (they could describe no ad accurately) to 2 (they could describe the ad and recall the theme identified). Credit was given only for "truth" advertisements, although the sequence included ads that were not part of the "truth" campaign. Three Philip Morris "Think. Don't Smoke" advertisements ran before and during the interviewing. Even though these ads were the most current, only 3.6% of respondents mentioned any of them as one of their two favorites.

We had to rely on self-reports to measure cognitive reactions to specific advertisements and the extent to which these reactions were tied to the general campaign message. In making these assessments, we asked respondents who confirmed that they were aware of the campaign whether a particular advertisement made them think about whether or not they should smoke. This question was asked as part of the sequence for each ad confirmed. A code of 0 was assigned to respondents not confirming awareness; those confirming awareness were assigned a code of 1 if they reported that one advertisement made them think about whether or not they should smoke and a code of 2 if they reported that both advertisements had this effect.

To measure whether the campaign's advertisements influenced the (behavior) decision matrix of individuals, we used an item embedded in a sequence of 19 items. In this sequence, which occurred approximately 100 items after the ad awareness sequence, respondents were read a lead-in stating that we were going to read a list of things they might think about and consider in deciding whether or not to smoke. They were to respond by telling us whether each item influenced them not at all, a little, some, or a lot. The 16th item on the list, "You feel tobacco companies are just trying to use you," was specifically designed to capture the industry manipulation theme. It was carefully worded not to come from any specific advertisement but to tie the various ad-specific messages to the general message. Response codes (0=none/a little, 1=some/a lot) for this item were collapsed.

The advertisement effectiveness index was formed from these 3 variables. Respondents who did not confirm awareness of any advertisements were not asked whether an ad made them think about whether or not they should smoke, but they were asked whether they felt tobacco companies were just trying to use them. Fewer than 2% of respondents who did not confirm awareness of "truth" ads gave a positive reply to this item. A code of 0 was assigned to all time 1 nonsmokers who did not confirm awareness (37.1%) of any ads, indicating that the advertising campaign had no effect on them. A code of 2 was assigned to time 1 nonsmokers who confirmed awareness of 2 ads, indicating that both made them think about whether or not they should smoke, and reported that the feeling that tobacco companies were just trying to use them influenced their decisions some or a lot (25.8%). The advertising campaign had a significant effect on these individuals. A code of 1 was assigned to all other time 1 nonsmokers (37.1%), and these individuals were treated as having been affected at a low level by the campaign.

Five additional variables were included: time 1 survey month, age, sex, susceptibility, and whether a parent smoked. These data were based on self-reports. Age was dichotomized (less than 16 years vs 16 years or older). Susceptibility was measured as having a best friend who smoked. Respondents were also asked separately whether they had a female and male parent or guardian in their household and whether each of these individuals smoked. If the respondent reported that either smoked, they were coded as having a parent smoker. SPSS (SPSS Inc, Chicago, Ill) was used in conducting statistical analyses.

Results

Smoking initiation rates per 100 time 1 nonsmokers at follow-up are shown in Table 1. Overall, for the 1480 time 1 nonsmokers, the smoking initiation rate (according to the CDC criterion) per 100 was 8.8. If we consider the established user definition, the rate was 5.2 per 100 time 1 nonsmokers. Estimated rates per year among young people aged 12 to 17 years at time 1 were 11.1 and 7.2, respectively.

Table 1 also shows the association between the advertisement effectiveness index and smoking initiation as well as the association of 5 other independent variables with initiation. Neither month of time 1 survey nor sex was significantly related to smoking initiation. Each of the other variables was related regardless of which definition of smoking was used. For each variable other than susceptibility, larger differentials were seen with the established user criterion.

For example, according to the CDC definition, those younger than 16 years had an initiation rate (7.8) 24.3% lower than the rate (10.3) for those older than 16 years. The comparable difference in rates for established smokers (3.6 and 8.3, respectively) was 56.6%. In regard to susceptibility, the CDC-defined initiation rate for time 1 nonsusceptible nonsmokers was 5.2, as compared with a rate of 16.7 for susceptible nonsmokers (a difference of 68.9%). The comparable rates for established smokers were 2.3 and 6.7 (a difference of approximately 65%).

Finally, the advertisement effectiveness index was similarly related to smoking initiation. According to the CDC definition, those with low scores on the ad effectiveness index and those with high scores were 22.0% and 40.4%, respectively, less likely to take up smoking than those not affected by the media campaign. The comparable rates for progression to established smoking were 51.3% and 62.5%. For both definitions, smoking initiation rates were lower among those scoring high as opposed to low on the ad effectiveness index, and there was no differential (23.2% vs 23.9%) between the definitions.

We used 2 logistic regression equations to determine whether the ad campaign had an effect on behavior independent of other variables. In each equation, the dependent variable (change in smoking status) was coded 0 for time 1 nonsmokers who became smokers and 1 for nonsmokers who remained nonsmokers at time 2. Table 2 shows estimated odds ratios depicting the associations between each independent variable and the likelihood of smoking initiation for each definition of smoking. The patterns were similar. Month of time 1 survey, age, and sex were not related to smoking initiation. Not being susceptible and not having a parent who smoked reduced the odds of a nonsmoker's becoming a smoker, and those who scored low and those who scored high on the ad effectiveness index were more likely to remain nonsmokers than those who were not affected by the campaign.

When the CDC definition was used, those scoring low on the ad effectiveness index were 1.3 times more likely to remain nonsmokers than those not affected by the campaign; those scoring high were 1.7 times more likely to remain nonsmokers. The comparable ratios for the definition of established smoking were 1.8 and 2.4.

Although no significant interactions were detected, we wanted to further validate these results. Table 3 shows adjusted odds ratios for the ad effectiveness index and smoking initiation by categories of the independent variables, after control for the other independent variables. These data largely confirmed the results already reported. All of the patterns were maintained, and most of the odds ratios remained significant. When the CDC definition was used,

TABLE 1—Smoking Initiation Rates for Time 1 Nonsmokers (per 100) at Follow-Up Using 2 Criteria to Measure Transitions in Smoking Behavior: Florida, 1998–1999

	Persons Who Smoked a Minimum of Puff or 2	Established Smokers
All persons	8.8	5.2
Time 1 survey		
April	9.0	5.4
June	9.4	5.1
September	8.4	5.2
Age, y		
<16	7.8*	3.6**
≥16	10.3	8.3
Sex		
Female	9.1	5.4
Male	8.6	5.0
Susceptibility		
Susceptible	16.7**	6.7**
Nonsusceptible	5.2	2.3
Parent smokes		
Yes	12.8**	8.8**
No	7.5	3.8
Ad effect index		
No ad effect	10.9**	8.0**
Low score	8.5	3.9
High score	6.5	3.0

**P*=.01; ***P*=.001.

TABLE 2—Odds Ratios Showing Effects of Independent Variables on the Likelihood of Time 1 Nonsmokers Remaining Nonsmokers at Time 2, After Control for Other Independent Variables: Florida, 1998–1999

	Persons Who Smoked a Minimum of Puff or 2			Established Smokers		
	OR	*P*	95% CI	OR	*P*	95% CI
Time 1 survey						
April	...			...		
June	0.964	.486	0.21, 2.72	1.043	.451	0.73, 2.07
September	0.983	.491	0.17, 3.14	1.091	.432	0.67, 2.19
Age	0.801	.257	0.34, 2.96	0.526	.011	0.23, 1.96
Sex	1.053	.397	0.41, 2.99	1.001	.487	0.41, 2.21
Susceptibility	0.290	.000	0.08, 2.13	0.278	.000	0.11, 1.14
Parent smoker	0.583	.003	0.33, 1.21	0.408	.001	0.16, 1.73
Ad effect index						
No ad effect	...	...	...	...	...	...
Low score	1.295	.047	0.97, 2.31	1.800	.010	1.19, 3.01
High score	1.720	.013	1.19, 2.92	2.379	.041	1.57, 4.12

Note. OR=odds ratio; CI=confidence interval.

the effect of the ad index was significant among those without a parent who smoked but not among those with a parent who smoked. Among youths 16 years or older and among male youths, having a low score on the ad effectiveness index did not produce a significant effect, but having a high score did. The association between the ad index and progression to established smoking held in all categorical comparisons with 1 exception; among male youths, a low score on the ad effectiveness index produced no effect, but a high score did.

Discussion

The present analysis suggests that an intense media campaign can help prevent youth smoking initiation. We used 2 definitions of smoking. The first treated any use of cigarettes in the 30 days before an interview as smoking. The second defined smoking as cigarette use on 6 or more days and more than 5 cigarettes smoked on days on which smoking occurred. The basic campaign effect on each type of smoking was maintained in adjusted odds ratios within age, sex, susceptibility, and parent smoking categories and when the remaining variables were taken into account.

The stronger implied effect of the advertising program on progression to established smoking than on any use may be important. The difference and its consistency suggest that the campaign may operate at 2 levels. First, it may prevent young nonsmokers from beginning any use. Second, it may affect young people who do take up smoking by making them more conscious of how often and how much they smoke. We cannot explore the link directly with the data available, but most of the ads produced for the Florida industry manipulation campaign had subthemes related to the addictive and health/mortality effects of tobacco.

As encouraging as these results appear, they need to be interpreted within at least 3 constraints. First, they are short-term findings. The work reported was designed to assess the 10-month effects of the "truth" campaign. Control for month of first survey within the context of this time frame showed no effect. Youth smoking behavior can be erratic; however, the fact that the time 1 measurements were derived from 3 different months and had no effect on either dependent variable suggests that the short-term effects observed captured real differences. We do not know whether the campaign's prevention effects will be maintained, but 2 recent reports involving different measurement techniques suggest long-term effects.[13,14] Moreover, even though the "truth" campaign had youths as its target, mass media campaigns reach persons outside their targets. In this case, we are most interested in younger people who are moving into high-risk age groups and who are likely to have been exposed to the campaign. These people will enter the target ages already exposed to a substantial dose of the "truth" message. If campaign effects are cumulative, we should observe lower risks of smoking initiation for these cohorts at later points in time. The data demonstrate that it is possible to achieve a significant effect from a media program in a relatively short time frame. They do not demonstrate, however, that this effect can be sustained.

Second, our results cannot be generalized to all anti-tobacco ad campaigns. The Florida campaign was unique in several respects. It was well funded, permitting an intense advertising dose resulting in nearly a 90% confirmed awareness of television ads by the time of the follow-up. Also, the campaign had a focused industry manipulation theme communicated through particularly hard-hitting, blatant, and direct advertisements. Furthermore, steps were taken to involve youths directly in decisions related to the campaign. These issues are im-

TABLE 3—Adjusted Odds Ratios Showing Effects of the Advertising Index on the Likelihood of Time 1 Nonsmokers Remaining Nonsmokers at Time 2, by Various Characteristics: Florida, 1998–1999

	Persons Who Smoked a Minimum of Puff or 2			Established Smokers		
	OR	*P*	95% CI	OR	*P*	95% CI
Aged <16 y						
No ad effect						
Low score	2.61	.004	1.31, 3.72	1.44	.041	0.87, 3.63
High score	2.68	.003	1.49, 3.98	1.69	.037	1.16, 3.59
Aged ≥16 y						
No ad effect						
Low score	1.20	.069	0.89, 2.41	1.42	.042	0.95, 2.65
High score	1.63	.032	1.09, 2.63	1.83	.029	1.19, 2.88
Female						
No ad effect						
Low score	1.68	.029	1.11, 3.01	2.68	.017	1.24, 4.12
High score	1.72	.022	1.24, 3.46	2.38	.029	1.21, 3.96
Male						
No ad effect						
Low score	0.95	.411	0.27, 2.22	1.16	.073	0.34, 2.94
High score	2.12	.012	1.07, 3.73	2.53	.026	1.33, 4.09
Nonsusceptible						
No ad effect						
Low score	1.59	.031	1.03, 3.12	2.55	.021	1.23, 4.31
High score	2.09	.020	1.16, 4.21	3.29	.001	1.97, 6.02
Susceptible						
No ad effect						
Low score	1.76	.021	1.07, 3.19	1.24	.052	0.43, 3.18
High score	1.87	.017	1.19, 3.65	1.38	.043	0.91, 3.22
No parent smokes						
No ad effect						
Low score	1.36	.046	0.87, 2.43	1.64	.040	1.19, 2.89
High score	2.04	.022	1.07, 4.17	1.79	.029	1.26, 3.01
Parent smokes						
No ad effect						
Low score	1.21	.073	0.53, 3.32	1.99	.017	1.19, 3.33
High score	1.29	.079	0.61, 3.36	2.10	.011	1.24, 4.11

Note. The remaining independent variables were controlled. OR = odds ratio; CI = confidence interval.

portant, because we do not know what might have occurred if any of the campaign characteristics had been altered. For example, the same effect might not have been achieved with a different message theme or less youth involvement. The data demonstrate that, within the context of the campaign's parameters, significant outcomes were achieved.

Third, our measurements of the outcome variable were different from those used in other recent analyses examining much longer term effects.[13,14] Yet, our results are consistent with the results reported in these investigations. Both recent studies documenting media effects have assessed these effects over a period of several years using time 1 data collected over a longer period of time. Both studies used the 100-cigarettes-in-a-lifetime criterion (at time 2) to measure progression to dependence. Our measure of established use captures movement toward dependence in a clearly defined time frame; it approximates the measures used in these studies, with the major difference being our shorter term period of observation. Given this, and the somewhat different ages observed, one would expect our effects to be larger than those reported in the earlier studies, and this is the case. Along with these differences in measurement of outcome variables, differences in measurement of advertisements might have contributed to the effect differences observed.

Finally, the adjusted odds ratios showed that although the campaign had an effect on both sexes, less of an effect was required to influence young women than young men. While we do not have data to directly address this issue, it is possible that the effect of the "truth" campaign on young men continues to be weakened, in part, by the influence of cigarette advertising that emphasizes male images and legitimates masculinity in terms of risk taking. The adjusted odds ratios also suggest that the campaign was more effective in preventing smoking initiation among youths without parents who smoked than among youths with a parent who smoked. However, the data show that progression to established smoking was affected by the campaign independently of whether or not a parent smoked. This suggests that the availability of cigarettes (in the home) or the role modeling of parents offset the campaign's effects on experimentation but not on progression to established use. □

Contributors

D. F. Sly designed the follow-up survey methodology, participated in data analysis, and prepared the original draft manuscript. R. S. Hopkins participated in the study design, data analysis, and final draft preparation. E. Trapido assisted in questionnaire development and data analysis. S. Ray assisted in questionnaire construction and coordinated the data collection and statistical analysis teams.

Acknowledgments

This research was supported by contracts from the Office of Tobacco Control, Florida Department of Health.

We wish to express our appreciation to Jeffrey McKenna and Terry F. Pechacek for comments on an earlier version of this paper.

References

1. *Best Practices for Comprehensive Tobacco Control Programs.* Atlanta, Ga: National Center for Chronic Disease Prevention and Health Promotion, Office on Smoking and Health; 1999.
2. Columbia Marketing Panel. Tobacco counter-marketing strategy recommendations. Paper presented at: Fifth Annual National Conference on Tobacco and Health; August 1999; Kissimmee, Fla.
3. Simon-Morton BG, Davis CA, Haynie DL, Saylor KE, Eitelp P, Yu K. Health communication in the prevention of alcohol, tobacco, and drug use. *Health Educ Behav.* 1995;5:544–554.
4. *The National Youth Anti-Drug Media Campaign: Communication Strategy Statement.* Washington, DC: Office of National Drug Control Policy; 1998.
5. McKenna J, Williams K. Crafting effective tobacco counter-advertisements: lessons from a failed campaign directed at teenagers. *Public Health Rep.* 1993;108(suppl 1):85–89.
6. Sly DF, Heald G, Hopkins RS, Moore T, McClosky M, Ray S. The industry manipulation attitudes of smokers and nonsmokers. *J Public Health Manage Pract.* 2000;6:49–56.
7. McKenna J, Gutierrez K, McCall K. Strategies for an effective youth counter-marketing program: recommendations from commercial marketing experts. *J Public Health Manage Pract.* 2000;6:7–13.
8. Goldman L, Glantz S. Evaluation of antismoking advertising campaigns. *JAMA.* 1998;297: 772–777.
9. Flay B. *Selling the Smokeless Society: Fifty-Six Evaluated Mass Media Programs and Campaigns Worldwide.* Washington, DC: American Public Health Association; 1987.
10. Bauman K, Padgett C, Koch G. A media based campaign to encourage personal communication among adolescents about not smoking cigarettes: participation, selection and consequences. *Health Educ Res.* 1989;4:35–44.

11. Murray D, Price P, Luepker RV, Pallonen U. Five- and six-year follow-up results from four seventh grade smoking prevention strategies. *J Behav Med.* 1989;12:207–218.
12. Bauman K, Laprelle J, Brown J, Koch G, Padgett C. The influence of three mass media campaigns on variables related to adolescent cigarette smoking: results of a field experiment. *Am J Public Health.* 1991;81:597–604.
13. Popham W, Potter L, Hetrick M, Muthen L, Duerr J, Johnson M. Effectiveness of the California 1990–1991 tobacco education media campaign. *Am J Prev Med.* 1994;10:319–326.
14. Siegel M, Biener L. The impact of an antismoking media campaign on progression to established smoking: results of a longitudinal youth study. *Am J Public Health.* 2000;90: 380–386.
15. *Florida v American Tobacco Company,* Civil Action 95–1466 AH (Fl Cir 1997).
16. Zucker D, Hopkins RS, Sly DF, Urich J, Kershaw JM, Solari S. Florida's "truth" campaign: a counter-marketing, anti-tobacco media campaign. *J Public Health Manage Pract.* 2000; 6:1–6.
17. Sly DF, Heald G. *Florida Anti-Tobacco Media Evaluation: One Year Assessment With National Comparisons.* Miami, Fla: Tobacco Research and Evaluation Coordinating Center, University of Miami; 1999.
18. Sly DF, Heald G, Ray S. The Florida "truth" anti-tobacco media evaluation: design, first year results and implications for planning future state media evaluations. *Tob Control.* In press.
19. Bauer UE, Johnson TM, Hopkins RS, Brooks RG. Changes in youth cigarette use and intentions following implementation of a tobacco control program: findings from the Florida Youth Tobacco Survey, 1998–2000. *JAMA.* 2000;284: 723–728.
20. Sly DF, Heald G. *Smoking-Related Behavioral Change and Maintenance During the "Truth" Campaign: Follow-Up Survey Results.* Miami, Fla: Tobacco Research and Evaluation Coordinating Center, University of Miami; 1999.

The Relation Between Community Bans of Self-Service Tobacco Displays and Store Environment and Between Tobacco Accessibility and Merchant Incentives

| Rebecca E. Lee, PhD, Ellen C. Feighery, RN, MS, Nina C. Schleicher, PhD, and Sonia Halvorson, BA

Objectives. These studies investigated (1) the effect of community bans of self-service tobacco displays on store environment and (2) the effect of consumer tobacco accessibility on merchants.

Methods. We counted cigarette displays (self-service, clerk-assisted, clear acrylic case) in 586 California stores. Merchant interviews (N = 198) identified consumer tobacco accessibility, tobacco company incentives, and shoplifting.

Results. Stores in communities with self-service tobacco display bans had fewer self-service displays and more acrylic displays but an equal total number of displays. The merchants who limited consumer tobacco accessibility received fewer incentives and reported lower shoplifting losses. In contrast, consumer access to tobacco was unrelated to the amount of monetary incentives.

Conclusions. Community bans decreased self-service tobacco displays; however, exposure to tobacco advertising in acrylic displays remained high. Reducing consumer tobacco accessibility may reduce shoplifting. (*Am J Public Health.* 2001;91:2019–2021)

In-store self-service tobacco displays are aimed at increasing product availability, visibility, and brand awareness and stimulating trial and purchase of products.[1] Self-service displays ensure direct consumer access to products while featuring tobacco advertisements. In addition to branding on products, cigarette displays show an average of 4 branded advertising signs[2] and usually are located by the checkout counter, exposing all shoppers to tobacco advertising.

Many communities have adopted self-service display bans to limit youth access to tobacco via illegal sales and shoplifting.[3,4] Bans are viewed unfavorably by some merchants who fear loss of incentives from tobacco companies.[5] Nearly two thirds of the merchants who own small stores reported receiving tobacco industry incentives.[6] Tobacco companies pay incentives for the placement of displays to increase sales.[3,7] Despite the potential loss of incentives, some merchants support elimination of self-service displays to reduce losses from shoplifting.[3] Up to 50% of youth smokers have shoplifted cigarettes at least once.[8] Stores with counter self-service displays may be nearly 40% more likely to experience shoplifting than are those without counter displays.[8]

Self-service display bans may reduce youth access; however, little is known about the effect of the bans on the in-store advertising environment. A study of 3 communities found that clear acrylic, Plexiglas-like displays replaced self-service displays in stores in communities with a self-service display ban.[5] The acrylic displays are the same size as self-service displays, sit on the checkout counter, display "packs" of cigarettes, and feature multiple branded advertising signs. However, these displays do not serve the same function as self-service displays, because the cigarette packs are enclosed in a clear acrylic case, which renders them inaccessible. Acrylic displays comply with self-service bans by eliminating direct consumer access to cigarettes, yet they ensure in-store tobacco brand advertising.[9]

The 2 studies presented here, first, documented the relation between community self-service display bans and the in-store environment and, second, investigated the relation of the in-store environment to merchant incentives and shoplifting. In study 1, we counted and coded tobacco displays in a sample of stores in California communities with and without self-service tobacco display bans. The purpose of the study was to document how bans affect the use of tobacco displays. Tobacco industry documents have asserted that merchants who allow direct consumer access to tobacco (e.g., self-service displays) receive tobacco company incentives; thus, despite merchant concerns about shoplifting, it may be *less* profitable for merchants to limit consumer access to tobacco cigarettes.[7] In study 2, we interviewed merchants to compare, in terms of tobacco incentives and shoplifting, stores that offer direct consumer access to tobacco products with stores in which merchants kept all tobacco products behind the counter.

STUDY 1: SELF-SERVICE VS ACRYLIC DISPLAYS

Methods

Tobacco advertising observations were completed in 586 stores drawn from a random sample of California stores that sold tobacco as part of a previous investigation of tobacco marketing in retail outlets.[10] The sample included 69 large markets, 164 small stores (3 or fewer cash registers), 148 convenience stores with or without gasoline, 53 gasoline stations, 113 liquor stores, and 39 drug stores or pharmacies. Displays were defined as free-standing racks provided by cigarette manufacturers containing cigarettes and branded signs. Displays were coded as self-serve if the consumer could directly access the cigarettes without clerk assistance, clerk-assist if clerk assistance was required to access cigarettes, or acrylic if the display was enclosed in clear acrylic and neither consumer nor clerk could access the cigarettes. A list of communities with self-service tobacco display bans was secured from the Americans for Non-Smokers Rights (http://www.no-smoke.org).

Analyses examined how bans affected cigarette display use. All stores were classified by

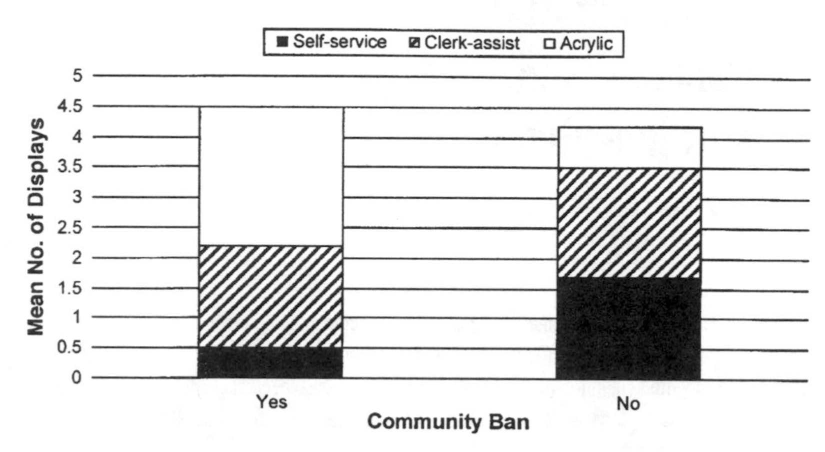

FIGURE 1—Type of tobacco display in stores, by community ban status: California, 2000.

their community ban status (no ban vs ban). A χ^2 analysis determined whether the proportion of stores featuring self-service displays was lower in communities with self-service display bans compared with communities without bans. We performed *t* tests to determine the relation between community self-service display policy and different kinds of displays.

Results

Fourteen percent (n=82) of the stores were located in communities with self-service display bans, and 86% (n=504) were located in communities without bans. Of those stores in communities with bans, 16% (n=13) had at least 1 self-service display, in violation of local bans. In communities without bans, significantly more (40%, n=200) stores featured self-service displays (χ^2_1=8.4, P<.05).

Figure 1 presents the mean number of displays per store by self-service ban status. Stores in communities with bans had significantly fewer self-service displays (mean=0.5) than did stores in communities without bans (mean=1.7, t_{584}=3.6, P<.001). Stores in communities with bans had about the same number of clerk-assist displays (mean=1.7) as stores in communities without bans (mean=1.8, P=.723). In contrast, stores in communities with bans had significantly more acrylic displays (mean=2.3) than did stores in communities without bans (mean=0.7, t_{584}=7.9, P<.001). Community self-service ban status was not related to the overall number of displays in a store; stores in both ban (mean=4.5) and no-ban (mean=4.2) communities had about the same number of total displays (P=.576).

STUDY 2: TOBACCO PLACEMENT AND MERCHANT INCENTIVES

Methods

Following completion of the in-store advertising surveys described in study 1, stores were contacted by telephone, and research staff interviewed the store employee who was responsible for negotiating contracts with sales representatives. If store negotiations were performed at the corporate level, then the store was ineligible for the merchant interview. Calls eliminated 466 stores that either did not meet eligibility criteria or whose responsible employee was not available for an interview, so the in-store advertising survey sample was augmented with 78 merchant interviews drawn from a list of 461 stores obtained from a leading provider of store lists for the marketing research industry. Interviews were completed at a total of 198 stores that represented large markets (n=11), small stores (n=65), convenience stores with or without gasoline (n=62), gasoline stations (n=20), and liquor stores (n=40).

Trained staff members conducted merchant interviews in English. A university internal review board approved all procedures. Merchants reported whether they stocked cigarettes and tobacco on self-service displays or on shelves accessible to consumers or whether they kept all cigarettes and tobacco products behind the counter, inaccessible to consumers. Merchants reported whether they received any incentives from tobacco companies, including discounted products, free goods with an order, "buy downs" (the manufacturer refunds the merchant for products they have on hand to lower prices of current stock), or money. If merchants received money, they were asked how much money they had received in the past 3 months. Merchants also reported the amount of money lost in a typical month from shoplifting of tobacco.

We performed *t* tests and χ^2 analyses to assess the relation of direct consumer access to tobacco products to merchant incentives and shoplifting.

Results

Most merchants (57%) reported receiving incentives and money (37%) from tobacco companies. Table 1 presents incentives, money received, and shoplifting by placement of tobacco. Merchants in stores with self-service tobacco displays were more likely to receive incentives (χ^2_1=8.0, P=.005) and money (χ^2_1=5.9, P=.015) than were merchants in stores with all tobacco behind the counter. However, the amount of money received from tobacco companies did not differ for merchants with and without self-service tobacco (t_{71}=1.2, P=.233). The amount of money lost to shoplifting was more than 3 times greater in stores with self-service tobacco (t_{70}=–4.9, P<.001).

DISCUSSION

The goals of the 2 studies were to document the relation of community self-service tobacco display bans to the in-store environment and to investigate the relation of the in-store environment to merchant incentives and shoplifting. Community bans limit self-service displays; however, our findings suggest that bans do not reduce the amount of tobacco brand advertising on acrylic displays. In study 2, more stores with consumer-accessible tobacco received incentives; however, actual amounts of money that stores received did

TABLE 1—Incentives, Money Received, and Shoplifting in Stores With Self-Service Tobacco vs All Tobacco Behind the Counter[a]: California, 2000

	Self-Service Tobacco (n = 57)	Tobacco Behind the Counter (n = 141)	Total Sample (N = 198)
Received tobacco incentives**	73.2%	51.1%	56.6%
Received tobacco money*	54.9%	35.2%	36.9%
Amount of money received in past 3 months, mean (SD)	$258 ($449)	$226 ($489)	$236 ($477)
Money lost to shoplifting in typical month,** mean (SD)	$100 ($100)	$29 ($57)	$50 ($78)

[a]Self-reported.
*$P < .05$; **$P < .01$.

not differ as a function of the location of tobacco products, and losses from shoplifting were substantially higher in stores with direct consumer access to tobacco.[3,7,8]

Tobacco industry documents state that visibility and brand awareness are important goals of tobacco advertising,[1] and tobacco control policies are needed to effectively combat these goals. The amount of advertising on displays in stores remains unchanged in the face of bans, because acrylic displays replace the advertising typically found on self-service displays. Acrylic displays function solely as advertising, accomplishing key goals of the tobacco industry. This finding suggests that brand displays are designed to spur sales to stimulate and maintain use of cigarettes.

Policymakers who regulate the in-store environment will need to partner with merchants to ameliorate concerns that may arise from the higher reported frequency of incentives given to merchants with direct access to tobacco. Despite these reports, actual *amounts* of money received were not related to tobacco access. Consistent with other reports,[3,8] another important benefit of community bans was that stores without direct consumer access to tobacco lost far less (more than 3 times less) money from shoplifting than did stores with consumer access. Merchants report that tobacco industry advertising produces a "cluttered" appearance in their stores.[3] A desire for reduced shoplifting losses and a clean-looking store may outweigh incentives from tobacco companies. These positive points may be useful in persuading merchants to eliminate tobacco displays.

These data were drawn from California, and our surveys had a high refusal or unreachable rate. Our data may not be generalizable to tobacco promotion in other locations, and inferences must be made with caution. We were unable to examine the direct relation between community bans and merchant incentives, because we excluded many corporately owned stores in study 2. Research is needed to document this relation and to investigate how corporate negotiations may affect tobacco advertising and merchant incentives. Last, our merchant incentive interviews relied on self-reports that may have overestimated or underestimated incentives or shoplifting.

The use of acrylic displays appears to be a strategy by tobacco companies to satisfy self-service display bans while maintaining advertising exposure. We found that acrylic displays provide a mechanism for prominent tobacco advertising at the point of sale. Research is needed to document and define other effects of acrylic displays on shoppers. Our results call into question claims that self-service bans will reduce net profits by reducing tobacco industry paid incentives and suggest that greater regulation may be needed to reduce unwitting exposure to tobacco advertising. ■

About the Authors

Rebecca E. Lee is with the Department of Preventive Medicine, University of Kansas School of Medicine, Kansas City. Ellen C. Feighery is with the Public Health Institute, Half Moon Bay, Calif. Nina C. Schleicher is with the California Polytechnic State University, San Luis Obispo. Sonia Halvorson is with the Stanford Center for Research in Disease Prevention, Stanford University School of Medicine, Stanford, Calif.

Requests for reprints should be sent to Rebecca E. Lee, PhD, Department of Preventive Medicine, University of Kansas School of Medicine, 3901 Rainbow Blvd, Kansas City, KS 66160 (e-mail: relee@kumc.edu).

This article was accepted June 29, 2001.

Contributors

E.C. Feighery conceived of the study and supervised all aspects of its implementation. S. Halvorson assisted with the study and completed the analyses. R.E. Lee synthesized analyses and led the writing of the paper. N.C. Schleicher assisted with the study and analyses. All authors helped to conceptualize ideas, interpret findings, and review drafts of the paper.

Acknowledgments

This study was made possible by funds received from the Tobacco Tax Health Protection Act of 1988—Proposition 99 through the California Department of Health Services under contract 94-20967-A04 and supported in part by an institutional grant (HL 58914) from the National Heart, Lung, and Blood Institute.

The authors gratefully acknowledge Kurt Ribisl, PhD, for his thoughtful comments and suggestions on the paper.

References

1. RJ Reynolds Tobacco Co. *New Product Introduction Through Point-of-Purchase.* Bates #500164188-500164208; 1978. Available at: http://www.tobaccodocuments.org. Accessed October11, 2001.
2. Feighery EC. A study of tobacco ads, retailer incentives and sales to minors in four central California communities. Report to the California Department of Health Services, Tobacco Control Section; 2000.
3. Wildey MB, Woodruff SI, Pampalone SZ, Conway TL. Self-service sale of tobacco: how it contributes to youth access. *Tob Control.* 1995;4:355–361.
4. *Reducing Tobacco Use: A Report of the Surgeon General.* Atlanta, Ga: National Center for Chronic Disease Prevention and Health Promotion, Office on Smoking and Health; 2000.
5. Bidell MP, Furlong MJ, Dunn DM, Koegler JE. Case study of attempts to enact self service tobacco display ordinances: a tale of three communities. *Tob Control.* 2000;9:1–77.
6. Feighery EC, Ribisl KM, Achabal DD, Tyebjee T. Retail trade incentives: how tobacco industry practices compare with those of other industries. *Am J Public Health.* 1999;89:1564–1566.
7. RJ Reynolds Tobacco Co. *Pilferage Presentation.* Bates #51434-8983; 1976. Available at: http://www.tobaccodocuments.org. Accessed October11, 2001.
8. Caldwell MC, Wysell MC, Kawachi I. Self-service tobacco displays and consumer theft. *Tob Control.* 1996;5:160–161.
9. UICC GLOBALink The International Tobacco Control Network. Legislation on underage sales of tobacco [bulletin board posting]. Available at: http://www.globalink.org. Accessed March 15, 2000.
10. Feighery EC, Ribisl KM, Schleicher N, Lee RE, Halvorson S. The tobacco industry's use of retail advertising and promotions: a statewide survey of California stores. *Tob Control.* 2001;10:184–188.

Counteracting Tobacco Motor Sports Sponsorship as a Promotional Tool: Is the Tobacco Settlement Enough?

Michael Siegel, MD, MPH

ABSTRACT

Objectives. This study sought to quantify television advertising exposure achieved by tobacco companies through sponsorship of motor sports events and to evaluate the likely effect of the Master Settlement Agreement on this advertising.

Methods. Data from *Sponsors Report*, which quantifies the exposure that sponsors of selected televised sporting events receive during broadcasts of those events, were compiled for all motor sports events covered by the service for the period 1997 through 1999.

Results. From 1997 through 1999, tobacco companies achieved 169 hours of television advertising exposure and \$410.5 million of advertising value for their products by sponsoring motor sports events. If tobacco companies comply with the Master Settlement Agreement and maintain their advertising at 1999 levels, they will still be able to achieve more than 25 hours of television exposure and an equivalent television advertising value of \$99.1 million per year.

Conclusions. Despite a federal ban on tobacco advertising on television, tobacco companies achieve the equivalent of more than \$150 million in television advertising per year through their sponsorship of motor sports events. The Master Settlement Agreement likely will do little to address this problem. (*Am J Public Health.* 2001;91:1100–1106)

Corporate sponsorship of special events is well recognized in the marketing literature as an important component of product promotion.[1–3] Sports sponsorship, in particular, is an important and effective promotional tool.[2,4–8] The tobacco industry has used sports sponsorship effectively to promote its products, largely by achieving television advertising exposure for its cigarette and smokeless tobacco brands in a way that circumvents the federal prohibition of tobacco advertising on television.[9–28] The sponsorship of televised motor sports events has been the primary tool used by tobacco companies to achieve continued television exposure for their brands in the presence of the television advertising ban.[20–28]

In 1998, US cigarette companies spent \$125.6 million on sports sponsorship and related promotional efforts.[29] The sponsorship of motor sports events constitutes approximately 70% of tobacco sponsorship expenditures.[30] The multistate settlement with the tobacco industry attempted to contain the promotion of tobacco through sports sponsorships by limiting each tobacco company to 1 brand-name sponsorship of a sporting event or series per year.[31] This restriction goes into effect on November 23, 2001.

In this article, I evaluate the likely effectiveness of the tobacco settlement in counteracting the effects of tobacco motor sports sponsorship by describing and analyzing the television advertising value achieved by tobacco companies through motor sports sponsorship from 1997 through 1999 and analyzing the television advertising value that tobacco companies would achieve by complying with the provisions of the Master Settlement Agreement.

In the marketing literature, the primary reason given for corporations to undertake sports sponsorships is to achieve television exposure for their companies or brands.[4] Among the established techniques for evaluating the effect of sports sponsorships is studying the extent of media coverage, including the dollar equivalent of free advertising achieved.[2,5–8] The *Sponsors Report*, based in Ann Arbor, Mich, specializes in valuing motor sports sponsorships by analyzing televised events and quantifying the amount of in-focus exposure time and number of verbal mentions for each company and brand sponsor.[32] Multiplying the in-focus exposure time by the individual broadcast's commercial advertising rate yields a dollar value for the television advertising each sponsor achieves. *Sponsors Report* clients use this information to evaluate the effect of their sponsorships.[32]

Although cigarette advertising on television has been prohibited since 1971,[33] and smokeless tobacco advertising on television has been prohibited since 1984,[34] several studies have reported that tobacco companies have circumvented these bans by sponsoring motor sports events and achieving television exposure of their brand names or logos.[20–24,28] However, the existing data have 2 major limitations. First, no recent data are available. The most recent published data on tobacco advertising through televised motor sports events are for the year 1993,[20,24] and only a newspaper article mentions data for 1 automobile race from 1996.[28] Second, previous studies have tended to report overall exposure data; data broken down by specific race series as well as specific brands have been limited.

A considerable body of research suggests that tobacco sports sponsorship may influence youth smoking attitudes and behavior.[35–43] This research has found that cigarette sports sponsorship has profound effects on brand awareness,[35,36,39–41] perceived connections between brands and sport,[35–38,40,42] associations between

Requests for reprints should be sent to Michael Siegel, MD, MPH, Boston University School of Public Health, Social and Behavioral Sciences Department, 715 Albany St, TW2, Boston, MA 02118 (e-mail: mbsiegel@bu.edu).

This article was accepted February 23, 2001.

cigarette brands and excitement,[35] attitudes about smoking,[39,42,43] and smoking behavior.[41,42]

Given the widespread television advertising exposure achieved by tobacco companies through sponsorship of motor sports, and given the evidence for an effect of this sponsorship on youth smoking attitudes and behavior, addressing tobacco motor sports sponsorship should be an important public health strategy. The attorneys general who negotiated the multistate settlement with the tobacco companies addressed this issue, and the resulting Master Settlement Agreement contains provisions that limit tobacco companies to a single brand-name sponsorship of a racing series per year.[31] But few, if any, published data are available to evaluate the likely effect of this provision on exposure to television advertising for tobacco products. For example, it is not clear how much television advertising is currently achieved by tobacco companies through sponsorship of a single racing series.

In this article, I present a current, comprehensive analysis of tobacco motor sports sponsorship in the United States. I provide (1) a complete picture of brand-specific television advertising exposure achieved by cigarette and smokeless tobacco companies through sponsorship of motor sports events during the period 1997 through 1999 and (2) data on tobacco advertising achieved through motor sports sponsorship, broken down by brand and racing series, to evaluate the likely effect of the Master Settlement Agreement's limitations on tobacco company sponsorship.

Methods

Data Sources

A service of Joyce Julius and Associates (Ann Arbor, Mich), *Sponsors Report* quantifies the exposure that sponsors of selected televised sporting events receive during broadcasts of those events.[32] The service covers most nationally televised motor sports events for racing series that originate in the United States.

Sponsors Report measures the national television exposure achieved by event sponsors by calculating the clear, in-focus exposure time (the time that a sponsor's name or logo can be readily identified by an unbiased viewer) during the event broadcast for each sponsor's company or brand name or logo. The number of verbal mentions of each sponsor during the broadcast is also recorded. The dollar value of the advertising exposure realized through the appearance and verbal mention of sponsor names and logos on television is estimated by multiplying the clear, in-focus exposure time by the individual broadcast's nondiscounted or estimated cost for commercial advertising. The broadcast's advertising cost per 30 seconds is used to generate a value per second, and this figure is multiplied by the number of seconds of in-focus exposure time. Verbal mentions are valued at 10 seconds each, and this time is combined with the in-focus exposure time in deriving an advertising dollar value.

Thus, the exposure value determined by *Sponsors Report* is an approximation of the amount a sponsor would have to pay to achieve the same exposure time via a paid television advertisement during that broadcast. *Sponsors Report* also estimates race attendance and total television viewing audience. The data in *Sponsors Report* have become the industry standard for measuring the television exposure value of sports sponsorship. No other service provides this information.

We obtained from *Sponsors Report* the comprehensive motor sports packages for 1997, 1998, and 1999. The package includes all *Sponsors Report* event issues that the research staff compiled during this time. These reports include data for 11 automobile racing series during each of the 3 years. The total number of automobile racing events covered in our data was 205 for 1997, 216 for 1998, and 211 for 1999 (632 races for all 3 years combined), and the total number of television broadcasts was 599 for 1997, 547 for 1998, and 600 for 1999 (1746 broadcasts for all 3 years combined). The number of broadcasts exceeds the number of events because some networks air replays of the events.

Data Extraction

We extracted from the *Sponsors Report* data the event audience and television viewing audience for each race in each of the racing series. We also extracted the total in-focus exposure time, number of verbal mentions, and equivalent advertising dollar value for each tobacco sponsor reported for each racing series. We summed these values over each racing series and year to obtain estimates of the brand-specific advertising value achieved for each cigarette and smokeless tobacco brand for each racing series and year and of the total event audience and television viewing audience for each racing series and year.

Note that the sum of event audiences given for each racing series likely represents unduplicated audiences (i.e., distinct individuals) because the events tended to take place in different geographic locations. However, the sum of event audiences across different racing series and the sum of television audiences represent a duplicated audience estimate (i.e., not distinct individuals). Many of the same individuals probably view multiple automobile races; thus, for example, a total viewing audience of 50 million for a racing series does not mean that 50 million different people viewed an event but that the total of the individual viewing audiences for each event is 50 million.

Results

In 1999, the 11 racing series in our study comprised 211 events and 600 broadcasts that were televised by 10 networks (3 broadcast and 7 cable stations). The races were attended by a total of 17.3 million people (average of approximately 82 000 per race) and watched on television by an average of 2.4 million viewers per race (Table 1). The average television audience per race ranged from 300 000 for the Indy Lights Championship to 6.8 million for the National Association of Stock Car Auto Racing (NASCAR) Winston Cup series. Tobacco companies achieved a total of $156.8 million of advertising exposure through these races. The highest tobacco advertising value achieved within a single racing series was $100.0 million for the NASCAR Winston Cup series.

During 1999, nine brands of cigarettes and smokeless tobacco products achieved a total television exposure time of 56 hours and 54 minutes and a total of 8408 verbal mentions through the 11 racing series in our study (Table 2). The greatest exposure time (22 hours, 11 minutes, 44 seconds) and number of verbal mentions (3462) were achieved through the NASCAR Winston Cup series. The greatest advertising exposure achieved by a single brand within a single racing series was the 19 hours, 29 minutes, and 40 seconds of advertising exposure; 3345 verbal mentions; and $87.9 million of advertising value achieved by Winston through the NASCAR Winston Cup series.

During the period 1997 through 1999, tobacco products achieved between 55 and 57 hours of television exposure per year and between $123 million and $157 million in television advertising value per year through motor sports sponsorship, for a total of 169 hours of exposure and $410.5 million of advertising value during the 3-year period (Table 3). Brands with the highest achieved television advertising value during this period were Winston ($305.8 million), Skoal ($32.2 million), Marlboro ($22.1 million), and Kool ($18.1 million).

The analysis of the effect of the Master Settlement Agreement on achieved television advertising of cigarettes showed that if the 3 cigarette companies that currently sponsor motor sports comply with the settlement by restricting themselves to the sponsorship of 1

TABLE 1—Televised Motor Sports Series: Audience Statistics and Equivalent Dollar Value of Tobacco Advertising, 1999

Racing Series	Networks	No. of Races (No. of Telecasts)	Total Viewing Audience, Millions	Average Viewing Audience per Race, Millions	Total Attendance, Millions	Average Attendance per Race	Equivalent Dollar Value of Tobacco Advertising, Millions	Tobacco Advertising Value as Percentage of Total Value for All Sponsors
NASCAR Winston Cup	ABC, CBS, NBC, TNN, TBS, ESPN/2	34 (108)	230.6	6.8	4.4	130088	100.0	7.0
NASCAR Busch	ABC, CBS, NBC, TNN, TBS, ESPN/2	32 (81)	81.6	2.5	1.9	58208	18.3	3.1
CART Championship	ABC, ESPN, ESPN2	20 (40)	42.5	2.1	2.5	126208	11.5	5.4
Special events[a]	CBS, TNN, SUN, FOXSP, ESPN/2	8 (13)	14.1	1.8	0.4	52625	11.3	19.7
NHRA Winston Drag Racing	ABC, TNN, FOXSP, SPDV, ESPN/2	23 (108)	30.3[b]	1.3[b]	2.3	101172	10.6	10.0
NASCAR Truck	ABC, CBS, ESPN/2	25 (66)	33.5	1.3	0.9	34184	2.9	1.5
ARCA Series	TNN, TBS, SPDV, FOXSP, ESPN/2	20 (48)	19.8	1.0	0.6	29455	1.4	3.7
Indy Racing League	ABC, FOXSP, ESPN/2	12 (17)	18.8	1.6	0.8	67500	0.7	0.5
Indy Lights Championship	ESPN2	12 (25)	3.9	0.3	1.4	112775	0.1	2.9
SCCA Trans-Am	TNN, FOXSP, SPDV	13 (50)	18.4	1.4	1.1	81304	0.01	0.1
Barber Dodge Pro Series	ESPN2	12 (44)	4.7	0.4	1.1	89213	0.006	0.4
Total (11 series)	10 networks	211 (600)	498.3	2.4	17.3	81954	156.8	5.6

Note. NASCAR=National Association of Stock Car Auto Racing; ESPN/2=ESPN and ESPN2; SPDV=Speedvision; FOXSP=Fox Sports Network; SUN=Sunshine Network; CART=Championship Auto Racing Team; NHRA=National-Hot Rod Association; ARCA=Automobile Racing Club of America; SCCA=Sports Car Club of America.

[a]Includes The Winston and selected races from the NASCAR Slim Jim All Pro Series, Featherlite Modified Tour Series, and Busch North Series.

[b]Viewer audience figures for NHRA Winston Cup Series indicate the number of households viewing the event; data on number of individual viewers were not available for this series.

racing series per year (and choose as their brand-name sponsorship the event series for which they achieved the greatest advertising value in 1999), the total achieved television advertising value per year by the 3 companies will be $99.1 million, or 70.4% of the actual 1999 advertising value achieved by these companies (Table 4). R.J. Reynolds, through Winston sponsorship of the NASCAR Winston Cup series, could continue to achieve a television advertising value of $87.9 million, or 68.1% of the company's current achieved advertising value. Brown & Williamson, through Kool sponsorship of a Championship Auto Racing Team, could continue to achieve a television advertising value of $8.4 million, or 99.3% of the company's current achieved advertising value. Philip Morris, through Marlboro sponsorship of a Championship Auto Racing Team, could continue to achieve a television advertising value of $2.8 million, or 86.8% of the company's current achieved advertising value. The companies would still achieve more than 25 hours of exposure and 3408 verbal mentions for their cigarette brands per year. This analysis assumes, of course, that companies do not increase their advertising presence at these racing series.

Discussion

To the best of my knowledge, this is the first systematic evaluation since 1993 of tobacco television advertising achieved through motor sports sponsorship in the United States. Despite a federal ban on the advertising of tobacco products on television, during the period 1997 through 1999, tobacco companies were able to achieve 169 hours of television advertising exposure and $410.5 million of advertising value for their products by sponsoring televised motor sports events. Although the Federal Trade Commission (FTC) does not collect data on this embedded television advertising, the $123.3 million in television advertising achieved by tobacco companies in 1997 represents 21% of the total reported cigarette advertising expenditures through newspapers, magazines, outdoor advertisements, and transit advertisements for that same year ($575.7 million).[29] The $156.8 million in television advertising value achieved by tobacco companies in 1999 represents 76% of their television advertising budget in 1970 in nominal dollars ($205.0 million)[29] and 18% of their 1970 television advertising budget in real dollars.

Not only are tobacco companies successful in achieving a high level of tobacco advertising for their products, but also the potential exposure to this advertising is great. In 1999, a total of 17.3 million people (average of 82000 per race) attended the 211 races in our sample, and these events were viewed on television by an average of 2.4 million people per race.

The Master Settlement Agreement limits each cigarette company to 1 brand-name sponsorship of a racing series per year, beginning in November 2001.[31] Although the settlement was widely reported to have limited each company to sponsorship of a single event,[44,45] the text of the agreement states that "sponsorship of a single national or multi-state series or tour . . . constitutes one Brand Name Sponsorship."[31] My analysis of the potential effect of this settlement provision indicates that if the cigarette companies comply with the provision and also do not increase their advertising presence at races from 1999 levels, the companies still will be able to achieve a combined total of more than 25 hours of television exposure, more than 3000 verbal mentions, and an equivalent annual television advertising value that represents over 70% of the 1999 advertising value. Thus, the tobacco settlement is unlikely to have any major effect on the marketing of cigarettes

TABLE 2—Televised Motor Sports Series Achieved Tobacco Advertising, Total and by Most Advertised Brand: 1999

Racing Series	Tobacco Brands Advertised	Total Achieved Exposure Time, All Brands[a]	Total No. of Verbal Mentions, All Brands	Total Equivalent Advertising Dollar Value, All Brands, Millions	Two Most Heavily Advertised Brands	Total Achieved Exposure Time[a]	Total No. of Verbal Mentions	Total Equivalent Advertising Dollar Value, Millions
NASCAR Winston Cup	Camel, Kodiak, Levi Garrett, Marlboro, Skoal, Winston	22:11:44	3462	100.0	Winston	19:29:40	3345	87.9
					Skoal	01:50:05	53	7.9
NASCAR Busch	Marlboro, Red Man, Skoal, Winston	06:48:13	1506	18.3	Winston	05:43:11	1431	16.0
					Red Man	00:57:50	75	2.1
CART Championship	Camel, Kool, Marlboro, Winston	06:01:30	113	11.5	Kool	04:29:50	61	8.4
					Marlboro	01:28:37	2	2.8
Special events[b]	Skoal, Winston	01:10:40	356	11.3	Winston	01:07:15	353	10.8
					Skoal	00:03:23	0	0.4
NHRA Winston Drag Racing	Copenhagen, Kodiak, Marlboro, Skoal, Winston	14:55:03	2480	10.6	Winston	13:17:48	2369	9.9
					Copenhagen	01:20:32	111	0.6
NASCAR Truck	Kool, Marlboro, Red Man, Skoal, Winston	03:47:32	180	2.9	Winston	03:16:10	180	2.5
					Marlboro	00:10:59	0	0.1
ARCA Series	Copenhagen, Red Man, Skoal, Winston	00:47:19	264	1.4	Winston	00:46:59	261	1.4
					Red Man	00:00:00	3	0.009
Indy Racing League	Marlboro, Skoal, Winston	00:19:14	21	0.7	Winston	00:13:57	21	0.5
					Skoal	00:03:05	0	0.08
Indy Lights Championship	Kool, Marlboro, Winston	00:43:46	20	0.1	Marlboro	00:23:29	0	0.06
					Kool	00:19:37	16	0.06
SCCA Trans-Am	Marlboro, Winston	00:04:11	6	0.01	Marlboro	00:04:11	0	0.009
					Winston	00:00:00	6	0.002
Barber Dodge Pro Series	Kool, Marlboro, Red Man, Winston	00:04:48	0	0.006	Winston	00:02:32	0	0.003
					Marlboro	00:01:20	0	0.002
Total (11 series)	9 brands	56:54:00	8408	156.8	Winston	44:01:13	8020	129.1
					Skoal	02:11:02	53	8.6

Note. NASCAR = National Association of Stock Car Auto Racing; CART = Championship Auto Racing Team; NHRA = National Hot Rod Association; ARCA = Automobile Racing Club of America; SCCA = Sports Car Club of America.
[a]Exposure time is recorded in units of hours:minutes:seconds.
[b]Includes The Winston and selected races from the NASCAR Slim Jim All Pro Series, Featherlite Modified Tour Series, and Busch North Series.

TABLE 3—Tobacco Advertising Achieved Through Televised Motor Sports Events, by Brand: 1997–1999

Value, Brand	1997 Achieved Exposure Time[a]	1997 Equivalent Dollar Value, Millions	1998 Achieved Exposure Time[a]	1998 Equivalent Dollar Value, Millions	1999 Achieved Exposure Time[a]	1999 Equivalent Dollar Value, Millions	Total (1997–1999) Achieved Exposure Time[a]	Total (1997–1999) Equivalent Dolla Millions
Camel	03:12:51	11.4	00:01:05	0.05	00:00:14	0.05	03:14:10	11.5
Kool	03:35:23	1.9	06:54:04	7.8	04:49:54	8.5	15:19:21	18.1
Marlboro	12:24:17	11.9	06:38:49	7.0	02:11:29	3.2	21:14:35	22.1
Winston	31:16:22	80.4	33:25:18	96.2	44:01:13	129.1	108:42:53	305.8
Copenhagen	00:46:19	0.5	01:10:12	1.5	01:20:33	0.6	03:17:04	2.7
Kodiak	01:17:27	4.8	01:06:28	3.4	00:39:23	3.1	03:03:18	11.3
Red Man	00:19:24	0.3	00:50:50	1.2	01:03:42	2.2	02:13:56	3.7
Skoal	04:26:50	11.9	04:04:01	11.7	02:11:02	8.6	10:41:53	32.2
R.J. Reynolds	00:00:21	0.2	00:00:12	0.3	00:00:17	0.3	00:00:50	0.8
US Tobacco	00:00:00	0	00:58:46	1.2	00:36:09	1.1	01:34:55	2.2
Total[b]	57:19:26	123.3	55:09:57	130.4	56:54:00	156.8	169:23:23	410.5

[a]Exposure time is recorded in units of hours:minutes:seconds.
[b]Total slightly exceeds sum of entries in table because small amounts of advertising for Doral, Newport, and Levi Garrett are not included as table entries.

through motor sports sponsorship. Moreover, the assumption that cigarette companies would maintain advertising at current levels is unlikely to hold; even without a restriction on sponsorship, Winston has steadily increased its annual television advertising value achieved through the Winston Cup series from $57.1 million in 1997 to $87.9 million in 1999.

The Master Settlement Agreement actually may allow cigarette companies to sponsor multiple racing series, because it lists NASCAR as an example of a single racing series.[31] If this interpretation is correct, then the Master Settlement Agreement would have even less of an effect on cigarette marketing through motor sports sponsorship. For example, R.J. Reynolds could choose to continue Winston sponsorship of the NASCAR Winston Cup,

TABLE 4—Analysis of Effect of Master Settlement Agreement on Realized Television Advertising Through Motor Sports Sponsorship (Assuming No Increase in Brand-Specific Television Advertising Exposure From 1999 Levels)[a]

Company	Probable Brand Chosen	Probable Racing Series Chosen	Nature of Sponsorship	Estimated Achieved Exposure Time[b]	Estimated No. of Verbal Mentions	Estimated Equivalent Dollar Value of Advertising, Millions	Estimated Advertising Value as Percentage of Actual 1999 Value for Company[c]
R.J. Reynolds	Winston	NASCAR Winston Cup	Series/Event	19:29:40	3345	87.9	68.1
Brown & Williamson	Kool	CART Championship	Team	04:29:50	61	8.4	99.3
Philip Morris	Marlboro	CART Championship	Team	01:28:37	2	2.8	86.8
Total				25:28:07	3408	99.1	70.4

Note. NASCAR = National Association of Stock Car Auto Racing; CART = Championship Auto Racing Team.

[a]This table presents the exposure time, number of verbal mentions, and equivalent dollar value of television advertising for cigarettes that would be achieved through motor sports sponsorship if cigarette companies comply with the Master Settlement Agreement (by limiting themselves to 1 brand-name sponsorship per year) and continue their advertising presence for allowed sponsorships at their 1999 levels. It is assumed that companies would choose as their brand-name sponsorship the event series for which they achieved the greatest advertising value in 1999.

[b]Exposure time is recorded in units of hours:minutes:seconds.

[c]Actual 1999 advertising value is the total achieved television advertising value for all cigarette brands produced by that company that gained advertising exposure through televised motor sports events (R.J. Reynolds: Camel and Winston; Brown & Williamson: Kool; Philip Morris: Marlboro).

NASCAR Busch, and NASCAR Truck series. At 1999 advertising levels, the company would achieve annual television exposure of 28 hours and an advertising value of $106 million for its Winston product by sponsoring these 3 series. This represents 82% of the advertising value R.J. Reynolds achieved in 1999 for all its cigarette products through all racing series covered by *Sponsors Report.*

This study probably underestimated the true amount of television advertising value achieved by tobacco companies through sponsorship of motor sports, for several reasons. First, not every racing event or series is covered by *Sponsors Report.* For example, none of the international Formula One races are included, even though many of these races are broadcast in the United States.

Second, television shows about racing were not included in the study. For example, Blum[22] reported that during a single month (January 1989), Winston achieved more than 58 minutes of exposure through the "Inside Winston Cup" television show alone.

Third, exposure of cigarette brand names and logos through sports and racing magazines was not captured by this study. For example, a spring 2000 special issue of *ESPN The Magazine* featured a front-page picture of 2 race-car drivers with the words "Winston Cup 2000."[46] This amounted to the equivalent of a free front-page advertisement for the Winston product.

Fourth, exposure to on-site promotions and advertising that accompany tobacco-sponsored racing events was not captured by this study. The Master Settlement Agreement allows tobacco companies to continue the marketing, distribution, and sale of specialty item merchandise at the site of their chosen brand-name sponsorships and to continue outdoor and billboard advertising at the site of a brand-name sponsorship for a 3-month period around each sponsored event.[31]

Fifth, the advertising dollar equivalents reported in this article refer to only broadcasts in the United States. In some cases, motor sports events are recorded and broadcast in other countries, so that additional advertising value for the sponsorship dollar is obtained.

The results of this study are particularly alarming in light of the effect tobacco motor sports sponsorship has on youth smoking attitudes and behaviors[35–43] and the growing popularity of car racing among youths.[8,47,48] According to the *Washington Post,* "NASCAR is targeting young customers with everything from amusement parks to NASCAR Barbie, grooming its next generation of fans even as TV ratings and race-day attendance soar."[47]

One potential criticism of this research is that short, repeated exposures to brand logos on race cars may not be as effective as an uninterrupted 30-second television commercial. However, a recent study that compared brand recall following exposure to a television clip of a NASCAR race or a 30-second commercial found that brand recall and attitudes toward advertised brands were significantly better for products that appeared prominently on race cars.[49] Multiple brief exposures during a race may be more powerful than uninterrupted exposure during a commercial because people may leave the room during a commercial or may enter into conversation or become distracted.[8] In addition, people generally do not recognize sponsorship as a tool of persuasion, so they are not likely to generate counterarguments, as they may do in response to a recognized advertisement. Several studies have documented high levels of brand awareness, brand recall, and brand loyalty for sponsoring products among automobile racing fans.[8,11,50–52]

Several strategies could be used to counteract the tobacco industry's use of motor sports sponsorship as a promotional tool. As early as 1986, legislation was introduced into Congress that would have eliminated brand-name sponsorship of sporting events by tobacco companies.[24] The recently overturned Food and Drug Administration tobacco regulations also would have eliminated tobacco brand-name sponsorship of sporting events.[19] Several states in Australia have enacted legislation that eliminates tobacco sponsorship of sport and allocates a portion of cigarette tax revenues to provide an alternative source of funding for sports sponsorship.[10,53–55] Sports sponsorship itself has been used as a tool to promote health messages.[56,57] Several organizations have used automobile races to counterpromote tobacco.[23,58] A California-based project has created a tobacco-free racing car and team that competes in motor sports events.[59]

An alternative approach that does not involve the enactment of new legislation or funding of new programs is simply enforcing the provisions of the Cigarette Labeling and Advertising Act. A strong precedent exists for this: in 1996 and 1997, the Department of Justice used the act to force tobacco companies to remove cigarette billboards from more than a dozen stadiums and arenas throughout the country.[60–62] The Department of Justice obtained court orders against Philip Morris in 1995 to prevent it from placing cigarette advertisements in arenas and stadiums so that they would be in view of television cameras, and the company entered into a 10-year consent agreement to remove all signs from locations in professional baseball, basketball, football, and hockey arenas that may reasonably be expected to appear on television programs.[60–62] There is no reason that the Department of Justice could not also use the Cigarette Labeling and Advertising Act to force the removal of cigarette logos and advertisements from locations likely to appear on television during automobile racing events. A legal ruling exists that supports the authority of the Department of Justice to address the problem of tobacco company circumvention of the Cigarette Labeling and Advertising Act through embedded television commercials.[63]

A precedent also exists for the FTC to enforce the ban on television advertising of smokeless tobacco products contained in the Comprehensive Smokeless Tobacco Health Education Act of 1986.[64,65] In 1991, the FTC entered into a consent agreement with Pinkerton Tobacco Company, in which the company agreed to discontinue advertising smokeless tobacco products on television by placing its brand name and logo in areas likely to be viewed by television cameras during sponsored truck and tractor events.[64,65] There appears to be no reason that the FTC could not take similar action with regard to the widespread smokeless tobacco product advertising on television achieved through motor sports sponsorship documented in this study.

This study found that despite a federal ban on tobacco advertising on television, tobacco companies achieve the equivalent of more than $150 million in television advertising per year through their sponsorship of televised motor sports events and that the Master Settlement Agreement likely will do little to address this problem. If public health practitioners are serious about reducing tobacco use, they must find an effective way to counteract this major form of tobacco product promotion. □

Acknowledgments

This work was supported by Research Project Grant RPG-98-264-01-PBP from the American Cancer Society.

References

1. Gardener MP, Shuman PJ. Sponsorship: an important component of the promotions mix. *J Advertising.* 1987;16:11–17.
2. Mescon TS, Tilson DJ. Corporate philanthropy: a strategic approach to the bottom line. *Calif Manage Rev.* 1987;29:49–61.
3. Ukman L. The special event: finding its niche. *Public Relations J.* 1984;40:21.
4. Abratt R, Clayton BC, Pitt LF. Corporate objectives in sports sponsorship. *Int J Advertising.* 1987;6:299–311.
5. Abratt R, Grobler PS. The evaluation of sports sponsorships. *Int J Advertising.* 1989;8:351–362.
6. Mihalik BJ. Sponsored recreation: a look at sponsors' program objectives and tactics, and guidelines for administration. *Public Relations J.* 1984;40:22–25.
7. Nothing sells like sports. *Business Week.* August 31, 1987;59:48–53.
8. Hagstrom RG. *The NASCAR Way: The Business That Drives the Sport.* New York, NY: John Wiley & Sons Inc; 1998.
9. Blum A. Tobacco industry sponsorship of sports: a growing dependency. In: Durston B, Jamrozik K, eds. *Tobacco and Health 1990—The Global War: Proceedings of the Seventh World Conference on Tobacco and Health.* Perth, Australia: Health Department of Western Australia; 1990: 882–884.
10. Holman CDJ, Donovan RJ, Corti B, Jalleh G, Frizzell SK, Carroll AM. Banning tobacco sponsorship: replacing tobacco with health messages and creating health-promoting environments. *Tob Control.* 1997;6:115–121.
11. Buchanan DR, Lev J. *Beer and Fast Cars: How Brewers Target Blue-Collar Youth Through Motor Sport Sponsorships.* San Rafael, Calif: Marin Institute for the Prevention of Alcohol and Other Drug Problems and AAA Foundation for Traffic Safety; 1990.
12. Dewhirst T. Tobacco sponsorship is no laughing matter. *Tob Control.* 1999;8:82–84.
13. Epps RP, Lynn WR, Manley MW. Tobacco, youth, and sports. *Adolesc Med.* 1998;9: 483–490.
14. Bates C. Tobacco sponsorship of sport. *Br J Sports Med.* 1999;33:299–300.
15. *Preventing Tobacco Use Among Young People: A Report of the Surgeon General.* Atlanta, Ga: National Center for Chronic Disease Prevention and Health Promotion, Office on Smoking and Health; 1994.
16. *Tobacco Use Among US Racial/Ethnic Minority Groups—African Americans, American Indians and Alaska Natives, Asian Americans and Pacific Islanders, and Hispanics: A Report of the Surgeon General.* Atlanta, Ga: National Center for Chronic Disease Prevention and Health Promotion, Office on Smoking and Health; 1998.
17. Lynch BS, Bonnie RJ, eds. *Growing Up Tobacco Free: Preventing Nicotine Addiction in Children and Youths.* Washington, DC: National Academy Press; 1994.
18. US Food and Drug Administration. Regulations restricting the sale and distribution of cigarettes and smokeless tobacco to protect children and adolescents; proposed rule. 60 *Federal Register* 41314–41786 (1995) (codified at 21 CFR Part 801, et al).
19. US Food and Drug Administration. Regulations restricting the sale and distribution of cigarettes and smokeless tobacco to protect children and adolescents; final rule. 61 *Federal Register* 44396–45318 (1996) (codified at 21 CFR Part 801, et al).
20. Slade J. Tobacco product advertising during motor sports broadcasts: a quantitative assessment. Paper presented at: Ninth World Conference on Tobacco and Health; October 10–14, 1994; Paris, France.
21. Madden PA, Grube JW. The frequency and nature of alcohol and tobacco advertising in televised sports, 1990 through 1992. *Am J Public Health.* 1994;84:297–299.
22. Blum A. The Marlboro Grand Prix: circumvention of the television ban on tobacco advertising. *N Engl J Med.* 1991;324:913–917.
23. Connolly GN, Orleans CT, Blum A. Snuffing tobacco out of sport. *Am J Public Health.* 1992; 82:351–353.
24. Locke DA. Counterspeech as an alternative to prohibition: proposed federal regulation of tobacco promotion in American motorsport. *Ind Law J.* 1994;70:217–253.
25. Longaker RA. Comment: warning: your tobacco sponsorship may be hazardous to our nation's health. *Villanova Sports Entertainment Law J.* 1998;5:105–195.
26. Patrick BJ. Comment: snuffing out the First Amendment: the FDA regulation of tobacco company advertising and sports sponsorships under the Federal Food, Drug, and Cosmetic Act. *Marquette Sports Law J.* 1997;8:139–179.
27. Matthews SD. Note: will NASCAR have to put on the brakes? The constitutionality of the FDA's ban on brand-name tobacco sponsorship in motor sports. *Ind Law Rev.* 1998;31:219–258.
28. Alm R. Cigarette ban may hurt auto racing most. *Dallas Morning News.* August 25, 1996:F1.
29. *Federal Trade Commission Report to Congress for 1998: Pursuant to the Federal Cigarette Labeling and Advertising Act.* Washington, DC: Federal Trade Commission; 2000.
30. *IEG Custom Research Report for Boston University School of Public Health.* Chicago, Ill: IEG Inc; 1998.
31. National Association of Attorneys General. *Multistate Settlement With the Tobacco Industry.* Boston, Mass: Tobacco Control Resource Center Inc and the Tobacco Products Liability Project; 2000. Available at: http://tobacco.neu.edu/Extra/multistate_settlement.htm#MASTER. Accessed June 7, 2000.
32. *What Is the Sponsors Report?* Ann Arbor, Mich: Joyce Julius & Associates Inc; 1998.
33. The Federal Cigarette Labeling and Advertising Act, 15 USC §1335 (1998).
34. The Comprehensive Smokeless Tobacco Health Education Act of 1986, 15 USC §4402 (1998).
35. Aitken PP, Leathar DS, Squair SI. Children's awareness of cigarette brand sponsorship of sports and games in the UK. *Health Educ Res.* 1986;1:203–211.
36. Ledwith F. Does tobacco sports sponsorship on television act as advertising to children? *Health Educ J.* 1984;43:85–88.
37. Meier KS. Tobacco truths: the impact of role models on children's attitudes toward smoking. *Health Educ Q.* 1991;18:173–182.
38. Aitken PP, Leathar DS, O'Hagan FJ. Children's perceptions of advertisements for cigarettes. *Soc Sci Med.* 1985;21:785–797.
39. Hoek J, Gendall P, Stockdale M. Some effects of tobacco sponsorship advertisements on young males. *Int J Advertising.* 1993;12:25–35.
40. Nelson E, While D. Children's awareness of cigarette advertisements on television. *Health Educ J.* 1992;51:34–37.
41. Charlton A, While D, Kelly S. Boys' smoking and cigarette-brand-sponsored motor racing. *Lancet.* 1997;350:1474.
42. Vaidya SG, Naik UD, Vaidya JS. Effect of sports sponsorship by tobacco companies on children's experimentation with tobacco. *BMJ.* 1996;313:400.
43. Vaidya SG, Vaidya JS, Naik UD. Sports sponsorship by cigarette companies influences the adolescent children's mind and helps initiate

smoking: results of a national study in India. *J Indian Med Assoc.* 1999;97:354–359.
44. Bloomberg News. Advertising & marketing: Reynolds to end race sponsorship. *Los Angeles Times.* October 13, 1999:C5.
45. Flynn A. Deal would curb tobacco sponsors. *The Arizona Republic.* November 13, 1998:A24.
46. *ESPN The Magazine* (Special Issue: Winston Cup 2000 Preview). Spring 2000.
47. Clarke L. To attract kids, stock car racing shifts gears. *Washington Post.* May 22, 1998:A1.
48. Whiting A, Verma R. Health: watching tobacco-sponsored sports can harm your health. *Inter Press Service World News.* November 20, 1997. Available at: http://www.oneworld.org/ips2/nov/tobacco2.html. Accessed February 9, 1999.
49. Brand recall: NASCAR sponsorship versus 30-second commercials. *A Second Look at Sponsorship Exposure in Sports Marketing.* 2000; 10(1):3–4.
50. Hassell G. Speed sells. Firms race to sponsor Grand Prix: growing following makes sponsorships lucrative. *Houston Chronicle.* October 2, 1998:D1.
51. NASCAR sells products—but which ones? *Motorsports Marketing News.* 1992;8(2):2.
52. NASCAR brand loyalty: top 25. *Motorsports Marketing News.* 1992;8(2):2–3.
53. Powles JW, Gifford S. Health of nations: lessons from Victoria, Australia. *BMJ.* 1993;306: 125–127.
54. Musk AW, Shean R, Walker N, Swanson M. Progress on smoking control in Western Australia. *BMJ.* 1994;308:395–398.
55. World no-tobacco day targets sports and the arts [Medical News and Perspectives]. *JAMA.* 1996; 275:1220.
56. Corti B, Donovan RJ, Holman CDJ, Coten N, Jones SJ. Using sponsorship to promote health messages to children. *Health Educ Behav.* 1997; 24:276–286.
57. Hastings GB, MacAskill S, McNeill REJ, Leathar DS. Sports sponsorship in health education. *Health Promotion.* 1988;3:161–169.
58. Blom ED. Tobacco free at the Indianapolis 500. *Ind Med.* 1996;89:207–209.
59. Olson CK. Countering pro-tobacco influences at the racetrack. *Am J Public Health.* 1999;89: 1431–1432.
60. Farhi P. Tobacco moving out of spotlight: Philip Morris agrees to reposition arena ads away from TV cameras. *Washington Post.* June 7, 1995:F1.
61. Vicini J. Philip Morris to curb cigarette ads at sports stadiums. *Chicago Sun-Times.* June 7, 1995:61.
62. Justice takes steps to ensure smoke-free Super Bowl broadcast [press release]. Washington, DC: US Dept of Justice; January 22, 1997. Available at: http://www.usdoj.gov/opa/pr/1997/January97/028civ.htm. Accessed December 20, 1998.
63. *Action for Children's Television v Federal Communications Commission, et al,* 999 F2d 19 (1st Cir 1993).
64. Pinkerton Tobacco Co. Proposed consent agreement with analysis to aid public comment. 56 *Federal Register* 57009–57011 (1991).
65. Pinkerton Tobacco Co. Prohibited trade practices and affirmative corrective actions. 57 *Federal Register* 4634 (1992).

Getting to the Truth: Evaluating National Tobacco Countermarketing Campaigns

| Matthew C. Farrelly, PhD, Cheryl G. Healton, DrPH, Kevin C. Davis, MA, Peter Messeri, PhD, James C. Hersey, PhD, and M. Lyndon Haviland, DrPH

Objectives. This study examines how the American Legacy Foundation's "truth" campaign and Philip Morris's "Think. Don't Smoke" campaign have influenced youths' attitudes, beliefs, and intentions toward tobacco.

Methods. We analyzed 2 telephone surveys of 12- to 17-year-olds with multivariate logistic regressions: a baseline survey conducted before the launch of "truth" and a second survey 10 months into the "truth" campaign.

Results. Exposure to "truth" countermarketing advertisements was consistently associated with an increase in anti-tobacco attitudes and beliefs, whereas exposure to Philip Morris advertisements generally was not. In addition, those exposed to Philip Morris advertisements were more likely to be open to the idea of smoking.

Conclusions. Whereas exposure to the "truth" campaign positively changed youths' attitudes toward tobacco, the Philip Morris campaign had a counterproductive influence. (*Am J Public Health.* 2002;92:901–907)

In early February 2000, the American Legacy Foundation (Legacy) launched "truth," a national tobacco countermarketing campaign conducted by an alliance of advertising firms led by Arnold Communications, Legacy staff, and nationwide youths. "truth" targets primarily 12- to 17-year-olds who are susceptible to smoking.[1–3] The core strategy of the campaign is to market its message as a brand, like other youth brands (e.g., Nike, Sprite), to appeal to youths most at risk of smoking. "truth" TV and print commercials feature what advertising experts call "edgy" youths (i.e., those who are on the cutting edge of trends), promotional items (e.g., T-shirts, stickers), street marketing, and a Web site (www.thetruth.com). Although "truth" is a national multiethnic campaign, special components were developed to reinforce its appeal to African Americans, Hispanics, and Asians.

While drawing youths to "truth," the campaign delivers stark facts about tobacco and tobacco industry marketing practices, rather than sending directive "just say no" messages such as those used in the Philip Morris Company's "Think. Don't Smoke." campaign, which began in 1998. Specifically, many of the "truth" advertisements are based on historical statements from the industry itself that reveal its youth marketing and obfuscation of tobacco's health effects. In unmasking these practices, "truth" seeks to replace the attractive identity portrayed by tobacco advertising with a "truth" alternative identity.[4]

The "truth" brand builds a positive, tobacco-free identity through hard-hitting advertisements that feature youths confronting the tobacco industry. This rebellious rejection of tobacco and tobacco advertising channels youths' need to assert their independence and individuality, while countering tobacco marketing efforts. For example, one well-known "truth" commercial, known as "Body Bags," features youths piling body bags outside of a tobacco company's headquarters and broadcasting loudly via megaphones that these represent the 1200 people killed daily by tobacco.

Empirical evidence for the potential benefits of the national "truth" campaign's approach comes from the dramatic decline in youth tobacco use associated with the Florida[5,6] and Massachusetts[7] campaigns, as well as from other studies that have found campaigns focusing on tobacco industry practices to be effective.[8–10]

Legacy's model is that "truth" will change youths' attitudes toward smoking, and that this in turn will change their smoking behavior, prevent them from initiating smoking, or both.[11] Thus, attitude shifts are an intermediate outcome on the path to changing smoking behavior. A telephone survey of youths in Florida and nationwide demonstrated that attitudes toward tobacco changed dramatically among Florida youths compared with youths in the rest of the United States after the first year (1998) of Florida's "truth" campaign, compared with a national sample of youths whose attitudes remained relatively constant.[12] The accompanying change in smoking prevalence was at first statistically nonsignificant, but results from the Florida Youth Tobacco Survey showed drops in smoking among middle-school and high-school students of 18% and 8%, respectively, after year 1 and of 40% and 18% after year 2.[5]

Some assert that a portion of this decline can be attributed to the November 1998 $0.45-per-pack price increase.[13] Cigarette prices increased by roughly 30% during 1998, year 1 of the Florida program, and by 7% during year 2.[14] With price increases of this magnitude, economic studies projected a 10% to 20% decline in youth smoking prevalence for 1998 and a 2% to 5% decline for 1999.[15–17] This suggests that although a significant fraction of the decline in smoking after the first year of Florida's program may have been due to price increases, the price increases alone cannot account for all of the 1998 decline or for the continued decline in smoking in 1999.

In the present study, we used the results of 2 national youth surveys to compare exposures to Legacy's "truth" and Philip Morris's "Think. Don't Smoke." campaigns. We then analyzed changes in youths' attitudes, beliefs, and intentions regarding the tobacco industry and tobacco use 10 months into the "truth" campaign as a function of levels of exposure to each campaign.

METHODS

To monitor the impact of the "truth" campaign on attitudes and behavior, in 1999 Legacy began sponsoring the Legacy Media

Tracking Surveys (LMTSs), which were designed to yield nationally representative samples of youths aged 12 to 17 and of young adults aged 18 to 24. We limited our analysis to 12- to 17-year-olds, the target audience for "truth." These 2-stage stratified-design surveys measured exposure to environmental tobacco smoke, access to tobacco products, knowledge and attitudes about tobacco, awareness of pro- and anti-tobacco advertising, and self-reported tobacco use and intentions. Before the "truth" campaign was launched (on February 7, 2000), the baseline telephone survey (LMTS-I) was conducted between December 6, 1999, and February 6, 2000. The next telephone survey (LMTS-II) was conducted between September 8, 2000, and December 23, 2000.

We enhanced representation of African Americans, Asians, and Hispanics by oversampling telephone exchanges concentrated in areas with high proportions of each of these racial/ethnic groups. Furthermore, Asian and Hispanic households were oversampled by supplementing the random-digit telephone dialing with lists of households with Asian and Hispanic surnames. Finally, the sample was drawn to ensure national representation in both urban and nonurban areas and in states with and without state-funded countermarketing campaigns. All analyses include an individual weighting factor that adjusts for age and oversampling by racial/ethnic group and residence in states with funded countermarketing campaigns. To adjust the standard error calculations for the clustered design, we used Stata Version 7 (Stata Corp, College Station, Tex).

To maximize the chances of finding adolescents and their parents at home, telephone calls were spread across all days of the week and times of day, including evenings and weekends. For each case, up to 12 callbacks were made, with a minimum of 2 daytime attempts per case. Finally, up to 2 refusal-conversion attempts per case were made unless the respondent or parent was adamant about not participating in the survey.[18]

Tobacco Attitudes, Beliefs, and Counteradvertising Exposure

The LMTS asked youths how strongly they agreed or disagreed (on a 5-point scale) with a series of attitude, belief, and behavioral-intent statements about the tobacco industry, youths' perceptions of tobacco's social acceptability, and youths' intentions to smoke during the next year. Nonsmokers were asked to report their likelihood of smoking any time in the next year. To show how these attitudes, beliefs, and intentions changed between the baseline and the follow-up surveys, we report the percentage (with 95% confidence intervals) of 12- to 17-year-olds who agreed or strongly agreed with the targeted attitudes.

The LMTS contained questions to measure awareness of television advertisements from "truth" and "Think. Don't Smoke." First, respondents were asked in an open-ended question to report any antismoking or anti-tobacco campaigns of which they were aware. This measure of unaided recall allows us to track which campaigns are most prominent in the minds of youths over time. We then queried youths about their awareness of specific campaign advertisements by asking them whether they had "recently seen an anti-smoking or anti-tobacco ad on TV that ———," followed by a brief description of the beginning of the advertisement. Questions were crafted to provide respondents with enough information to recognize the advertisement in question but not enough for them to "fake" awareness of it.[12] A respondent who indicated recognition was then asked to report further ad details to confirm awareness. Confirmed awareness of 1 or more advertisements indicated campaign awareness or exposure. Questions pertaining to the various advertisements were presented in random order to control for order effects and included all advertisements from both campaigns aired within 6 weeks of the survey's start. For each youth surveyed, we quantified the exposure dose by measuring the total number of advertisements seen for each campaign.

Statistical Analyses

We combined the 2 LMTSs and used a cross-section time-series approach to elucidate the relationship between shifts in attitudes and beliefs and exposure to the "truth" and "Think. Don't Smoke." campaigns.[19] The attitudes and beliefs in the LMTS address tobacco industry behavior, the social acceptability of tobacco use, and intentions to smoke during the next year. We estimated separate multivariable logistic regressions to assess how "truth" and "Think. Don't Smoke." have affected these outcomes. For these regressions, the outcomes were dichotomized so that 1 represented an anti-tobacco attitude—indicated by a reply of "strongly agrees" or "agrees" (or "strongly disagrees" or "disagrees" as appropriate)—and 0 represented no anti-tobacco attitude. The cross-section time-series models were used to estimate the odds that respondents agreed with a given attitude, belief, or intention as a function of their exposure to the "truth" and "Think, Don't Smoke." campaigns and other variables. The other control variables included sociodemographics (age, gender, race/ethnicity, weekly available spending money, working status, and religiousness), household environment (lives in a 2-parent household, hours of television watched per day, lives with a smoker, has parents who discourage smoking, household smoking restrictions), and perceptions of the prevalence of peer and adult smoking. To assess dose–response effects, we estimated a second set of regression models using number of campaign advertisements seen.

To control for the possibility that the changes in attitudes are part of a secular trend, we included an indicator variable (0/1) for respondents in the LMTS-II. This variable captures influences on national attitudes, such as news about lawsuits against tobacco companies. Because youths' responses may be influenced by parents or others household members, we controlled for interviewer perception that someone else was listening on the telephone during the survey (yes/no indicator). Finally, we controlled for the potential influence of state tobacco control programs and policies by including state-specific indicator variables. We calculated odds ratios for agreeing (or disagreeing) with an attitude or a belief, according to exposure to media campaigns and controlling for other influences noted above. To calculate 95% confidence intervals to account for probability sampling and stratification reflected in the LMTS design, we used Stata Version 7 (Stata Corp, College Station, Tex).

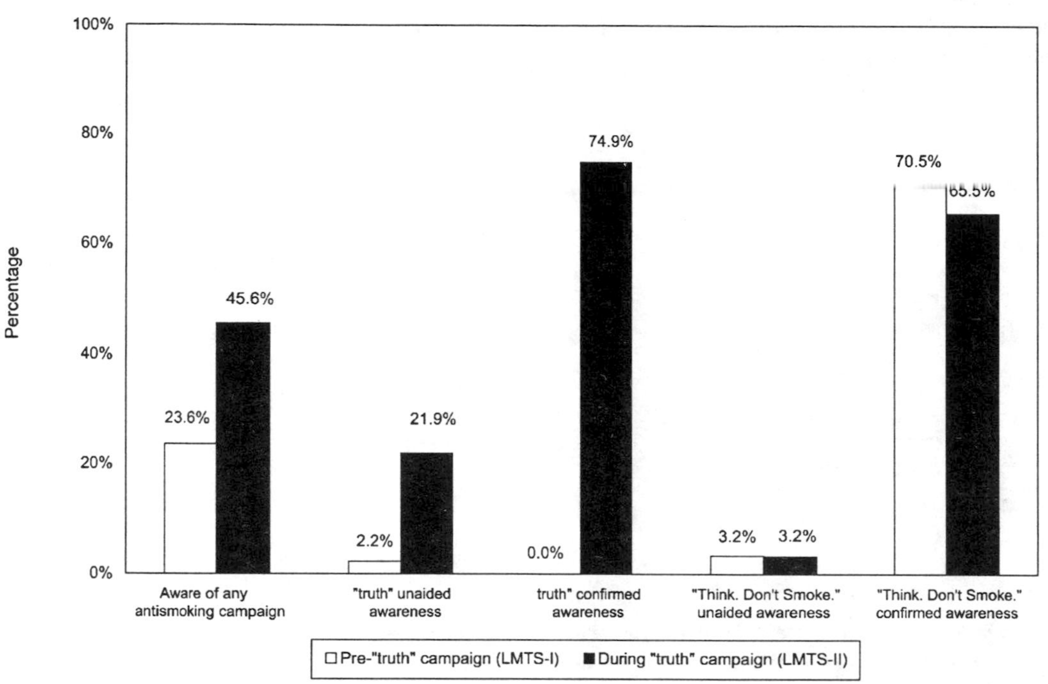

Note. LMTS = Legacy Media Tracking Survey.

FIGURE 1—Aided and unaided awareness of the American Legacy Foundation's "truth" campaign and Philip Morris's "Think. Don't Smoke." campaign among 12- to 17-year-olds.

RESULTS

The total sample size for the LMTS-I was 6897 (3439 12- to 17-year-olds and 3458 18- to 24-year-olds). The LMTS-II was larger and focused more on 12- to 17-year-olds, with 10692 surveyed (6233 12- to 17-year-olds and 4459 18- to 24-year-olds). The response rates for LMTS-I and LMTS-II were 52.5% and 52.3%, respectively, based on a standardized response rate calculation (American Association of Public Opinion Research response rate calculation no. 4).[20] Discovery Research Group (Salt Lake City, Utah) and Issues and Answers (Virginia Beach, Va) collected data for the LMTS-I, and Discovery Research Group collected data for the LMTS-II.

Changes In Exposure to Tobacco Countermarketing Campaigns

The percentage of 12- to 17-year-olds who reported awareness of any tobacco countermarketing campaign (Figure 1) doubled during the first 10 months of the "truth" campaign—from 23.6% to 45.6% ($P<.05$). Awareness of the "truth" campaign accounted for much of this increase. With no prompting (unaided awareness), 22% of 12- to 17-year-olds in the LMTS-II indicated that they were aware of the "truth" campaign, compared with 3% who indicated awareness of "Think. Don't Smoke." Confirmed awareness of specific campaign advertisements among 12- to 17-year-olds was 75% for "truth" and 66% for "Think. Don't Smoke." The distribution of exposure to 1, 2, 3, and 4 or more advertisements was 23%, 19%, 14%, and 19% for "truth" and 37%, 21%, 6%, and 1% for "Think. Don't Smoke." in the LMTS-II.

Attitudes and Beliefs About Tobacco and Intentions to Smoke

Between surveys, the percentage of 12- to 17-year-olds who agreed with several attitudes and beliefs that are central to the "truth" campaign changed by an amount that ranged from 6.6% to 26.4% (Table 1). These attitudes and beliefs center on tobacco industry behavior (e.g., denying the health effects and addictive nature of tobacco), attitudes toward the tobacco industry (e.g., "should go out of business"), social acceptability of tobacco use (e.g., "not smoking is a way to express your independence" and "smoking makes you look cool"), and intention to smoke during the next year. The prevalence of youths who agreed (or disagreed if that was the target direction of attitudinal change) increased ($P<.05$) for all of these statements. The percentage of current nonsmokers who said that they probably or definitely would not smoke 1 year from the time of the survey also increased, but the change was not statistically significant. To clarify how changes in attitudes, beliefs, and intentions are related to exposure to the "truth" and "Think. Don't Smoke." campaigns, we estimated logistic regression models for each outcome by using 2 key independent variables representing expo-

TABLE 1—Percentages (With 95% Confidence Intervals) of 12- to 17-Year-Olds Who Agreed With Indicated Attitudes at Baseline and 10-Month Surveys

Attitude	LMTS-I (95% CI)	LMTS-II (95% CI)	% Change
Cigarette companies try to get young people to start smoking.	74.0 (71.3, 76.7)	83.0 (81.4, 84.6)	12.2
Cigarette companies lie.	74.7 (72.0, 77.3)	83.8 (82.2, 85.4)	12.3
Cigarette companies deny that cigarettes cause cancer and other harmful diseases.	48.4 (45.3, 51.5)	58.6 (56.4, 60.8)	21.0
Cigarette companies deny that cigarettes are addictive.	57.9 (54.8, 60.9)	64.0 (61.8, 66.1)	10.6
I would like to see cigarette companies go out of business.	70.4 (67.6, 73.2)	78.9 (77.0, 80.7)	12.0
I want to be involved in efforts to get rid of smoking.	65.2 (62.2, 68.1)	82.4 (80.7, 84.2)	26.4
Taking a stand against smoking is important to me.	72.1 (69.4, 74.9)	83.2 (81.4, 85.0)	15.4
Not smoking is a way to express your independence.	57.4 (45.9, 52.1)	70.1 (53.8, 58.6)	22.2
Smoking cigarettes makes people your age look cool or fit in.[a]	86.4 (84.2, 88.6)	92.1 (90.9, 93.3)	6.6
Do you think you will smoke a cigarette at any time during the next year?[b]	94.3 (92.8, 95.9)	95.9 (95.0, 96.8)	1.6

Note. LMTS = Legacy Media Tracking Survey; CI = confidence interval.
[a]Disagreed or strongly disagreed.
[b]Definitely not or probably not.

TABLE 2—Logistic Regression Models Showing Effect of Exposure to American Legacy Foundation's "truth" Campaign and Philip Morris's "Think. Don't Smoke." (TDS) Campaign on Attitudes, Beliefs, and Intentions Among 12- to 17-Year-Olds

Outcome	Confirmed Awareness, OR (*P*)		Dose,[a] OR (*P*)	
	"truth"	TDS	"truth"	TDS
Cigarette companies try to get young people to start smoking.	1.292 (0.097)	1.154 (0.224)	1.107 (0.005)	1.026 (0.694)
Cigarette companies lie.	1.972 (0.000)	1.123 (0.321)	1.280 (0.000)	0.971 (0.659)
Cigarette companies deny that cigarettes cause disease.	1.354 (0.015)	0.755 (0.003)	1.045 (0.119)	0.864 (0.003)
Cigarette companies deny that cigarettes are addictive.	1.153 (0.252)	0.953 (0.619)	1.036 (0.194)	0.970 (0.557)
I would like to see cigarette companies go out of business.	0.987 (0.936)	0.792 (0.044)	1.014 (0.670)	0.901 (0.072)
I want to be involved in efforts to get rid of smoking.	1.353 (0.077)	1.086 (0.483)	1.053 (0.198)	0.998 (0.971)
Taking a stand against smoking is important to me.	2.633 (0.000)	1.082 (0.520)	1.213 (0.000)	1.047 (0.482)
Not smoking is a way to express independence.	1.459 (0.003)	1.329 (0.004)	1.082 (0.007)	1.102 (0.066)
Smoking makes people your age look cool or fit in.[b]	1.521 (0.047)	1.343 (0.065)	1.099 (0.063)	1.106 (0.299)
Do you think you will smoke a cigarette at any time during the next year?[c]	1.657 (0.088)	0.644 (0.050)	1.076 (0.347)	0.770 (0.017)

Note. OR = odds ratio.
[a]Number of advertisements seen.
[b]Disagreed or strongly disagreed.
[c]Definitely not or probably not.

sure—simple awareness (yes/no) and dose (the total number of advertisements seen, including 0) (Table 2). Exposure to "truth" was associated with youths' attitudes toward the tobacco industry's marketing practices, its efforts to conceal tobacco's harmful effects, and the industry as a whole; for example, youths exposed to "truth" were more likely to agree that "cigarette companies try to get young people to start smoking" (odds ratio [OR]= 1.29; $P<.097$). Furthermore, a significant dose–response effect was seen with increased exposure to "truth"(OR=1.2; $P<.005$). There was no association between this belief and either measure of exposure for "Think. Don't Smoke."

Exposure to "truth" was associated with a doubling of the odds that youths would agree that "cigarette companies lie" (OR=1.97; $P<.001$), and increases in exposure to additional advertisements were associated with concomitant increases in the odds of agreeing with this statement (OR=1.28 per additional advertisement; $P<.001$). Exposure to "Think. Don't Smoke." advertisements showed no such associations (Table 2). Although neither campaign influenced the percentage of youths who were aware of cigarette companies' past efforts to conceal tobacco's addictive properties, exposure to "truth" increased youths' awareness of how the industry concealed tobacco's deleterious health effects (OR=1.35; $P<.02$) whereas exposure to "Think. Don't Smoke." had the opposite effect (OR=0.755; $P<.003$).

In contrast, the odds of agreeing that cigarette companies have denied that cigarettes cause disease declined by 24% with exposure to any "Think. Don't Smoke." advertisement ($P<.003$), and exposure to additional advertisements reinforced this effect ($P<.003$). Although no association was seen between exposure to "truth" and the opinion "I would like to see cigarette companies go out of business," the odds ratio for exposure to any "Think. Don't Smoke." for this attitude was 0.79 ($P<.04$), and each additional advertisement decreased the odds of agreeing to this statement by 10% ($P<.07$).

We constructed 4 models of youths' intentions and attitudes toward smoking (Table 2). The first model examined youths' endorsement of the statement "I want to get involved in efforts to get rid of smoking" and the second examined their agreement that "taking a stand against smoking [was] important" to them. Exposure to the "truth" campaign was associated with a 35% ($P<.08$) and a 163% ($P<.01$) increase, respectively, in the odds of agreement with either of these statements. In addition, the more "truth" advertisements seen, the greater the odds of wanting to take a stand against smoking ($P<.01$). Exposure to "Think. Don't Smoke." advertisements did not influence youths' level of agreement with either of these statements.

In the 2 other models, youths were asked whether they agreed that "not smoking is a way to express independence" and disagreed with the assertion that smoking makes youths "look cool or fit in." The odds ratios for "truth" campaign exposure were 1.46 and 1.52, respectively. The results for "Think. Don't Smoke." were similar, but the result for "looking cool" was only marginally statistically significant ($P<.07$). Logistic regressions that include the number of advertisements (i.e., the dose effect) generally confirm these results.

Exposure to "truth" was associated with a marginally statistically significant decrease in the odds of current nonsmokers' expressing an intention to smoke any time in the next year (OR=1.66; $P<.09$); however, the dose–response relationship was not statistically significant. In contrast, exposure to "Think. Don't Smoke." was associated with an increase in the odds of youths' intending to smoke in the next year ($P<.05$), and the dose–response relationship was statistically more robust ($P<.02$).

TABLE 3—Association Between Attitudes and Beliefs and Intention to Smoke in 1 Year Among 12- to 17-Year-Olds

Belief Item	Odds Ratio (*P*)
Cigarette companies try to get young people to start smoking.	1.225 (.413)
I want to be involved with efforts to get rid of cigarette smoking.	3.542 (.000)
Cigarette companies lie.	0.836 (.490)
Cigarette companies deny that cigarettes cause disease.	1.95 (.002)
Cigarette companies deny that cigarettes are addictive.	0.988 (.953)
I would like to see cigarette companies go out of business.	1.801 (.013)
Taking a stand against smoking is important to me.	2.223 (.000)
Not smoking is a way to express independence.	1.542 (.038)
Smoking makes people your age look cool or fit in.[a]	2.459 (.000)

Note. Intention not to smoke is coded as 1 and intention not to smoke as 0.
[a]Disagreed or strongly disagreed.

We estimated a logistic regression model of intention to smoke among nonsmokers as a function of each attitude reported in Table 2, with intention to smoke coded 0 and no intention to smoke coded 1. We found that 6 of the 9 attitudes were strongly associated with smoking intentions ($P<.05$), with odds ratios ranging from 1.54 for "not smoking is a way to express independence" to 3.54 for "I want to be involved with efforts to get rid of cigarette smoking" (Table 3). Respondents' attitudes toward the tobacco industry that were associated with smoking intentions were wanting to see cigarette companies go out of business (OR=1.80) and agreeing that cigarette companies deny the harmful effects of tobacco (OR=1.95). Attitudes about smoking and youth activism were all strongly and negatively associated with intention to smoke. The largest odds ratios were for agreement with the statements "I want to be involved in efforts to get rid of smoking" (OR=3.54) and "taking a stand against smoking is important" (OR=2.22) and disagreement with the assertion that "smoking cigarettes makes people [my] age look cool or fit in" (OR=2.46). These findings suggest that if "truth" continues to affect attitudes toward smoking and the tobacco industry, the prevalence of smoking is likely to decline as the campaign progresses.

DISCUSSION

Results from the 2 nationally representative surveys demonstrate that 10 months into the "truth" campaign, tobacco was more prominent in the minds of youths. Unaided awareness of tobacco countermarketing campaigns has nearly doubled. The "truth" campaign resonates more with youths than "Think. Don't Smoke," even though the "Think. Don't Smoke." campaign began in 1998 and aired for more than 12 months before the initial 10-month run of the "truth" campaign reported here.

Exposure to the "truth" campaign also appears to have changed the way youths think about tobacco. The percentage of youths who held anti-tobacco attitudes and beliefs increased by an amount that ranged from 6.6% to 26.4% during the first 10 months of the campaign, which compares favorably with the 10% average increase in Florida during the first year of the campaign.[12] Our results parallel the experience of Florida's "truth" campaign, in which strong shifts in attitudes preceded changes in behavior, despite a somewhat lower level of campaign awareness than was achieved in Florida.[12]

The attitudes that changed most dramatically were "taking a stand against smoking is important," "not smoking is a way to express independence," and "cigarette companies deny that cigarettes cause cancer and other harmful diseases." These concepts are central to the strategy of "truth" and underlie advertisements such as "Body Bags," which featured teens challenging the tobacco industry by dragging body bags in front of a cigarette company's offices to remind them that they market a product that kills. These attitudinal changes were shown to be associated with youths' exposure to the "truth" campaign.

We believe that Philip Morris's "Think. Don't Smoke." campaign is clearly designed not to draw attention to tobacco industry marketing tactics or behavior; thus, the attitudes that relate to the tobacco industry do not represent a test of the success of its campaign. Interestingly, however, we found that exposure to "Think. Don't Smoke." engendered more favorable feelings toward the tobacco industry than we found among those not exposed to "Think. Don't Smoke." advertisements. This discovery lends support to the assertion of tobacco control activists that the purpose of the Philip Morris campaign is to buy respectability and not to prevent youth smoking.[21] In addition, the campaign slogans "Think. Don't Smoke." (Philip Morris) and "Tobacco Is Whacko, if You Are a Teen" (Lorillard) are distinctly counter to recommendations made by the Columbia Expert Panel on youth tobacco countermarketing. This panel advises against directive messages such as those telling youths not to smoke and that smoking is uncool and for adults only.[10]

Although the way in which exposure to "Think. Don't Smoke." affects young people's attitudes toward the tobacco industry may not be an appropriate measure by which to judge the performance of the campaign, the attitudes toward smoking included in our analyses are relevant to "Think. Don't Smoke." Our analyses indicate that although the level of confirmed awareness for both campaigns is roughly equal, "truth" has had a more consistent impact on attitudes toward smoking. Our quantitative analysis supports the findings of a focus-group study of 120 12- to 16-year-olds in Arizona, California, and Massachusetts. This study indicated that "Think. Don't Smoke." advertisements were the least effective among a group of advertisements including 10 representing several state campaigns.[9] Youths rated advertisements that graphically, dramatically, and emotionally portrayed the serious consequences of smoking highest in terms of making them "stop and think about not using tobacco."[9]

The current study uses a quasi-experimental cross-sectional design. Thus, youths who recall tobacco countermarketing messages may be different in some way from those who do not. As a result, some of the association between changes in attitudes and exposure to the "truth" campaign may reflect the possibility that those who have stronger anti-tobacco attitudes may be more attentive to the campaign. In addition, those with favorable attitudes toward the tobacco industry may be more attentive to Philip Morris's efforts to curb youth smoking.

Another possible limitation may be the difficulty in separating the independent effects of each campaign if there is insufficient variation in exposure to both campaigns (i.e., multicollinearity). This possibility could explain why we find that "Think. Don't Smoke." appears to move youths' attitudes in a pro-tobacco direction. Our examination of this question through changing model specifications suggested that multicollinearity across the 2 campaign exposures was not present. To determine whether or not this multicollinearity is a concern, we dropped the "truth" exposure variable from the logistic regression models and examined whether the odds ratios were influenced. Results showed that all of the odds ratios remained stable.

In summary, our findings suggest that an aggressive national tobacco countermarketing campaign can have a dramatic influence within a short period of time on attitudes toward tobacco and the tobacco industry. These attitudinal changes were also associated with reduced intentions to smoke among those at risk. If these changes in attitude are predictive of future changes in tobacco use, as demonstrated in Florida,[6,12] they indicate that the "truth" campaign is on its way to curbing tobacco use among youths. ■

About the Authors

Matthew C. Farrelly and Kevin C. Davis are with Research Triangle Institute, Research Triangle Park, NC. Cheryl G. Healton, Peter Messeri, and M. Lyndon Haviland are with the American Legacy Foundation, Washington, DC. James C. Hersey is with Research Triangle Institute, Washington, DC.

Requests for reprints should be sent to Matthew C. Farrelly, PhD, Research Triangle Institute, 3040 Cornwallis Rd, PO Box 12194, Research Triangle Park, NC 27709 (e-mail: mcf@rti.org).

This article was accepted January 30, 2002.

Contributors

M.C. Farrelly designed the survey questionnaire and methodology, directed the data analysis, and prepared the original draft manuscript. C.G. Healton participated in preparation of the final draft. K.C. Davis participated in preparing the original draft manuscript and conducted all analyses. P. Messeri participated in the data analysis and in preparation of the final draft. J.C. Hersey participated in survey questionnaire development and methodology and data analysis. M.L. Haviland participated in preparation of the final draft.

Acknowledgments

We express our appreciation to David Sly for his contributions to the design of the survey questionnaire and methodology. We are also grateful to Rachel Royce for insightful comments on the final draft, Don Akin for sample design and variance estimation, and Susan Murchie for editorial review.

References

1. Leventhal H, Cleary PD. The smoking problem: a review of the research and theory in behavior risk modification. *Psychol Bull.* 1980;88:370–405.

2. Flay BR. Youth tobacco use: risks, patterns, and control. In: Slade J, Orleans CT, eds. *Nicotine Addiction: Principles and Management.* New York, NY: Oxford University Press; 1993:365–385.

3. Pierce JP, Choi WS, Gilpin EA, Farkas AJ. Validation of susceptibility as a predictor of which adolescents take up smoking in the United States. *Health Psychol.* 1996;15:511–515.

4. Biener L, Siegel M. Tobacco marketing and adolescent smoking: more support for a causal inference. *Am J Public Health.* 2000;90:407–411.

5. Bauer UE, Johnson TM, Hopkins RS, Brooks RG. Changes in youth cigarette use and intentions following implementation of a tobacco control program: findings from the Florida Youth Tobacco Survey, 1998–2000. *JAMA.* 2000;284:723–728.

6. Sly DF, Heald GR, Ray S. The Florida "truth" anti-tobacco media evaluation: design, first year results, and implications for planning future state media evaluations. *Tob Control.* 2001;10:9–15.

7. Siegel M, Biener L. The impact of an antismoking media campaign on progression to established smoking: results of a longitudinal youth study. *Am J Public Health.* 2000;90:380–386.

8. Goldman LK, Glantz SA. Evaluation of antismoking advertising campaigns. *JAMA.* 1998;279:772–777.

9. *Counter-Tobacco Advertising Exploratory Summary Report.* Northbrook, Ill: Teenage Research Unlimited; 1999.

10. Columbia University Tobacco Counter-Advertising Expert Panel. Research synthesis on the effects of tobacco advertising and counter-advertising on youth tobacco use behavior: report to the Office on Smoking

and Health, Centers for Disease Control and Prevention. New York: Columbia University; 1996.

11. Fishbein MG, Azjen I. *Belief, Attitude, Intention and Behavior: An Introduction to Theory and Research.* Reading, Mass: Addison Wesley; 1975.

12. Sly DF, Hopkins RS, Trapido E, Ray S. Influence of a counteradvertising media campaign on initiation of smoking: the Florida "truth" campaign. *Am J Public Health.* 2001;91:233–238.

13. Healton C. Who's afraid of the truth? *Am J Public Health.* 2001;91:554–558.

14. The Tax Burden on Tobacco: Historical Compilation. Arlington, Va: Orzechowski and Walker. vol34; 1999.

15. Chaloupka FJ, Grossman M. Price tobacco control policies and youth smoking. Paper presented at: Economics of Substance Abuse Session II of the 71st Annual Conference of the Western Economic Association International; July 1996; San Francisco, Calif.

16. Evans WN, Huang LX. Cigarette taxes and teen smoking: new evidence from panels of repeated cross-sections. Working paper. Department of Economics, University of Maryland; 1998. Available at: http://www.bsos.umd.edu/econ/evans/wpapers/teensmk3.pdf. Accessed March 18, 2002.

17. Gruber J. Tobacco at the crossroads: the past and future of smoking regulation in the United States. *J Econ Perspect.* 2001;15:193–212.

18. Farrelly MC, Davis KC, Hersey JC, Pendergast KB. *Legacy Media Tracking Baseline Survey Summary Final Report.* Research Triangle Park, NC: Research Triangle Institute; 2001.

19. Greene WH. *Econometric Analysis.* New York, NY: Macmillan Publishing; 1990.

20. *Standard Definitions: Final Dispositions of Case Codes and Outcome Rates for RDD Telephone Surveys and In-Person Household Surveys.* Ann Arbor, Mich: American Association for Public Opinion Research; 1998.

21. Novelli WD. Don't smoke, buy Marlboro. *BMJ.* 1999;318:1296.

Smooth Moves: Bar and Nightclub Tobacco Promotions That Target Young Adults

| Edward Sepe, MS, Pamela M. Ling, MD, MPH, and Stanton A. Glantz, PhD

Objectives. This article describes the tobacco industry's use of bars and nightclubs to encourage smoking among young adults.

Methods. Previously secret tobacco industry marketing documents were analyzed.

Results. Tobacco industry bar and nightclub promotions in the 1980s and 1990s included aggressive advertising, tobacco brand-sponsored activities, and distribution of samples. Financial incentives for club owners and staff were used to encourage smoking through peer influence. Increased use of these strategies occurred concurrently with an increase in smoking among persons aged 18 through 24 years.

Conclusions. The tobacco industry's bar and nightclub promotions are not yet politically controversial and are not regulated by the 1998 Master Settlement Agreement between the industry and the states. Tobacco control advocates should include young adults in research and advocacy efforts and should design interventions to counter this industry strategy to solidify smoking patterns and recruit young adult smokers. (*Am J Public Health.* 2002;92:414-419)

During the 1990s, tobacco industry sponsorship of bars and nightclubs increased dramatically,[1,2] accompanied by cigarette brand paraphernalia, advertisements, and entertainment events in bars and clubs.[3–7] Young adults are not immune to late smoking initiation, and they are vulnerable to concentrated tobacco industry marketing. The 1998 National Household Survey on Drug Abuse shows a steady increase in the smoking rate among young adults (aged 18–25 years) from 34.6% in 1994 to 41.6% in 1998.[8(p22)] Wechsler et al. reported an increase in smoking prevalence among college students from 22.3% in 1993 to 28.5% in 1998.[9]

These results are consistent with the association found in other studies between changes in tobacco marketing and parallel increases in smoking in the target population (e.g., women in the 1930s and 1960s and youth in the 1980s and 1990s[10–13]). In contrast to the view that smoking initiation occurs only before age 18, smoking initiation in young adults (18–24 years) occurred frequently during the early and mid 20th century and continues to be high among young adults in some ethnic groups.[8,14–18]

We used previously secret tobacco industry documents to describe why and how the industry uses bars to encourage smoking among young adults. (We use the term "bars" to include bars and nightclubs.) We sought to answer the following questions: (1) How did bar promotions develop, and what were the concomitant marketing benefits? (2) How did these promotions benefit the industry in the research, social, and political arenas? (3) What are the connections between bar promotions and other industry marketing programs, including advertising in the alternative press and studies of peer influence?

METHODS

We used standard techniques[19] to search tobacco industry document archives made available by tobacco litigation during the 1990s. The documents came from 4 sources: the Mangini collection of RJ Reynolds marketing documents at the University of California, San Francisco (http://www.library.ucsf.edu/tobacco/mangini), tobacco industry document Internet sites (Philip Morris, http://www.pmdocs.com; Brown & Williamson, http://www.brownandwilliamson.com; RJ Reynolds, http://www.rjrtdocs.com), and Tobacco Documents Online (http://www.tobaccodocuments.org).

We started with keyword searches on "bars," "nightclubs," "young adults," and "promotions," then searched for related documents, using authors, titles, dates, and Bates document numbers. Initial searches yielded thousands of documents; approximately 250 had content relevant to bar and nightclub promotional activities, the alternative press, and young adult peer influence. While the industry often uses the term "young adult" to refer to teenagers, it was clear from the context that the documents we identified were genuinely discussing young adults.

RESULTS

Development of Bar and Nightclub Promotions

Early plans for bar promotions were prepared for RJ Reynolds in the mid-1980s as part of a general industry trend toward increasing use of promotions[20] to reach young adults. RJ Reynolds' 1983 marketing plan strategy discusses the benefits of a "field marketing" strategy using person-to-person interaction at parties, concerts, and nightclubs to "reinforce Camel's masculine psychological image within the context of programs which are lifestyle oriented" and to integrate smoking with nightlife, music, and sports.[21] A proposal by Entertainment Marketing and Communications International submitted to RJ Reynolds in the mid-1980s emphasized the value of the bar setting to reach young people starting to smoke: "In general, this showcase nightclub audience targets perfectly new and current users at a time when brand loyalty is being tested and established."[22] A Romann & Tannenholz proposal to Philip Morris also described how its bar and nightclub program would compete with Camel's for the "entry-level" smoker.[23]

At a 1989 brainstorming session for the Camel Smooth Moves campaign, many of the elements of bar promotions "to elicit consumer involvement," including cigarette sampling, free Camel accessories, amateur band talent contests, comedy clubs, races, beaches, winter resorts, and "cruising," were presented.[24] A memorandum between RJ Reynolds executives described details of the promotional activities at Florida nightclubs during US universities' spring break in 1989:

> The Camel night club entertainment really was "cool." As you entered the club smokers received cigarettes, lighters, Camel t-shirts and a key which you brought over to the Camel tent for a chance to win the car. Once inside the club the classy Smooth Character girls, dressed in bright blue, sang and danced. The crowd was alive when the girls performed. Also, there was a really hip guy with sun glasses who led the girls.[25]

A detailed report from a marketing firm describes how RJ Reynolds' spring break promotions at Daytona Beach nightclubs used live music, contests, games, and distribution of free cigarette samples:

> The centerpiece of Camel's Spring Break program is the "Smooth Moves." Essentially the Smooth Moves consists of a male emcee and three very attractive and talented women who perform a professionally produced vocal/dance routine in Daytona's most popular clubs. . . . At each of the individual club promotions involving the Smooth Moves performance, several additional promotions will also be executed.
> 1. Smooth Moves Photoboard. . . .
> 2. Find Your Smooth Character Game. . . . All males entering will receive a male card. . . . All females entering receive a female card. . . . The objective is for both males and females to find their Smooth Character. If they find 2, 3, or 4 correct matches (tips) for the Smooth Move they have, they visit a prize center located in the club to receive a Camel prize.
> 3. Sampling will occur at each club promotion. Samplers will be distributing Camel Lights and Camel Filters along with a car key to smokers only. The key is an entry into a localized Smooth Car Sweepstakes where smokers have a chance to win a Nissan 300 ZX Turbo, or a variety of beach related Camel premiums.[26]

Brown & Williamson's bar promotions training manual outlines similar activities, such as a "Kool Theme Song Sing Along," a dance contest, and cigarette sample distribution.[27] Philip Morris events also included provocative games and cigarette sampling.[28]

Benefits of Bar Promotions to Tobacco Companies and to Bars

The tobacco industry cultivated brand presence in bar environments; this advertising grew more aggressive over time. Tobacco companies first provided bars with supplies to saturate the environment during events and provide a lasting presence. A 1989 marketing report for RJ Reynolds included a description of a "Bar/Nightclub Presence Kit" including Camel-branded items for patrons and staff:

> Establishments participating in Camel promotional activities will be supplied with the following items for special Camel nights and permanent brand presence:
> Cork lined bar trays
> Bar towels
> Simulated neon-lit write-on boards
> Napkin/Coaster/Stirrer Holders
> Ash Trays
> Coasters
> Napkins
> Table tents with write-in area[29]

Brown & Williamson used these tactics to promote Kool cigarettes in nightclub events during 1992[30]; its training manual instructs employees to remove the promotional materials belonging to competing tobacco companies during Kool events.[27] Philip Morris' 1990 bar promotions used Marlboro bar supplies, racing jackets, and pants for staff; in 1991 neon message boards and cocktail trays were added, to be "left behind as mementos from Marlboro."[31,32]

Tobacco companies also attracted bar owners with financial incentives. In 1991, RJ Reynolds hired Compel Marketing to conduct a survey of bar owners on their views of tobacco bar promotion. Compel recommended the following:

> I. A "bar paraphernalia" program should be tested incorporating a variety of Camel logo items.
> Over 40 percent of respondents were very interested and 70% were somewhat to very interested in purchasing from this type of program. . .
> II. A bar cigarette rack/sales program should be tested. . . . Discussions with attendants at the show strongly indicated that those bars who had established their own cigarette sales programs felt it represented a significant profit center. . . .
> III. A program of bar promotion kits should be tested. . . . Approximately 50 percent of respondents indicated a willingness to share the costs of these programs. It should be noted, however, that the level of cost sharing was modest; perhaps due to the $1500 estimated cost mentioned.[33]

A 1994 report to RJ Reynolds from KBA, an advertising firm that ran the RJ Reynolds Camel Club Program, addressed bar owners' cost concerns. "Using our Camel Club crew, we will approach clubs with promotional opportunities that will not only be cool and exciting, but also cost saving. . . . Being a Camel Club will make the venue eligible for valuable goods and services, both tangible and intangible."[34]

KBA recommended providing "premiums" worth $12 000 to bar owners and managers,[34] as well as offering promotional incentives to bar owners to display advertisements:

> In exchange for promotional support that we will provide for nightclubs, we will require the club to allow us to install in-club displays. These displays will be designed and coordinated keeping club aesthetics in mind. Nothing produced will be obtrusive, bright or out of the ordinary looking for a nightclub. Some of these items will be bar cigarette dispensers, cash register lights, and display marquees.[34]

A 1994 Philip Morris contract with a participating club guaranteed Parliament signage at the entrances, on the roof, and in at least 50% of available space during the events.[35] Memos from Brown & Williamson and Philip Morris indicate that these practices were expanded through 1995 to promote Lucky Strike and Parliament cigarettes.[28,36,37] In a 1996 operating plan, RJ Reynolds also stressed the importance of bartenders' selling cigarettes to bar patrons.[38]

Other Benefits to the Tobacco Companies

Research. Tobacco companies used promotions to build their name databases and collect information for marketing profiles, direct marketing, and potential political organizing.[39] A 1994 report to RJ Reynolds described how cigarette brand market research fit with promotional activities in bars and nightclubs:

> In order to monitor our success and evaluate strategies, market research will be a valuable tool. To maintain consistency with underlying discreet feel of the Camel Club Program, it is essential that market research is completed in non obtrusive fashion.
> In nightclubs, it is very common for an individual hired by the club to mingle with patrons, while obtaining names and information for the

> club's mailing list data base. As another perk for the nightclubs, we may hire and supervise this mailing list in person for them and use the information they collect for the purposes of Camel Club research. . . .[34]

A handwritten note on the document says, "This is also a service to the club—provide them with a general list—don't link back to the club—covert name-catching. . . . Can tailor a questionnaire for smoking with date of birth with signature."[34]

Brown & Williamson also designed smoker survey cards to profile smokers during nightclub promotions in 1988.[40] In a 1992 report, National Field Marketing Corporation advised the company to present the surveys as entries for a prize drawing.[30] Philip Morris documents list "name generation" for the company's consumer database as a primary objective of Parliament and Marlboro promotions.[41–43] Philip Morris used gifts, luxury car sweepstakes, and interactive video racing games to encourage patrons to fill out marketing surveys.[31,44,45] These 1993 promotions generated approximately 1.3 million new names for the Philip Morris database.[46] These databases were used to generate smoker profiles, direct mailing campaigns, and conduct telephone research studies after the bar events.[47]

Minority targeting. Bar promotions were also used to target specific communities, as was the case with RJ Reynolds' 1989 Camel Hispanic Program[29] and Philip Morris' Inner City Bar Night Program:

> To achieve trial, awareness and conversion objectives among Black smokers, Brand recommends an expansion of the Marlboro Menthol Inner City Bar Night Program developed during the second half of 1988. Given that we have limited tools to reach Black smokers, this represents an attempt to penetrate the audience via an aggressive event program which will work in combination with targeted in-store and media efforts.[48]

Philip Morris planned a $1.2 million expansion of this 1989 program.[48] A 1989 Brown & Williamson document also noted Philip Morris' pursuit of the "Black consumer" in bars.[40] Brown & Williamson's Kool Festival bar promotion events included a cocktail party for retailers to build awareness of Kool's "involvement in the community."[49]

A shield from social and political pressures. In the 1990s, bars provided a safe place to continue to promote cigarettes despite increasing social pressures against smoking. Reports from Brown & Williamson and Philip Morris note the "non hostile, festive lifestyle atmosphere"[30] and "smoker friendly environment" of bars.[50] Bar promotions also conferred protection against clean indoor air laws. In a 1994 report, Philip Morris consultant Romann and Tannenholz observed, "[f]acing increasing restrictions on smoking in public places, parties represent one of the last refuges—a place where smoking is not only permissible but part of the shared experience."[23]

Bar promotions also avoided the controversy around tobacco marketing to children. RJ Reynolds' 1996 operating plan mentions keeping marketing strategies "under the radar."[38] A Romann and Tannenholz 1994 market research report for Philip Morris recommends the company avoid political pressure by "develop[ing] a comprehensive below-the-line marketing program." The same report points out that bar promotions would "prevent potential public-relations issues [and] anticipate future restrictions on advertising."[23] Romann and Tannenholz correctly anticipated that marketing restrictions would likely be limited to youth and that bar and nightclub promotions would be immune, as they were in the 1998 Master Settlement Agreement.

Bar Promotions and the Alternative Press

The alternative press was an essential element of new tobacco industry advertising strategies to promote bar programs.[1,2,24] RJ Reynolds appears to have been the first to launch such an advertising campaign in the alternative press.[1,51] Other tobacco companies followed throughout the 1990s. The Ruxton Group, which managed alternative-press advertising in several major cities, recommended placing a "Smooth Character Column" on young adult entertainment in alternative newspapers in 1991:

> The Objective
> - To increase Camel's visibility with urban young adult smokers.
> - To identify Camel with young-adult entertainment in priority markets.
> - To maximize reader involvement with Camel ads . . .
> - To associate Camel with what's fun to do in town.
>
> The Concept
> Introducing The Smooth Character: a column of colorful banter about what's doing in town and who's been doing it with whom . . .
> The Benefits
> - Reaches young-adult smokers in priority markets.
> - Provides unique creative for each market on a weekly basis at a low cost.
> - Associates Camel with what's hot, what's fun, what's local.
> - Provides opportunities for promotional, and merchandising tie-ins.
> - Reaches research documented full- and part-time smokers.[52]

KBA advertising, in a 1994 marketing proposal, also recommended the alternative press as media support for bar promotions. The company noted how this technique was used by Girbaud jeans to reach young adults who frequent nightclubs:

> Every major city in the nation has a number of alternative media outlets. These newspapers and magazines appeal to the urban, progressive trend setters and often have gossip columns that speak of trendy happenings, such as art openings, nightclub events, underground parties, and benefits. These free periodicals are distributed at most trendy nightclubs and are found in the stores and coffeehouses that the club crowd frequents.
> Developing an alternative advertising campaign geared towards the club goers, would be ideal. In the past year, Girbaud jeans, a trendy high profile clothing company has sponsored a full-page calendar of hip events for the week in New York's Village Voice. The placement of this particular ad is directly adjacent to the nightclub gossip column. This has aligned Girbaud with every trend setting event in New York City for the past year. Girbaud clothing first became prominent seven years ago in the club scene and has sustained its hip image through its affiliation with the trend setting scene. Aligning Camel with certain publications by way of advertising lends immediate hip credibility to the brand.[34]

The 1996 operating plan for RJ Reynolds suggests placement of tobacco advertisements in the alternative press by the "use of club page local media to hype event."[38] An analysis of tobacco promotions in the alternative press shows that these strategies were implemented, with the highest concentration of tobacco advertisements in entertainment-focused sections.[1]

Bar Promotions and Young Adult Peer Influence

Bar promotions also provided a tool with which to engineer peer influence among young adults. The tobacco industry studied peer influence for years and considered it to be a major factor in promoting smoking initiation among both adolescents and young adults.[22,53–55] The industry worked to identify "social leaders" or "trendsetters,"[53,55] believing that changing the smoking behavior of social leaders would, in turn, influence a large number of potential smokers.[54]

In 1992, Philip Morris conducted extensive research in its "Social Networks Project":

> If data from brief questionnaires can distinguish between leaders and other group members, this capability could be applied to:
> - Marketing efforts to communicate more extensively with leaders than other group members.
> - Screening for subsequent research, given leaders' importance in the diffusion process.[53]

Philip Morris attempted to design questionnaires that could differentiate leaders from nonleaders in a short telephone survey.[55] In the mid-1980s an RJ Reynolds contractor, Entertainment Marketing & Communications International (EMCI), attempted to reach "trendsetters" through make-your-own music videos in bars.[22] Brown & Williamson sought to market Lucky Strike cigarettes to social leaders in 1995.[36]

The relationships between bar owners, club promoters, employees, and patrons provided an ideal social structure for the use of leaders to encourage smoking. In 1994, the KBA advertising firm reported to RJ Reynolds on "trend influence marketing," a strategy that capitalized on clearly defined "leaders": bar owners, bar workers, club promoters, and bar patrons. KBA's "Camel Club Program" sought to influence 3 "tiers": bar owners, workers, and patrons. KBA recommended providing premiums totaling $12 000 to bar owners and managers (the first tier).[34] The tobacco-sponsored entertainment events also helped bar owners financially by encouraging patronage and defraying the cost of live entertainment. KBA observed that club promoters were another source of influence:

> A very important entity in the nightclub scene is the nightclub promoter. Most nightclubs utilize these individuals or groups to promote special events. Promoters are generally the trend setters of the nightclub scene. They define what is hip. A promoter will generate an idea for an event, usually something thematic that involves some sort of entertainment.
> In many cases, promoters use their own funds to produce events. In these cases, where promoters are self-financed, our financial support in the form of printing reimbursements and premium giveaway packages will win their loyalty with relative ease. . . .
> We will use the same techniques for club owners and managers to make promoters part of Camel Trend Influence Marketing effort, i.e. Camel jackets, premiums, event sponsorship funds, etc.[31]

Bar employees constituted the second tier of KBA's plan. The plan described how to influence bar employees to become allies in marketing cigarettes:

> Tier Two: Utilize our "foot in the door" to influence bar employees and convert them to Camel brand smokers and promote the brand. . . .
> The crux of Tier Two is to convert the bar staff to Camel. We will do so by offering top notch premiums such as leather motorcycle jackets, with the employees name embroidered on the front. Embroidering the employee's name will make the jacket a more valuable tool to reinforce and enhance our relationship with this influential segment. . . . In addition, our "Camel Club Crew" will develop relationships with these employees, always tip well at the bar (very important!) And occasionally schmooze the employees with other Camel gifts as well as dinner packages at local restaurants. Of course, Camel Club employees will have an ample supply of Camel cigarettes for personal use and to present to patrons.[34]

Bar employees were also slated to receive $12 000 in premiums, according to KBA's start-up budget.[34] Camel's 1996 operating plan also recommended cultivating a relationship with bar workers, stressing that it was "critical to convert bar staff to Camel [so they could] act as selling agents."[38]

The third tier consisted of trend-setting patrons who would be influenced by the bar management and staff to smoke Camels:

> Tier Three: Work with the bar employees to influence the trend setting patrons, which will then start to make smoking Camel a recognized trend . . .
> Once our relationship is solidified with club owners, management and bar staff, we will begin to subtly train the employees on how to influence smokers of competitive brands to sample Camel with the goal of eventually switching brands. Because we are making Camel "trendy" as well as formulating a positive and productive relationship with the staff . . . the process of generating trial among patrons will appear quite natural and uncontrived.[34]

Ideally, hip young bar patrons would also recruit their non–club-going friends who viewed them as leaders.

DISCUSSION

Bar and nightclub promotions started as part of an increase in promotional events that integrated tobacco marketing with young adult activities and reached beginning smokers. They were later expanded to increase consumer involvement and to create smoke-friendly promotional environments. These promotions are also used for marketing research, to target minorities, and as a haven from social pressures. They protect the industry from advertising regulations, clean indoor air laws, and accusations of marketing to adolescents. Bar promotions help the industry engineer peer influence to encourage tobacco use among young adults.

The volume of tobacco industry documents (more than 40 million pages) and the inefficiency with which many are indexed makes it difficult to know whether we located all relevant documents. Those we did analyze, however, provide a consistent picture of industry marketing activities that were still observable in bars and clubs in 2001. The fact that these practices have been duplicated over time and replicated by several tobacco companies increases our confidence in these findings. The relationship between tobacco and alcohol use in these venues is beyond the scope of this study, but it is a fertile topic for future inquiry.

Bar and nightclub promotions are an example of the tobacco industry's shift from traditional advertising to promotional activities. Tobacco promotional allowances tripled between 1988 and 1998, while spending on advertising remained constant.[20] The industry has taken affirmative steps to protect bar promotional venues. The 1998 Master Settlement Agreement between the tobacco industry and many states' attorneys general explicitly exempts marketing in "adult-only facilities" from its limitations on industry activities.[56] The industry opposes bar provisions of clean indoor air laws with particular vigor[57,58] and has fought hard (if unsuccessfully) to repeal the provisions in California's smoke-free workplace law that apply to bars and clubs.[59–61]

The industry's penetration into bars may have serious implications for smoking initiation among the young adults who frequent bars. The industry's manipulation of peer influence through incentives to "social leaders" can encourage nonsmoking young adults to initiate smoking as well as move experimenters toward addiction.[22,23,34] The increase in smoking rates among young adults indicates that their smoking behavior is still amenable to outside influences and suggests the success of the tobacco industry's strategy.[8,9]

The fact that it is legal for young adults to smoke does not mitigate the public health burden of disease and suffering that will be incurred later in life by these young smokers and the nonsmokers who will be exposed to their secondhand smoke. Tobacco control advocates should include young adults in research and advocacy efforts and should design interventions to counter the tobacco industry's bar promotion strategy.

The industry's use of this strategy can also provide a guide for public health practitioners working with young adults. Bars' association with the tobacco industry should be portrayed as negative exploitation of social and cultural institutions. Rather than stressing resistance skills to counter peer pressure, public health educators should seek to identify social leaders and encourage them to promote and defend smoke-free lifestyles. Creation of smoke-free bars—with appropriate groundwork and public education—may be a key to undermining the tobacco industry's efforts to use bars to reestablish the social acceptability of smoking and secondhand smoke. ■

About the Authors

The authors are with the Institute for Health Policy Studies and the Center for AIDS Prevention Studies, University of California, San Francisco.

Requests for reprints should be sent to Stanton A. Glantz, PhD, Division of Cardiology, Box 0130, University of California, San Francisco, CA 94143-0130 (e-mail: glantz@medicine.ucsf.edu).

This article was accepted October 14, 2001.

Contributors

All authors contributed to the design of the study and writing and editing of the paper. E. Sepe and P.M. Ling collected the data.

Acknowledgments

This work was supported by National Cancer Institute grants CA-61021 and CA-87472 and by the Richard and Rhoda Goldman Fund.

This work was presented at the Annual Meeting of the American Public Health Association, Atlanta, Ga, October 21–25, 2001.

References

1. Sepe E, Glantz SA. Tobacco promotions in the alternative press: targeting young adults. *Am J Public Health.* 2002;92:75–78.

2. Cruz T, Weiner M, Schuster D, Unger J. Growth of tobacco-sponsored bars and clubs from 1996–2000. Paper presented at: Annual Meeting of the American Public Health Association; November 12–16, 2000; Boston, Mass.

3. Carreon C. Cigarette clubs waft into Portland scene. *The Oregonian.* July 31, 1998:C01.

4. Davis HL. A Party to Die For? *Buffalo News.* July 27, 1998:A4–A5.

5. Gellene D. Joining the clubs: tobacco firms find a venue in bars. *Los Angeles Times.* September 25, 1997: D1–D3.

6. Scholtes PS. You're not invited. *City Pages.* September 22, 1999. Available at: http://www.citypages.com/databank/20/981/article8000.asp. Accessed December 27, 2001.

7. Graham C. Tobacco companies heat up the nightclub scene. *St. Petersburg Times.* August 16, 1998. Available at: http://www.sptimes.com. Accessed December 27, 2001.

8. Summary of findings from the 1998 National Household Survey on Drug Abuse. August 1999. Available (in PDF format) at: http://www.samhsa.gov/oas/NHSDA/NHSDAsumrpt.pdf. Accessed December 31, 2001.

9. Wechsler H, Rigotti NA, Gledhill-Hoyt J, Lee H. Increased levels of cigarette use among college students: a cause for national concern. *JAMA.* 1998;280: 1673–1678.

10. Pierce JP, Lee L, Gilpin EA. Smoking initiation by adolescent girls, 1944 through 1988. An association with targeted advertising. *JAMA.* 1994;271:608–611.

11. Gilpin E, Pierce J. Trends in adolescent smoking initiation in the United States: is tobacco marketing an influence? *Tobacco Control.* 1997;6:122–127.

12. Pierce JP, Choi WS, Gilpin EA, Farkas AJ, Berry CC. Tobacco industry promotion of cigarettes and adolescent smoking [published correction appears in *JAMA.* 1998;280:422]. *JAMA.* 1998;279:511–515. (See comments.)

13. Pollay RW, Siddarth S, Siegel M, et al. The last straw? Cigarette advertising and realized market shares among youths and adults, 1979–1993. *J Marketing.* 1996;60(2):1.

14. Burns D, Lee L, Vaughn J, Chiu Y, Shopland D. Rates of smoking initiation among adolescents and young adults, 1907–1981. *Tobacco Control.* 1995; 4(suppl 1):S2–S8.

15. Centers for Disease Control and Prevention. Surveillance for selected tobacco-use behaviors—United States, 1900–1994. *MMWR CDC Surveill Summ.* 1994;43: no. SS-03.

16. Escobedo LG, Anda RF, Smith PF, Remington PL, Mast EE. Sociodemographic characteristics of cigarette smoking initiation in the United States: implications for smoking prevention policy. *JAMA.* 1990;264: 1550–1555.

17. Gilpin EA, Lee L, Evans N, Pierce JP. Smoking initiation rates in adults and minors: United States, 1944–1988. *Am J Epidemiol.* 1994;140:535–543.

18. Centers for Disease Control and Prevention. Differences in the age of smoking initiation between blacks and whites—United States. *MMWR Morb Mortal Wkly Rep.* 1991;40:754–757.

19. Malone RE, Balbach ED. Tobacco industry documents: treasure trove or quagmire? *Tobacco Control.* 2000;9:334–338. (See comment in: *Tobacco Control.* 2000;9:261–262).

20. Federal Trade Commission. 2000 Report on Cigarette Sales, Advertising and Promotion. Available (in PDF format) at: http://www.ftc.gov/reports/cigarettes/cig98rpt.pdf. Accessed December 31, 2001.

21. RJ Reynolds. Camel 1983 marketing plan strategy. Document no. 501255159/5163. Available at: http://www.library.ucsf.edu/tobacco/mangini. Accessed December 13, 2000.

22. Entertainment Marketing and Communications International. Camel's make your own music video. Document no. 507366721/6731. Available at: http://www.library.ucsf.edu/tobacco/mangini. Accessed December 16, 2000.

23. Romann and Tannenholz. Cigarette concepts for young adult male smokers. June 10, 1994. Document no. 2041601862-2041601885. Available at: http://www.pmdocs.com. Accessed October 27, 2000.

24. Topline summary of Camel 1989 brainstorming sessions. 1989. Document no. 507244940/4966. Available at: http://www.library.ucsf.edu/tobacco/mangini. Accessed December 13, 2000.

25. Layne S, Murphy K. Daytona Promotions. March 27, 1989. Document no. 506868845/8847. Available at: http://www.library.ucsf.edu/tobacco/mangini. Accessed December 22, 2000.

26. Promotional Marketing I. Camel spring resort program Daytona Beach, 1989. 1988. Document no. 507240802-507240812. Available at: http://www.library.ucsf.edu/tobacco/mangini. Accessed December 15, 2000.

27. Kool promotion crew training manual. Document no. 300119790/9806. Available at: http://www.tobaccodocuments.org. Accessed December 27, 2000.

28. GMR Marketing. Parliament party zone 1995 program. August 11, 1994. Document no. 2040575026/5043. Available at: http://www.pmdocs.com. Accessed February 14, 2001.

29. Promotional Marketing Inc. Camel Hispanic program. February 15, 1989. Document no. 507133229/3239. Available at: http://www.library.ucsf.edu/tobacco/mangini. Accessed December 15, 2000.

30. Butcher J, Zito F, National Field Marketing Corporation. Virginia test market final report summer 1992. Document no. 300119873/9928. Available at: http://www.tobaccodocuments.org. Accessed December 27, 2000.

31. Berner V. Marlboro target marketing Phoenix blitz program/March 2 and April 8, 1990. February 1, 1990. Document no. 2048626715/6722. Available at: http://www.pmdocs.com. Accessed February 13, 2001.

32. Howe K. Special markets '91 Marlboro regional event marketing. February 15, 1991. Document no. 2043685428/5441. Available at: http://www.pmdocs.com. Accessed February 13, 2001.

33. Compel Marketing Inc. Top shelf B.A.R. show Camel survey analysis. October 16, 1991. Document

no. 507647227/7241. Available at: http://www.library.ucsf.edu/tobacco/mangini. Accessed December 13, 2000.

34. KBA. Trend influence marketing program. April 14, 1994. Document no. MB(2)25655–MB(2)25687. Available at: http://www.library.ucsf.edu/tobacco/mangini. Accessed December 13, 2000.

35. Reynolds GM. Re: Parliament party zone '94 Program. January 4, 1994. Document no. 2042021610/1613. Available at: http://www.pmdocs.com. Accessed February 14, 2001.

36. Barclay C. Lucky Strike–Promotion materials. March 3, 1995. Document no. 325000013/0017. Available at: http://www.tobaccodocuments.org. Accessed December 27, 2000.

37. Parliament party zone. June 1995. Document no. 2045562051/2080. Available at: http://www.pmdocs.com. Accessed February 14, 2001.

38. Camel 1996 operation plan. Document no. 514757323/7327. Available at: http://www.library.ucsf.edu/tobacco/mangini. Accessed December 22, 2000.

39. Samuels B, Glantz SA. The politics of local tobacco control. *JAMA.* 1991;266:2110–2117.

40. Paulley B. Potential Kool bar kit items. February 7, 1989. Document no. 300102450/2451. Available at: http://www.tobaccodocuments.org. Accessed December 27, 2000.

41. Parliament creative brief. September 1993. Document no. 2040556561/6563. Available at: http://www.pmdocs.com. Accessed February 12, 2001.

42. Marlboro racing bar nights. August 1993. Document no. 2040993113/3116. Available at: http://www.pmdocs.com. Accessed February 13, 2001.

43. Marlboro Country 1994 dance club night program. 1993. Document no. 2041942879/2885. Available at: http://www.pmdocs.com. Accessed February 13, 2001.

44. DiJulio A. Re: Marlboro event card topline response: fourth quarter 93. February 9, 1994. Document no. 2042050103-2042050105. Available at: http://www.pmdocs.com. Accessed February 13, 2001.

45. Briefing format for Marlboro dance showdown '94. May 19, 1994. Document no. 2041943026/3028. Available at: http://www.pmdocs.com. Accessed February 13, 2001.

46. von Germeten A. Re: Marlboro database management. August 17, 1994. Document no. 2042045416/5425. Available at: http://www.pmdocs.com. Accessed February 13, 2001.

47. Resman T. Parliament party zone research. January 9, 1995. Document no. 2045173494/3529. Available at: http://www.pmdocs.com. Accessed February 15, 2001.

48. Menthol-event sponsorship Marlboro menthol inner city bar nights. 1989. Document no. 2048678695/8697. Available at: http://www.pmdocs.com. Accessed February 13, 2001.

49. Kool Festival 1986 revised promotions plan. April 1986. Document no. 697005957/5967. Available at: http://www.bw.aalatg.com. Accessed December 27, 2000.

50. Gennaro MJ. Marlboro Country Nights Dance Showdown '94. May 31, 1994. Document no. 2061803735-2061803737. Available at: http://www.pmdocs.com. Accessed February 13, 2001.

51. Orlowsky M. Younger Adult Smoker Newspapers. May 11, 1981. Document no. 500126859. Available at: http://www.pmdocs.com. Accessed December 16, 2000.

52. Ruxton Group. Media/Presentation Opportunities for Camel: The Ruxton Group Proposes The Camel "Smooth Character" Column. RJ Reynolds. Document no. 508824458C-508824461. Available at: http://www.library.ucsf.edu/tobacco/mangini. Accessed December 22, 2000.

53. Social networks and adventure team promotions: summary of findings. April 1, 1993. Document no. 2045170995/1040. Available at: http://www.pmdocs.com. Accessed September 19, 2000.

54. Bittner B. Draft Syllabus of Research Conducted Under the Auspices of W.M. Bittner, March 1990 to Present. Philip Morris. December 1, 1992. Document no. 2047918063-2047918070. Available at: http://www.pmdocs.com. Accessed December 20, 2000.

55. Philip Morris. 3 Years in Review. 1991. Document no. 2045173702-3710. Available at: http://www.pmdocs.com. Accessed December 20, 2000.

56. National Association of Attorneys General. Master Settlement Agreement. 1998. Section II c and III c–g. Available at: http://www.naag.org/tobac/cigmsa.rtf. Accessed December 20, 2000.

57. Macdonald HR, Glantz SA. Political realities of statewide smoking legislation: the passage of California's Assembly Bill 13. *Tobacco Control.* 1997;6:41–54.

58. Glantz SA, Balbach ED. *Tobacco War: Inside The California Battles.* Berkeley: University of California Press; 2000.

59. Magzamen S, Glantz SA. The new battleground: California's experience with smoke-free bars. *Am J Public Health.* 2001;91:245–252.

60. Magzamen S, Charlesworth A, Glantz S. Print media coverage of the California smokefree bar law. *Tobacco Control.* 2001;10:154–160.

61. University of California San Diego, Cancer Prevention and Control Program. Tobacco control in California: who's winning the war? 1998. Available at: http://jukebox.ucsd.edu/tobacco/reports/.

Why and How the Tobacco Industry Sells Cigarettes to Young Adults: Evidence From Industry Documents

| Pamela M. Ling, MD, MPH, and Stanton A. Glantz, PhD

Objectives. To improve tobacco control campaigns, we analyzed tobacco industry strategies that encourage young adults (aged 18 to 24) to smoke.

Methods. Initial searches of tobacco industry documents with keywords (e.g., "young adult") were extended by using names, locations, and dates.

Results. Approximately 200 relevant documents were found. Transitions from experimentation to addiction, with adult levels of cigarette consumption, may take years. Tobacco marketing solidifies addiction among young adults. Cigarette advertisements encourage regular smoking and increased consumption by integrating smoking into activities and places where young adults' lives change (e.g., leaving home, college, jobs, the military, bars).

Conclusions. Tobacco control efforts should include both adults and youths. Life changes are also opportunities to stop occasional smokers' progress to addiction. Clean air policies in workplaces, the military, bars, colleges, and homes can combat tobacco marketing. (*Am J Public Health.* 2002;92:908–916)

Virtually all tobacco control programs emphasize primary prevention for children and teens or smoking cessation for adult smokers. Tobacco control efforts aimed at young adults (aged 18–24 years) are generally limited to cessation for pregnant women,[1–8] military personnel,[9–14] or college students.[15–17] Despite the widely accepted view that smoking initiation occurs only before age 18, smoking frequently began during young adulthood in the early and mid-20th century and still does among some ethnic groups.[18–21] Rates of current cigarette use among young adults increased steadily, from 34.6% in 1994 to 41.6% in 1998,[20] and then declined slightly, to 39.7% in 1999 and to 38.3% in 2000.[22] The prevalence of current smoking among college students increased from 22.3% in 1993 to 28.5% in 1998.[23]

The number of young people at moderate to high risk for established smoking increases throughout the teen years, with more people in the early stages of smoking initiation (open to smoking, experimenting, and nonregular smoking) at ages 14 to 19 than at 11 to 14.[24] The number of 18- to 19-year-olds in the early stages of smoking initiation is more than twice the number of 18-year-old established smokers.[24] These youths are at risk to become established smokers as young adults and thus are prime targets for interventions to make them nonsmokers again.

Since 1998, more than 40 million pages of previously secret tobacco industry documents have been made available to the public. Previous investigations with these documents concentrated on proving that tobacco industry marketing targeted youths.[25–27] We analyzed the documents to find why and how the tobacco industry markets to young adults and drew 3 conclusions. First, the industry views the transition from smoking the first cigarette to becoming a confirmed pack-a-day smoker as a series of stages[28–30] that may extend to age 25,[31] and it has developed marketing strategies not only to encourage initial experimentation (often by teens) but also to carry new smokers through each stage of this process.[28,32–36] Second, industry marketers encourage solidification of smoking habits and increases in cigarette consumption by focusing on key transition periods when young adults adopt new behaviors—such as entering a new workplace, school, or the military—and, especially, by focusing on leisure and social activities.[33,37,38] Third, tobacco companies study young adults' attitudes, social groups, values, aspirations, role models, and activities and then infiltrate both their physical and their social environments.[37,39–43] Understanding this process can help public health practitioners to develop better tobacco control programs and physicians to encourage nonsmoking among young adult patients.

METHODS

We searched tobacco industry document archives from the University of California–San Francisco's collection of R.J. Reynolds (RJR) and British American Tobacco marketing documents (http://www.library.ucsf.edu/tobacco), tobacco industry document Web sites (Philip Morris: http://www.pmdocs.com; Brown and Williamson: http://www.brownandwilliamson.com; RJR: http://www.rjrtdocs.com; Lorillard: http://www.lorillarddocs.com), and Tobacco Documents Online (http://www.tobaccodocuments.org). Initial search terms included the following: young adults, younger adult, new smokers, marketing, advertising, college, bars, military, Generation X, industry terms for young adult smokers (such as "YAFS," a Philip Morris abbreviation for Young Adult Female Smokers), lifestyle, motivation, strategy, and brand names.

Initial searches yielded thousands of documents. Applying standard techniques,[44] we repeated and focused the searches. We also conducted further searches for contextual information on relevant documents by using their names, locations, dates, and reference (Bates) numbers. This analysis is based on a final collection of approximately 200 marketing research reports, questionnaires, memorandums, and plans. We found most of the documents in the Philip Morris, Lorillard, and RJR collections; these companies also own the brands most popular among young people (Marlboro, Camel, and Newport).[22,45] Although the tobacco industry has used "younger adult smoker" as a code word to disguise efforts to recruit teenage smokers,[46] we limited this analysis to tobacco industry docu-

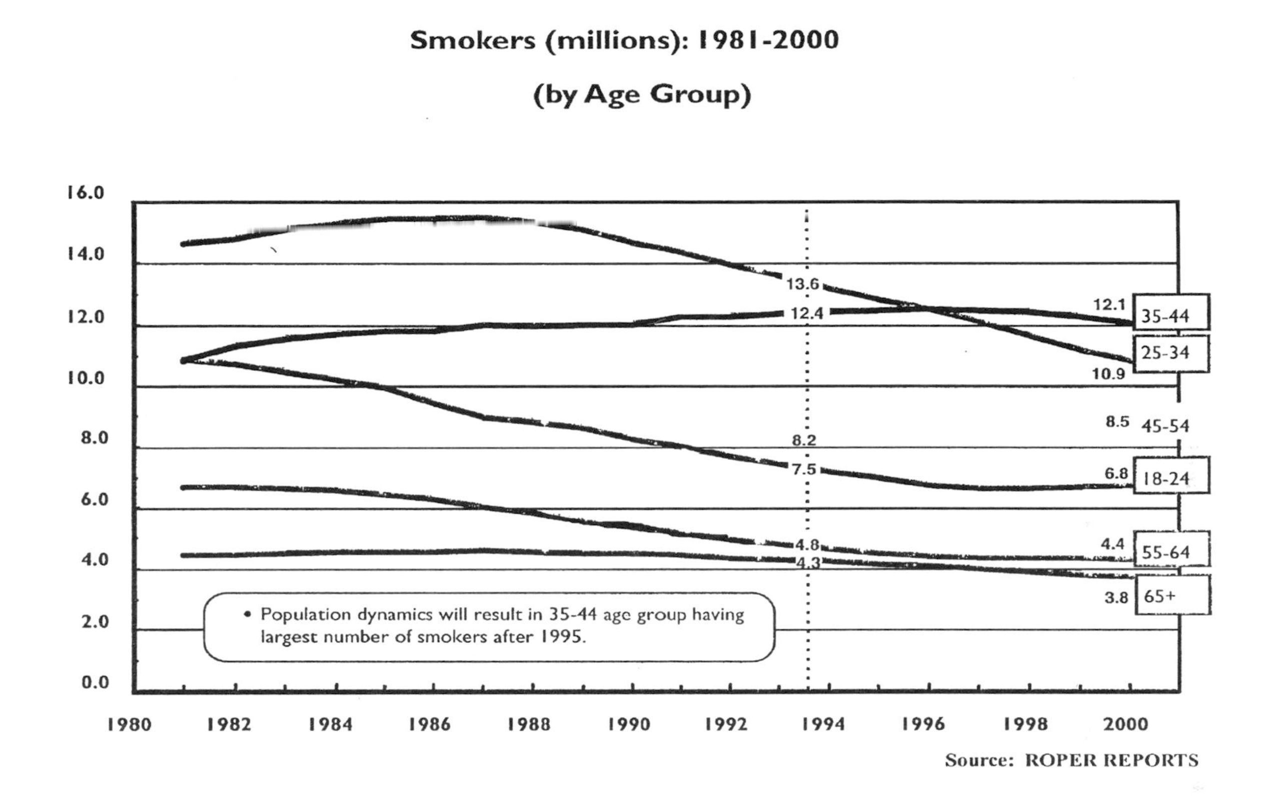

FIGURE 1—A 1993 Philip Morris document showing numbers of smokers by age group from 1981 to 2000 (projected).

ments that explicitly discussed 18- to 24-year-olds or young adult activities, such as military service, college, or going to bars.

RESULTS

Tobacco Industry Efforts to Encourage Smoking Span Youth and Adulthood

Tobacco marketers regard smoking initiation as a process that begins among teenagers but that must be cultivated among young adults. Not only does the tobacco industry encourage youths to start smoking, but its efforts to reinforce smoking continue well into adulthood.[34] In contrast to public health's concentration on youth, the tobacco industry tracks smokers in every age group (Figure 1). Philip Morris's 1993 projections of the smoking population estimated that there would be 6.8 million young adult smokers in 2000—more than double the number of teen smokers in public health estimates.[24,47]

Like tobacco marketers, public health researchers portray smoking initiation as a progression of stages.[45,48] For more than 30 years, tobacco industry researchers have also used models presenting the creation of an addicted smoker in a series of stages, each with different needs and motivations, and have developed marketing strategies to move people through this process. For example, in 1973, RJR strategist Claude Teague illustrated how the young smoker progresses from "pre-smoker" to "learner" to "confirmed smoker" in a model less sophisticated than but similar to later public health models (Figure 2). He advised that tobacco marketing should match each stage in this process.[28]

Another 1985 report written for RJR explained how smoking evolves from a social means of connecting with peers in the teenage years to become a habitual response to stress or boredom in adulthood (Figure 3).[33] The report illustrates the changing role of smoking for young adults:

> These years of transition represent a shift between the comfort of the high influence of the peer group, and relative structure in life, to the development of one's own personal, social and occupational goals. For some, smoking seems to fulfill the function during teens of uniting one with the all-important peer group. In adulthood, it may be used to ease the feelings of stress created by the pursuit of one's goals. Smoking, for a young adult, may fulfill both roles, providing a concrete balance at a time when life is chaotic and stressful. It represents both the ties with the "old days" and "old friends," as well as the more mature instrument for relaxing.[33]

Similar strategies based on stage models of smoking were developed by several tobacco companies and their consultants in the 1970s, 1980s, and 1990s.[30,32,34,37,39] One Philip Morris researcher noted in a 1981 report that "the overwhelming majority of smokers first begin to smoke while still in their teens. In addition, the ten years following the teenage years is the period during which average daily consumption per smoker increases to the average adult level."[29] Both RJR and

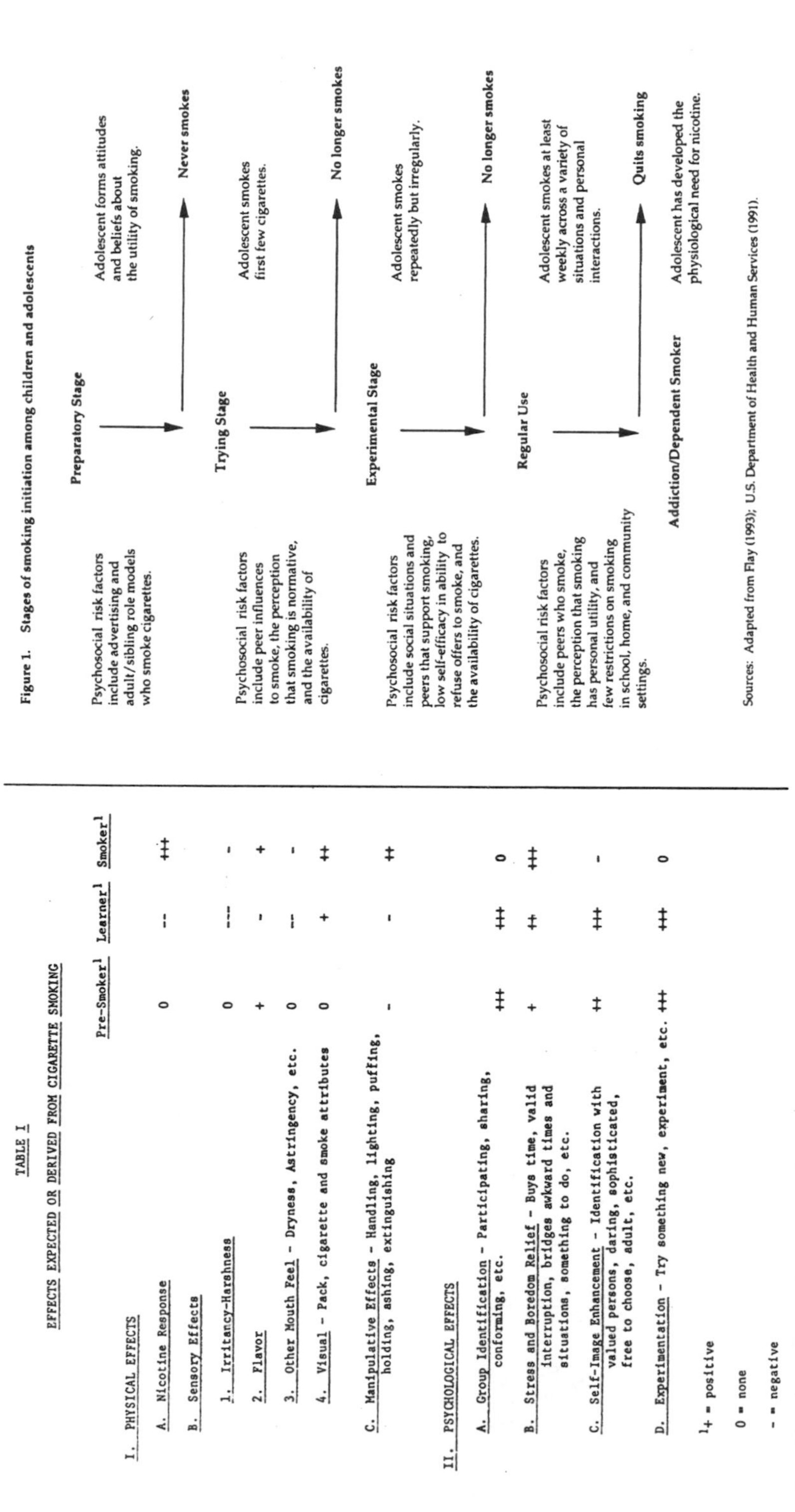

TABLE I

EFFECTS EXPECTED OR DERIVED FROM CIGARETTE SMOKING

	Pre-Smoker[1]	Learner[1]	Smoker[1]
I. PHYSICAL EFFECTS			
A. Nicotine Response	0	--	+++
B. Sensory Effects			
1. Irritancy-Harshness	0	---	-
2. Flavor	+	-	+
3. Other Mouth Feel - Dryness, Astringency, etc.	0	--	-
4. Visual - Pack, cigarette and smoke attributes	0	+	++
C. Manipulative Effects - Handling, lighting, puffing, holding, ashing, extinguishing	-	-	++
II. PSYCHOLOGICAL EFFECTS			
A. Group Identification - Participating, sharing, conforming, etc.	+++	+++	0
B. Stress and Boredom Relief - Buys time, valid interruption, bridges awkward times and situations, something to do, etc.	+	++	+++
C. Self-Image Enhancement - Identification with valued persons, daring, sophisticated, free to choose, adult, etc.	++	+++	-
D. Experimentation - Try something new, experiment, etc.	+++	+++	0

[1]+ = positive

0 = none

- = negative

FIGURE 2—Comparison of tobacco industry model (1973 R.J. Reynolds document[28]) and public health model (1994 Surgeon General's Report[45]) of smoking initiation.

Philip Morris developed cigarette brands for each stage of smoking, including these later stages.[32,34,49] For example, in 1994, Philip Morris's advertising agency, Young & Rubicam, presented the following model to illustrate evolution of brand choice as the young adult smoker matures:

> Choice of "starter" brand→youthful conformity/rebellion
> "Break-away" brand→early maturation: individuation and self-assertion
> Choice of "mature" brand(s)→later maturation: self-management/tradeoffs[32]

Young & Rubicam recommended that Philip Morris position Chesterfield to appeal to young adults who were approaching a life transition that involved increasing "individuation and self-assertion":

> Who Are We Talking To: Young Adult Male Smoking Enthusiasts, 18–24, who no longer want to be labeled as one of the crowd. They resist peer group pressure, and therefore are open to an alternative to Marlboro. As smokers, our target lives in a climate of exile and disapproval. They view smoking as part of their *choice*, their *individuality*, their *self-expression*. *"Not Your First"* capitalizes on our target's desire for individualistic style—and intense experiences—while dramatizing Chesterfield's superior smoking pleasure.[32] [Emphasis in original]

Not only is tobacco marketing designed to cultivate smokers throughout the process of smoking initiation; brands are also positioned for established smokers who are thinking seriously about quitting, such as those who are concerned about health and the financial costs of smoking.[50,51] Examination of an RJR 1981 segmentation study presentation reveals how brands were positioned for each life stage (Figure 4).[34] RJR attempted to match a brand image—such as "macho, strong and masculine" or "low tar, health concerned"—to the smoker's life stage.[34]

Young Adulthood Provides Opportunities to Solidify Addiction

Young adults are particularly important to the industry for several reasons. First, the progression from "experimenter" to "mature" smoker is accompanied by an important increase in consumption.[29] Second, young adults face multiple life transitions that provide opportunities for adoption and solidification of smoking as a regular part of new

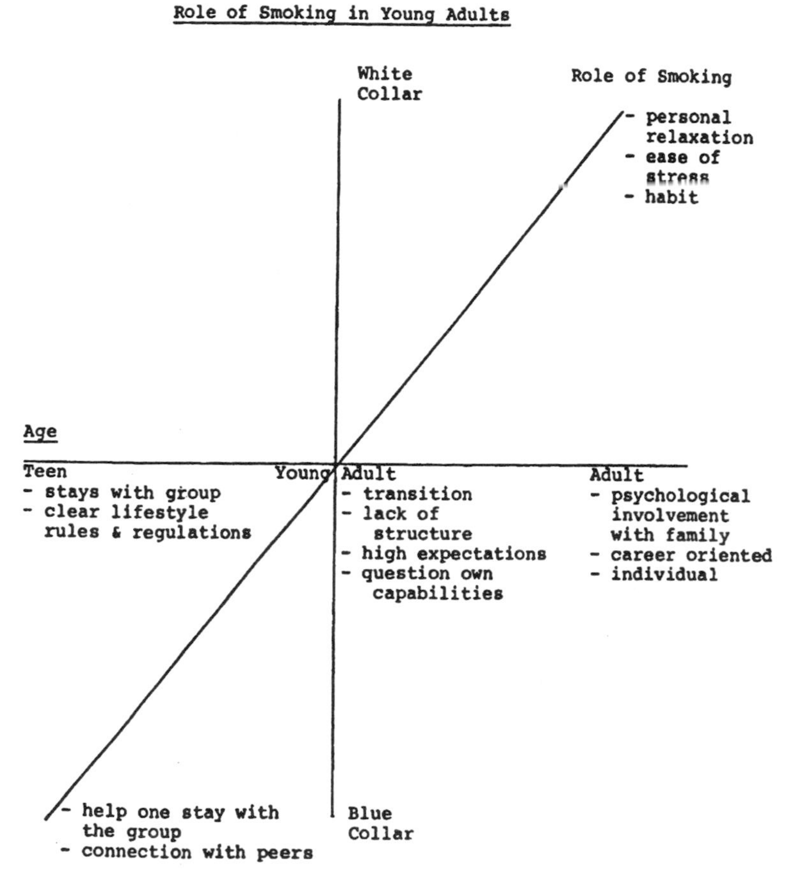

Note. This report also explored the role of smoking among young adult blue- and white-collar workers.[33]

FIGURE 3—A 1985 R.J. Reynolds document illustrating different roles of smoking for teens, young adults, and adults.

activities.[36] Third, the stresses of these life transitions invite the use of cigarettes for the drug effects of nicotine.[36]

Tobacco marketers investigated how changes in friends, family, and work are linked to smoking among young adults. In 1982, a Philip Morris researcher described how changes in young people's lives make them more likely to switch brands and to increase cigarette consumption:

> Life passages are major, milestone events in a person's life which can significantly affect the quality and content of the person's life from that day forward. One can imagine a young man or woman experiencing these changes as they age and mature. . . . a significant number of people are experiencing changes in their lives, and these people are volatile in their smoking behavior: They are more likely to switch and increase consumption.[52]

Each "life passage" provides an opportunity for the tobacco marketer to introduce and solidify smoking. As Philip Morris advertising consultants Young & Rubicam noted in 1994, "significant choice moments in cigarette smoking tend to coincide with critical transition stages in life."[32]

In addition, tobacco marketers knew that such "life passages" were stressful and that these periods were an opportune time to take advantage of the pharmacological effects of nicotine. In young adulthood, smoking increasingly becomes a way to deal with the stresses of life:

> A young adult is leaving childhood on his way to adulthood. He is leaving the security and regiment of high school and his home. He is taking a new job; he is going to college; he is enlisting in the military. He is out on his own, with less support from his friends and family. These situations will be true for all generations of younger adults as they go through a period of transition from one world to another. . . . Dealing with these changes in his life will create increased levels of uncertainty, stress and anxiety. . . . During this stage in life, some younger adults will choose to smoke and will use smoking as a means of addressing some of these areas.[36]

The tobacco industry has known since at least the 1960s that the pharmacological effects of nicotine are "most rewarding to the individual under stress"[53] and that nicotine is "an addictive drug effective in the release of stress mechanisms."[54]

A 1976 Philip Morris internal memorandum summarizing secondary sources of data on smoking initiation noted that stress may encourage nonsmokers to start smoking and may prompt occasional smokers to smoke more:

> Stressful situations occurring in an environment favorable to smoking may contribute to the starting of the smoking habit, as well as to its continuation. For instance, some men begin smoking in the tense days of their first job. Smokers consistently report that they tend to smoke more when under tension.[35]

Tobacco company research has also shown that people use cigarettes "as a tranquilizer" during stressful times.[30,35]

While they are learning to smoke, young adults may increasingly use cigarettes in response to stress, a practice that invites higher consumption:

> For young adults who smoke, the use of cigarettes is seen as a mechanism to help ease the stress of transition from teen years to adulthood. The psychological role smoking plays for these young adults can be compared and contrasted with its use for teens and also for adults.
>
> • Smoking is now used to help meet the stresses of daily life,
> • Many are smoking more cigarettes now than they did in their teens.[33]

Ironically, much of the stress that cigarettes relieve is caused by nicotine withdrawal; it is common for people who stop smoking, once

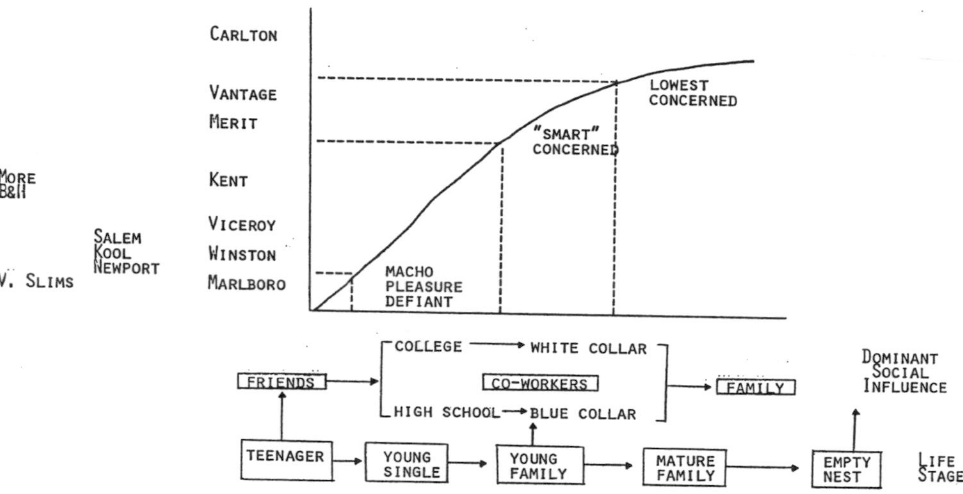

FIGURE 4—A 1981 R.J. Reynolds document that positions cigarette brands to match each stage of life.

they are past withdrawal, to feel less stress than they experienced while smoking.[55] The use of smoking for "stress relief" as supported by tobacco marketing is really self-medication for nicotine withdrawal.

Importance of the Physical and Social Environment in Appeal to Young Adults

A 1993 study for Philip Morris elucidated the importance of the environment in promoting smoking among young adults. In this study, 1564 smokers aged 18 to 24 years were surveyed about their concerns, beliefs, norms, values, leisure activities, and socialization patterns. Participants' responses were analyzed to identify common behavioral groups and the major forces affecting smoking behavior.[37] The report noted that for young smokers, activities may be more important "drivers" of behavior than attitudes:

> For instance among youngsters, *males or females indifferently, the high level of involvement in activities* obviously constitutes the driver. **No matter what they think, no matter how they are perceived, [young people] act first.** The behavior overwhelmingly shapes values, so that norms do not even show up. The engagement in specific situations (parties, beach . . .) is the only thing which counts. As a result, *the concept of goodness and badness is not even relevant at this age,* which translates it as Fun and Sex vs the rest.[37] [Emphasis in original]

The author of this report emphasized that activities are particularly important "in a new environment (away from where one grew up, in a larger city, at college, in the army…)" because although the old rules of childhood have ceased to operate, the young person has not yet developed a new set of rules to direct his or her behavior. At this time, the immediate environment is a powerful influence:

> Briefly said, the role of the environment appears determinant since it leads to and designs behaviors, which by itself implies a certain type of socialization, a natural selection of whom smokers socialize with. *Classically, repeated accidental marketing exposure would be very efficient at favoring contexts where those behaviors can then take place.*[37] [emphasis in original]

Tobacco marketers were also aware that social environments can encourage increased consumption; one researcher noted that the friendly social ambiance of a pub or social club "contributes a great deal to enjoyment of smoking and also encourages smokers to smoke more heavily than usual."[30] This understanding of young adult behavior helps to explain why tobacco marketing strategies for young adults emphasize integration with the activities and environments of young adults, including work, military service, college, and especially bars and nightclubs.[33,38,56–59]

Philip Morris, RJR, and Lorillard's studies of young adult smokers all emphasize smokers' social activities and leisure interests. For example, the profiles of young adult male smokers ("YAMS") aged 18 to 24 years developed for Philip Morris in 1990 explored how smoking different cigarette brands corresponded to 46 different social activities and

22 kinds of music.[43] Detailed tobacco industry studies of the goals, aspirations, activities, and psychology of young adult smokers were used to target advertising at groups with similar attitudes.[51] In addition, tobacco industry advertising agencies have conducted extensive research on young adult trends, music, icons, language, media usage, politics, and purchasing habits for Philip Morris, RJR, and Lorillard.[30,32,49,56,60–66]

Integration of their products with young adult activities provides tobacco companies with critical currency among their target audience. RJR focused on music and social activities in its brainstorming efforts to reach 18- to 20-year-olds.[67] A 1994 proposal for Lorillard for an advertising campaign aimed at young adults also acknowledged the importance of the physical environment in a list of concepts expected to elicit a positive response in the target audience:

> • Irreverence and sassiness. Fun, hip and honest communications that say "we know." Communications must VIOLATE THE RULES.
> • Escapist fantasies. Travel and entertainment are key themes.
> • Instant gratification: they want what they want—NOW!
> • Interactivity: talk with them, not at them. 800# promotions do well with this group.
> • "Egonomics"—marketing to the "me," which means that anything personalized or customized to the individual does very well; the implications for direct marketing and place-based marketing are clear. Brands must be where their audience is—physically as well as emotionally.[61]

Tobacco industry sponsorship of music and sporting events, bar promotions, and parties all work to associate smoking with normal adult life.[38,59] A 1985 proposal written for Lorillard targeted young adult smokers in Boston through their physical environment and social activities by focusing on Kenmore Square, where the ballpark and nightclubs formed "a social nerve center for the target demographic."[63] Feedback from Newport smokers suggested to Lorillard that portrayal of realistic and aspirational activities in Newport advertisements would heighten their relevance to this audience.[68]

DISCUSSION

During the critical years of young adulthood, public health efforts dwindle at the same time that tobacco industry efforts intensify. Young adults are an important target for the tobacco industry, particularly because they face major changes in their lives. The industry studies young adult attitudes, lifestyles, values, aspirations, and social patterns with a view toward making smoking a socially acceptable part of young adults' new activities.

In spite of the industry's claim that it does not market to nonsmokers, the marketing plans for young adults enable the industry to recruit new smokers between the ages of 18 and 24 years and to encourage light, occasional, or experimenting smokers to smoke more regularly.[28,33,34] Young adults are also the youngest legal marketing target in an industry that depends on beginning smokers,[69] and they vastly outnumber teen smokers.[22,24,29,47] Furthermore, young adult marketing promotes smoking to older teens, who see young adults as their primary role models.[28,30,70]

Beginning in the 1990s, the tobacco industry increased the use of age-specific promotions, such as bar promotions and sponsored activities aimed at young adults.[38,59] It has also opposed smoke-free bars to protect bars as promotional venues[71]; in addition, the 1998 Master Settlement Agreement (which resolved state lawsuits against the tobacco industry) included provisions that explicitly exempted marketing in "adult-only facilities" from its limitations on industry activities.[72]

These industry strategies suggest new directions for tobacco control. Young adult life events such as beginning a new job, going away to college, starting a family, entering the military, or starting to socialize in bars are opportunities for the tobacco industry to encourage smoking. These transitions are also opportunities for public health programs to intervene and block the process leading to creation of confirmed daily smokers. To date, however, the public health community has left tobacco marketing in these arenas largely unopposed. Most smoking prevention efforts for young adults have focused on pregnant women smokers, who make up less than 2% of young adults and less than 12% of young adult female smokers.[22,73,74]

Public health efforts should apply successful tobacco control strategies to match the tobacco industry's interest in young adults and should develop new interventions to discourage occasional or light smokers from progressing to addiction. Although not specifically targeted toward young adults, some of the regulatory interventions have affected this important group. For example, cigarette taxes also decrease smoking rates, and they have their greatest effect on teens and young adults.[75,76] Smoke-free workplaces encourage smokers to quit or cut down[77–79]; they probably also prevent young-adult occasional smokers entering the workforce from progressing to addiction. Smoke-free bars and nightclubs can help to break the associations between adult social patterns, alcohol use, and smoking cultivated by tobacco promotions. Smoke-free campus housing is associated with lower smoking rates among college students.[80] Smoke-free homes are associated with increased quitting, decreased relapse, and lighter cigarette consumption,[79,81] particularly when a nonsmoking adult or a child resides in the home.[82,83] Educating young adults about the dangers of secondhand smoke may be especially effective because they are starting new households and new families. Educating young adult parents (and parents-to-be) about the dangers of secondhand smoke not only will provide benefits for the new child (who will avoid the morbidity associated with involuntary smoking[84]) but also may prompt cessation among the adults.

Although our analysis concentrates on industry efforts to solidify the smoking habit among young adults, it does not dispute the worth of smoking cessation and addiction treatment among smokers of all ages. Tobacco control efforts should be tailored to each age, as are tobacco marketing efforts. Media campaign messages about secondhand smoke and tobacco industry manipulation are effective for adults and youths[85] and have played an important role in reducing both smoking and heart disease death rates in California.[86,87] Countermarketing campaigns developed with careful attention to the audience's underlying motivations, such as those used in the Florida and American Legacy Foundation truth campaigns,[88] may also be useful in developing messages for adults. Media messages supporting clean air policies may also erode the social acceptability of smoking that tobacco companies so carefully work to build and protect.[89,90]

The tobacco industry has for many years appreciated the importance of the period of young adulthood in establishing the addicted pack-a-day smoker. Public health programs targeting children and adolescents may only delay smoking initiation,[91,92] leaving these people vulnerable to industry marketing as young adults. The tobacco industry has long been aware that "anti-smoking attitudes the [children] have learned in school and elsewhere can be unlearned or replaced by pro-smoking norms held by others their own age or a little older."[70] Working to delay smoking initiation among youths while allowing it to continue among young adults has little long-term benefit. Although important, primary prevention is not the only way to reduce the damage tobacco causes; while never smoking is obviously the most desirable situation, stopping smoking before age 30 eliminates virtually all of the long-term mortality effects.[93] It is time for the medical and public health communities to follow the tobacco industry's lead and develop individual and communitywide interventions to block the process of initiating and solidifying smoking among young adults. The same life situations that have proven so fruitful for the tobacco industry are equally promising targets for health interventions. ■

About the Authors

Pamela M. Ling is with the Traineeships in AIDS Prevention Studies, Center for AIDS Prevention Studies, University of California, San Francisco. Stanton A. Glantz is with the Center for Tobacco Control Research and Education, Institute for Health Policy Studies, Cardiovascular Research Institute, University of California, San Francisco.

Requests for reprints should be sent to Stanton A. Glantz, PhD, Professor of Medicine, Box 0130, University of California, San Francisco, CA 94143 (e-mail: glantz@medicine.ucsf.edu).

This article was accepted February 9, 2002.

Contributors

All authors contributed to the conception and writing of the manuscript. P.M. Ling located most of the industry documents.

Acknowledgments

This work was supported by the National Institutes of Health (grant T32 MH-19105), and the National Cancer Institute (grant CA-87472).

References

1. Orleans CT, Johnson RW, Barker DC, Kaufman NJ, Marx JF. Helping pregnant smokers quit: meeting the challenge in the next decade. *West J Med.* 2001; 174:276–281.

2. Ershoff DH, Mullen PD, Quinn VP. A randomized trial of a serialized self-help smoking cessation program for pregnant women in an HMO. *Am J Public Health.* 1989;79:182–187.

3. Hartmann KE, Thorp JM Jr, Pahel-Short L, Koch MA. A randomized controlled trial of smoking cessation intervention in pregnancy in an academic clinic. *Obstet Gynecol.* 1996;87:621–626.

4. Gielen AC, Windsor R, Faden RR, O'Campo P, Repke J, Davis M. Evaluation of a smoking cessation intervention for pregnant women in an urban prenatal clinic. *Health Educ Res.* 1997;12:247–254.

5. Secker-Walker RH, Solomon LJ, Flynn BS, Skelly JM, Mead PB. Reducing smoking during pregnancy and postpartum: physician's advice supported by individual counseling. *Prev Med.* 1998;27:422–430.

6. Lando HA, Valanis BG, Lichtenstein E, et al. Promoting smoking abstinence in pregnant and postpartum patients: a comparison of 2 approaches. *Am J Manage Care.* 2001;7:685–693.

7. Wisborg K, Henriksen TB, Jespersen LB, Secher NJ. Nicotine patches for pregnant smokers: a randomized controlled study. *Obstet Gynecol.* 2000;96: 967–971.

8. Solomon LJ, Secker-Walker RH, Flynn BS, Skelly JM, Capeless EL. Proactive telephone peer support to help pregnant women stop smoking. *Tob Control.* 2000;9(suppl 3):III72–III74.

9. Hurtado SL, Conway TL. Changes in smoking prevalence following a strict no-smoking policy in US Navy recruit training. *Mil Med.* 1996;161:571–576.

10. Bushnell FK, Forbes B, Goffaux J, Dietrich M, Wells N. Smoking cessation in military personnel. *Mil Med.* 1997;162:715–719.

11. Helyer AJ, Brehm WT, Gentry NO, Pittman TA. Effectiveness of a worksite smoking cessation program in the military. Program evaluation. *AAOHN J.* 1998; 46:238–245.

12. Carpenter CR. Promoting tobacco cessation in the military: an example for primary care providers. *Mil Med.* 1998;163:515–518.

13. Conway TL. Tobacco use and the United States military: a longstanding problem. *Tob Control.* 1998;7: 219–221.

14. Clements-Thompson M, Klesges RC, Haddock K, Lando H, Talcott W. Relationships between stages of change in cigarette smokers and healthy lifestyle behaviors in a population of young military personnel during forced smoking abstinence. *J Consult Clin Psychol.* 1998;66:1005–1011.

15. Black DR, Loftus EA, Chatterjee R, Tiffany S, Babrow AS. Smoking cessation interventions for university students: recruitment and program design considerations based on social marketing theory. *Prev Med.* 1993;22:388–399.

16. Walsh MM, Hilton JF, Masouredis CM, Gee L, Chesney MA, Ernster VL. Smokeless tobacco cessation intervention for college athletes: results after 1 year. *Am J Public Health.* 1999;89:228–234.

17. Christie-Smith D. Smoking-cessation programs need to target college students. *Am J Health Syst Pharm.* 1999;56:416.

18. Gilpin EA, Lee L, Evans N, Pierce JP. Smoking initiation rates in adults and minors: United States, 1944–1988. *Am J Epidemiol.* 1994;140:535–543.

19. Differences in the age of smoking initiation between blacks and whites—United States. *MMWR Morb Mortal Wkly Rep.* 1991;40:754–757.

20. *Summary of Findings From the 1998 National Household Survey on Drug Abuse.* Rockville, Md: Substance Abuse and Mental Health Services Administration, Office of Applied Studies; August 1999. Available at: http://www.samhsa.gov/oas/NHSDA/NHSDAsumrpt.pdf. Accessed November 1, 2001.

21. Centers for Disease Control and Prevention. MMWR CDC Surveillance Summaries. Surveillance for Selected Tobacco-Use Behaviors—United States, 1900–1994. *MMWR Morb Mortal Wkly Rep.* 1994; 43:18, 34.

22. *Summary of Findings From the 2000 National Household Survey on Drug Abuse.* Rockville, Md: Substance Abuse and Mental Health Services Administration, Office of Applied Studies; September 2001. Report No. SMA 01–3549. Available at: http://www.drugabusestatistics.samhsa.gov. Accessed November 1, 2001.

23. Wechsler H, Rigotti NA, Gledhill-Hoyt J, Lee H. Increased levels of cigarette use among college students: a cause for national concern [published erratum appears in *JAMA.* 1999;281:136]. *JAMA.* 1998;280: 1673–1678.

24. *First Look Report 3. Pathways to Established Smoking: Results From the 1999 National Youth Tobacco Survey.* Washington, DC: American Legacy Foundation; October 2000. Report No. 3.

25. Pollay RW. Targeting youth and concerned smokers: evidence from Canadian tobacco industry documents. *Tob Control.* 2000;9:136–147.

26. Perry CL. The tobacco industry and underage youth smoking: tobacco industry documents from the Minnesota litigation. *Arch Pediatr Adolesc Med.* 1999; 153:935–941.

27. Hastings G, MacFadyen L. A day in the life of an advertising man: review of internal documents from the UK tobacco industry's principal advertising agencies [see comments]. *BMJ.* 2000;321:366–371.

28. Teague CE. Research planning memorandum on some thoughts about new brands of cigarettes for the youth market. R.J. Reynolds Tobacco Company. February 2, 1973. Bates No. 502987357 -7368. Available at: http://www.rjrtdocs.com, www.library.ucsf.edu/tobacco/mangini. Accessed December 1, 2000.

29. Johnston ME, Daniel BC, Levy CJ. Young smokers prevalence, trends, implications, and related demographic trends. Philip Morris USA. March 31, 1981. Bates No. 1000390803/0855. Available at: http://www.pmdocs.com. Accessed December 5, 2000.

30. Hugh Bain Research. The psychology and significant moments and peak experiences in cigarette smoking. British American Tobacco Company. November 1993. Bates No. 500237804–7890. Available at: http://www.library.ucsf.edu/tobacco. Accessed April 16, 2001.

31. Hall LW. Early warning system input—reasons for smoking, initial brand selection, and brand switching. R.J. Reynolds Tobacco Company. October 25, 1976. Bates No. 501103147 -3150. Available at: http://www.rjrtdocs.com. Accessed February 4, 2002.

32. Young & Rubicam. Chesterfield. Philip Morris Tobacco Company. March 24, 1994. Bates No. 2500086977/7024. Available at: http://www.pmdocs.com. Accessed June 7, 2001.

33. Business Information Analysis Corporation. RJR young adult motivational research. R.J. Reynolds Tobacco Company. January 10, 1985. Bates No. 502780379 -0424. Available at: http://www.rjrtdocs.com, www.library.ucsf.edu/tobacco/mangini. Accessed December 12, 2000.

34. Author unknown. 1981 segmentation study. R.J. Reynolds Tobacco Company. 1981. Bates No. 501233021 -3038. Available at: http://www.rjrtdocs.com. Accessed March 5, 2001.

35. Udow A. Why people start to smoke. Philip Morris Tobacco Company. June 2, 1976. Bates No. 2042789380/9387. Available at: http://www.pmdocs.com. Accessed December 15, 2000.

36. Harden RJ. A perspective on appealing to younger adult smokers. R.J. Reynolds Tobacco Company. February 2, 1984. Bates No. 502034940 -4943. Available at: http://www.rjrtdocs.com, www.library.ucsf.edu/tobacco/mangini. Accessed December 12, 2000.

37. Author unknown. Young adult male smokers and young adult female smokers. Philip Morris Tobacco Company. November 1993. Bates No. 2045180640/0775. Available at: http://www.pmdocs.com. Accessed August 30, 2000.

38. Sepe E, Ling PM, Glantz SA. Smooth moves: bar and nightclub tobacco promotions that target young adults. *Am J Public Health.* 2002;92:414–419.

39. Author unknown. 1985 segment description study–aging issues. R.J. Reynolds Tobacco Company. 1985. Bates No. 508550616–0667. Available at: http://galen.library.ucsf.edu/tobacco/mangini/html/j/005/otherpages/allpages.html. Accessed August 17, 2000.

40. R.J. Reynolds Tobacco Company. RJRTC 1991–1995 strategic plan. August 1990. Bates No. 513330214 -0338. Available at: http://www.rjrtdocs.com. Accessed August 24, 2000.

41. Fields TF. Working class vs apirational mindsets: influence of demographics. R.J. Reynolds Tobacco Company. January 15, 1986. Bates No. 504098434. Available at: http://www.rjrtdocs.com. Accessed July 26, 2001.

42. Harden RJ. First usual brand younger adult smoker media and promotion exploratory. R.J. Reynolds Tobacco Company. February 20, 1985. Bates No. 507174907 -4951. Available at: http://www.rjrtdocs.com. Accessed October 17, 2001.

43. Michael Normile Marketing. Young adult smokers opportunity profiles. Philip Morris Tobacco Company. August 1990. Bates No. 2043102805/2944. Available at: http://www.pmdocs.com. Accessed September 7, 2000.

44. Malone RE, Balbach ED. Tobacco industry documents: treasure trove or quagmire? [comment in: *Tob Control.* 2000;9:261–262]. *Tob Control.* 2000;9:334–338.

45. *Preventing Tobacco Use Among Young People: A Report of the Surgeon General.* Atlanta, Ga: US Dept of Health and Human Services; July 1994.

46. Cummings KM, Morley C, Horan J, Steger C, Leavell N. Marketing to America's youth: evidence from corporate documents. *Tob Control.* 2002; 11(suppl 1):i5–i17.

47. Author unknown. Conjoint simulation model. Philip Morris Tobacco Company. February 23, 1993. Bates No. 2045199142/9311. Available at: http://www.pmdocs.com. Accessed September 15, 2000.

48. US Dept of Health and Human Services. A model of smoking initiation: cigarette advertising as a shaping force of an adolescent's ideal self-image. Philip Morris Tobacco Company. 1994. Bates No. 2048711844. Available at: http://www.pmdocs.com. Accessed November 28, 2000.

49. Ansberry C, Oboyle T, Roberts J. Today's adult young male smoker. Philip Morris Tobacco Company. August 1992. Bates No. 2060127742/7919. Available at: http://www.pmdocs.com. Accessed August 24, 2000.

50. R.J. Reynolds. 1985 Segment Description Study. Overview Presentation. 1985. Bates No. 506203246 -3327. Available at: http://www.rjrtdocs.com. Accessed January 28, 2001.

51. Ling PM, Glantz SA. Using tobacco industry marketing research to design more effective tobacco control campaigns. *JAMA.* In press.

52. Fields TF. Correlation of brand switching with life passages. R.J. Reynolds Tobacco Company. January 19, 1982. Bates No. 501745636 -5637. Available at: http://www.rjrtdocs.com. Accessed December 3, 2000.

53. Wakeham H. Dr H. Wakeham R & D presentation to the board of directors (691126). Philip Morris USA. November 26, 1969. Bates No. 1000276678/6690. Available at: http://www.pmdocs.com. Accessed April 29, 2002.

54. Yeaman A. Implications of Battelle Hippo I & II and the Griffith Filter. Brown and Williamson Tobacco Company. July 17, 1963. Bates No. 1802.05. Available at: http://www.library.ucsf.edu/tobacco/docs/html/1802.05/index.html. Accessed October 12, 2001.

55. Parrott AC. Nesbitt's Paradox resolved? Stress and arousal modulation during cigarette smoking. *Addiction.* 1998;93:27–39.

56. Himmelfarb S. Beyond "X"–a different look at 18–29s. Philip Morris Tobacco Company. November 1992. Bates No. 2045199377–9394. Available at: http://www.pmdocs.com. Accessed September 15, 2000.

57. Heironimus J. Impact of workplace restrictions on consumption and incidence. Philip Morris Tobacco Company. January 21, 1992. Bates No. 2045447779–7806. Available at: http://www.pmdocs.com. Accessed December 21, 2000.

58. Author unknown. Summary of segmentation among Marlboro smokers. R.J. Reynolds Tobacco Company. No date [content suggests document date is 1984]. Bates No. 506190133–0139. Available at: http://www.library.ucsf.edu/tobacco/mangini. Accessed November 30, 2000.

59. Sepe E, Glantz SA. Bar and club tobacco promotions in the alternative press: targeting young adults. *Am J Public Health.* 2002;92:75–78.

60. Author unknown. Younger adult smoker opportunity. Purpose. R.J. Reynolds Tobacco Company. April 1988. Bates No. 506653159 -3218. Available at: http://www.rjrtdocs.com. Accessed March 11, 2001.

61. Heller & Cohen. Proposal program concepts for Kent International. Lorillard Tobacco Company. April 5, 1994. Bates No. 93347305/7326. Available at: http://www.lorillarddocs.com. Accessed October 29, 2001.

62. Young & Rubicam. Brand X: a qualitative exploratory among young adult male smokers. Philip Morris Tobacco Company. February 1994. Bates No. 2040174998/5045. Available at: http://www.pmdocs.com. Accessed August 30, 2000.

63. Taylor Shain Inc. Proposal for a Boston tactical plan targeted for the young adult segment using the "tunnels of influence" strategic construct. Lorillard Tobacco Company. April 10, 1985. Bates No. 85003058/3074. Available at: http://www.lorillarddocs.com. Accessed October 29, 2001.

64. Bruce Eckman Inc. The viability of the Marlboro Man among the 18–24 segment. Philip Morris Tobacco Company. March 1992. Bates No. 2045060177/0203. Available at: http://www.pmdocs.com. Accessed October 13, 2000.

65. Brainreserve. Final presentation for Philip Morris USA. Philip Morris Tobacco Company. December 22, 1988. Bates No. 2044328997/9058. Available at: http://www.pmdocs.com. Accessed October 16, 2000.

66. Leo Burnett Agency. The young adult woman smoker. Philip Morris Tobacco Company. June 1991. Bates No. 2050900002/0115. Available at: http://www.pmdocs.com. Accessed September 6, 2000.

67. Nassar SC. Marlboro vulnerability–idea generation. R.J. Reynolds Tobacco Company. January 21, 1985. Bates No. 503043738–3746. Available at: http://www.library.ucsf.edu/tobacco/mangini. Accessed November 30, 2000.

68. RIVA Market Research Inc. Final report on eight focus groups with black and white users of Newport, Salem, and Kool Cigarettes on issues related to Newport cigarettes and its advertising campaign. Lorillard Tobacco Company. January 1994. Bates No. 82875399/5507. Available at: http://www.lorillarddocs.com. Accessed May 2001.

69. Tindall J. Cigarette market history and interpretation and consumer research. Philip Morris Tobacco Company. February 13, 1992. Bates No. 2057041153/1196. Available at: http://www.pmdocs.com. Accessed July 5, 2001.

70. Friedman LR, Lazarsfeld PF, Meyer AS. Motivational conflicts engendered by the on-going discussion about cigarette smoking. Philip Morris Tobacco Company. January 1972. Bates No. 1003291740/1916. Available at: http://www.pmdocs.com. Accessed December 15, 2000.

71. Magzamen S, Glantz SA. The new battleground: California's experience with smoke-free bars. *Am J Public Health.* 2001;91:245–252.

72. National Association of Attorneys General. Master settlement agreement. 1998. Available at: http://www.naag.org/tobac/cigmsa.rtf. Accessed February 15, 2001.

73. Matthews TJ. Smoking during pregnancy in the 1990s. *Natl Vital Stat Rep.* August 28, 2001;49(7).

74. Ventura SJ, Mosher WD, Curtin SC, Abma JC, Henshaw S. Highlights of trends in pregnancies and pregnancy rates by outcome: estimates for the United States, 1976–96. *Natl Vital Stat Rep.* December 15, 1999;47(29).

75. Chaloupka FJ. Macro-social influences: the effects of prices and tobacco-control policies on the demand for tobacco products. *Nicotine Tob Res.* 1999; 1(suppl 1):S105–S109.

76. Biener L, Aseltine RH Jr, Cohen B, Anderka M. Reactions of adult and teenaged smokers to the Massachusetts tobacco tax. *Am J Public Health.* 1998;88:1389–1391.

TABLE 1—Characteristics of Communities and Retailers

Characteristic	Retailers, % (n = 3462)
Population density	
Large city	16.3
Midsize city	11.0
Urban fringe, large city	33.0
Urban fringe, midsize city	12.7
Large/small town	15.9
Rural	11.0
Tobacco control	
States without programs	70.5
States with programs[a]	29.5
Store type	
Convenience	12.4
Convenience/gas	34.5
Gas station	7.5
Mom/pop store	3.3
Grocery store	9.1
Supermarket	9.0
Drug store	9.6
Liquor store	8.5
Tobacco store	2.0
Other	4.1
Store size, No. of cash registers	
1	61.0
2	17.2
≥3	21.7

[a]Arizona, California, Florida, Massachusetts, Maine, Oregon.

marketing than are adults.[4] Research shows that tobacco advertising has both predisposing and reinforcing effects on youth smoking, acting as an inducement to experimentation with smoking as well as reinforcing continued progression toward regular smoking.[12] For example, one study showed that, in comparison with students who saw pictures of stores with no tobacco advertising, students exposed to photographs of stores with tobacco ads perceived that tobacco was significantly easier to acquire, believed more of their peers had tried and approved of smoking, and expressed weaker support for tobacco control policies such as advertising restrictions and cigarette price increases.[16]

Also, a merchant intervention study conducted in Baltimore, Md, showed that youths were more likely to attempt cigarette purchases in stores with exterior cigarette advertising depicting models who were youthful in appearance than in stores without similar ads.[17] In that 3 of 4 teenagers visit a convenience store at least once per week,[18] these research studies suggest that the point-of-purchase environment may have important influences on youths in terms of making tobacco use seem normative and, ultimately, increasing the likelihood of smoking initiation.

In conclusion, evidence suggests that point-of-purchase advertising and promotions have increased since implementation of the MSA billboard tobacco advertising ban. These increases, at least in part, are likely to have resulted from the shifting of resources once spent on billboard advertising to other marketing efforts. As a result of this shift, the intended effect of the billboard advertising ban may not be realized, because overall exposure to advertising and promotions may not be reduced. Further research is needed to examine the impact of the billboard ban and other MSA restrictions on tobacco company marketing strategies and on youth and adult smoking. ■

About the Authors

Melanie A. Wakefield is with the Center for Behavioral Research in Cancer, Anti-Cancer Council of Victoria, Melbourne, Victoria, Australia. Yvonne M. Terry-McElrath is with the Institute for Social Research, University of Michigan, Ann Arbor. Frank J. Chaloupka and Sandy J. Slater are with the Health Research and Policy Centers, University of Illinois at Chicago. Frank J. Chaloupka is also with the Department of Economics, University of Illinois at Chicago. Dianne C. Barker is with Barker Bi-Coastal Health Consultants, Calabasas, Calif. Pamela I. Clark is with Battelle Centers for Public Health Research and Evaluation, Baltimore, Md. Gary A. Giovino is with the Department of Cancer Prevention, Epidemiology, and Biostatistics, Roswell Park Cancer Institute, Buffalo, NY.

Requests for reprints should be sent to Melanie A. Wakefield, PhD, Center for Behavioral Research in Cancer, Anti-Cancer Council of Victoria, 1 Rathdowne St, Carlton, Victoria 3053, Australia (e-mail: melanie.wakefield@cancervic.org.au).

This article was accepted March 19, 2001.

***Note.** The views expressed in this article are those of the authors and do not necessarily reflect the views of the Robert Wood Johnson Foundation.*

Contributors

M.A. Wakefield contributed to developing the survey instruments, supervised the analysis, and wrote the article. Y.M. Terry-McElrath undertook the data analysis and contributed to the writing of the article. F.J. Chaloupka and D.C. Barker conceived the study. F.J. Chaloupka, D.C. Barker, S.J. Slater, P.I. Clark, and G.A. Giovino contributed to developing the survey instruments and analyzing the data and assisted in the writing of the article.

Acknowledgments

This research was supported by a grant from the Robert Wood Johnson Foundation to the University of Illinois at Chicago, as part of the foundation's Bridging the Gap Initiative.

We wish to thank members of the ImpacTeen Research Group for input into instrument design, Jaana Myllyluoma and the team at Battelle Centers for Public Health Research and Evaluation for data collection, and Erin Ruel for advice on data analysis.

References

1. *Report to Congress for 1997, Pursuant to the Federal Cigarette Labeling and Advertising Act.* Washington, DC: Federal Trade Commission; 1999.

2. Warner KE. *Selling Smoke: Cigarette Advertising and Public Health.* Washington, DC: American Public Health Association; 1986.

3. *Reducing the Health Consequences of Smoking: 25 Years of Progress. A Report of the Surgeon General.* Rockville, Md: Public Health Service; 1989.

4. Pollay RA, Siddarth S, Siegel M, et al. The last straw? Cigarette advertising and realized market shares among youth and adults, 1979–1993. *J Marketing.* 1996;60:1–16.

5. Saffer H. Economic issues in cigarette and alcohol advertising. *J Drug Issues.* 1998;28:781–793.

6. Saffer H, Chaloupka F. Tobacco advertising: economic theory and international evidence. *J Health Economics.* 2000;19:1117–1137.

7. Wakefield MA, Terry YM, Chaloupka FJ, et al. Changes at the point-of-sale for tobacco following the 1999 tobacco billboard ban. Available at: http://www.uic.edu/orgs/impacteen/pub_fs/htm. Accessed February 26, 2001.

8. *Promo Sourcebook Supplement.* Englewood, NJ: Point of Purchase Advertising Institute; 1999.

9. Pierce JP, Lee L, Gilpin EA. Smoking initiation among adolescent girls, 1988 through 1994: an association with targeted advertising. *JAMA.* 1994;271:608–611.

10. Pierce JP, Gilpin E. A historical analysis of tobacco marketing and the uptake of smoking by youth in the United States: 1890–1977. *Health Psychol.* 1995;14:1–9.

11. Feighery EC, Borzekowski DLG, Schooler C, Flora J. Seeing, wanting, owning: the relationship between receptivity to tobacco marketing and smoking susceptibility in young people. *Tob Control.* 1998;7:123–128.

12. *Preventing Tobacco Use Among Young People: A Report of the Surgeon General.* Rockville, Md: Public Health Service; 1994.

13. Pierce JP, Choi WS, Gilpin EA, Farkas AJ, Berry CC. Tobacco industry promotion of cigarettes and adolescent smoking. *JAMA.* 1998;279:511–515.

14. Biener L, Seigel M. Tobacco marketing and ado-

TABLE 2—Regression Analyses: Association of Tobacco Advertising and Promotion Variables With Date of Ban

Dependent Variable	No. of Stores	Preban, %	Postban, %	Unadjusted OR (95% CI)	*P*	Adjusted OR[a] (95% CI)	*P*
Interior ads, any vs none	3424	76.0	79.6	1.23 (1.05, 1.45)	.012	1.27 (1.06, 1.52)	.011
Interior ads	3424			1.09 (0.95, 1.25)	.210	1.08 (0.94, 1.25)	.292
Free of any ads		24.0	20.4				
Ads limited to where sold		57.5	62.1				
High levels of ads[b]		18.6	17.6				
Low-height tobacco ads	2646	44.3	43.3	0.96 (0.82, 1.12)	.592	1.02 (0.86, 1.20)	.846
Exterior ads, any vs none	3401	55.2	59.9	1.22 (1.06, 1.40)	.006	1.22 (1.03, 1.44)	.020
Exterior ads	3401			1.29 (1.13, 1.46)	.000	1.30 (1.12, 1.50)	.001
Free of any ads		44.8	40.1				
<5 ads, each <30 cm in any dimension		20.3	17.5				
High levels of ads[c]		34.9	42.4				
Parking lot ads, any vs none[d]	1421	41.1	39.8	0.95 (0.76, 1.17)	.613	1.02 (0.81, 1.27)	.877
Parking lot ads[d]	1421			1.10 (0.89, 1.35)	.396	1.19 (0.95, 1.47)	.128
Free of any ads		58.9	60.3				
<5 ads, each <30 cm in any dimension		15.6	6.2				
High levels of ads[c]		25.5	33.6				
Promotions, any vs none	3414	43.3	52.0	1.42 (1.24, 1.63)	.000	1.65 (1.42, 1.92)	.000
Promotions, specific types							
Multipack promotions, 1 or more	3424	23.4	27.1	1.22 (1.04, 1.43)	.014	1.38 (1.17, 1.64)	.000
Gift-with-purchase promotions, 1 or more	3423	3.8	8.5	2.36 (1.73, 3.23)	.000	2.51 (1.81, 3.47)	.000
Cents-off promotions, 1 or more	3415	32.3	40.4	1.43 (1.24, 1.64)	.000	1.65 (1.41, 1.92)	.000
Functional objects, any vs none	3434	65.9	72.8	1.38 (1.19, 1.60)	.000	1.63 (1.38, 1.93)	.000
Functional objects	3434			1.36 (1.20, 1.54)	.000	1.57 (1.38, 1.79)	.000
None		34.1	27.2				
1-2		33.7	33.6				
3-4		17.7	20.9				
≥5		14.6	18.2				

Note. OR = odds ratio; CI = confidence interval.
[a]Adjusted for store type, number of cash registers (proxy for store size), urbanicity of community, and presence of statewide tobacco control program in April 1999.
[b]Combination of "has ads in sections of the store distinctly separate from where product sold" and "has ads covering almost all available space throughout the store."
[c]Combination of "had less than 5 ads, but one or more is larger than 30 cm in any dimension" and "has 5 or more ads."
[d]Includes only stores with parking lots (gas stations and convenience stores selling gas), n = 1454.

lescent smoking: more support for a causal inference. *Am J Public Health.* 2000;90:407–411.

15. Schooler C, Feighery E, Flora JA. Seventh graders' self-reported exposure to cigarette marketing and its relationship to their smoking behavior. *Am J Public Health.* 1996;86:1216–1221.

16. Henriksen L, Jackson C. Reliability of children's self-reported cigarette smoking. *Addict Behav.* 1999;24:271–277.

17. Voorhees CC, Yanek LR, Stillman FA, Becker DM. Reducing cigarette sales to minors in an urban setting: issues and opportunities for merchant intervention. *Am J Prev Med.* 1998;14:138–142.

18. *The Point of Purchase Advertising Industry Fact Book.* Englewood, NJ: Point of Purchase Advertising Institute; 1992.

| SECTION III |

Tobacco & The Environment

The Smoke You Don't See: Uncovering Tobacco Industry Scientific Strategies Aimed Against Environmental Tobacco Smoke Policies

| Monique E. Muggli, MPH, Jean L. Forster, PhD, MPH, Richard D. Hurt, MD, and James L. Repace, MSc

Objectives. This review details the tobacco industry's scientific campaign aimed against policies addressing environmental tobacco smoke (ETS) and efforts to undermine US regulatory agencies from approximately 1988 to 1993.

Methods. The public availability of more than 40 million internal, once-secret tobacco company documents allowed an unedited and historical look at tobacco industry strategies.

Results. The analysis showed that the tobacco industry went to great lengths to battle the ETS issue worldwide by camouflaging its involvement and creating an impression of legitimate, unbiased scientific research.

Conclusions. There is a need for further international monitoring of industry-produced science and for significant improvements in tobacco document accessibility. (*Am J Public Health.* 2001;91:1419–1423)

Concerns regarding the health effects of environmental tobacco smoke (ETS) began as early as 1973 when the US Civil Aeronautics Board required nonsmoking areas on all commercial airplanes. Arizona and Minnesota became the first US states to restrict indoor smoking to designated areas with the enactment of clean indoor air acts in 1973 and 1975, respectively. The US surgeon general's 1979 report concluded that ETS exposure should be considered a separate scientific issue from active smoking.[1]

Investigation of ETS as a source of indoor air pollution and a potential carcinogen increased throughout the 1980s.[2–5] An early 1990s investigation of the association between heart disease and ETS showed that approximately 37 000 annual heart disease deaths among nonsmokers occur in the United States owing to ETS exposure,[6] a finding supported by subsequent research.[7] In January 1990, 2 years after airliner cabin air quality was addressed, the US Environmental Protection Agency (EPA) released a draft risk assessment reporting that 3800 lung cancer deaths per year were attributable to ETS.[8]

The final EPA report, *Respiratory Health Effects of Passive Smoking: Lung Cancer and Other Disorders,* was released on January 13, 1993, and attributed 3700 annual US lung cancer deaths to ETS exposure.[8] (The EPA report was completed in December 1992; therefore, it is commonly referred to as the "1992 EPA report.") Five months after the release of the report, representatives of the tobacco industry filed suit against the EPA in an attempt to force withdrawal of the conclusion that ETS was a group A carcinogen. In 1998, after a 5-year court battle, Judge William L. Osteen voided EPA's classification of ETS as a group A carcinogen. The judge did not, however, vacate other EPA findings regarding ETS and various respiratory disorders.[9]

METHODS

Approximately 618 boxes of industry documents were reviewed by one of the authors (Monique E. Muggli) from May 1998 to February 1999. The Minnesota Tobacco Document Depository estimated that each of the boxes included 2500 pages. The number of document pages reviewed from the other sources described subsequently (the British American Tobacco Document Depository and the tobacco industry's Web site, the Tobacco Archives) was estimated to be fewer than 2000.

Minnesota Tobacco Document Depository

On May 8, 1998, the tobacco companies announced a settlement exceeding $6 billion with the State of Minnesota and BlueCross BlueShield of Minnesota. The Minnesota settlement required the US tobacco companies to maintain a public document depository in Minneapolis to house more than 32 million pages of internal documents. The 4(b) index is a database that categorizes documents by specific fields such as author, recipient, copyee, document date, title keyword(s), plaintiff request number, and document type. The 4(b) index used at the Minnesota depository was created by the US defendants named in *State of Minnesota et al. v Philip Morris et al.* to catalog the documents.

British American Tobacco Document Depository

The Minnesota settlement also required the British American Tobacco Co to provide public access to its approximately 8 million internal documents in a depository located near Guildford, England. A limited search of documents related to ETS was performed at the British American Tobacco document depository. The depository index was searched via the fields *file user* and *file owner.* Files owned or used by key British American Tobacco scientists and public relations personnel were reviewed.

Tobacco Archives

The Tobacco Archives Web site was created in 1998 by Philip Morris, RJ Reynolds, Lorillard, Brown and Williamson, the US Tobacco Institute, and the Council for Tobacco Research, Inc. The index used at the Web site is referred to as the National Association of Attorneys General Index. This index is operationally similar to the 4(b) index but contains 2 additional fields: *named organization* and *named person.*

Search Strategy

The search for documents at the depository involved the following: (1) searching the 4(b) index, (2) requesting the box(es) that contained the found document(s), and (3) reviewing the contents of the box(es) in a public viewing area. Several measures were implemented to ensure as thorough a search as possible. The selected topic (i.e., ETS) and related terms (e.g., EPA) were searched as *title keywords*. With broad keywords such as ETS or EPA, a time frame limit (e.g., 1988–1993) was placed on the search to reduce the number of documents produced. Results of the document searches were reviewed. The title keyword search allowed identification of key scientists, public relations staff, attorneys, and consultants and assisted in the development of a chronology of events from 1988 to 1993 relating to the ETS issue.

Once key persons, dates, and keywords were identified, the 4(b) index was searched by *author, recipient, copyee,* and *date*. Finally, a combined search using the 4(b) index and the National Association of Attorneys General Index allowed us to review boxes not found in the former because of differences in, for example, the fields used in the 2 indexes.

RESULTS

The ETS Threat

The tobacco industry's expansive campaign to produce scientific research and influence public opinion on the health consequences associated with ETS was developed to protect the financial and political interests of the companies. The documents reveal that the industry feared the ETS issue and any governmental regulation of smoking in public places, because both would have a profound effect on industry profits owing to (1) decreases in consumption, (2) increases in litigation, and (3) weakened support from business owners and politicians.

Philip Morris's longtime public relations firm, Burson Marsteller, warned in one document that consumers would be "deprived of more and more locations in which they can smoke, and psychologically given more incentive to quit."[10] In addition, the vice chairman of the board of Philip Morris, Inc, identified the ETS issue as the "single most important challenge we currently face" and went on to state:

> ETS is the driving force behind smoking restrictions in the workplace, on airlines and other forms of public transportation, and in virtually all areas offering public access. If present trends continue, smokers will have fewer and fewer opportunities to enjoy a cigarette. This will have a very direct and major impact on consumption.[11]

Industry-retained attorneys feared that fallout from the ETS issue would result in an increase in product liability, workers' compensation, and other ETS exposure litigation surrounding secondhand smoke.[12] The EPA's 1993 ETS risk assessment was a focus for this fear, because an increase in smoking bans could be initiated if ETS were classified as a carcinogen.

Finally, the ETS issue and the EPA report could instigate a potential loss of political support from merchandisers, business owners, and politicians. In a 1992 speech to the Philip Morris Board of Directors, Craig L. Fuller, the senior vice president of corporate affairs of Philip Morris and former chief of staff to Vice President George Bush, noted that the risk assessment would be challenging as a result of the inevitable negative political effect the report would have on business communities.

> [I]f . . . the Administrator of the EPA . . . issues the Risk Assessment which asserts that secondary tobacco smoke [ETS] is carcinogenic, we have a very difficult problem. Our allies who have held the line in buildings, restaurants, shopping areas, sports complexes and other areas will almost certainly be forced to rethink their position.[13]

Not only would businesses, restaurants, and bars be forced to choose between smoking bans and the installation of costly ventilation systems, business owners would be forced into the political arena. As long as the industry could deny any health risk associated with ETS, it could continue to count on its traditional political support. However, if the EPA were to proclaim that ETS caused cancer, employers and politicians alike would be less likely to openly show support for the tobacco industry. For the first time, the industry and its supporters could no longer simply respond to tobacco's health effects on smokers who were "making a personal choice" to smoke. The ETS issue would effectively remove the umbrella of personal choice under which the industry had hidden for decades.

Philip Morris's fear of the ETS issue was justified. In 1993, an industry-funded group estimated that 3 to 5 fewer cigarettes smoked per day as a result of smoking restrictions would reduce annual manufacturer profits by more than $1 billion per year.[14] Consequently, during the year between the release of the first and second drafts of EPA's risk assessment, Philip Morris spent more than $16.5 million on their "scientific campaign" against the ETS issue.[15] The industry's concern over this issue is also evidenced by the 1996 Philip Morris media affairs ETS–EPA budget, which was almost twice that for youth access initiatives and US Food and Drug Administration regulatory issues.[16]

Industry Science: The ETS Disinformation Campaign

During the 1980s, the industry's primary argument against health consequences associated with ETS was simple: there were other agents responsible for poor indoor air quality.[11] As the next decade approached, the industry knew that ETS and related health issues would persist. They quickly began to recognize that more effective strategies to counter ETS arguments were needed. The Philip Morris vice chairman of the board told industry attorneys in 1989 that the old industry messages regarding ETS were failing and that they "must find stronger arguments to support our position on ETS."[11]

The Center for Indoor Air Research (CIAR), a nonprofit organization funded by the tobacco industry, played an essential role in developing "stronger arguments" to support the industry's position that ETS represented an insignificant health risk.[11] CIAR was founded in March 1988, allegedly for the purpose of "sponsoring high quality research on indoor air issues and to facilitate the communication of research findings to the broad scientific community."[17] Founding members of CIAR included Philip Morris, R. J. Reynolds, and Lorillard.[17] From 1989 to 1999, CIAR funded at least 244 published studies,[18] some of which, documents suggest, were central to the industry's efforts aimed against the EPA and the US Occupational Safety and Health Administration (OSHA). In 1995, Philip Morris and R.J. Reynolds paid CIAR annual dues of $5.3 million and $1 million, respectively.[19]

Since its inception in 1988, CIAR had acted as a buffer between the tobacco industry and scientists. An attorney from the Washington, DC–based law firm Covington and Burling (counsel to the Tobacco Institute and Philip Morris) made the following statement in regard to CIAR:

> [W]e all know that many scientists will not accept funding directly from the industry but will accept funding from entities like CIAR. We need to have access to the best qualified researchers at the most prominent institutions worldwide when deciding who should conduct research for which funds have been made available. CIAR should provide us with that access, now and into the future.[20]

This buffer allowed industry-funded scientists to produce seemingly independent results aimed at contradicting ETS findings and disclaiming the EPA report while keeping such research under industry control. Covington and Burling attorney John Rupp reported to another tobacco company that the industry indeed had ultimate control over CIAR-funded projects:

> The responsibility for "ensur[ing] effective use" of the findings of funded research remains, in the final analysis, the responsibility of those who have funded the research. With published reports of funded research in hand, the industry has to decide how and when to make use of the findings—whether through mailings of one sort or another, filings in regulatory proceedings, inclusion of the funded research in review articles or presentations by consultants...or in other statements that may be made on the industry's behalf. We have found in the past that CIAR grantees often are prepared to assist with such efforts. As noted, however, the responsibility for ensuring the effective use of the findings of funded research is a responsibility that remains ultimately with the industry.[20]

CIAR studies designed to rebut regulatory agency activities. OSHA was also considered a threat to the industry's ETS efforts because if the EPA ruled that secondhand smoke was a group A carcinogen, OSHA would then have the authority to regulate workplace smoking. Documents disclose that there were 2 projects in particular that were developed to provide industry support against the threat of the EPA and OSHA initiating further smoking restrictions: the "US Exposure Study" and the "US Confounders Study."[21] According to a Philip Morris document titled *CIAR Applied Project*, CIAR paid $1.2 million for the exposure study, carried out by Drs Michael Guerin and Roger Jenkins at the Oak Ridge National Laboratory, and $1.3 million for the confounders study, conducted by Dr Genevieve Matanoski at Johns Hopkins University.[22]

In addition to the Matanoski study, the industry was also interested in producing research that considered other confounding factors, such as genetic predisposition,[23] diet,[24] and stress,[25] that would lessen the important role that ETS played in lung cancer etiology. In fact, over an 8-year period, Philip Morris provided more than $7 million to the Friedman Institute for various studies on topics such as unsuccessful stress management as a causal factor in cancer.[25]

> The Friedman project could play a key role in getting the cancer monkey off the cigarette industry's back, by showing that unsuccessful stress management could account for the large amount of cancer mortality currently attributed to cigarette smoking.[25]

Exposure studies were also planned in Germany, Sweden, Spain, France, and Italy, as were confounder studies in Germany, Sweden, the United Kingdom, and Hong Kong.[26] Japan was a proposed site as well, and a handwritten Philip Morris document suggests that the studies were to be conducted by "'fresh faces'; not the same old industry consultants."[27] It is difficult to evaluate from the documents the total amount spent on the exposure studies; however, one document recorded that CIAR budgeted approximately $2.4 million for exposure studies conducted outside the United States in 1994.[19]

After almost 10 years of funding research that "remain[ed] ultimately with the industry," CIAR is no longer in operation. The recent master settlement agreement between the US tobacco companies and the US state attorneys general, announced on November 16, 1998, required CIAR to disband.[28]

Use of scientific consultants. Similar to CIAR, an industrywide ETS consultant program was also fully functioning in the United States by 1988; however, its operation and funding were apparently somewhat different from those of CIAR. Funded by the American, Japanese, and European tobacco companies,[29] ETS consultant programs were created in the Latin American, Australian, Middle Eastern, Asian, US, Nordic, and European markets. Although some scientists would conduct research similar to that funded by CIAR, their role would focus more on public endorsement of such research[30] in an effort to "keep the [ETS] controversy alive."[31]

ETS consultants embarked on various activities under the industry's direction, including (1) attending and presenting papers at selected ETS symposia and conferences[32–34]; (2) writing op-ed pieces in top-tier newspapers and magazines such as *The New York Times*, *The Washington Times*, and *Newsweek*[33,35,36]; (3) submitting comments to the EPA and the CIAR Scientific Advisory Board on the draft 1990 EPA report[33]; and (4) engaging in media tours (labeled "Truth Squad" tours) designed, seemingly, to discredit the EPA and its ETS risk assessment.[32,33,37–39]

Industry scientific consultants were also used to infiltrate international public health conferences addressing ETS, including the 6th and 8th World Conferences on Tobacco or Health.[40,41] Documents show that Japan Tobacco, Inc, sought to "change the very nature and tone" of the 1987 world conference by having approximately 40 scientists attend and present "neutral" papers:

> Since 300 scientists are expected to attend, 40/300 of the papers presented would represent a [neutral] position [on] smoking [and] health, thereby exerting influence on the general tone of the conference.[40]

Although the use of scientists to spread industry messages was widespread, documents suggest that some industry leaders did recognize that the industry was jeopardizing its credibility by paying the ETS consultants. A Philip Morris document titled *Environmental Tobacco Smoke: S. Parrish* [Steve Parrish] *Dictation* reported the following:

> [W]e should push the notion that these people are of such stature that they cannot be corrupted by receiving a few thousand dollars from the tobacco industry. . . . Also, we should attempt to get some high-powered spokespersons or reputable scientists to do the job for nothing—this may not be impossible.[42]

DISCUSSION

This review of internal tobacco company documents has expanded the existing knowledge of industry tactics against EPA policies and the industry's use of both science and scientific consultants. It has also provided support for previously suspected strategies and outlined previously undisclosed industry approaches aimed at the public health community.

The documents reviewed show that the tobacco industry went to great lengths to battle the ETS issue by camouflaging its involvement and creating an impression of legitimate, unbiased scientific research. The industry put forth considerable effort to discredit ETS science and US regulatory agencies such as the EPA and OSHA by creating organizations and programs such as CIAR and the ETS consultant program.

The facade of the public pronouncements of the tobacco industry has been partially exposed in earlier reports.[43–47] For example, Barnes and Bero found that of 106 published ETS articles reviewed, 37% concluded that ETS was not harmful to one's health, and almost 75% of these articles were authored by scientists known to be associated with the tobacco industry.[48] A similar trend was found on examination of written submissions received by the EPA after the release of the June 20, 1990, draft risk assessment. Sixty-four percent of the written submissions asserted that the conclusion of the draft was groundless, and 71% of these submissions were authored by individuals known to be associated with the tobacco industry.[49] This report expands the earlier findings with support from additional internal documents.

Critical to understanding tobacco industry scientific tactics is the realization of how CIAR and scientific consultants operated. For example, in the United States, documents show that the consulting scientists were paid to disseminate industry messages against the EPA and OSHA via symposia, scientific publications, and submissions to EPA and the media. In Europe, however, scientists were used in an attempt to infiltrate the World Health Organizations' cancer research arm, the International Agency for Research on Cancer, which had published a study corroborating the EPA's finding that ETS is a carcinogen.[50,51] It appears that the industry tailored its use of scientists to fit the markets in which the companies operated.

While the media and US public policy initiatives have refuted any industry claims of CIAR's being an independent nonprofit organization, internal industry strategies operating under CIAR have not been widely reported.[52,53] Documents reveal that CIAR was used in an attempt to publicly demonstrate to US regulatory agencies that the industry was making a concerted effort to study ETS and its health effects, yet CIAR studies were actually developed to discredit EPA and OSHA agendas. It is equally important to note that internal documents certify that research funded by CIAR was ultimately under the control of the industry and mostly controlled by industry-retained attorneys.

This review shows that the industry strategy is to take the long and wide view. Even as the industry loses a battle, it buys time—a Philip Morris strategy referred to as "sand in the gears."[13] For each year of delay, an estimated 4 million people die around the globe from tobacco-related diseases.[54] It is apparent from this review and recent events that the ETS battle is far from over. Once again, the tobacco industry has bought more time.

If global public health gains against the ETS issue are to be realized, efforts to promote financial disclosure of scientific presentations in the literature, in symposia, and in the media must be strengthened in developing nations such as those of South and Central America and the Asian Pacific region. It is probable that consulting tobacco industry scientists will flood the scientific literature in those countries as they did in the United States. The consultants may be more difficult to identify as affiliated with the tobacco industry, however, because "fresh faces" are being sought.

Initiatives to improve document accessibility and searching capability are important to ensure that all documents housed at the Minnesota Tobacco Document Depository and at the British American Tobacco document depository in Guildford, England, are available worldwide on the Internet. Disclosure of internal tobacco documents has opened opportunities never before imagined. Obtaining access to these documents, however, can be an arduous process owing to indexing inefficiencies, lack of document standardization, and unreasonable limits to public access to documents not yet on the Internet.

Although the internal, once-secret tobacco industry documents provide an invaluable source of information, there are inherent limitations to their acquisition and use, including the following:

1. Full-text searching is not available; therefore, researchers must rely on certain fields only. Searching by these fields only can generate erroneous information and does not capture all of the documents produced related to ETS.
2. In our case, only about 1.5 million pages of more than 40 million available documents housed at the Minnesota and Guildford depositories were reviewed. This represents only 3.75% of the estimated document population. In the interest of conciseness, only a fraction of the searched pages have been cited here.
3. There are large gaps in knowledge of the industry's activities with respect to the ETS issue because of privileged documents that were unavailable at the time of document acquisition.
4. Time and financial resources represent a limitation in that the documents are spread across the globe in different depositories and across multiple Web sites.
5. The physical state of the documents can be problematic owing to missing attachments or illegibility caused by multiple photocopying.
6. Access to the British American Tobacco depository in Guildford remains extremely limited.
7. In our case, it was not possible to interview the persons who authored, received, or were named within the documents cited in this article. ■

About the Authors

Monique E. Muggli is an independent consultant in Minneapolis, Minn. Jean L. Forster is with the School of Public Health, Division of Epidemiology, University of Minnesota, Minneapolis. Richard D. Hurt is with the Nicotine Dependence Center, Mayo Clinic Foundation, Rochester, Minn. James L. Repace is with Repace Associates, Second Hand Smoke Consultants, Bowie, Md.

Requests for reprints should be sent to Jean Forster, PhD, MPH, 1300 S Second St, Suite 300, Minneapolis, MN 55454 (e-mail: forster@epi.umn.edu).

This article was accepted March 7, 2001.

Contributors

M.E. Muggli conducted all document research and drafted the manuscript. J.L. Forster acted as an advisor for the master's thesis from which this paper was developed, and she contributed to the writing of the paper. R.D. Hurt assisted in reviewing critical documents and contributed to the writing of the paper. J.L. Repace provided background information and contributed to the writing of the paper.

Acknowledgment

We would like to thank Dr Anne Joseph and the BlueCross BlueShield Foundation of Minnesota for initiating and funding this project.

References

1. *Smoking and Health: A Report of the Surgeon General.* Washington, DC. US Dept of Health, Education, and Welfare; 1979. DHEW publication DHS 79-50066.

2. Repace JL, Lowrey AH. Indoor air pollution, tobacco smoke, and public health. *Science.* 1980;208: 464–476.

3. Hirayama T. Non-smoking wives of heavy smokers have a higher risk of lung cancer: a study from Japan. *BMJ.* 1981;282:183–185.

4. Repace JL, Lowrey AH. A quantitative estimate of nonsmokers' lung cancer risk from passive smoking. *Environment Int.* 1985;11:3–22.

5. *The Health Consequences of Involuntary Smoking: A Report of the Surgeon General.* Washington, DC: US Dept of Health and Human Services; 1986. DHHS publication CDC 87-8398.

6. Glantz SA, Parmley WW. Passive smoking and heart disease—epidemiology, physiology and biochemistry. *Circulation.* 1991;83:1–12.

7. Steenland K. Passive smoking and the risk of heart disease. *JAMA.* 1992;267:94–99.

8. *Respiratory Health Effects of Passive Smoking: Lung Cancer and Other Disorders.* Washington, DC: Environmental Protection Agency; 1993.

9. Tobacco Resource Center Inc. Mistaken ruling, unmistakable facts: how Judge Osteen got it wrong when he vacated the EPA's finding that secondhand smoke is a known carcinogen and why his ruling may not matter. Available at: http://www.tobacco.neu.edu/extra. Accessed November 24, 1998.

10. Humber T. *ETS Media Strategy.* Undated. Philip Morris Inc. Document 2023920090-0101 at 0090. Minnesota Tobacco Document Depository, Minneapolis.

11. *Remarks by William Murray, Vice Chairman of the Board, Philip Morris Companies Inc., at the 1989 Philip Morris Legal Conference; Ritz-Carlton Hotel, Naples, Florida.* April 4, 1989. Philip Morris Inc. Document 2023265282-5295 at 5284. Minnesota Tobacco Document Depository, Minneapolis.

12. *ETS, Indoor Smoking and Indoor Air Quality: Planning for the 1990s* [confidential attorney-client communication, draft]. April 22, 1992. Philip Morris Inc. Document 2023371119-1157 at 1142-1143. Minnesota Tobacco Document Depository, Minneapolis.

13. *Presentation for the Board of Directors-June 24, 1992: Craig L. Fuller, Senior Vice President, Corporate Affairs; Kathleen Linehan, Vice President, Government Affairs.* June 24, 1992. Philip Morris Inc. Document 2047916000-6012 at 6010. Minnesota Tobacco Document Depository, Minneapolis.

14. *Confidential-A Smokers' Alliance* [draft]. July 1, 1993. Philip Morris Inc. Document 2025771934-1995 at 1937. Minnesota Tobacco Document Depository, Minneapolis.

15. *The ETS Program for 1991 Is Divided Into Four Major Categories.* Philip Morris Inc. Document 2023856052-6057 at 6053. Minnesota Tobacco Document Depository, Minneapolis.

16. *Philip Morris USA Media Affairs 1996 Original Budget.* 1996. Philip Morris Inc. Document 2048226919. Minnesota Tobacco Document Depository, Minneapolis.

17. Pages R. *Center for Indoor Air Research (CIAR)-Background.* May 14, 1992. Philip Morris Inc. Document 2021528170. Minnesota Tobacco Document Depository, Minneapolis.

18. *Published Results for CIAR Supported Research, January 1999.* January 1999. Philip Morris Inc. Document 2063813820-3837. Minnesota Tobacco Document Depository, Minneapolis.

19. Center For Indoor Air Research. *Presentation At R.J. Reynolds, November 1995.* November 1995. R.J. Reynolds Tobacco Co. Document 517550005-0025 at 0023. Minnesota Tobacco Document Depository, Minneapolis.

20. Rupp J. *Privileged and Confidential Attorney Work Product.* March 12, 1993. Philip Morris Inc. Document 2023053695-3700 at 3697-3698. Minnesota Tobacco Document Depository, Minneapolis.

21. Pages R. *FYI RE: CIAR.* September 16, 1993. Philip Morris Inc. Document 2023694870. Minnesota Tobacco Document Depository, Minneapolis.

22. *CIAR Applied Project.* Undated. Philip Morris Inc. Document 20235219994-9995. Minnesota Tobacco Document Depository. Minneapolis.

23. Pages R. *Wynder Proposal to VdC.* January 29, 1992. Philip Morris Inc. Document 2023222815-2816 at 2815. Minnesota Tobacco Document Depository, Minneapolis.

24. Rylander R. *Studies of Confounders for ETS With Particular Reference to the Possibility to Perform Studies in Sweden.* May 23 1994. Philip Morris Inc. Document 2023711168-1172 at 1168. Minnesota Tobacco Document Depository, Minneapolis.

25. Lincoln J. *Final Friedman Points and Reduced Funding Requirements.* September 27, 1991. Philip Morris Inc. Document 2023223204-3205 at 3204. Minnesota Tobacco Document Depository, Minneapolis.

26. *IARC Planning Meeting, Wednesday, June 15, 1994; Richmond, VA.* June 15, 1994. Philip Morris Inc. Document 2023711156-1160 at 1157-1158. Minnesota Tobacco Document Depository, Minneapolis.

27. *CIAR Meeting.* February 22, 1994. Philip Morris Inc. Document 2023899211-9213 at 9211. Minnesota Tobacco Document Depository, Minneapolis.

28. Master settlement agreement. Available at: http://www.naag.org/tob2.htm, Accessed March 1999.

29. *Preliminary 1994 Consultants Programs Proposal.* Undated. Philip Morris Inc. Document 2023590685-0687 at 0685. Minnesota Tobacco Document Depository, Minneapolis.

30. Whist A. *Update-ETS Consultant Project.* May 18, 1988. Philip Morris Inc. Document 2021546791-6792. Minnesota Tobacco Document Depository, Minneapolis.

31. Boyse S. *Note on Special Meeting of the UK Industry on Environmental Tobacco Smoke; London, February 17th, 1988.* February 17, 1988. R.J. Reynolds Tobacco Co. Document 516038933-8938 at 9835-9838. Minnesota Tobacco Document Depository, Minneapolis.

32. Whist A. *ETS.* July 11, 1989. Philip Morris Inc. Document 2023034623-4946 at 4629-4632. Minnesota Tobacco Document Depository, Minneapolis.

33. *TI ETS/IAQ Consultant Activity: 1988-1990.* Undated. R.J. Reynolds Tobacco Co. Document 507850594-0613. Minnesota Tobacco Document Depository, Minneapolis.

34. *Industry ETS Consultancy Programmes.* Undated. British American Tobacco Co. Document 300515335-5340 at 5338. Guildford Document Depository, Guildford, England.

35. Fleiss J. Untitled document. June 1, 1990. Philip Morris Inc. Document 2028396805-6809 at 6805. Minnesota Tobacco Document Depository, Minneapolis.

36. Gross A. *Charges on Simon Turner et al. Paper and Letter.* January 1992. Philip Morris Inc. Document 2001020014-0015. Minnesota Tobacco Document Depository, Minneapolis.

37. *"Truth Squad" Media Tours. Jack Peterson, Ph.D and David Weeks, M.D.* Undated. Philip Morris Inc. Document 2021179904-9906. Minnesota Tobacco Document Depository, Minneapolis.

38. *"Truth Squad" Media Tours. Dr. David Weeks.* Undated. Philip Morris Inc. Document 2015024370. Minnesota Tobacco Document Depository, Minneapolis.

39. *"Truth Squad" Media Tours. Dr. Jack Peterson.* Undated. Philip Morris Inc. Document 2015024413. Minnesota Tobacco Document Depository, Minneapolis.

40. Egawa M. Untitled document. April 25, 1986. Philip Morris Inc. Document 2021654119-4123. Minnesota Tobacco Document Depository, Minneapolis.

41. Dastugue JB. *8th World Conference on Smoking & Health.* June 14, 1991. Document 304004077-4078. British American Tobacco Co. Guildford Document Depository.

42. *Environmental Tobacco Smoke: S. Parrish Dictation.* Undated. Philip Morris Inc. Document 2021183691-3692 at 3691. Minnesota Tobacco Document Depository, Minneapolis.

43. Marshall E. Tobacco science wars. *Science.* 1987; 236:250–251.

44. Marshall E. Tobacco industry does slow burn over EPA advisor. *Science.* 1991;250:203.

45. Ernster V, Burns D. A rebuttal to the tobacco industry's paper "Cigarette smoke and the nonsmoker." *J Public Health Policy.* 1984;5:368–375.

46. Glantz SA, Slade J, Bero LA, Hanauer P, Barnes DE. *The Cigarette Papers.* Berkeley, Calif: University of California Press; 1996.

47. Barnes DE, Bero LA. Industry-funded research and conflict of interest: an analysis of research sponsored by the tobacco industry through the Center for Indoor Air Research. *J Health Polit Policy Law.* 1996;21:515–542.

48. Barnes D, Bero L. Why review articles on the health effects of passive smoking reach different conclusions. *JAMA.* 1998;279:1566–1570.

49. Bero L, Glantz S. Tobacco industry response to a risk assessment of environmental smoke. *Tob Control.* 1993;2:103–113.

50. Cerioli A. Untitled document. May 26, 1995. Philip Morris Inc. Document 2502251076. Minnesota Tobacco Document Depository, Minneapolis.

51. Reif H. *Visit to IARC, Lyon–July 19, 1993.* July 19, 1993. Philip Morris Inc. Document 2025470309–0312 at 0309. Minnesota Tobacco Document Depository, Minneapolis.

52. Shane S. Center tied to tobacco industry; indoor air research funding is questioned. *Baltimore Sun.* May 17, 1998:A1.

53. Shane S. Tobacco deal would disband controversial research center; organization that gives money for pollution study considered a tobacco front. *Baltimore Sun.* November 14, 1998:A3.

54. World Health Organization. Tobacco free initiative. Available at: http://www.who.org/toh. Accessed July 2000.

Boards of Health as Venues for Clean Indoor Air Policy Making

| Joanna V. Dearlove, BA, and Stanton A. Glantz, PhD

Objectives. This study sought to determine the tobacco industry's strategies for opposing health board actions and to identify elements necessary for public health to prevail.

Methods. Newspaper articles, personal interviews, and tobacco industry documents released through litigation were reviewed.

Results. Twenty-five instances in which the tobacco industry opposed health board regulations were identified. It was shown that the tobacco industry uses 3 strategies against health boards: "accommodation" (tobacco industry public relations campaigns to accommodate smokers in public places), legislative intervention, and litigation. These strategies are often executed with the help of tobacco industry front groups or allies in the hospitality industry.

Conclusions. Although many tobacco control advocates believe that passing health board regulations is easier than the legislative route, this is generally not the case. The industry will often attempt to involve the legislature in fighting the regulations, forcing advocates to fight a battle on 2 fronts. It is important for health boards to verify their authority over smoking restrictions and refrain from considering nonhealth factors (including industry claims of adverse economic impacts) so as to withstand court challenges. (*Am J Public Health.* 2002;92:257–265)

In the United States, many states and localities have boards of health that can issue regulations to protect public health independent of legislative approval. Most health boards are also designed to be insulated from the political pressures experienced by legislators, and often the regulations they issue must be based solely on health considerations. Most boards are appointed for fixed terms (only 29% of boards have elected members[1]), so members are generally not subject to reelection concerns or susceptible to the influence of campaign contributions.[2–4] These facts, combined with the overwhelming evidence that secondhand smoke causes disease in nonsmokers,[5–8] make health boards a logical venue to issue tobacco control measures.

There are 3 main strategies the tobacco industry uses against health board smoking regulations: "accommodation" (public relations campaigns to accommodate smokers in public places), legislative intervention, and litigation. (These strategies are in addition to the industry's overarching strategy of state preemption, which removes the authority of local governmental bodies to issue tobacco control policies.[9–15]) Although boards of health are designed to be insulated from political pressures, the industry, in certain of its strategies, relies on politics to oppose health board regulations.[16,17] In the present article, we examine the tobacco industry's strategies and provide case studies.

Despite industry opposition, some boards of health have successfully passed and defended regulations, while others have had their regulations repealed, amended, or weakened. Successful regulation of secondhand smoke by a board of health requires that the board acquire the public support necessary to withstand the political attack that the tobacco industry will mount, derive its authority from a statute and associated case law that will permit it to withstand a legal challenge by the tobacco industry, and carefully craft the regulation in anticipation of such a challenge.

METHODS

We obtained information from newspaper articles, the Americans for Nonsmokers' Rights Tobacco Industry Tracking Database, previously unreleased tobacco industry documents that have been made available through litigation against the tobacco industry and now can be viewed on the Internet at sites maintained by the industry, and public documents associated with litigation against boards of health. Search terms included "board of health," names of localities that had experienced health board challenges, and names of organizations and individuals involved on both sides of the issue. We also conducted interviews with individuals attempting to pass the selected health board actions and involved with the associated industry challenges, including grassroots tobacco control advocates, members of voluntary health organizations, and members of the boards of health. We did not interview tobacco industry representatives; we believed that the internal documents most credibly represented the industry perspective.

We identified 25 appointed boards of health in 7 states that possessed the authority to pass health regulations independently and that had issued or considered issuing regulations related to clean indoor air and consequently encountered industry opposition. Although additional communities passed or attempted to pass health regulations, we focused on these 25 communities because they clearly illustrated tobacco industry strategies. The cases we describe subsequently are not recent because information about recent cases is not available in internal industry documents, which usually date to 1995 or earlier. However, reports of health board actions and the opposition against them suggest that the strategies outlined in these cases were still being used in 2001.

RESULTS

Accommodation

In its accommodation strategy, the tobacco industry's attempts to convince decision makers that regulation of indoor smoking (specifically, smoke-free dining laws) is unnecessary and that establishments should take voluntary action to accommodate smokers and nonsmokers. These campaigns usually occur as a health board is considering a regulation. The industry rarely acknowledges its involvement in accommodation campaigns[18]; instead, it uses existing hospitality groups or coalitions or organizes and funds new ones to act as surrogates.[16,17,19–23] These organizations include beverage associations,[24,25] convenience store associations,[24,26] and tavern–restaurant associations.[20,22,27] Claims of adverse economic consequences for restaurants and bars form the centerpiece of the arguments advanced through accommodation programs.

Because boards of health are supposed to consider only health factors in their decision making, accommodation campaigns are generally unsuccessful. There have, however, been instances in which the industry used this approach successfully to pressure boards into rescinding smoking restrictions in restaurants and bars.

A case study involving Wake County, North Carolina, is illustrative of the accommodation strategy. In 1993, inspired by the 1992 US Environmental Protection Agency report[5] classifying secondhand smoke as a class A carcinogen, the Wake County Board of Health proposed smoking control rules that would phase out smoking in airports, workplaces, and restaurants over a 3-year period. By 1996, smoking areas were to be permitted in these establishments only when they were serviced by separate heating, ventilation, and air conditioning systems.

In May 1993, just after the board voted to hold public hearings on the proposed regulation, the Tobacco Institute, the tobacco industry's political and lobbying arm based in Washington, DC, developed a plan to defeat or stall the scheduled vote. Even in the tobacco-growing state of North Carolina, the Tobacco Institute recognized the need to create the false impression that opposition was not originating from the industry. The Tobacco Institute plan recommended the following:

> Identify core working group to develop and coordinate overall strategy. *As much as possible, it is essential for the tobacco industry (especially tobacco companies) to maintain a low profile for the strategy to work most effectively.* The coalition should be a broad-based group drawn from throughout the county. While we expect to see a fair number of growers and allied supporters at the hearing, *it is important for us to recruit for public activities supporters not obviously linked to the industry and who also live or work in Wake County.*[28] [italics added]

The Tobacco Institute specified how members of the coalition should be selected and trained:

> Individuals or associations should be contacted only if it is reasonably certain they will oppose WCSCR [Wake County Smoking Control Rules]. Brief allies, provide background materials and update regularly. Organize a broad-based coalition to take the lead in opposing WCSCR publicly; *identify one or two lay spokespersons for the groups who are not affiliated with the tobacco industry.*[28] [italics added]

Jerry Williams, executive vice president of the North Carolina Restaurant Association, was listed as one such ally. Williams later claimed credit for the industry-financed lawsuit against the health board and recruited plaintiffs, some of whom were unaware of industry involvement.[29] The Tobacco Institute also advised mobilization of the National Smokers Alliance, an organization created on the part of Philip Morris by the public relations firm Burson-Marstellar,[30] and distributed talking points, answers to common media questions, and fact sheets to the industry-generated coalition.[28]

The industry also wanted to redefine the issue from public health to government intrusion: "Fashion the issue not as a question of smoking or [environmental tobacco smoke] and health, but rather unfair, unreasonable and unnecessary government interference in private enterprise."[28] Williams often cited such arguments: "If the health department can [regulate smoking] because of the health implications they can come back and say, 'you can no longer serve chocolate cake.' It opens the door to endless possibilities of regulations."[29]

This accommodation strategy failed to stop the board of health from adopting the restrictions. Later, however, the tobacco industry shifted to a legal strategy and sued the board, which backed down and amended the ordinance to include much weaker provisions. Subsequent state legislation (House Bill [HB] 957) preempted the authority of Wake County to improve the inadequate regulation resulting from the tobacco industry lawsuit.

Legislative Intervention

When the accommodation strategy fails to prevent a health board from passing a smoking regulation, the industry will often turn to the legislative branch of government, where it exerts more influence. The industry lobbies the legislative body for 2 purposes: to use any authority possessed by the legislative body to limit health board actions and to pass legislation to remove the health board's authority over smoking.

Limiting health board actions. This goal can be accomplished in a variety of ways. For example, the health boards we examined were appointed by their local legislative bodies, and therefore legislators could be influenced to deny reappointment to board members supportive of smoking restrictions. This was the strategy explained by Philip Morris government affairs executive Chris Smiley in a memorandum regarding opposition to a health board smoking regulation in New York's Westchester County:

> Since the B.O.H. [board of health] is an appointed board of officials we need to put pressure on the legislator[s] even if they are not directly responsible. The only way we can beat this ban is if our accounts call their legislators and put the pressure on them in hope that they will in turn put the pressure on the B.O.H.[31]

The tobacco industry has used 3 variations of this strategy, pressuring legislatures to (1) cut health department budgets, (2) deny reappointments of board members in favor of smoking restrictions, and (3) deny health boards access to use of localities' legal counsel.

Another example involved Guilford County, North Carolina. In 1993, the county's legislature attempted to use its authority over the health board to limit the board's actions, considering the removal of board members who supported smoking restrictions and refusing the board the resources necessary to defend itself against a lawsuit filed by Lorillard Tobacco Co, located in Guilford County.

On September 27, 1993, the board of health voted 6–5 to pass regulations restricting smoking in workplaces and bars and ending smoking in restaurants.[32] Guilford's regulations were part of a statewide movement to pass local clean indoor air laws before implementation of state legislation (HB 957) that would preempt localities from imposing smoking restrictions. The matter came before the health board after the county's legislative body, the board of commissioners, sidestepped a local lawyer's petition to consider the issue and referred it to the board.[33]

Public criticism from the board of commissioners led the health board to place a moratorium on enforcement of the regulations and to consider alternatives.[34] Shortly after the board passed its regulations, County Commissioner Melvin Alston publicly encouraged county citizens to defy the new rules[35] and announced his plan to propose a board of commissioners resolution opposing the regulations.[35] Later, with Commissioner Joe Wood, he declared that he would oppose reappointing the 2 board members who most vocally supported the regulations: Lynn Snotherly and Dr Leon Holt.[36] The following day, Commissioner Robert Moores publicly called for removing all 6 health board members who voted for the regulations.[37]

Ultimately, the board of commissioners voted 6–4 against removing the 6 board members but refused to reappoint Snotherly; Holt left the board when his term expired. Former chairperson of the Guilford County ASSIST [tobacco control] Coalition Richard Rosen felt that the commissioner's vigorous attempt to undermine the health board's effort was the result of tobacco industry influence; Lorillard Tobacco Co was considered one of the county's outstanding corporate citizens (R. Rosen, verbal communication, April 2000).

Although the moratorium had been enacted on October 5, a group of plaintiffs including Lorillard sued the Guilford County Board of Health on October 29 to void the regulations. The board of health was prevented from responding to the suit when the board of commissioners denied it the \$70 000 needed to defend the suit and refused to allow the board access to the county attorney.[38] The commissioners also attacked Guilford County Health Director Ron Clitherow, who had encouraged the health board to pass the regulations. Clitherow resigned shortly thereafter. As health board members left, either voluntarily or for lack of reappointment, the county commissioners began appointing members opposed to smoking restrictions,[39] including a tobacco farmer.[40] As a result, opponents of smoking restrictions were in the majority.

The issue over legal fees ended when the health board agreed to extend the moratorium until a virtually identical legal challenge against nearby Halifax County's smoking regulations was resolved.[41] When the Halifax rules were overturned, Guilford's health board repealed its regulations.[42]

Removal of health board authority. In addition to pressuring local legislatures to use any authority they possess over the board of health to limit its actions, the industry sometimes also pressures legislatures to pass laws or resolutions restricting or removing the board's authority to enact regulations. This strategy is usually initiated during the debate over health board smoking restrictions, when opposition is mobilized in the legislature. Although these restrictive measures can sometimes be passed at the local level, the industry prefers they pass at the state level to preempt localities from adopting smoking regulations through their health boards.

The industry uses 3 major approaches to restrict health board authority through legislation: (1) requiring boards of health to obtain approval from local legislatures before enacting regulations, (2) requiring health boards to follow complicated and lengthy rule-making procedures to allow the industry more time to mobilize opposition and create more opportunities for procedural appeals, and (3) forbidding health boards from considering smoking restrictions or regulations that would have an economic impact. These measures discourage tobacco control advocates from using the regulatory process to pass restrictions and take the issue back to the legislature, where the industry exercises more influence.

A situation illustrating this strategy occurred in the state of Ohio. At a 1994 conference of Philip Morris lobbyists and other employees involved in government affairs, company executives reported on their efforts in Ohio to illustrate the approach of what they called "practical preemption"[26] to restrict the authority of local boards of health without openly attacking the politically popular concept of local government "home rule." Philip Morris drafted state legislation to transform the board of health rule-making process into a time-consuming, complicated operation. As Philip Morris executive Jim Pontarelli explained, "The legislation still respects the concept of home rule/control. It doesn't prevent boards of health from proposing bans, it just adds a bureaucratic nightmare of hoops they must jump through before they can get their proposal on the books."[26]

The legislation required elected officials to vote on any smoking regulation proposed by their health board before it became law. The health board was also required to adopt a "resolution of intent" as the first step of the rule-making process and to hold 3 hearings at least 7 days apart on this resolution before proceeding. The resolution was to be published in every newspaper within the health board's jurisdiction twice before each hearing. After the hearings, the board was required to issue a written report to the local legislature for review. A similarly convoluted process would then begin at the legislative level, and the legislative body could amend the proposal without the health board's approval. If the health board disagreed with the changes, the process started all over again. Pontarelli summarized the industry's goals:

> If, at any point, a single newspaper in some Godforsaken corner of an affected county is overlooked during the publishing of the notices, the whole process has to go back and start from scratch. You get the picture. This entire process would take—at the very least—three full months. This gives us lots of time to marshal our retailers and our other allies, to generate letters, opinion pieces, etc.
> It also gives us a solid shot at elected officials, who have to sign off on the proposal and take whatever political heat they have coming to them for doing so. And it gives us a chance to amend the proposal and make it more to our liking, if it looks like it's going to get passed anyway.
> This process won't stop every Board of Health smoking restriction from getting through, but it does place tremendous burdens on the other side, making it as difficult as possible and forcing them to expend resources.[26]

In 1995, Harry J. Lehman, a lobbyist for RJ Reynolds Tobacco Co,[43,44] circulated this proposed legislation, which eventually became known as HB 299. Following a similar industry strategy in which pro-tobacco legislation is presented as tobacco control legislation,[22,45] the bill included provisions nominally preventing youth access to tobacco, but the primary purpose was to reduce the power of boards of health. Youth access provisions, which generally are not effective in reducing youth smoking,[46] were inserted to discourage health advocates from opposing the bill. Ultimately, the bill expanded to a measure that would preempt all local smoking laws, whether passed by health boards or by local legislatures.

Although tobacco control advocates recognized that the tobacco industry was responsible for HB 299, the industry was hardly visible during the debate. Instead, Phil Craig, local lobbyist and executive director of the Ohio Licensed Beverage Association, led the opposition. Craig formed a coalition, Ohioans for Sensible Tobacco Regulations, whose publicly disclosed members consisted mainly of individuals involved with hospitality businesses. Craig regularly reported coalition activities to executives at Philip Morris, RJ Reynolds, and Brown & Williamson.[47–52] The bill was voted out of committee but never passed the full state assembly, because voluntary health organizations and other health advocates successfully mobilized against it.[53]

The idea of removing authority from boards of health resurfaced in 2000 when Republican State Representative Robert Schuler introduced a bill identical to the proposal drafted in 1995[44] after he met with a "coalition of hotel, motel, bar and restaurant owners" led by Phil Craig. Unlike HB 299, this legislation remained focused only on removing authority from health boards. It would require the legislative authority of a locality to approve any smoking rules issued by its board of health. On March 28, 2000, the Ohio General Assembly passed the bill by a vote of 76–18. The measure was expected to pass the Senate, but when Governor Robert Taft threatened to veto the bill, the Senate withdrew it from consideration.[54,55]

Litigation

When a health board smoking regulation passes or nears passage despite accommodation or legislative intervention, the tobacco industry often uses litigation or the threat of litigation to overturn the regulation or intimidate the board of health into repealing it. (Tobacco interests generally file litigation in federal court, where they have experienced more favorable decisions than in state courts, particularly in product liability, even though federal claims against boards of health are usually unsuccessful.) Similar to the accommodation strategy, the industry rarely acknowledges its involvement and acts through surrogates. Our research revealed only one instance in which a tobacco company was named as a plaintiff, in Guilford County, North Carolina. Nevertheless, the industry has always been heavily involved in recruiting plaintiffs, determining legal strategies, and financing legal costs.[20,56]

The industry relies on more than one argument in these legal challenges, but the most popular argument charges that the board of health does not possess the authority to enact the smoking regulations in question, either because the board exempted certain businesses from smoking restrictions (and thereby considered factors irrelevant to health) or because state law preempts the restrictions (a claim usually found to be untrue). The industry also often asserts that the health board failed to follow the correct procedure in adopting the rules.

Although the industry challenges regulations that contain exemptions, it is usually responsible for incorporation of these exemptions. Tobacco interests lobby boards of health to grant exemptions on the basis of economic impact—most typically for bars and bingo parlors—and then challenge regulations on the grounds that the boards inappropriately considered economic factors when they should have considered only health factors. The industry also claims that such exemptions violate the US Constitution's equal protection clause, because establishments that are allowed smoking areas are granted an alleged economic advantage over those that are not. This practice of lobbying for exemptions in order to challenge the legality of the regulations based on these exemptions may be a calculated strategy, or it may be the natural outcome of the separate strategies of attempting to weaken regulations and to legally revoke them.

Opinions from state or local legal officials can be helpful in withstanding industry litigation; when the industry sued the Mid-Ohio River Valley Health Department in West Virginia as a result of the smoking regulations passed by its health board, an opinion from the state attorney general was crucial in winning the case for the health department. According to the court:

> [T]he attorney general is a constitutional officer (W.Va. Const., Art.7, '1) whose express statutory duties include giving "written opinions and advice upon questions of law" . . . W.Va. Code, '5-3-1 (Michie Cum.Supp. 1995). . . . Furthermore, although such opinions are, without question, not precedent or binding as authority upon the Supreme Court of Appeals, they are considered particularly persuasive when issued rather contemporaneously with the adoption of a statute, rule or regulation in question. Walter v. Ritchie, 156 W.Va. 98, 191 S.E.2d 275 (1972).[57]

Likewise, an unfavorable opinion may save tobacco control advocates from wasting resources on a regulatory pathway that will ultimately fail when challenged in court. However, advocates should first consider an attorney general's previous positions on the issue and recognize that the office is highly politicized, a factor that may affect the attorney general's original stance.

The industry first realized health boards posed a serious threat when the New York State health board, known as the Public Health Council, considered strong (for the time) smoking restrictions in 1986.[20,58,59] The regulation ended smoking in most public places and workplaces and mandated that restaurants with more than 50 seats reserve 70% of seating for nonsmokers. Smaller restaurants, hotel rooms, tobacco stores, and bars were exempted from the regulations. The Tobacco Institute recognized that the regulations could set "an alarming precedent"[60] and began considering a legal challenge. Michael Irish, director of government affairs for Philip Morris, advised his superiors that "RJR Corporate Attorney Steven Heard (McGarrahan & Heard) feels that a lawsuit by aggrieved parties such as the State Legislature, Restaurant Association, etc., would 'be a winner.'"[60]

After an unsuccessful attempt to convince the state legislature to challenge the health council's regulations, the industry searched elsewhere for potential plaintiffs. On March 13, 1986, State Senator Thomas Bartosiewicz; State Assemblyman Robert Wertz; the Brooklyn Chamber of Commerce; the United Restaurant, Hotel, and Tavern Association; Dennis Paperman (president of the Brighton Beach Board of Trade); and Fred Boreali of Boreali's Restaurant Inc sued the Public Health Council and State Health Commissioner David Axelrod on the grounds that the council had exceeded its powers. Although no tobacco companies were named as plaintiffs, several of the named plaintiffs were identified in industry planning documents as potential litigants in an industry-organized lawsuit.[61] Furthermore, an industry law firm (Hinman, Straub, Pigors & Manning)[62–66] represented the plaintiffs.

On April 23, Justice Harold Hughes of the trial court (the State Supreme Court of Schoharie County) found in favor of the plaintiffs and ruled that the council regulation was null and void because the council had usurped the legislature's lawmaking authority (*Boreali v Axelrod,* Supreme Court of Schoharie County, 1987).[67,68]

The state appealed, and the Appellate Division of the Supreme Court ruled 3–2 to uphold Hughes' decision (*Boreali v Axelrod,* 130 AD2d 107).[69] The state then appealed to the highest court in New York, the Court of Appeals, which ruled 6–1 against the state (*Boreali v Axelrod,* 71 NY 2d 1).[70]

In its opinion, written by Judge Titone, the Court of Appeals found 4 indicators that the council had overstepped its authority. First, the Public Health Council exempted certain establishments (e.g., bars and small restaurants) from the regulations because of economic concerns. The court determined that these factors could be considered only by a legislative body. Second, the council created rules without legislative guidance; the court determined that the council's proper function should be instead to supplement legislation with details regarding implementation. Third, the council acted on an issue previously debated by the legislature. The court found that "the repeated failures by the Legislature to arrive at such an agreement do not automatically entitle an administrative agency to take it upon itself to fill the vacuum and impose a solution of its own."[70] Finally, the court ruled that no public health expertise was needed to develop the regulations.

This decision effectively prevented local boards of health in New York from passing smoking restrictions.[20] Every time a local health board took action and the industry challenged its smoking regulation by arguing that the board did not have authority to act, the court referred to *Boreali* and found for the plaintiffs. As of this writing, no New York health board has passed a 100%-smoke-free health regulation. Such a regulation might withstand a court challenge, because it renders the first indicator of the *Boreali* test (that the health board inappropriately considered economic factors by including exemptions) inapplicable.

Another case study, involving the state of Massachusetts, is illustrative of the litigation strategy. Local boards of health in Massachusetts have been successful in defending state health board smoking regulations against litigation. The Massachusetts Restaurant Association has been cooperating with the tobacco industry[27]; in June 1998, the association filed suit against the Boston Public Health Commission as a result of the commission's smoking regulations. Individual restaurants have filed lawsuits challenging health board regulations in 4 other Massachusetts localities: Amherst, New Bedford, Northampton, and Barnstable. All 5 localities passed regulations despite threats of litigation, although New Bedford's regulations were amended as a result of pressure from the legislature.

In all of these cases, the requests for preliminary injunctions suspending the rules were denied, allowing them to go into effect as scheduled. When the Barnstable case was appealed, the State Supreme Judicial Court (the highest court in Massachusetts) essentially ended this legal debate over the authority of Massachusetts health boards to regulate smoking by ruling in favor of the Barnstable Board of Health.[71–75]

Massachusetts' experience in defending these health board smoking restrictions indicates a successful approach for countering the tobacco industry's litigation strategy. One of the main factors in Massachusetts health boards' success in this litigation involved a unique element of the Massachusetts Tobacco Control Program: the Community Assistance Statewide Team (CAST). CAST, which consists of a team of attorneys from several organizations (the Massachusetts Tobacco Control Program/Department of Public Health, the Tobacco Control Resource Center based in the Northeastern University School of Law, the Massachusetts Association of Health Boards, and the Massachusetts Municipal Association[76]), provides local health advocates with the legal expertise needed to enact regulations in the appropriate manner and draft them to withstand industry challenges.

CAST reviews drafts of local health board regulations and ordinances to ensure legal viability and suggests appropriate changes. CAST members sometimes attend local public hearings and advise on the enactment process to avoid procedural errors that could form the basis of a legal challenge; they also review proposed changes in regulations as they are being developed. This legal expertise has not only produced regulations less vulnerable to industry litigation but has also made it more difficult for the industry to intimidate localities into rescinding, weakening, or avoiding clean indoor air policies.[76]

Another factor in the success of health boards' smoking regulations is that Massachusetts state law grants broad authority to local health boards, both in statute and in the court rulings interpreting this statute. These rulings, which afford health boards a great deal of discretion, are integral to Massachusetts' success in defending litigation against smoking regulations. According to the 1985 decision in *Arthur D. Little, Inc. v Commissioner of Health,* courts should strike a board of health regulation only if the challenger can prove "the absence of any conceivable ground upon which [the rule] may be upheld."[77] Likewise, if a public health issue is "fairly debatable," the court cannot substitute its own judgment for that of the board of health.[77] This situation contrasts starkly with that in New York when the court ruled in *Boreali* that "no special expertise or technical competence in the field of health was involved in the development of the antismoking regulations."[70]

DISCUSSION AND COMMENT

The 3 strategies of accommodation, legislative intervention, and litigation are the tools with which the tobacco industry has opposed health board (and other) smoking regulations (Table 1). They continue to be effective strategies for the industry: in August 2000 smoking regulations passed by the Princeton Health Commission in New Jersey were struck down after the National Smokers' Alliance filed suit,[78–80] and in November 2000 the Ohio State Legislature would have passed

TABLE 1—Tobacco Industry Strategies to Oppose Boards of Health and Subsequent Outcomes in 25 Localities

Outcome	Locality (or State)	Year	Accommodation	Legal Intervention		Litigation
				Limiting Health Board Actions	Removal of Authority	
Passed-upheld or unchanged	Amherst, Mass	1998				✓
	Barnstable, Mass	2000				✓
	Boston, Mass	1998	✓			✓
	Westchester County, NY	1996				✓
	Licking County, Ohio	1992	✓			✓
	Mid-Ohio Valley, WV	1994				✓
Passed-repealed						
	Halifax County, NC	1993				✓
	Princeton, NJ	2000				✓
	Dutchess County, NY	1999			✓	✓
	Nassau County, NY	1996	✓	✓		✓
	Niagara County, NY	1998	✓		✓	✓
	New York State	1987		✓	✓	✓
	Delaware County, Ohio	1998				✓
	Franklin County, Ohio	1993	✓			✓
	Knox County, Ohio	1994				✓
Passed-amended						
	Falmouth, Mass	1998	✓			
	New Bedford, Mass	1999		✓		✓
	Wakefield, Mass	1997	✓	✓		
	Forsythe County, NC	1994		✓		
Passed-rescinded						
	Bourne, Mass	1996	✓			
	Guilford County, NC	1993		✓		✓
	Wake County, NC	1993	✓			✓
	Monongalia County, WV	1998	✓			✓
Unknown as of yet						
	State of Arkansas	2001	✓		✓	
	Putnam County, NY	2000				✓

a bill (HB 298) removing authority from local health if not for a threatened gubernatorial veto.[55,81] Tobacco control advocates were able to counter these strategies successfully in other areas of the country: in January 2001 the highest court in Massachusetts ruled (in a lawsuit against health board smoking regulations brought by restaurant owners) that health boards possessed broad authority over regulating smoking in public places,[71,72,74,75] and in February 2001 the Arkansas State Board of Health passed regulations ending smoking in restaurants even as the state legislature considered a bill removing the board's authority over regulating smoking.[82,83]

Because the legislative intervention strategy involves influencing the legislative body, advocates must realize that pursuing health board regulations will not necessarily allow them to avoid a political fight within the legislative body. Advocates may believe that because a health board is generally composed of health advocates, grassroots support is less important for the success of a smoking regulation than when clean indoor air is pursued through legislation. However, even when health advocates work through boards of health, grassroots support is crucial in order to neutralize the industry's legislative strategy to oppose the health board action. Strong grassroots support remains pivotal to the success of clean indoor air policies, regardless of venue.

In its litigation strategy, the industry usually challenges the authority of health boards on the basis of exemptions from smoke-free regulations. The industry typically fights for exemptions based on economic arguments and then uses these exemptions to challenge regulations on the grounds that consideration of such factors is beyond the authority of health boards. Advocates should persuade health boards not to consider any testimony relating to topics outside of health, particularly in that the negative economic impact predicted by the tobacco industry has never been substantiated in objective studies.[84–90]

Health boards also provide exemptions to avoid the implementation problems inherent in any sudden transition. They, therefore, restrict smoking in places where most of the population is exposed and exempt establishments, such as bars, in which implementation may be particularly difficult and that serve a limited population. They may also craft limited regulations based on the sensitivity of children to secondhand smoke (i.e., justifying regulations allowing smoking in bars on the basis that it would not affect the health of children). As discussed earlier, however, such exceptions may cause legal difficulties; the tobacco industry and its allies will argue in court that if secondhand smoke poses such a significant health threat, it should be restricted everywhere. If health board authority is interpreted narrowly to preclude the board from allowing exemptions, advocates may be forced to recommend an all-inclusive smoke-free workplace regulation if they choose to use the regulatory pathway. However, an incremental approach that begins with general workplaces, moves to restaurants, and ends with bars is often most effective from a perspective of implementing smoke-free environments.[91]

If advocates determine that health board authority is interpreted narrowly in their state, they may decide to pursue smoking restrictions outside of the health board venue. It should be remembered, however, that even if health regulations are defeated or challenged and repealed, the effort may not be in vain. Often, the policy battles are highly publicized because the tobacco industry wants to create a public controversy over the issue and exaggerate possible negative effects of the proposed policy. If advocates stay focused on health issues, these campaigns can serve to educate the public about the health hazards of secondhand smoke and may elicit action in the legislature.[20]

Before advocates attempt to use the regulatory pathway, they should assume that the industry will sue, and they should analyze the state authorizing statute, as well as applicable case law, to make certain that a board of health has the authority to pass the smoking restrictions in question. Most state authorizing statutes are broad, and court interpretation and case law are the determinants of a health board's authority. Despite similar laws, state courts have interpreted authority broadly in some states (e.g., West Virginia, Massachusetts) and narrowly in others (e.g., New York).

Massachusetts' experience illustrates that a strong state tobacco control program offering legal expertise to health boards can facilitate advocacy by providing information, legal guidance, and assistance in drafting viable regulations. Although Massachusetts has experienced much success against attacks on health board regulations, it should be noted that the state's strong tobacco control infrastructure contributes greatly to its success and that the methods Massachusetts uses in enacting clean indoor air policies may not be relevant outside of this infrastructure.

Boards of health can be effective venues for tobacco control, but the regulatory approach is not the easy path that public health advocates often expect. As with local ordinances pursued legislatively, success requires public health advocates to anticipate and prepare for aggressive tobacco industry opposition at every step. ■

About the Authors

The authors are with the Institute for Health Policy Studies, Department of Medicine, University of California, San Francisco.

Requests for reprints should be sent to Stanton A. Glantz, PhD, Box 0130, University of California, San Francisco, CA 94143-0130 (e-mail: glantz@medicine.ucsf.edu).

This article was accepted October 7, 2001.

Contributors

Both authors conceived the paper, organized the research, and wrote and revised the manuscript. J. V. Dearlove collected most of the primary data.

Acknowledgments

This work was supported by National Cancer Institute grants CA-61021 and CA-87472 and by the Richard and Rhoda Goldman Fund.

We thank Edward L. Sweda of the Tobacco Control Resource Center at Northeastern University School of Law for his comments on the manuscript and consultation on legal issues related to Massachusetts regulations. We also thank Elva Yanez of Americans for Nonsmokers' Rights for helpful discussions and comments on a draft of the manuscript.

References

1. *National Profile of Local Boards of Health.* Atlanta, Ga: Centers for Disease Control and Prevention; 1997.
2. Glantz SA, Begay ME. Tobacco industry campaign contributions are affecting tobacco control policymaking in California. *JAMA.* 1994;272:1176–1182.
3. Monardi F, Glantz SA. Are tobacco industry campaign contributions influencing state legislative behavior? *Am J Public Health.* 1998;88:918–923.
4. Moore S, Wolfe S, Lindes D, Douglas C. Epidemiology of failed tobacco control legislation. *JAMA.* 1994;272:1171–1175.
5. *Respiratory Health Effects of Passive Smoking: Lung Cancer and Other Disorders.* Washington, DC: US Environmental Protection Agency; 1992.
6. *Environmental Tobacco Smoke: Measuring Exposures and Assessing Health Effects.* Washington, DC: National Research Council; 1986.
7. *The Health Consequences of Involuntary Smoking: Report of the Surgeon General.* Washington, DC: US Dept of Health and Human Services; 1986. DHHS publication PHS 87-8398.
8. California Environmental Protection Agency. *Health Effects of Exposure to Environmental Tobacco Smoke.* Sacramento, Calif: Office of Environmental Health Hazard Assessment; 1997.
9. Siegel M, Carol J, Jordan J, et al. Preemption in tobacco control: review of an emerging public health problem. *JAMA.* 1997;278:858–863.
10. Conlisk E, Siegel M, Lengerich E, Kenzie WM, Malek S, Eriksen M. The status of local smoking regulations in North Carolina following a state preemption bill. *JAMA.* 1995;273:805–807.
11. Jacobson P, Wasserman J, Raube K. The politics of antismoking legislation. *J Health Polit Policy Law.* 1993; 273:787–819.
12. Ellis G, Hobart R, Reed D. Overcoming a powerful tobacco lobby in enacting local smoking ordinances: the Contra Costa County experience. *J Public Health Policy.* 1996;17:28–46.
13. Davis R. The ledger of tobacco control: is the cup half empty or half full? *JAMA.* 1996;275:1281–1284.
14. Freyman R. Butting in: the tobacco lobby shows no sign of flickering in its push to move smoking regulation out of city halls and into statehouses. *Governing.* 1995;9:55–57.
15. *Preemption: Tobacco Control's Enemy #1.* Berkeley, Calif: Americans for Nonsmokers' Rights; 1996.
16. Samuels B, Glantz SA. The politics of local tobacco control. *JAMA.* 1991;266:2110–2117.
17. Traynor MP, Begay ME, Glantz SA. New tobacco industry strategy to prevent local tobacco control. *JAMA.* 1993;270:479–486.
18. Samuels BE, Begay ME, Hazan AR, Glantz SA. Philip Morris's failed experiment in Pittsburgh. *J Health Polit Policy Law.* 1992;17:329–351.
19. Philip Morris. The accommodation program "flip book" talking points: draft for review. Bates no. 2045517326/7336. Available at: http://www.pmdocs.com. Accessed November 29, 2001.
20. Dearlove JV, Glantz SA. *Tobacco Industry Political Influence and Tobacco Policy Making in New York.* San Francisco, Calif: Institute for Health Policy Studies, University of California, San Francisco; 2000.
21. Philip Morris. 1994 accommodation program draft. Bates no. 2044317469/7529. Available at: http://www.pmdocs.com. Accessed November 29, 2001.
22. Glantz SA, Balbach ED. *Tobacco War: Inside the California Battles.* Berkeley, Calif: University of California Press; 2000.
23. Mangurian CV, Bero LA. Lessons learned from the tobacco industry's efforts to prevent the passage of a workplace smoking regulation. *Am J Public Health.* 2000;90:1926–1929.
24. Tobacco Institute. The Tobacco Institute 1996

budget: Lorillard Tobacco Company. Bates no. 91891283/1293. Available at: http://www.pmdocs.com. Accessed November 29, 2001.

25. Philip Morris. Local hospitality groups embrace "the accommodation program" [press release]. Bates no. 2063433609/3610. Available at: http://www.pmdocs.com. Accessed November 29, 2001.

26. Pontarelli J. [Transcript: Philip Morris]. Bates no. 2040235925/5949. Available at: http://www.pmdocs.com. Accessed November 29, 2001.

27. Ritch WA, Begay ME. Strange bedfellows: the history of collaboration between the tobacco industry and the Massachusetts Restaurant Association. *Am J Public Health.* 2001;91:598–603.

28. Tobacco Institute. Client confidential working plan: Lorillard Tobacco Company. Bates no. 93779701/9706. Available at: http://www.pmdocs.com. Accessed November 29, 2001.

29. Ruley M. Tobacco goes a-courtin': Wake County restaurants try to stub out smoking regulations. *Independent Weekly.* February 23, 1993:10–11.

30. Stauber J, Rampton S. *Toxic Sludge Is Good for You!* Monroe, Maine: Common Courage Press; 1995.

31. Smiley C. [Memo: Philip Morris]. Bates no. 2061838186. Available at: http://www.pmdocs.com. Accessed November 29, 2001.

32. State of North Carolina. Complaint: Mana's Foods, Inc., et al. v. Wade, et. al. Bates no. 88025746/5759. Available at: http://www.pmdocs.com. Accessed November 29, 2001.

33. Smoking rules shadow debate on unfilled jobs. *Greensboro News & Record.* November 9, 1993:A8.

34. Smoking ban on hold in wake of protests/second thoughts: board delays ban. *Greensboro News & Record.* October 6, 1993:B1.

35. Defy Guilford ban, Alston tells smokers. *Greensboro News & Record.* September 29, 1993:B1.

36. Commissioners divided on debate over health board. *Greensboro News & Record.* October 27, 1993:B4.

37. Official wants health board members out. *Greensboro News & Record.* September 30, 1993:B2.

38. Nag JA. Politics cloud indoor smoking ban. *Greensboro News & Record.* November 17, 1994:A1.

39. Finn DT. Officials meddle in selection process for health board. *Greensboro News & Record.* February 18, 1994:A12.

40. Leaf farmer is on health panel. *Greensboro News & Record.* January 14, 1994:B1.

41. Guilford health board votes to delay smoking regulations. *Winston-Salem Journal.* November 17, 1994:B2.

42. Grossman M. Group to propose new smoking law; suggested legislation would permit local agencies to regulate smoking in public buildings. *Greensboro News & Record.* May 3, 1999:B1.

43. Hawthorne M. Industry lobbyist influenced original tobacco bill. *Cincinnati Enquirer* [newspaper on-line]. July 4, 1999. Available at: http://enquirer.com/editions/1999/07/04/loc_industry_lobbyist.html. Accessed May 2, 2000.

44. Radel C. Ohio tobacco bill threatens public health. *Cincinnati Enquirer.* March 31, 2000:C3.

45. Macdonald H, Aguinaga S, Glantz SA. The defeat of Philip Morris' "California Uniform Tobacco Control Act." *Am J Public Health.* 1997;87:1989–1996.

46. Glantz SA. Preventing tobacco use–the youth access trap [editorial]. *Am J Public Health.* 1996;86:156–157.

47. Fisher S. Upcoming hospitality events [Philip Morris memorandum]. Bates no. 2063417256. Available at: http://www.pmdocs.com. Accessed November 29, 2001.

48. Craig P. Proposal for continued grassroots efforts [Philip Morris document]. Bates no. 2063422773. Available at: http://www.pmdocs.com. Accessed November 29, 2001.

49. Craig P. Upcoming coalition meetings [Philip Morris memorandum]. Bates no. 2063422746. Available at: http://www.pmdocs.com. Accessed November 29, 2001.

50. Craig P. Columbus Dispatch editorial board meeting [Philip Morris memorandum]. Bates no. 2063422755/2756. Available at: http://www.pmdocs.com. Accessed November 29, 2001.

51. Craig P. Cleveland Plain Dealer editorial board meeting [Philip Morris memorandum]. Bates no. 2063422757/2758. Available at: http://www.pmdocs.com. Accessed November 29, 2001.

52. Craig P. Current coalition activities [Philip Morris memorandum]. Bates no. 2063422807. Available at: http://www.pmdocs.com. Accessed November 29, 2001.

53. Monardi FM, Glantz SA. *Tobacco Industry Political Activity and Tobacco Control Policy Making in Ohio: 1981–1998.* San Francisco, Calif: Institute for Health Policy Studies; 1998.

54. Bradshaw J. Bill stalls that would restrict authority to ban smoking. *Columbus Dispatch.* November 17, 2000:B7.

55. Bradshaw J. Taft's veto threat sidetracks measure that would stymie smoking bans. *Columbus Dispatch.* November 16, 2000:A1.

56. Agenda: working group meeting on smoking ordinances in North Carolina: Lorillard Tobacco Company. Bates no. 87596439. Available at: http://www.pmdocs.com. Accessed November 29, 2001.

57. Hill GW. *Goldsmit-Black & Mark W. Ray vs. Mid-Ohio Valley Health Department (95-C-381)* [Court document]. Wood County, WVa: Wood County Circuit Court; 1996.

58. Boman S. Powers of state boards of health [Tobacco Institute memorandum]. Bates no. TIOK0019132. Available at: http://www.pmdocs.com. Accessed November 29, 2001.

59. Sullivan R. New York adopts wide restrictions on public smoking. *New York Times.* February 7, 1987:A1.

60. Irish M. New York/Public Health Council [Philip Morris memorandum]. Bates no. 2024272134/2135. Available at: http://www.pmdocs.com. Accessed November 29, 2001.

61. Irish M. Public Health Council [Philip Morris memorandum]. Bates no. 2025857755/7756. Available at: http://www.pmdocs.com. Accessed November 29, 2001.

62. Supplemental memorandum of law [Philip Morris legal document]. Bates no. 2025875684/5715. Available at: http://www.pmdocs.com. Accessed November 29, 2001.

63. 1988 state of the state message [Philip Morris memorandum]. Bates no. 2024274183. Available at: http://www.pmdocs.com. Accessed November 29, 2001.

64. Butta D. Lawyer faults smoking-ban notice. Bates no. 2024200769. Available at: http://www.pmdocs.com. Accessed November 28, 2001.

65. Philip Morris Management Corp. *FYI* [Philip Morris newsletter]. Bates no. 2024200778/0779. Available at: http://www.pmdocs.com. Accessed November 29, 2001.

66. Irish M. New York/Public Health Council [Philip Morris memorandum]. Bates no. 2024959639/9643. Available at: http://www.pmdocs.com. Accessed November 29, 2001.

67. Hughes HJ. Memorandum decision–PHC [Philip Morris document]. Bates no. 2024959525/9532. Available at: http://www.pmdocs.com. Accessed November 29, 2001.

68. Arneberg M. NY ban on smoke rejected; judge says panel ruling was illegal. *Newsday.* April 25, 1987:6.

69. Weiss J. Opinion–appeal of Fred Boreali et al. v. David M. Axelrod. 130 A.D. 2d 107 July 23, 1987. *Supreme Court of New York, Appellate Division, Third Department.* Dayton, Ohio: Lexis-Nexis Academic Universe; 1987.

70. Titone J. Opinion–appeal of Fred Boreali et al. v. David M. Axelrod et al. 71 NY 2d 1 November 25, 1987. *Court of Appeals of New York.* Dayton, Ohio: Lexis-Nexis Academic Universe; 1987.

71. Lasalandra M. SJC upholds public smoking bans. *Boston Herald.* January 20, 2001:8.

72. Finucane M. Supreme Judicial Court upholds local smoking bans. Available at: http://web.lexis-nexis.com/universe. Accessed November 28, 2001.

73. Pratt D. Windjammer's challenge to ban put out. *Barnstable Patriot* [newspaper on-line]. January 25, 2001. Available at: http://www.barnstablepatriot.com/01-25-01-news/smoke.html. Accessed November 28, 2001.

74. Jeffrey K. Bans on smoking in restaurants, bars upheld by Supreme Judicial Court. *Cape Cod Times* [newspaper on-line]. January 19, 2001. Available at: http://www.capecod on-line.com. Accessed January 20, 2001.

75. Kibbe D. Court rejects challenge to local smoking bans. *Standard-Times* [newspaper on-line]. January 20, 2001. Available at: http://www.s-t.com/daily/01-01/01-20-01/a01sr004.htm. Accessed November 28, 2001.

76. Kelder G. *Partnerships Between Attorneys and Public Health Professionals to Support Local Tobacco Control Efforts.* Boston, Mass: Tobacco Control Resource Center; 1999.

77. *Clearing the Air: A Resource Manual for Environmental Tobacco Smoke for Massachusetts.* Boston, Mass: Tobacco Control Resource Center Inc; 1998.

78. Barrett Carter K. Judge extinguishes Princeton's strict ban on smoking. *Star-Ledger.* August 30, 2000:23.

79. Henry D. Princeton smoking ban hits a legal snag. *Star-Ledger.* July 21, 2000:30.

80. Stern R. Panel won't fight ruling against its smoking ban. *Times of Trenton.* September 20, 2000:A6.

81. Leonard L. Smoke screen: the debate on local control of tobacco rules. *Columbus Dispatch.* April 3, 2000:A7.

82. Yee D. Health board opts to pursue smoking ban; regulation to prohibit lighting up in restaurants needs public hearing, legislative support. *Arkansas Democrat Gazette.* January 26, 2001:A1.

83. Yee D. Board of health to consider ban on smoking in eateries; alternate proposal would allow segregated area until July 2006. *Arkansas Democrat Gazette.* January 25, 2001:B3.

84. Glantz SA, Smith LRA. The effect of ordinances requiring smoke-free restaurants on restaurant sales. *Am J Public Health.* 1994;84:1081–1085.

85. Glantz SA, Smith LRA. The effect of ordinances requiring smoke-free restaurants and bars on revenues: a follow-up. *Am J Public Health.* 1997;87:1687–1693.

86. Hyland A, Cummings KM, Nauenberg E. Analysis of taxable sales receipts: was New York City's Smoke-Free Air Act bad for restaurant business? *J Public Health Manage Pract.* 1999;5:14–21.

87. Hyland A, Cummings KM. Restaurant employment before and after the New York City Smoke-Free Air Act. *J Public Health Manage Pract.* 1999;5:22–27.

88. Hyland A, Cummings KM. Consumer response to the New York City Smoke-Free Air Act. *J Public Health Manage Pract.* 1999;5:28–36.

89. Hyland A, Cummings KM. Restaurateur reports of the economic impact of the New York City Smoke-Free Air Act. *J Public Health Manage Pract.* 1999;5:37–42.

90. Bartosch WJ, Pope GC. The economic effect of smoke-free restaurant policies on restaurant business in Massachusetts. *J Public Health Manage Pract.* 1999;5:53–62.

91. Magzamen S, Glantz SA. The new battleground: California's experience with smokefree bars. *Am J Public Health.* 2001;91:245–252.

Clean Indoor Air: Advances in California, 1990–1999

Elizabeth A. Gilpin, MS, Arthur J. Farkas, PhD, Sherry L. Emery, PhD, Christopher F. Ake, PhD, and John P. Pierce, PhD

Objectives. This study assessed progress in achieving clean indoor air in California.

Methods. Data were from large, cross-sectional population-based surveys (1990–1999).

Results. Indoor workers reporting smoke-free workplaces increased from 35.0% (95% confidence interval [CI]=33.7, 36.3) in 1990 to 93.4% (95% CI=92.6, 94.2) in 1999. Exposure of nonsmoking indoor workers to secondhand tobacco smoke decreased from 29.0% (95% CI=27.2, 30.8) to 15.6% (95% CI=14.1, 17.1). Adults with smoke-free homes increased from 37.6% (95% CI=35.1, 40.1) in 1992 to 73.7% (95% CI=73.2, 74.2) in 1999; nearly half of smokers in 1999 had smoke-free homes. In 1999, 82.2% (95% CI=81.5, 82.9) of children and adolescents (0–17 years) had smoke-free homes, up from 38.0% (95% CI=35.1, 40.9) in 1992.

Conclusions. California's advances highlight an important opportunity for tobacco control. (*Am J Public Health.* 2002;92:785–791)

The health hazards of secondhand smoke to nonsmokers were first recognized in the 1972 US surgeon general's report.[1] Following numerous population and laboratory investigations, the 1986 surgeon general's report reviewed all of the accumulated evidence and confirmed the health threat.[2] Ordinances restricting smoking in public places, including the workplace, became increasingly common.[3] Advocacy for clean air came largely from private organizations such as Americans for Nonsmokers' Rights.

The first comprehensive state governmental tobacco control program was initiated in California in 1988, funded by the $0.25 per pack excise tax increase passed by voters as Proposition 99.[4] This program was based on accumulated knowledge concerning the most effective tobacco use prevention strategies documented to date, as eventually outlined by the National Cancer Institute.[5] Although the importance of clean indoor air was recognized, smoking restrictions in public places, including worksites, were mainly viewed as a means for promoting smoking cessation and for establishing societal antismoking norms. Worksites were seen as a venue for delivery of smoking cessation assistance, and smoking restrictions were promoted as economically beneficial to the employer.[5] Another early study suggested that smoke-free workplaces and college settings might interrupt smoking initiation.[6]

Initially, the California Tobacco Control Program did not include nonsmokers among its "target populations" for whom it established goals.[7] Prompted by the release in 1992 of the US Environmental Protection Agency report on the dangers of secondhand smoke,[8] protection of nonsmokers from secondhand smoke in the workplace became a program goal.[9] A further review published in 1995 by the California Environmental Protection Agency[10] and later more widely circulated as a National Cancer Institute monograph[11] implicated secondhand smoke not only as a cause of cancer but also as a cause of heart disease and as a contributing cause of respiratory and auricular morbidity in young children. In 1997, clean indoor air in the workplace *and* for children at school and in the home were touted as program accomplishments, and protection of all nonsmokers from secondhand smoke became a clearly articulated program goal.[12]

The first statewide law (Assembly Bill 13) mandating clean air in indoor workplaces was enacted in California in 1994; however, application of this law to gaming clubs, bars and taverns, and bar areas of restaurants was delayed until January 1, 1998. Compliance with this law may be problematic in some settings, so monitoring exposure of nonsmokers to secondhand smoke in the workplace is important.

Whereas smoke-free workplaces are now mandated by law in California, smoking restrictions in the home are by agreement among household members. National data indicate that smokers who have smoke-free workplaces are more likely to live in smoke-free homes.[13] Workplace smoking restrictions may help establish norms against smoking around nonsmokers and make people more aware of the dangers of secondhand smoke. Having a smoke-free home is the most effective step parents can take to reduce their children's exposure to secondhand smoke.[14] A recent study indicated that protection of adolescents with smoking parents occurred in smoke-free homes but not in homes with lesser or no restrictions.[15]

In this article, we present trends from large population-based surveys of Californians, conducted in 1990, 1992, 1993, 1996, and 1999, indicating that the California Tobacco Control Program has been highly successful in its goal of promoting clean indoor air both in the workplace and in the home.

METHODS

The California Tobacco Surveys

The California Tobacco Surveys are random-digit-dialed telephone surveys conducted periodically to evaluate the California Tobacco Control Program. A 5-minute screening interview with a household adult (18 years or older) enumerates all household residents and obtains demographic information, including age and smoking status. For the 1990, 1992, 1996, and 1999 California Tobacco Surveys, some adults listed were randomly selected for an extended interview (approximately 25 minutes), with selection probability lower for persons who had not smoked in the last 5 years. Table 1 presents the details of the various California Tobacco Surveys, and more information is available in summary and technical reports.[16]

In 1993, because of budgetary constraints, no adult extended interview was done; instead, a brief interview (approximately 5 min-

TABLE 1—Characteristics of California Tobacco Surveys (1990, 1992, 1993, 1996, and 1999)

	1990	1992	1993	1996	1999
Households					
Sample	42790	14736	44172	71989	91174
Successfully screened	32135	10774	30910	39674	46590
Response rate	75.1%	73.1%	70.0%	55.1%	51.1%
Adult extended interview					
Enumerated[a]	65139	21870	61848	78337	93555
Targeted[b]	32266	11532	30910[c]	25546 26372[c]	21538
Successfully interviewed	24296	7263	30716[c]	18616 25812[c]	14729
Response rate	75.3%	71.3%	99.4%[c]	72.9% 97.9%[c]	68.4%

[a]Persons aged 18 years or older in household as enumerated by screening respondent.
[b]Persons targeted for an extended interview.
[c]Brief interview with screening respondent.

utes) was conducted with the screener respondent. In 1996, in addition to the adult extended interview, the brief interview was conducted with the screener respondent (if not selected for an extended interview) so that the methodology would be comparable to that of 1993. Subsequent analyses showed that the estimates from the 1996 adult extended and brief interviews (for the common questions) were very close. Consequently, the 1999 California Tobacco Survey used the same design as the 1990 and 1992 California Tobacco Surveys.

Each survey was weighted so that population estimates could be computed. First, base weights were computed from the probability of household selection and the probability of being selected for an extended interview.[16] These base weights were then ratio adjusted to the latest available California census data.

Survey Questions Analyzed

Survey items analyzed for this study included demographics, smoking status, employment status, exposure to smoking in the workplace, presence of smoking restrictions in the home, and exposure to secondhand smoke in places other than the workplace and home. These questions had slight differences in some years, which are delineated in the following paragraphs. However, it is highly unlikely that the observed changes in secondhand smoke exposure were because of these differences.

Smoking status. In 1990, 1992, and 1993, respondents to the adult extended interview were asked, "Do you smoke cigarettes now?" In 1996 and 1999, the question was changed ("Do you currently smoke cigarettes every day, some days, or not at all?") to be consistent with national surveys.[17,18] Respondents to the 1990, 1992, and 1993 adult extended interviews were classified as current smokers if they answered "yes" to the smoke-now question, and respondents to the 1996 and 1999 adult extended interviews were classified as current smokers if they responded "every day" or "some days." The remaining respondents were classified as nonsmokers. In 1996, the screener interview retained the older smoke-now question. The new smoking status question was expected to produce slightly higher population smoking prevalence estimates because some respondents who might not admit to smoking now (i.e., being a current smoker) might admit to smoking some days. Screening data on smoking status (including proxy reports) were used to assess whether there were adult smokers in the household.

Smoke-free workplaces and exposure to secondhand smoke. In 1990 and 1992, respondents were asked, "Which of the following best describes your current employment status? Self-employed, employed by someone else, not employed, or retired." Those self-employed or employed by someone else were asked, "Do you currently work outside your home?" Those answering "yes" were asked, "Do you work primarily indoors or outdoors?" Indoor workers outside the home were asked, "Do you/does your employer have an official policy that restricts smoking in any way?" If the answer to that question was "yes," respondents were asked 2 further questions: "Which of the following best describes (your/your employer's) smoking policy for indoor public or common areas, such as lobbies, rest rooms, and lunch rooms?" and "Which of the following best describes (your/your employer's) smoking policy for areas in which employees work?" The response choices for these 2 questions were (1) not allowed in any, (2) allowed in some, and (3) allowed in all. For the current analysis, we report the percentage of indoor workers who answered "not allowed in any" to both questions. Such workplaces are considered smoke-free. Indoor nonsmoking workers also were asked, "During the past 2 weeks, has anyone smoked in the area in which you work?"

In 1993, only nonsmokers were asked about workplace smoking restrictions. Because previous research indicated that smokers and nonsmokers answer differently,[19] the 1993 data were not analyzed for this study. However, as in the 1990 and 1992 surveys, nonsmoking indoor workers in 1993 were asked the question about anyone smoking in their work area in the past 2 weeks.

In 1996 and 1999, all respondents were asked, "Do you currently work for money in an indoor setting, such as an office, plant, or store, outside of your home?" Because nearly all indoor workplaces (except bars and game rooms) should have been smoke-free by law, those who answered "yes" were asked, "Is your place of work completely smoke-free indoors?" Again, nonsmokers were asked the question about exposure to anyone smoking in their work area in the past 2 weeks.

To assess compliance with the smoke-free workplace law, the 1999 California Tobacco Survey asked, "What best describes where you currently work outside your home for money? Do you work (1) in an office, (2) in a plant or factory, (3) in a store or warehouse, (4) in a classroom, (5) in a hospital, (6) in a restaurant or bar, (7) in a vehicle, or (8) in some other indoor setting?" Indoor workers who stated that their workplace was not smoke-free were asked, "For each of the following indoor areas in your building, is smoking allowed in: (1) any indoor work areas, (2) a special smoking room or lounge, (3) a break room or cafeteria, or (4) a hallway or lobby?"

Smoke-free homes. The 1992 California Tobacco Survey was the first to include a question about smoking restrictions in the home. In that survey, adults who answered the extended interview were asked, "What are the smoking rules or restrictions in your household, if any?" Respondents could answer as follows: (1) smoking is completely banned, (2) smoking is generally banned with few exceptions, (3) smoking is allowed in some rooms only, or (4) there are no restrictions on smoking. The first answer choice defined a smoke-free home. The 1993, 1996, and 1999 California Tobacco Surveys asked this question of the screener respondent, and the 1996 and 1999 California Tobacco Surveys also asked the question on the adult extended interview. To compute the rate of report of smoke-free homes for smokers, their response was the one considered, but to establish the overall percentage of smoke-free homes or the percentage of children and adolescents living in smoke-free homes, the screener respondent's answer was used. In 1992, only households that had at least 1 completed adult interview could be analyzed, and the least stringent response was used.

Exposure to secondhand smoke outside of work or the home. The 1999 California Tobacco Survey included the question, "In California, in the past 6 months, that is, since [date computed], have you had to put up with someone smoking near you at any other place besides your home or your workplace?" Respondents answering "yes" were asked, "The last time this happened in California, where were you?" The question was open ended, but the interviewer had precoded categories for the following answers: (1) restaurant, (2) restaurant bar, (3) bar or tavern, (4) pool hall, (5) shopping mall, (6) public park/outdoors, (7) community event, (8) sports event, (9) another person's home, (10) another person's automobile, (11) game room/casino/bingo hall, or (12) other–specify. For the current analysis, we grouped pool hall with game room/casino/bingo hall and community event with sports event.

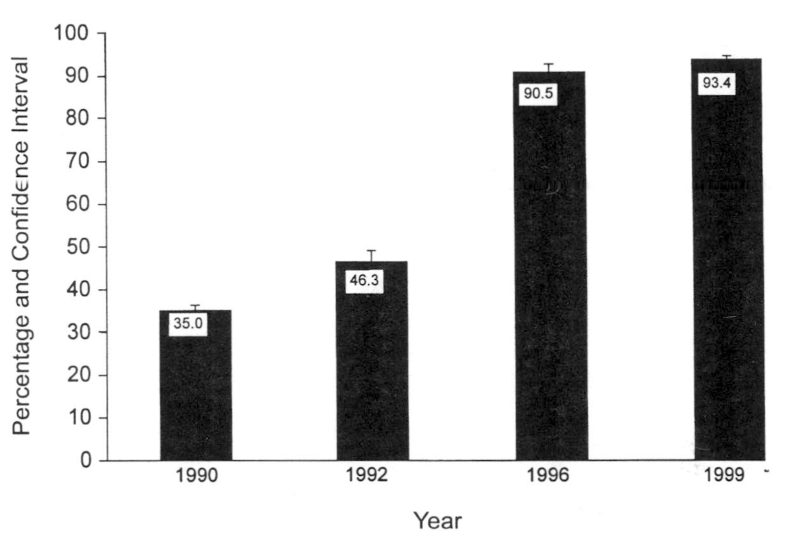

FIGURE 1—Indoor workers reporting smoke-free workplaces (1990, 1992, 1996, and 1999 California Tobacco Surveys).

Statistics

All analyses were performed with the WesVarPC statistical package,[20] which takes into account the survey sample designs and uses a jackknife procedure for variance estimation.[21] All percentages are reported with 95% confidence intervals (CIs).

RESULTS

Clean Indoor Air in the Workplace

Figure 1 shows the increase from 1990 to 1999 in the percentage of California indoor workers reporting smoke-free workplaces. In 1990, only 35.0% (95% CI=33.7, 36.3) of California indoor workers reported working in a clean air environment, but this percentage increased to 93.4% (95% CI=92.6, 94.2) by 1999. In 1999, indoor workers not reporting smoke-free workplaces could have answered affirmatively about more than 1 of the following workplace policies: 2.4% (95% CI=1.9, 2.9) perceived that their employer's smoking policy allowed smoking in indoor work areas, 1.5% (95% CI=1.1, 1.9) perceived that smoking was allowed in special smoking rooms or lounges, 0.9% (95% CI=0.7, 1.1) said that it was allowed in a break room or cafeteria, and 1.1% (95% CI=0.8, 1.4) said that it was allowed in a hall or lobby.

As expected, a concomitant decrease in work area exposure to secondhand smoke occurred. From 1990 to 1996, the percentage of nonsmoking indoor workers who reported that someone had smoked in their work area within the previous 2 weeks declined by a factor of nearly 60%–from 29.0% (95% CI=27.2, 30.8) in 1990 to 11.8% (95% CI=10.3, 13.3) in 1996 (Table 2). From 1996 to 1999, the percentage reporting exposure increased to 15.6% (95% CI=14.1, 17.1).

Despite the increase in smoke-free workplaces, clean air working environments have not been established equally in all demographic groups. Table 2 shows that some of the inequities in exposure that existed in 1990 persisted through 1999. In general, males, younger workers, minorities, and the less educated still have higher rates of work area exposure to secondhand smoke. Nonetheless, females, young adults (18–24 years), African Americans, and the more

TABLE 2—Exposure of Nonsmokers to Secondhand Smoke in the Past 2 Weeks in Indoor Work Areas, by Demographic Characteristics (1990, 1993, 1996, and 1999 California Tobacco Surveys)

	1990 (n = 7293)	1993 (n = 12 888)	1996 (n = 5393)	1999 (n = 4588)
Overall	29.0 (27.2, 30.8)	22.4 (21.1, 23.7)	11.8 (10.3, 13.3)	15.6 (14.1, 17.1)
Sex				
Male	35.6 (32.7, 38.5)	27.6 (25.8, 29.4)	16.4 (14.0, 18.8)	18.0 (16.1, 19.9)
Female	22.7 (20.7, 24.7)	17.1 (15.5, 18.7)	7.0 (5.5, 8.5)	13.2 (10.9, 15.5)
Age, y				
18–24	41.6 (36.9, 46.3)	31.1 (27.4, 34.8)	17.8 (13.3, 22.3)	29.8 (25.0, 34.6)
25–44	28.0 (25.7, 30.6)	22.7 (21.1, 24.3)	12.3 (10.4, 14.2)	15.3 (13.2, 17.4)
45–64	23.3 (20.7, 25.9)	16.3 (18.4, 18.4)	8.6 (6.0, 11.2)	10.5 (7.4, 13.6)
≥65	16.6 (7.3, 25.9)	17.9 (12.1, 23.7)	9.7 (3.1, 16.3)	11.9 (5.0, 18.8)
Race/ethnicity				
Non-Hispanic White	25.9 (24.1, 27.7)	19.0 (17.6, 20.4)	9.0 (7.3, 10.7)	12.2 (10.7, 13.7)
Hispanic	39.8 (34.9, 44.7)	32.2 (28.4, 36.0)	19.5 (15.7, 23.3)	20.5 (17.4, 23.6)
African American	22.9 (15.4, 30.4)	19.5 (15.1, 23.9)	7.9 (2.7, 13.1)	16.0 (10.1, 21.9)
Asian or Pacific Islander	27.8 (22.2, 33.4)	26.4 (21.1, 31.7)	11.9 (7.9, 15.9)	19.4 (11.9, 26.9)
Other	29.9 (7.4, 52.4)	19.7 (10.5, 28.9)	6.3 (1.0, 11.6)	12.0 (2.1, 21.9)
Education				
< 12 y	42.1 (33.5, 50.7)	35.6 (30.4, 40.8)	28.7 (21.5, 35.9)	27.4 (19.8, 35.0)
High school graduate	33.7 (30.2, 37.2)	28.0 (25.7, 30.3)	17.1 (13.7, 20.5)	19.3 (16.3, 22.3)
Some college	30.0 (26.8, 33.2)	21.6 (19.7, 23.5)	9.4 (7.3, 11.5)	15.1 (12.8, 17.4)
College graduate	18.5 (16.8, 20.2)	13.6 (12.3, 14.9)	5.1 (3.9, 6.3)	10.2 (8.2, 12.2)

Note. Table entries are weighted percentages and 95% confidence intervals. Weights are computed based on the probability of selection for interview and then ratio adjusted to population demographic totals so that estimates are representative of the California population.

highly educated showed recent increases in exposure.

In 1999, the level of reported exposure to secondhand smoke differed according to workplace type. Nonsmoking workers in hospitals and classrooms reported the least exposure (6.9% [95% CI=3.4, 10.4] and 7.1% [95% CI=3.9, 10.3], respectively). Offices also had a relatively low exposure rate of 11.6% (95% CI=9.8, 13.4). Exposure was much higher for workers in plants and factories (17.9% [95% CI=9.7, 26.1]), stores and warehouses (24.5% [95% CI=20.0, 29.0]), and restaurants and bars (31.5% [95% CI=22.9, 40.1]). Workers whose workplace was a vehicle had an even higher exposure rate: 50.7% (95% CI=32.0, 69.4). Also, nonsmokers' exposure was related to worksite size. Exposure was 11.8% (95% CI=10.1, 13.5) in workplaces with more than 50 workers, 17.5% (95% CI=12.4, 22.6) at very small worksites with fewer than 5 employees, 17.8% (95% CI=14.9, 20.7) in workplaces with 5 to 24 employees, and 20.6% (95% CI=15.6, 25.6) in workplaces with 25 to 50 employees.

Clean Indoor Air in the Home

The percentage of Californians reporting smoke-free homes was 73.7% (95% CI=73.2, 74.2) in 1999, almost a 2-fold increase since 1992 (Figure 2), when this question was first included in the California Tobacco Survey. Not surprisingly, in each year, nonsmokers were much more likely than smokers to report smoke-free homes, but the margin narrowed over time from nearly a factor of 3 in 1992 to less than a factor of 2 by 1999. In 1999, more than 3 times as many smokers reported living in smoke-free homes as in 1992.

This increase in smoke-free homes has resulted in increased protection of children and adolescents from exposure to secondhand smoke at home. Figure 3 shows the increase in protection at home from 1992 to 1999 in all California households with children and adolescents (white bars), in homes with at least 1 adult smoker (striped bars), and in homes in which all adults were smokers (black bars). These categories are not mutually exclusive. In 1999, more than 80% of California's children and adolescents were

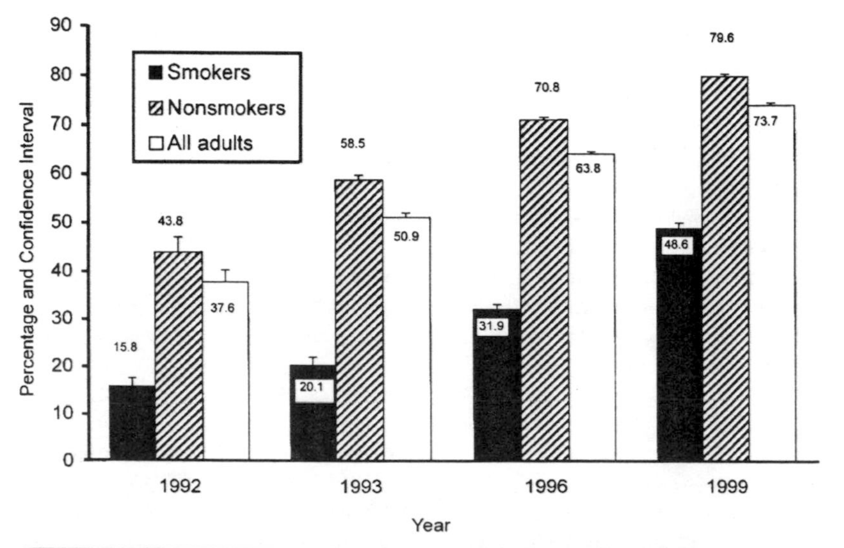

FIGURE 2—Californians reporting smoke-free homes (1992, 1993, 1996, and 1999 California Tobacco Surveys).

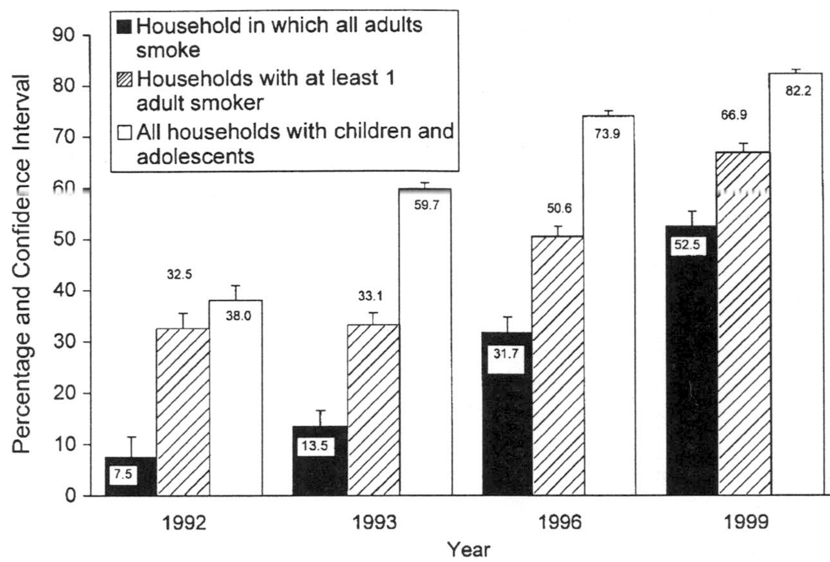

FIGURE 3—Children and adolescents living in smoke-free homes (1992, 1993, 1996, and 1999 California Tobacco Surveys).

TABLE 3—Children and Adolescents Living in Smoke-Free Homes, by Race/Ethnicity (1992, 1993, 1996, and 1999 California Tobacco Surveys)

	1992 (n[a] = 3756)	1993 (n = 21 698)	1996 (n = 25 264)	1999 (n = 32 511)
Non-Hispanic White	37.4 (33.9, 40.9)	58.2 (56.7, 59.7)	70.9 (69.3, 72.5)	80.4 (79.4, 81.4)
Hispanic	39.5 (35.1, 43.9)	62.1 (56.7, 64.7)	78.0 (77.3, 79.5)	85.1 (84.2, 86.0)
African American	32.6 (21.9, 43.3)	55.0 (49.4, 60.6)	65.7 (61.8, 69.6)	75.6 (72.4, 78.8)
Asian or Pacific Islander	43.2 (29.1, 57.3)	65.4 (60.2, 70.6)	78.2 (75.7, 80.7)	82.9 (80.8, 85.0)
Other	33.5 (14.4, 52.6)	53.0 (41.9, 64.1)	70.0 (66.4, 73.6)	78.4 (73.4, 83.4)

Note. Table entries are weighted percentages and 95% confidence intervals. Weights are computed based on the probability of selection for interview and then ratio adjusted to population demographic totals so that estimates are representative of the California population.

[a]In 1992, only children and adolescents from households in which an adult completed an extended interview could be included.

protected from secondhand smoke at home, an increase from just over a third in 1992. Importantly, fewer than 10% of California's children and adolescents were protected from secondhand smoke in homes in which all adults smoked in 1992, whereas more than half were protected in 1999.

As with exposure to secondhand smoke in the workplace, advances in clean air at home were seen in some groups more than in others. Table 3 indicates that in 1999, Hispanic children and adolescents were more protected from secondhand smoke than were other racial/ethnic groups. However, all groups have shown impressive increases in protection since 1992 and even since 1996.

Protection in Places Other Than Work or Home

Because of gains in home and workplace protection from secondhand smoke, a new category of nonsmokers is emerging: those who rarely (if ever) are exposed to secondhand smoke. Among nonsmoking adults in 1999, 37.2% (95% CI=35.7, 38.7) had smoke-free homes, had no workplace exposure in the past 2 weeks, and did not encounter any other situation in the past 6 months in California where they had to put up with someone smoking around them.

The other approximately two thirds of nonsmoking Californians who did report an instance of being around a smoker sometime in the past 6 months in California were most likely to report that the last time such exposure occurred indoors was in a restaurant (13.4% [95% CI=12.0, 14.8]). Reports of exposure in restaurant bars (2.1% [95% CI=1.6, 2.6]) and bars or taverns (8.1% [95% CI=6.9, 9.3]) were relatively lower, reflecting that more people go to restaurants to eat than go to bars. The most frequent place identified was public parks and other outdoor areas (31.8% [95% CI=30.1, 33.5]). Shopping malls (4.1% [95% CI=3.4, 4.8]), community and sports events (5.4% [95% CI=4.5, 6.3]), and game room/casino/bingo hall/pool hall venues (3.2% [95% CI=2.6, 3.8]) were not frequently mentioned. Reports of exposure to a smoker in other people's homes (12.4% [95% CI=10.9, 13.9]) were more frequent, but reports of exposure in others' automobiles (3.7% [95% CI=2.9, 4.5]) were less so.

DISCUSSION

The evidence presented here shows that during the California Tobacco Control Program from 1990 to 1999, marked advances were made in guaranteeing clean indoor air for nonsmokers. In 1999, about 95% of California's indoor workers reported that their workplace was smoke-free. Nearly three quarters of Californians have smoke-free homes, including nearly half of all current smokers, and more than 80% of children and adolescents are protected from exposure at home. Furthermore, more than a third of nonsmoking Californians reported that they had not had to put up with anyone smoking in their presence, outside of work or the home, in the past 6 months.

Despite these impressive gains, further steps are needed to improve the rate of compliance with the clean indoor air law (Assembly Bill 13). The 6.6% of indoor workers who failed to report that their indoor workplace was smoke-free and the 15.6% of indoor workers reporting exposure to secondhand smoke in their work area in the past 2 weeks in 1999 indicate that compliance is not complete. This study cannot determine whether lack of compliance is due to lack of knowledge of the law or lack of enforcement. It also cannot validate self-reports of exposure at work with a biomarker; actual exposure at work may be greater than is reported because of lack of recall. The few workers who stated that their employer's policy allowed smoking in indoor work areas and common areas, such as break rooms, cafeterias, hallways, or lobbies, either have misinformed or noncompliant employers or are themselves misinformed. Although nonsmoking workers in large workplaces (>50 employees) reported less exposure than did workers in smaller workplaces, there was little difference in exposure for different sized workplaces in the 50-or-fewer-employees group. In particular, no evidence showed that very small workplaces disregard the clean indoor air law more than do moderate-sized workplaces.

Nonsmokers in workplace settings such as stores and warehouses, plants and factories, and restaurants and bars reported particularly high rates of exposure to someone smoking in their work area in the past 2 weeks. Interestingly, nonsmokers protected at work and at home frequently named restaurants as the setting where they most recently had to put up with someone smoking around them. Some of the exposure in restaurants may have occurred in outdoor patios or eating areas. Nevertheless, increased enforcement efforts aimed at restaurant working environments are called for to protect Californians who are still most exposed to secondhand tobacco smoke. Steps to bring these work settings into greater compliance also might serve to address the racial/ethnic and other disparities in protection from secondhand smoke in the workplace. Stores and restaurants frequently employ younger, less educated workers.

The original impetus for workplace smoking restrictions was to encourage smoking cessation, and increasing evidence indicates that such restrictions do affect smoking behavior. A recent review[22] of studies addressing the effect of workplace smoking restrictions indicated that 12.5% of the 76.5 billion decrease in annual cigarette consumption in the United States between 1988 and 1994 can be attributed to smoke-free workplaces. Many studies showed declines in smoking prevalence, daily smoking, or cigarette consumption.[22] A report from a large national survey indicated that smoking prevalence was 6% lower among indoor workers who worked where smoking was completely banned and that consumption among daily smokers was 14% less than among indoor workers without workplace smoking restrictions.[23] However, such effects may not be fully realized if workplaces with smoke-free policies do not actively or consistently enforce them[24] or if the bans are not total.[23]

Heightened public awareness of the dangers of secondhand smoke may be partly responsible for the steadily increasing numbers of Californians reporting that their homes are smoke-free. An analysis of data from the 1996 California Tobacco Survey indicated that current smokers who believed that secondhand smoke causes cancer in nonsmokers and harms the health of children and babies or who lived in households with nonsmoking adults or with children were more likely to report smoke-free homes.[25]

The findings about nonsmoking adults and children also were present in national data.[13] In the California study, female smokers, older smokers, and African American smokers were less likely to report having smoke-free homes.[25] Hispanics were more likely to have smoke-free homes than were other racial/ethnic groups. There was little difference by educational level. Hispanic women have low smoking rates,[26] and as a group, Hispanics are more likely to be occasional smokers[27] who possibly do not need to smoke indoors at home. Thus, the higher rates of smoke-free homes and protection of children and adolescents in this ethnic group are not surprising.

Promoting awareness of the dangers of secondhand smoke through the mass media is a focus of the California Tobacco Control Program. Mass media campaigns appear to reach a large segment of the population, regardless of educational level.[28]

Both the national and the California studies[13,25] found that smokers who live in smoke-free homes smoke less and show more quit attempts than do smokers who live in homes that are not smoke-free. These studies were not longitudinal, so it is not known whether smokers who are trying to quit adopt smoking bans or whether smoking bans lead to quitting behavior. However, it is logical that consumption might be reduced if a smoker can no longer smoke right after awakening or while sitting at the table after a meal; the effort to go outside would be a deterrent to smoking. For smokers trying to quit, not being able to smoke indoors at home may facilitate success by eliminating some of the stimuli to relapse.[29,30] The 1996 California Tobacco Survey indicated that smokers abstained from cigarettes longer during their most recent quit attempt if they had smoke-free homes.[25]

The California Tobacco Control Program goals for 2000 to 2003 include a call to "continue to press for smokefree workplaces, public places, events, schools, and homes."[31] Specific recommendations urge that efforts be directed at increasing the number of clean air outdoor locations (e.g., toddler play lots, bus stops, amusement parks, fairgrounds, concerts, sporting events) and the number of clean air shared living facilities (apartments, townhouses, condominiums); they also suggest that teenagers be educated to be less accepting of secondhand smoke. The racial/ethnic differences in protection from secondhand smoke among indoor workers in the workplace and in the protection of children and adolescents in the home suggest an important opportunity for the special statewide ethnic networks to support and work within these communities to address this issue. Education of parents in culturally sensitive ways about the effects of secondhand smoke on their children and family and encouragement of the adoption of smoke-free homes and cars would be an important contribution for these groups. One recent program by the African American Tobacco Education Network—"Not in Mama's Kitchen"—is an example.[31]

In contrast to earlier government recommendations for tobacco control strategies,[5] a recent report by the Centers for Disease Control and Prevention—*Best Practices for Comprehensive Tobacco Control Programs*—now mentions eliminating nonsmokers' exposure to environmental tobacco smoke as a goal.[32] However, it makes few concrete recommendations, merely stating that programs should promote governmental and voluntary policies to advocate clean indoor air and calling for "strict enforcement of laws against smoking in public places." The importance of educating the public about the dangers of secondhand smoke and of promoting smoke-free homes is given scant attention. The results from the California Tobacco Control Program suggest that this omission represents a missed opportunity for tobacco control policy development. ■

About the Authors

The authors are with the Cancer Prevention and Control Program, Cancer Center, University of California, San Diego, La Jolla, Calif.

Requests for reprints should be sent to John P. Pierce, PhD, Cancer Prevention and Control Program, Cancer Center, University of California, San Diego, La Jolla, CA 92093-0645 (e-mail: jppierce@ucsd.edu).

This article was accepted June 18, 2001.

Contributors

E.A. Gilpin specified analyses and wrote the paper. A.J. Farkas reviewed drafts and quality-checked analyses. S.L. Emery reviewed and commented on early preliminary analyses and drafts. C.F. Ake conducted analyses. J.P. Pierce reviewed drafts and helped frame issues discussed in the introduction and literature review.

Acknowledgments

Preparation of this paper was supported by the Cancer Prevention Research Unit (grant CA72092) funded by the National Institutes of Health. Data for the California Tobacco Surveys were collected under contracts 89-97872 (1990 and 1992), 92-10601 (1993), 95-23211 (1996), and 98-15657 (1999) from the California Department of Health Services, Tobacco Control Section, Sacramento.

References

1. *The Health Consequences of Smoking: A Report of the Surgeon General; 1972.* Washington, DC: Public Health Service and Mental Health Administration, US Dept of Health, Education and Welfare; 1972. DHEW publication HSM 72-7516.

2. *The Health Consequences of Involuntary Smoking: A Report of the Surgeon General.* Atlanta, Ga: Centers for Disease Control; 1986. DHHS publication CDC 87-8398.

3. *Major Local Tobacco Control Ordinances in the United States.* Smoking and Tobacco Control Monograph No. 3. Bethesda, Md: National Cancer Institute; 1993. NIH publication 93-3532.

4. Bal DG, Kizer KW, Felten PG, Mozar HN, Niemeyer D. Reducing tobacco consumption in California. *JAMA.* 1990;264:1570–1574.

5. *Strategies to Control Tobacco Use in the United States: A Blueprint for Public Health Action in the 1990's.* Smoking and Tobacco Control Monograph No. 1. Bethesda, Md: National Cancer Institute; 1991. NIH publication 92-3316.

6. Pierce JP, Naquin M, Gilpin E, Giovino G, Mills S, Marcus S. Smoking initiation in the United States: a role for worksite and college smoking bans. *J Natl Cancer Inst.* 1991;83:1009–1013.

7. Tobacco Education Oversight Committee. *Toward a Tobacco-Free California: A Master Plan to Reduce Californians' Use of Tobacco.* Sacramento: California Department of Health Services, Tobacco Control Section; January 1, 1991.

8. *Respiratory Health Effects of Passive Smoking: Lung Cancer and Other Disorders.* Washington, DC: Office of Research and Development and Office of Air and Radiation, US Environmental Protection Agency; 1992. Publication EPA/600/6-90-006F.

9. Tobacco Education Oversight Committee. *Toward a Tobacco-Free California: Exploring a New Frontier 1993–1995.* Sacramento: California Department of Health Services, Tobacco Control Section; February 1993.

10. California Environmental Protection Agency (CalEPA). *Health Effects of Exposure to Environmental Tobacco Smoke: Final Report.* Sacramento, Calif: Office of Environmental Health Hazard Assessment; 1997.

11. *Health Effects of Exposure to Environmental Tobacco Smoke: The Report of the California Environmental Protection Agency.* Smoking and Tobacco Control Monograph No. 10. Bethesda, Md: National Cancer Institute; 1999. NIH publication 99-4645.

12. Tobacco Education Research Oversight Committee. *Toward a Tobacco-Free California: Renewing the Commitment 1997–2000.* Sacramento: California Department of Health Services, Tobacco Control Section; 1997.

13. Farkas AJ, Gilpin EA, Distefan JM, Pierce JP. The effects of household and workplace smoking restrictions on quitting behaviors. *Tob Control.* 1999;8: 261–265.

14. Mannino DM, Siegel M, Husten C, Rose D, Etzel R. Environmental tobacco smoke exposure and health effects in children: results from the 1991 National Health Interview Survey. *Tob Control.* 1996;5:13–18.

15. Biener L, Cullen D, Di ZX, Hammond SK. Household smoking restrictions and adolescents' exposure to environmental tobacco smoke. *Prev Med.* 1997;26: 358–363.

16. Pierce JP, Gilpin EA, Emery SL, et al. *Tobacco Control in California: Who's Winning the War? An Evaluation of the Tobacco Control Program, 1989–1996.* La Jolla: University of California, San Diego; 1998. Available at: http://ssdc.ucsd.edu/tobacco.

17. Benson V, Marano MA. Current estimates from the National Health Interview Survey, 1993. National Center for Health Statistics. *Vital Health Stat 10.* 1994; No. 1004:10.

18. *Current Population Survey, September 1992: Tobacco Use Supplement Technical Documentation.* Washington, DC: US Bureau of the Census, Data Users Services Division, Data Access and Use Staff; 1992.

19. Gilpin EA, Stillman FA, Hartman AM, Gibson JT, Pierce JP. An index for state tobacco control initial outcomes. *Am J Epidemiol.* 2000;152:727–738.

20. *A User's Guide to WesVarPC, Version 2.0.* Rockville, Md: Westat Inc; 1996.

21. Efron B. *The Jackknife, the Bootstrap and Other Resampling Plans.* CMBS Regional Conference Series in Applied Mathematics 38. Philadelphia, Pa: Society for Industrial and Applied Mathematics; 1982.

22. Chapman S, Borland R, Scollo M, Brownson RC, Woodward S. The impact of smoke-free workplaces on declining cigarette consumption in Australia and the United States. *Am J Public Health.* 1999;89: 1018–1023.

23. Farrelly MC, Evans WN, Sfekas AES. The impact of workplace smoking bans: results from a national survey. *Tob Control.* 1999;8:272–277.

24. Biener L, Nyman AL. Effect of workplace smoking policies on smoking cessation: results of a longitudinal study. *J Occup Environ Med.* 1999;41:1121–1127.

25. Gilpin EA, White MM, Farkas AJ, Pierce JP. Home smoking restrictions: which smokers have them and how they are associated with smoking behavior. *Nicotine Tob Res.* 1999;1:153–162.

26. Navarro AM. Cigarette smoking among adult Latinos: the California Tobacco Baseline Survey. *Ann Behav Med.* 1996;18:238–245.

27. Gilpin EA, Cavin SW, Pierce JP. Adult smokers who do not smoke daily. *Addiction.* 1997;92: 473–480.

28. Pierce JP, Macaskill P, Hill D. Long-term effectiveness of mass media led antismoking campaigns in Australia. *Am J Public Health.* 1990;80:565–569.

29. Best JA, Hakstian AR. A situation-specific model for smoking behavior. *Addict Behav.* 1978;3:79–92.

30. Shiffman S, Gnys M, Richards TJ, Paty JA, Hickcox M, Kassel JD. Temptations to smoke after quitting: a comparison of lapsers and maintainers. *Health Psychol.* 1996;15:455–461.

31. Tobacco Education Research Oversight Committee. *Toward a Tobacco-Free California: Strategies for the 21st Century 2000–2003.* Sacramento: California Department of Health Services, Tobacco Control Section; January 2000.

32. *Best Practices for Comprehensive Tobacco Control Programs–August 1999.* Atlanta, Ga: Office of Smoking and Health, National Center for Chronic Disease Prevention and Health Promotion; 1999.

Science, Politics, and Ideology in the Campaign Against Environmental Tobacco Smoke

| Ronald Bayer, PhD, and James Colgrove, MPH

The issue of environmental tobacco smoke (ETS) and the harms it causes to nonsmoking bystanders has occupied a central place in the rhetoric and strategy of antismoking forces in the United States over the past 3 decades. Beginning in the 1970s, anti-tobacco activists drew on suggestive and incomplete evidence to push for far-reaching prohibitions on smoking in a variety of public settings. Public health professionals and other antismoking activists, although concerned about the potential illness and death that ETS might cause in nonsmokers, also used restrictions on public smoking as a way to erode the social acceptability of cigarettes and thereby reduce smoking prevalence. This strategy was necessitated by the context of American political culture, especially the hostility toward public health interventions that are overtly paternalistic. (*Am J Public Health.* 2002;92:949–954)

PROTECTING BYSTANDERS

At the dawn of the public health movement against tobacco in the early 1960s, smoking was ubiquitous. Public spaces and sociability were defined by the presence of cigarettes. For nonsmokers, the presence of smoke was a part of the social environment. Although for many there was little or no annoyance, some found cigarette smoke irritating, and others found it frankly intolerable. For those who found smoking difficult to endure, the only solution was to withdraw from the public space into the protection afforded by privacy.

Over the next 3 decades, a profound social transformation was to occur. What had been a mark of sociability would become antisocial, and smoking would increasingly be restricted to private settings. Such shifts in social attitudes toward and policies regarding public smoking began in the early 1970s, advanced by public health officials and antismoking activists drawing on the first hints and suggestive evidence about the hazards posed by smoking for nonsmokers. The movement against public smoking was shaped by the broader emergent environmental movement, a new health consciousness, and the array of rights-based challenges to the status quo. As a consequence, the needs of the nonsmoking bystander assumed great salience. In the end, however, the most dramatic effect was on smokers themselves, who were forced to change their routines, came to endure increasing stigmatization, and felt mounting pressure to quit their habit because of the transformation in the public context within which smoking could occur.

The exceptional importance that has been accorded to the issue of environmental tobacco smoke (ETS) must be understood in light of the ideological constraints imposed by American culture and politics and the profound hostility occasioned by public policies that are explicitly paternalistic. It was within this context that antismoking policies and activism had to find subjects who were worthy of protection—nonsmokers—and on whose behalf restrictions on smoking could be justified. In this article, the claims of the bystander are the focus of analysis. We examine the ways in which the political and ideological context of the United States influenced evolving notions of the harm caused by secondhand smoke and the public health strategies created as a response.

FIRST GESTURES

In an address to a coalition of organizations concerned about smoking and health in 1971, Surgeon General Jesse L. Steinfeld voiced his concern for those placed at risk by smokers, innocents who could not protect themselves. "The mother who smokes," he said, "is subjecting the unborn child to the adverse effects of tobacco and as a result we are losing . . . and possibly handicapping babies." Just as he raised alarm about the dangers of fetal exposure, the surgeon general expressed his concern for those compelled to breathe air filled with smoke. "Evidence is accumulating that the nonsmoker may have untoward effects from the pollution his smoking neighbor forces upon him. Nonsmokers have as much right to clean air and wholesome air as smokers have to their so-called right to smoke, which I would redefine as a 'right to pollute.'" The surgeon general then went on to propose a policy agenda that would define the goals of the antismoking movement over the next 3 decades. "It is high time to ban smoking from all confined public spaces such as restaurants, theaters, airplanes, trains and buses. It is time that we interpret the Bill of Rights for the nonsmokers as well as the smoker."[1] The 1972 *Surgeon General's Report on Smoking* for the first time identified the exposure of nonsmokers to cigarette smoke as a health hazard.[2]

The newly apprehended hazard served as a catalyst for the nonsmokers' rights movement in the 1970s. Among the most prominent organizations was the evocatively named GASP (Group Against Smokers' Pollution). In its first newsletter, *The Ventilator*, the call went out to nonsmokers, "the innocent victims of tobacco smoke," to assert the "right to breathe clean air." That was a right that took precedence over "the right of the smoker to enjoy a harmful habit."[3] GASP and other groups began to press for policies to restrict public smoking.

They did so against the backdrop of considerable public support for such measures. As early as 1970 (before the surgeon general had spoken out about harm to nonsmokers), 58% of men who had never smoked and 72% of women who had never smoked agreed that lighting up should be allowed in fewer public spaces. More than three quarters of those who had never smoked felt that it was "annoying to be near" someone who was smoking.[4]

Some initial successes in this area showed how potentially effective the nonsmokers' rights movement—which by focusing on how smokers placed others at risk was able to counter the accusation of paternalism—could be. In 1973, the Civil Aeronautics Board ordered domestic airlines to provide separate seating for smokers and nonsmokers. In 1974, the Interstate Commerce Commission ruled that smoking be restricted to the rear 20% of seats in interstate buses.[5] States and localities also began to impose restrictions. In 1973, Arizona became the first state to restrict smoking in some public spaces. In 1974, Connecticut enacted the first statute to restrict smoking in restaurants. In 1975, Minnesota passed a comprehensive statewide law "to protect the public health, comfort, and the environment by prohibiting smoking in public spaces and at public meetings except in designated smoking areas."[6] In 1977, Berkeley, Calif, became the first local community to limit smoking in restaurants and other public settings.[2]

These successes occurred within a context of scientific uncertainty and some skepticism about the precise nature of the physical harms, if any, incurred by secondhand exposure to tobacco smoke. It was such skepticism that informed a 1975 editorial in the *New England Journal of Medicine.* Gary Huber,[7] who in later years would emerge as a sharp critic of the developing public health consensus on the risks of tobacco smoke to nonsmokers, concluded that beyond the "psychogenic" effect of exposure to ETS, the questions centering on the potential biological effect "remain unanswered." Writing 5 years later, when a study was published that found that ETS impaired respiratory function, Claude L'Enfant and Barbara Liu[8] of the National Heart, Lung, and Blood Institute asserted that until that time, "[t]he case against smoking in the environment has often been anecdotal, based on annoyances, feelings and sometimes more objective physical reactions such as eye and nose irritation." Even though there was solid evidence that maternal smoking had damaging effects on a fetus and that children could be harmed by secondhand smoke in the home, L'Enfant and Liu acknowledged, "Generally speaking, the evidence that passive smoking in a general environment has health effects remains sparse, incomplete, and sometimes unconvincing."

With such ambiguity in the available science, it is not surprising that those who were ideologically opposed to regulatory interventions would seek to characterize the efforts of the nonsmokers' rights movement as politically motivated and baseless—an expression of moralism.

The tobacco industry viewed the effect of the nonsmokers' rights movement as potentially ominous. As early as 1973, the *US Tobacco Journal,* an industry publication, expressed concern that because of the changing social climate, some smokers were beginning to enjoy their habit less and were forgoing it in some social situations. "The tobacco industry must begin to think about this phenomenon along with the groundwork for a countervailing strategy to defeat it."[5(p14)]

Most dramatic was a report prepared in the late 1970s by the Roper Organization for the Tobacco Institute.[9] The findings of the analysis were quite troubling. Almost 60% of those surveyed believed that smoking was probably hazardous to nonsmokers. Strikingly, 40% of smokers agreed that their smoking posed a danger to bystanders. Given these data, the Roper Organization concluded that the issue was no longer "what the smoker does to himself, but what he does to others." Writing to the industry that had commissioned the study, the Roper Organization painted a stark picture. "We believe it would be difficult to overemphasize the importance of [these] finding[s], indicating as [they do] that the battle to convince the public of the dangers of passive smoking is in the process of being lost, if indeed it is not already over." The Roper Organization concluded that the trend posed a hazard to the very viability of the tobacco industry. Although there was little support, suggested the report, for a total ban on smoking in public, there was support for the segregation of smokers and nonsmokers. This trend could transform itself from a "ripple to a tide." Furthermore, if segregation did not achieve the goal of the antismoking movement, if nonsmokers saw themselves as still at unacceptable risk, "the present sentiment . . . could become support for a total ban."

The industry had no alternative. It had to confront the proponents of restrictions on public smoking head-on, by "developing and widely publicizing clear-cut, credible medical evidence that passive smoking is not harmful to the nonsmoker's health."

A CHANGING CLIMATE

That effort was to become more difficult in the early 1980s. In 1980, a scientific article in the *New England Journal of Medicine* reported that the exposure of nonsmokers to tobacco smoke reduced breathing capacity.[10] That study led L'Enfant and Liu, in the above-cited editorial, to conclude, "Now for the first time we have a quantitative measurement of a physical change—a fact that may tip the scales in favor of the nonsmoker."[8(p743)] In 1981, two studies found that nonsmoking wives exposed to their husbands' cigarette smoking were at increased risk for lung cancer. Whatever their methodological limitations, the studies from Greece[11] and Japan[12] had a profound effect in shaping public perceptions and concerns.

Two editorials in the *New York Times* captured the new mood. In response to the study reporting the effect of passive smoking on breathing capacity, the *New York Times* wrote, "The case for restricting smoking in public rooms is getting stronger."[13] Although acknowledging that the clinical significance of reduced lung function was not known, the editorial concluded that unless smokers could be segregated so that they could not "jeopardize their neighbors . . . a prohibition on smoking in indoor places would be justified."[13] In response to the studies of exposed wives, the *New York Times,* with obvious allusions to violent spousal abuse, titled its editorial "Smoking Your Wife to Death."[14] The *New York Times* claimed that the new data "adds to the growing evidence that second-hand smoke kills. The result strengthens the case for banning smoking in public places, especially where abstainers are exposed to smoke for long periods."[14]

When the National Academy of Sciences addressed the issue of ETS in its 1981 report *Indoor Pollutants,* it provided an imprimatur to the goals set a decade earlier by the nonsmokers' rights movement. "Public policy should clearly articulate that involuntary exposure to tobacco smoke has adverse health effects and ought to be minimized or avoided where possible."[15]

The apparent emerging scientific consensus provided a weapon to antismoking forces, which skillfully used it to mobilize public opinion for greater restrictions despite the fierce opposition of the tobacco industry. In 1983, a Gallup poll found that 82% of nonsmokers believed that smokers should refrain from their habit in their presence and that smoking posed a health hazard for them; 64% of smokers held the latter view as well.[16]

By 1986, 41 states and the District of Columbia had enacted statutes that imposed restrictions on smoking. Only 8% of the US population resided in states with some restrictions in 1971, whereas 80% of the population resided in states with some restrictions by the mid-1980s. Although such laws varied in their scope, the trend over the 15 years since the surgeon general had called for such enactments in 1971 was in a more restrictive direction.[6] In addition to state laws, local jurisdictions began to enact prohibitions or limitations on public smoking. By the end of 1985, 89 cities and counties had done so, approximately 75% of which were in California, a measure of the effect of the Berkeley-based Americans for Nonsmokers Rights.[17]

In the 15-year-old struggle to impose ever-stricter controls on public smoking, 1986 represented a watershed year. Both the National Academy of Sciences and the surgeon general issued critically important reports that sought to document the dangers of exposing nonsmokers to tobacco smoke and, in so doing, propelled the movement for broader and more restrictive public smoking measures. The National Academy's Committee on Passive Smoking was the more limited of the 2 reports. Nevertheless, its message was clear and direct. "Considering the evidence as a whole, exposure to ETS increases the incidence of lung cancer in nonsmokers."[18] It was unable to come to a firm conclusion on a matter that would, in the next years, become of great concern: the effect of ETS on heart disease.[18(p11)]

The report of the surgeon general, *The Health Consequences of Involuntary Smoking*,[6] was broad in scope and sharp in its warnings. Data did not permit the report to provide a quantitative estimate of the numbers of lung cancers caused by passive smoking, but there was no question that such cases occurred and that whatever the number, it was "sufficiently large to generate substantial public health concern." Surgeon General C. Everett Koop was mindful of the controversy that surrounded the issue of passive smoking—a controversy fueled by the tobacco industry, which sought to focus attention on the limitations of the data—and confronted it directly. For the purposes of the public health, the data were good enough, and the costs of inaction were too great. "Critics often express that more research is required, that certain studies are flawed, or that we should delay action until more conclusive proof is produced," Koop declared. "As both a physician and a public health official it is my judgment that the time for delay is past, measures to protect the public health are required now." Strikingly, he went on to suggest that many of the measures that had been put into place were inadequate. Merely separating smokers and nonsmokers in rooms that shared a common ventilation system reduced, but did not eliminate, exposure. In the end, Koop returned to the moral foundation of the call for protective measures. "The choice to smoke cannot interfere with the nonsmoker's right to breathe air free of tobacco smoke. . . . [t]he right of smokers to smoke ends where their behavior affects the health and well-being of others."[6]

In the years following the publication of these 2 reports, efforts to further restrict smoking intensified, as did resistance on the part of the tobacco industry. In 1987, the US Department of Health and Human Services established a smoke-free environment in all of its buildings nationwide, extending protection to more than 100 000 federal employees. In 1988, Congress imposed a smoking ban on all US domestic flights of 2 hours or less. Two years later, the ban was extended to flights of 6 hours or less, in effect banning smoking on all domestic flights. By 1988, smoking restrictions had been imposed in 125 counties and cities in California; 118 required nonsmoking sections in restaurants, and 117 limited workplace smoking.[19] In all, by 1988, 400 local ordinances restricting smoking had been enacted in the United States.[20]

BATTLES OVER EVIDENCE

Confronted with a movement that enjoyed widespread popular support, the tobacco industry sought to thwart smoking restrictions through several strategies. Most significant was the effort to undermine the very basis of such efforts by challenging the scientific evidence that ETS represented a health hazard. In 1984, the Tobacco Institute issued a broadside critique of the scientific "misinformation" strengthening the emerging public health consensus. "We don't think [the harmful effect of exposure to tobacco smoke] has been shown," an industry publication claimed.[21] Seeking to undermine the claims of those who argued that the industry always denied that smoking posed a hazard, the Tobacco Institute was willing to embrace strategically those whom it typically denounced: "Many scientists who believe smoking is harmful to smokers have publicly stated there is not sufficient evidence to conclude [that] public smoking is harmful to nonsmokers."

Central to the industry's strategy was the perpetuation of controversy to preclude closure of the scientific discussion. In 1988, the industry created the Center for Indoor Air Research to fund studies that would attempt to undercut findings that ETS threatened the health of nonsmokers.[22]

A second element of the industry's strategy was to transform the issue of restrictive smoking policies from one centered on potential hazards to one focused on the core American values of liberty and choice. Hence, the industry fostered and then underwrote smokers' rights activities and publications.[23] Characterizing regulatory efforts to restrict smoking and smokers as intrusive and unnecessary, the industry proposed as an alternative the virtues of common sense, courtesy, and mutual respect by smokers and nonsmokers.

Finally, as it discovered that it could not match grassroots efforts in cities and counties to restrict smoking, the industry supported the enactment of state statutes that preempted legislation and regulation at the local level.

Reflecting on the significance of what had been achieved and what still needed to be done, antismoking activists recognized that the shift to an environmental perspective had been extraordinarily effective in providing justification for the imposition of measures to restrict public smoking, changing the public debate about the legitimacy of governmental efforts to limit the freedom of smokers, and permitting the movement to shed the taint of an intrusive paternalism. The executive director of Americans for Nonsmokers Rights thus said in 1987, "We're just telling smokers to step outside, not how to save their lives."[17] In addressing himself to other activists, Stanton Glantz,[24] who more than any other individual had defined the ETS issue as crucial, emphasized the strategic importance of the focus on protecting innocents. "Activists should state that they are not 'antismoker' but rather environmentalists concerned with clean air for everyone. The issue should be framed in the rhetoric of the environment, toxic chemicals, and public health rather than the rhetoric of saving smokers from themselves or the cigarette companies."[24]

However, despite that strategic posture, Glantz's vision was broader, concerned as it was with lifting the burden of smoking on American society. "Although the nonsmokers' rights movement concentrates on protecting the nonsmokers rather than on urging the smoker to quit for his or her own benefit, clean indoor air legislation reduces smoking because it undercuts the social support network for smoking by implicitly defining smoking as an anti-social act."[24(p746)] These remarks were included in an editorial titled "Achieving a Smokefree Society."[24] Glantz's aspirations were echoed in the mid-1980s by the director of the Office on Smoking and Health of the federal Department of Health and Human Services. "Of all the issues, [the issue of passive smoking] will propel the United States toward a smoke-free society."[25]

In the 1990s, the pivotal moment for those seeking to rid the public space of smoke and smokers came with publication in 1992 of the Environmental Protection Agency's *Respiratory Health Effects of Passive Smoking: Lung Cancer and Other Disorders.*[25] The agency placed numbers on those affected that previously had been only vaguely apprehended, and it did so with an apparent precision that made the published statistics politically electric. Many children and infants were being placed at risk. Between 150 000 and 300 000 annual cases of lower-respiratory-tract infections such as bronchitis and pneumonia were linked to ETS exposure in children younger than 18 months. Between 200 000 and 1 000 000 asthmatic children had their conditions exacerbated by exposure to tobacco. The Environmental Protection Agency's declaration that ETS was a class A carcinogen, placing it in the same category as asbestos, benzene, and radon, was even more damaging. Approximately 3000 annual lung cancer deaths were attributed to ETS.[26]

Newspapers across the United States responded to the report with a sense of urgency. In an editorial titled "No Right to Cause Death," the *New York Times* claimed that "the evidence is now overwhelming" that ETS was dangerous.[27] In the *New York Times'* view, the "toxic fumes" and "lethal clouds" generated by smokers made them "at least a small hazard to virtually all Americans—and a fitting target for tighter restrictions." The *New York Times* drew an analogy between secondhand smoke and other hazards regulated by the Environmental Protection Agency: "No one would grant his neighbor the right to blow tiny amounts of asbestos into a room or sprinkle traces of pesticide onto food."[27]

The antiregulatory *Wall Street Journal* remained a contrarian voice, openly questioning the antismoking science even after the government reports of 1986 and 1993. In a 1994 editorial,[28] the newspaper claimed that "the anti-smoking brigade relies on proving that secondhand smoke is a dangerous threat to the health of others. 'Science' is invoked in ways likely to give science a bad name. . . . [t]he health effects of secondhand smoke are a stretch."

Armed with science, activists, linked with their public health allies and sympathetic political figures, pressed for more extensive restrictions in the early and mid-1990s. Two measures that were proposed but not implemented illustrate how far-reaching the efforts to restrict smoking had become. The Occupational Safety and Health Administration proposed a rule that would have effectively banned smoking in most workplaces in the United States, and Congress considered the Smoke-Free Environment Act, which would have barred smoking in every building "entered by 10 or more people at least one day a week." Smoking in buildings open to the public could occur only in rooms restricted for that purpose and that permitted venting to the outside. Smoking also would have been prohibited outside building entrances.[29] Endorsed by the Clinton administration, the American Medical Association, and several former surgeon generals, the legislation failed to move forward when the Republicans took control of Congress in 1994.

A review of restrictions undertaken by the surgeon general noted that by the end of 1999, 45 states and the District of Columbia had enacted some legislation to protect indoor air. Forty-three states and the District of Columbia restricted smoking at government worksites; 29 of the 43 limited smoking to designated areas, and 11 imposed total bans. Despite the failure of the Occupational Safety and Health Administration to promulgate its workplace rule, 21 states had restricted smoking at private worksites. Twenty-one states regulated restaurant smoking.[2] The number of local ordinances restricting smoking also grew dramatically from the mid-1980s, when there had been some 400 such measures, to 1998, when there were more than 800.[30] Capturing the transformation that had occurred, historian Allan Brandt could say of smokers in the United States that they "literally had no place to hide."[31]

BYSTANDERS FIRST

Public health officials for almost 4 decades had been calling attention to the enormous toll exacted by cigarette smoking, generally estimated at close to 400 000 lives a year. The consensus about the effect of ETS on lung cancer was that 3000 to 4000 deaths a year could be traced to exposure of nonsmokers to tobacco smoke. Agreement eluded efforts to determine whether passive smoking also increased the risk of heart disease. Some proposed as early as 1991 that 37 000 deaths each year from heart disease were linked to ETS.[31] Those estimates served as a rallying cry for antismoking activists, who argued that with tens of thousands of deaths each year attributable to ETS, passive smoking was the "third leading preventable cause of death in the United States, behind active smoking and alcohol."[32(p10)]

However, by the end of the 1990s, uncertainty remained about the centrally important question of the effect of ETS on coronary heart disease. When a summary of epidemiological studies published in the *New England Journal of Medicine* in 1999 concluded that "passive smoking [was] associated with a *small* increase in the risk of heart disease [italics added],"[33] the accompanying editorial, written by a biostatistician who had previously been critical of the meta-analytic method used in the review, noted, "We still do not know, with accuracy, how much or even whether exposure to environmental tobacco smoke increases the risk of coronary heart disease."[34] To such doubt, the advocates of strict control over ETS continued to respond with new evidence buttressing the politics of certainty that defined their posture.[35] Forceful editorial commentaries urged the importance of protecting "everyone . . . from even short-term exposure to the toxins in second-hand smoke."[36]

Given the ongoing debate about the relation between ETS and heart disease, and the fact that the health burden in smoking-related death and disease is so much greater on smokers themselves than on nonsmokers, why had the plight of the bystander assumed such salience in the rhetoric and political strategy of the official and grassroots antismoking movements? Why did the addictive nature of tobacco not provide the foundation for strategies that directly targeted smokers themselves in the first decades of the anti-tobacco campaign? How can one explain the fact that in the 1970s and early 1980s, the efforts to restrict public smoking outstripped the scientific evidence on the effects of ETS? What can account for the alacrity with which efforts were made to extend the scope of restrictions from settings in which the evidence was clearest, such as exposure of infants and children in home environments, to those in which the evidence was at best suggestive, such as exposure in restaurants and other public spaces?[37]

The anti-tobacco movement was, of course, spurred by the degree to which ETS unfairly injured nonsmokers and by the preventable deaths and illnesses for which it was responsible. However, more was involved. By repositioning the bystander to center stage, public health advocates were able to press for changes that, if pursued directly, would have been politically unpalatable. Just as restrictions on advertising could most easily be justified in the name of protecting children from manipulation, restricting smoking could be justified by the claims of the bystanders. It was possible to pursue the goal of a smoke-free society without adopting the paternalistic posture that would have been necessitated by expressly seeking to regulate the choices adults made on their own behalf. This approach thus represented a public health equivalent of the Catholic doctrine of double effect, which holds that an outcome that would be morally wrong if caused intentionally would be permissible if unintended, even if foreseen.

Finally, the changing social class composition of smoking has facilitated the campaign against ETS. As tobacco consumption has become concentrated among those of lower socioeconomic status, it has become easier to stigmatize as undesirable behavior. In this way, efforts by public health activists to reduce smoking mirror campaigns by Progressive Era reformers to impose hygienic behavior on the "lower orders" in the name of public health. Unlike those earlier efforts, however, contemporary antismoking strategies have not been overtly paternalistic.

Some antismoking activists have exulted in the ever-more-stringent limitations on public tobacco consumption, lobbying to extend such restrictions because of their broad effects on the social acceptability of smoking. Others have begun to worry that their movement may have begun to take on the taint of moralism and authoritarianism. The debate over how far to push flared in the journal *Tobacco Control* in 2000, centering on the question of the legitimacy of imposing bans on outdoor smoking, efforts that could be justified only in terms of annoyance abatement, not of disease prevention. Two officials at the National Cancer Institute's tobacco program noted approvingly that some communities had chosen to restrict outdoor smoking for reasons other than health, including the reduction of fire risks, litter control, and the elimination of nuisances.[38] Antismoking activist James Repace, who was among the first to quantify the health burdens of ETS, asserted, "Even if outdoor environmental tobacco smoke were no more hazardous than dog excrement stuck to the bottom of a shoe, in many places laws require dog owners to avoid fouling public areas. Is this too much to ask of smokers?"[39] To all of this, *Tobacco Control's* editor Simon Chapman expressed his dismay: "We need to ask whether efforts to prevent people smoking outdoors risk besmirching tobacco control advocates as the embodiment of intolerant, paternalistic busybodies, who not content at protecting their own health want to force smokers not to smoke, even in circumstances where the effects of their smoking on others are immeasurably small."[40]

But it was precisely because restrictions on public smoking had important effects on smoking itself that many public health activists gave such emphasis to broadening the range of prohibitions. It would have been impossible to ignore the fact that measures initially pursued in the name of protecting nonsmokers had secondary benefits—restricting smoking itself—that far outweighed the contribution associated with limiting exposure to ETS.[41]

Only the risk of overreaching in a way that would have made clear the paternalistic impulse and the prospect of political resistance served as a restraint. In a nation where efforts to limit liberty in the name of public health can so readily provoke opposition, the shape of the anti-tobacco strategy was all too predictable.

The strictures imposed by the cultural and ideological antipathy to paternalism may serve as an impediment to the further development of policies designed to alter the normative and public context of smoking in America. To the extent that such a transformation is critical to reductions in smoking and to the death and disease to which smoking is linked, it may well be necessary to directly address public smoking as a matter of protecting not only nonsmokers, but smokers themselves. ■

About the Authors

The authors are with the Program in the History and Ethics of Public Health and Medicine, Division of Sociomed-

ical Sciences, Mailman School of Public Health, Columbia University, New York, NY.

Requests for reprints should be sent to Ronald Bayer, PhD, Columbia University, 600 W 168th St, New York, NY 10032 (e-mail: rb8@columbia.edu).

This article was accepted November 16, 2001.

Contributors

Both authors contributed to the conceptualization of, research for, and writing of this article.

Acknowledgments

Work on this article was supported by the Robert Wood Johnson Foundation through the grant Tobacco Control and the Liberal State: The Legal, Ethical, and Policy Debates.

References

1. Steinfeld JL. Women and children last? Attitudes toward cigarette smoking and nonsmokers' rights, 1971. *N Y State J Med.* 1983;83:1257–1258.

2. *Surgeon General's Report on Smoking and Health 2000.* Washington, DC: US Dept of Health and Human Services; 2000.

3. Nathanson C. Social movement as catalysts for policy change: the case of smoking and guns. *J Health Polit Policy Law.* 1999;24:420–488.

4. Markle G, Troyer R. Smoke gets in your eyes: cigarette smoking as deviant behavior. *Soc Problems.* 1979;26:611–625.

5. Schmidt RW. The U.S. experience in nonsmokers' rights. *Am Lung Assoc Bull.* 1975:11–15.

6. *The Health Consequences of Involuntary Smoking.* Washington, DC: US Dept of Health and Human Services; 1986.

7. Huber GL. Smoking and nonsmokers—what is the issue? *N Engl J Med.* 1975;292:858–859.

8. L'Enfant C, Liu BM. (Passive) smokers versus (voluntary) smokers. *N Engl J Med.* 1980;302:742–743.

9. *A Study of Public Attitudes Toward Cigarette Smoking and the Tobacco Industry in 1978.* Vol 1. The Roper Organization Inc; 1978.

10. White J, Froeb H. Small-airways dysfunction in nonsmokers chronically exposed to tobacco smoke. *N Engl J Med.* 1980;302:720–723.

11. Trichopoulos D, Kalandidi A, Sparros L, MacMahon B. Lung cancer and passive smoking. *Int J Cancer.* 1981;27:1–4.

12. Hirayama T. Non-smoking wives of heavy smokers have a higher risk of lung cancer: a study from Japan. *BMJ.* 1981;282:183–185.

13. Thy neighbor's lungs. *New York Times.* April 2, 1980:A26.

14. Smoking your wife to death. *New York Times.* January 21, 1981:22.

15. Committee on Indoor Pollutants. *Indoor Pollutants.* Washington, DC: National Academy Press; 1981.

16. Summary of results of the April 1983 survey by the Gallup Organization Survey of Attitudes Toward Smoking [news release]. New York, NY: American Lung Association; September 20, 1983.

17. Hamilton J, Smith ET, Angiolillo P, Rhein R. 'No smoking' sweeps America. *Business Week.* July 27, 1987.

18. National Academy of Sciences. *Environmental Tobacco Smoke: Measuring Exposures and Assessing Health Effects.* Washington, DC: National Academy Press; 1986.

19. Rigotti NA. Trends in the the adoption of smoking restrictions in public places and worksites. *NY State J Med.* 1989;89:19–26.

20. Brownson R, Eriksen MP, Davis RM, Warner KE. Environmental tobacco smoke: health effects and policies to reduce exposure. *Annu Rev Public Health.* 1997;18:163–185.

21. *Cigarette Smoke and the Nonsmoker.* The Tobacco Institute; 1984.

22. Barnes DE, Bero LA. Industry-funded research and conflict of interest: an analysis of research sponsored by the tobacco industry through the center for indoor air research. *J Health Polit Policy Law.* 1996;21:515–542.

23. Cardador MT, Hazan AR, Glantz SA. Tobacco industry smokers' rights publications: a content analysis. *Am J Public Health.* 1995;85:1212–1217.

24. Glantz SA. Achieving a smokefree society. *Circulation.* 1987;76:746–752.

25. Iglehart JK. The campaign against smoking gains momentum. *N Engl J Med.* 1986;314:1059–1064.

26. Environmental Protection Agency. *Respiratory Health Effects of Passive Smoking: Lung Cancer and Other Disorders.* Washington, DC: US Dept of Health and Human Services; 1992.

27. No right to cause death. *New York Times.* January 10, 1993:22.

28. No smoking. *Wall Street Journal.* June 7, 1994:A14.

29. Hilts PJ. Smoking ban wins Clinton's support. *New York Times.* February 8, 1994:16.

30. *Annual Report 1999: Appendix A.* New York, NY: American Lung Association; 2000.

31. Brandt A. Blow some my way: passive smoking, risk and American culture. In: Lock S, Reynolds L, Tansey M, eds. *Ashes to Ashes: The History of Smoking and Health.* Atlanta, Ga: Rodopi; 1998:164–187.

32. Glantz SA, Parmley WW. Passive smoking and heart disease: epidemiology, physiology and biochemistry. *Circulation.* 1991;83:1–12.

33. He J, Vupputuri S, Allen K, Prerost MR, Hughes J, Whelton PK. Passive smoking and the risk of coronary heart disease—a meta-analysis of epidemiologic studies. *N Engl J Med.* 1999;340:920–926.

34. Bailar J. Passive smoking, coronary heart disease, and meta-analysis. *N Engl J Med.* 1999;340:958–959.

35. Otsuka R, Watanabe H, Hirata K, et al. Acute effects of passive smoking on the coronary circulation in healthy young adults. *JAMA.* 2001;286:436–441.

36. Glantz SA, Parmley WW. Even a little secondhand smoke is dangerous. *JAMA.* 2001;286:462–463.

37. Rabin R. Review essay: some thoughts on smoking regulation. *Stanford Law Review.* 1991;43:475–496.

38. Bloch M, Shopland DR. Outdoor smoking bans: more than meets the eye. *Tob Control.* 2000;9:99.

39. Repace J. Banning outdoor smoking is scientifically justifiable. *Tob Control.* 2000;9:98.

40. Chapman S. Banning smoking outdoors is seldom ethically justifiable. *Tob Control.* 2000;9:95–97.

41. Task Force on Community Preventive Services. Recommendations regarding interventions to reduce tobacco use and exposure to environmental tobacco smoke. *Am J Prev Med.* 2001;20:10–15.

| SECTION IV |

Tobacco & Maternal and Child Health

Tobacco Marketing and Adolescent Smoking: More Support for a Causal Inference

Lois Biener, PhD, and Michael Siegel, MD, MPH

ABSTRACT

Objectives. This prospective study examined the effect of tobacco marketing on progression to established smoking.

Methods. Massachusetts adolescents (n = 529) who at baseline had smoked no more than 1 cigarette were reinterviewed by telephone in 1997. Analyses examined the effect of receptivity to tobacco marketing at baseline on progression to established smoking, controlling for significant covariates.

Results. Adolescents who, at baseline, owned a tobacco promotional item and named a brand whose advertisements attracted their attention were more than twice as likely to become established smokers (odds ratio = 2.70) than adolescents who did neither.

Conclusions. Participation in tobacco marketing often precedes, and is likely to facilitate, progression to established smoking. Hence, restrictions on tobacco marketing and promotion could reduce addiction to tobacco. (*Am J Public Health.* 2000;90:407–411)

Despite tobacco industry claims to the contrary, researchers have consistently implicated cigarette marketing activities as an important catalyst in the smoking initiation process.[1] Much of the evidence for a link between advertising and youth smoking is based on cross-sectional or correlational studies.[2–39] For example, some studies have found a correlation between trends in the intensity of cigarette marketing and trends in the rates of adolescent smoking initiation.[2,3] Others have shown increases in smoking rates among population subgroups specifically targeted by marketing campaigns.[4,5] Still others have shown correlations between the intensity of brand-specific cigarette advertising and brand awareness, preference,[6–14] or brand market shares[12,15,16] among youths. Many cross-sectional studies have reported associations between exposure to cigarette advertising or participation in promotional activities and attitudes toward smoking,[17] susceptibility to smoking,[18–23] and smoking behavior[6,9,11,17,19,21,22,24–39] among youths. Because of the cross-sectional nature of these studies, it is not possible to determine whether the exposure to tobacco marketing preceded and contributed to smoking initiation or whether smoking initiation preceded increasing receptivity to tobacco advertising and promotions.

Very few longitudinal studies that prospectively link exposure to tobacco advertising to smoking initiation have been done. Two Australian studies reported higher rates of smoking initiation among youth who 1 or 2 years earlier had indicated approval of cigarette advertising[40] or reported that cigarette advertisements made smoking appear attractive to them.[41] A Scottish study found that youths with higher awareness of, and liking for, cigarette advertisements at baseline were more likely to develop positive intentions to smoke after a 1-year follow-up period, but a significant effect on smoking behavior was not observed.[42] Only 1 relevant longitudinal study has been published in the United States. Pierce et al.[43] found that receptivity to cigarette promotional activities among California adolescents was associated 3 years later with progression along a 4-point smoking initiation continuum. One third (33%) of those who progressed increased their intentions to smoke, 59% actually experimented with cigarettes, and 7% became established smokers.

Although changes in intentions to smoke have been associated repeatedly with subsequent smoking initiation,[44–47] stronger evidence of the power of advertising requires the demonstration of a prospective link with smoking behavior. The present study investigated this link.

Methods

Sample

Data were from the 1993 Massachusetts Tobacco Survey of youths, which was based on a probability sample of Massachusetts housing units drawn by means of random-digit dialing. After conducting a household screening interview with an adult resident, interviewers selected a representative sample of youths. Interviews were completed with 75% of the eligible youths, yielding a final baseline sample of 1606 adolescents, 1069 of whom were between 12 and 15 years of age.[48]

Between November 1997 and February 1998, we attempted to recontact the 1069 youths. We were unable to trace 328 (30.7%) but completed interviews with 618 (83.4%) of the remaining 741 youths for an overall follow-up response rate of 57.8%. These 618 adolescents constituted our final youth cohort. For this research, a subset of the sample was used: those 529 respondents who indicated at baseline that they had smoked no more than 1 cigarette in their lifetime.

Measures

Outcome variable. The outcome measure was a dichotomous indicator of whether the respondent had become an established smoker by smoking 100 or more cigarettes

Lois Biener is with the Center for Survey Research, University of Massachusetts, Boston. Michael Siegel is with the Social and Behavioral Sciences Department, Boston University School of Public Health, Boston, Mass.

Requests for reprints should be sent to Lois Biener, PhD, Center for Survey Research, University of Massachusetts at Boston, 100 Morrissey Blvd, Boston, MA 02125 (e-mail: lois.biener@umb.edu).

This brief was accepted October 8, 1999.

by follow-up. This criterion is commonly used to define "ever smokers" among adults.

Predictors: receptivity to tobacco marketing. A 3-level indicator of receptivity to tobacco marketing was constructed from the following 2 survey questions: (1) "Some tobacco companies make clothing, hats, bags, or other things with the brand on it. Do you have a piece of clothing or other thing that has a tobacco brand name or logo on it?" and (2) "Of all the cigarette advertisements you have seen, which brand's ads do you think attract your attention the most?" The highest level of receptivity was assigned to those who reported owning a promotional item and who named a cigarette brand in response to the second question. Those who either owned an item or named a brand were scored as being moderately receptive to marketing. Those who neither owned an item nor named a brand were scored at the lowest level of receptivity.

Potential confounding variables. To rule out the possibility that some third factor could be responsible for causing both receptivity to tobacco marketing and subsequent progression to established smoking, we included, at baseline, measures of variables that have been associated with smoking initiation to determine whether they also were associated with receptivity to tobacco marketing. These variables included demographic characteristics (age, sex, race/ethnicity, socioeconomic status), social influences (smoking among family members and friends), psychological problems (rebelliousness and depression), and baseline smoking status.[1,46,47,49,50] If these variables also were associated with receptivity to advertising, failing to control for them in the analysis would leave open the possibility that the link between baseline receptivity to advertising and subsequent progression to established smoking was due to the fact that respondents who have friends or parents who smoke may be more likely to receive promotional items as gifts than those who do not. Rebelliousness or depression may increase the likelihood of both becoming a smoker and being attracted to the images and promotional items associated with particular cigarette brands. Likewise, nonsmoking youths who were ambivalent about smoking in the future, or those who had engaged in early experimentation, might be more receptive to tobacco marketing than those who, at baseline, had a firm commitment not to become a smoker.

To assess these variables, interviewers asked respondents about their age, sex, and race/ethnicity, as well as about the number of their close friends who smoked. The interview with the adult household informant provided information on the number of adult family members who smoked, the educational level of the adult informant, and the total annual household income. Rebelliousness was measured with 6 items that represent several domains related to problem behavior in adolescence: attraction to risk and danger (e.g., "I get a kick out of doing things that are a little risky or dangerous"[51]), poor relationships with family (e.g., "I have a lot of arguments with my family"[52]), and solidarity with deviant peers (e.g., "I don't mind lying to keep my friends out of trouble with the authorities"). These items have good face validity and moderate internal consistency (Cronbach $\alpha = .60$). Depression was measured with 6 items adapted from the Center for Epidemiologic Studies Depression Scale,[53] which ask how often in the past year the respondents felt hopeless, felt depressed, had trouble sleeping, and so on (Cronbach $\alpha = .71$).

Although the cohort consisted of youths who had smoked no more than 1 cigarette in their lifetime, they were differentiated into 3 smoking risk groups based on whether they had ever had a puff of a cigarette and on their responses to 3 items measuring "susceptibility to smoking," a measure previously shown to be a valid predictor of smoking initiation.[44-47] Respondents in the lowest risk group (confirmed nonsmokers) reported never having had even a puff of a cigarette and showed a firm commitment not to smoke in the future by answering "no" to the question "Do you think that you will try a cigarette soon?" and "definitely not" to the questions "If one of your best friends were to offer you a cigarette, would you smoke it?" and "Do you think you will smoke a cigarette during the next year?" Respondents in the moderate risk group (ambivalent nonsmokers) reported never having had a puff of a cigarette but answered "yes" to the question about trying a cigarette soon or gave less definitively negative responses to the other 2 questions. Respondents who reported that they had had a puff or a whole cigarette were classified in the highest risk group (early experimenters).

Data Analysis

To select variables to be included as covariates in the analysis, we examined the bivariate relationships between the potential confounding variables listed above and the main predictor and outcome variables. Any variable significantly associated with both receptivity to tobacco marketing and becoming an established smoker was included as a covariate. We performed a logistic regression analysis with progression to established smoking as the dependent variable, controlling for the selected covariates. We reported adjusted odds ratios (ORs) that reflect the ratio of the odds of progression to established smoking while controlling for the simultaneous effects of other variables. All analyses were conducted with the SPSS statistical package.[54]

The baseline survey data set included weights that reflected each respondent's probability of selection. Because the primary objective of this study was to draw conclusions about the effect of tobacco marketing on progression to established smoking among cohort members, rather than to generalize to the state as a whole, we conducted unweighted analyses.

Results

Attrition

To evaluate potential bias in the cohort, we compared the characteristics of baseline nonsmokers who were retained in the sample with those of subjects who were lost to follow-up. The youths who were lost to follow-up were significantly older and more likely to have reported owning a promotional item. They tended to be more rebellious and to have a close friend who smoked, but neither of these differences reached the .05 level of significance. The pattern of differences suggests that youths at higher risk for progression to established smoking were somewhat underrepresented in the cohort.

Characteristics of the Cohort

Table 1 presents the characteristics of the cohort overall and according to their receptivity to tobacco marketing and progression to established smoking. Receptivity was significantly associated with living in a household in which at least 1 adult smoked, having at least 1 close friend who smoked, being an early experimenter, and scoring above the median in rebelliousness.

Twenty-one percent (n = 110) of the 529 respondents became established smokers during the 4-year follow-up period. Progression to established smoking was significantly more likely among White than minority youths, among youths who lived with at least 1 adult smoker, among youths who had at least 1 close friend who smoked, among youths who were early experimenters, and among youths who scored high in rebelliousness.

Among those with high receptivity to tobacco marketing (owned a promotional item and named a cigarette brand as attracting their attention), 46% progressed from no smoking or early experimentation to established smoking. The rates for adolescents with moderate and low receptivity were 18% and 14%, respectively ($\chi^2_2 = 28.9$, $P < .001$).

TABLE 1—Baseline Distribution of Demographic Characteristics and Psychosocial Variables Among Massachusetts Youth Cohort,[a] by Receptivity to Tobacco Marketing in 1993 and Progression to Established Smoking by 1997

	Receptivity to Tobacco Marketing in 1993				Became Established Smoker by 1997			
	Low (n = 121)	Moderate (n = 342)	High (n = 66)	P^b	Yes (n = 110)	No (n = 419)	P^b	Total (n = 529)
Age group in 1993, y								
12–13	56.7	53.7	57.6	.759	49.1	56.4	.173	54.8
14–15	43.3	46.3	42.4		50.9	43.6		45.2
Sex								
Male	43.0	50.9	54.5	.224	45.5	50.6	.337	49.5
Female	57.0	49.1	45.5		54.5	49.4		50.5
Race/Ethnicity								
White, non-Hispanic	81.2	79.5	83.1	.777	88.0	78.3	.025	80.3
Other	18.8	20.5	16.9		12.0	21.7		19.7
Education of adult informant								
High school or less	40.0	43.1	38.5	.712	48.1	40.1	.131	41.8
More than high school	60.0	56.9	61.5		51.9	59.9		58.2
Household income, $								
≤50 000	42.3	42.2	35.3		40.7	41.5		41.3
>50 000	57.7	57.8	64.7	.644	59.3	58.5	.892	58.7
At least 1 adult smoker in household								
Yes	29.8	36.8	51.5	.013	50.0	33.7	.002	37.1
No	70.2	63.2	48.5		50.0	66.3		62.9
At least 1 close friend who smokes								
Yes	51.2	60.5	78.8	.001	79.1	55.8	.000	60.7
No	48.8	39.5	21.2		20.9	44.2		39.3
Baseline smoking status								
Confirmed nonsmoker	64.5	54.0	42.4	.000	31.2	61.1	.000	54.9
Ambivalent nonsmoker	24.0	21.1	15.2		18.3	21.7		21.0
Early experimenter	11.6	24.9	42.4		50.5	17.2		24.1
Rebelliousness								
Low	66.7	47.4	27.7	.000	32.1	53.8	.000	49.3
High	33.3	52.6	72.3		67.9	46.2		50.7
Depression								
Low	47.0	41.2	36.9	.285	36.1	43.6	.378	42.0
Medium	32.5	31.2	27.7		34.3	30.2		31.0
High	20.5	27.6	35.4		29.6	26.3		27.0

[a]Cohort includes adolescents who at baseline had smoked no more than 1 cigarette in their lifetime.
[b]Probability listed is for the χ^2 statistic.

Table 2 presents the results of a multiple logistic regression that examined the effect of receptivity while controlling for family and peer smoking, baseline smoking status, and rebelliousness—the variables significantly related to both receptivity to tobacco marketing and progression to established smoking. This analysis found that adolescents who were highly receptive to marketing in 1993 were more than twice as likely to become an established smoker by 1997 compared with those who had low receptivity (OR = 2.70, 95% confidence interval [CI] = 1.24, 5.85). Being an early experimenter and having a close friend who smoked also were significant independent predictors of progression to established smoking.

To examine the effect of tobacco marketing on youths who had not engaged in any experimentation with tobacco, we repeated the analyses with only the 402 respondents who, at baseline, had never taken a puff of a cigarette. Among these neversmokers, the rate of progression to established smoking was 29% for those who had high receptivity to tobacco marketing at baseline. The rates of smoking initiation among those who had moderate and low receptivity were 12% and 11%, respectively ($\chi^2_2 = 8.38$, $P < .02$).

We used the same multiple logistic regression model described above but substituted a 2-level indicator of susceptibility to smoking for the 3-level baseline smoking status; the magnitude of the effect of receptivity to tobacco marketing was essentially unchanged. The adjusted odds ratio for youths with high receptivity in relation to those with low receptivity was 2.32. However, the 95% confidence interval for the odds ratio included 1, most likely a result of lower statistical power because of the reduced sample size.

Discussion

To the best of our knowledge, this is only the second longitudinal study in the United States to examine the effect of tobacco advertising and promotional activities on smoking among a cohort of adolescents and the only longitudinal study to quantify the effect on progression from nonsmoking or early experimentation to established smoking. We found that attending to cigarette advertising and becoming involved in tobacco product promotions by obtaining an item of clothing, a sports bag, or some other piece of gear with a cigarette brand logo on it precede, and reliably predict, progression to established smoking, even when other factors that influence both smoking initiation and receptivity to marketing are controlled for. Thus, even though the group of youths who were highly receptive to tobacco marketing at baseline were more likely to be rebellious, to have experimented with ciga-

TABLE 2—Progression to Established Smoking Over 4 Years Among Cohorts[a] of Massachusetts Adolescents, by Ownership of a Tobacco Promotional Item, With Control for Significant Demographic and Psychosocial Factors

	Adjusted[b] Odds Ratio	95% Confidence Interval
Receptivity to tobacco marketing		
High	2.70	1.24, 5.85
Moderate	0.98	0.53, 1.83
Low	1.00	. . .
At least 1 adult smoker in household		
Yes	1.52	0.95, 2.42
No	1.00	. . .
At least 1 close friend who smokes		
Yes	1.80	1.03, 3.14
No	1.00	. . .
Baseline smoking status		
Early experimenter	3.82	2.19, 6.69
Ambivalent nonsmoker	1.48	0.79, 2.80
Confirmed nonsmoker	1.00	. . .
Rebelliousness		
High	1.29	0.77, 2.16
Low	1.00	. . .

[a]Cohort includes adolescents who at baseline had smoked no more than 1 cigarette in their lifetime.
[b]Adjusted odds ratios were derived from analyses in which all other listed variables were included in the model.

rettes, and to have been exposed to parental or peer smoking, these differences do not fully account for the observed differences in progression to established smoking.

The observed finding also cannot be explained by differential loss to follow-up. Among respondents who were lost to follow-up, those who owned a promotional item also scored higher on the covariates related to subsequent smoking. Had we been successful in interviewing the entire sample, we would most likely have found an even greater disparity in the proportion of established smokers between those with high and those with low receptivity, even if receptivity had no independent effect. Hence, if anything, our estimate of the effect of tobacco marketing activities is conservative.

This study found that the associations detected in prior studies were not solely a result of increased participation in tobacco promotions among youths who have already moved along the smoking initiation continuum. Also, our findings support those of Pierce et al.,[47] who found that among nonsmoking California adolescents who were not susceptible to smoking at baseline, the risk of progression to established smoking over a 3-year follow-up period was about 3 times higher for those who owned or were willing to use a tobacco promotional item at baseline. The fact that this outcome has been observed in the first 2 states to conduct population-based, longitudinal studies that examined factors associated with smoking initiation broadens the generalizability of the findings in both studies.

It is important to point out that we do not attribute the effect of tobacco marketing observed in this study to merely seeing cigarette advertisements and coming into possession of a tobacco promotional item. A better explanation of the process is that promotional items and the images they have come to represent through advertising campaigns are particularly attractive to adolescents who, for some reason, are looking for an identity that the images are carefully designed to offer. These are the youths who would retain the items, whereas those whose identity needs are met in other ways would likely lose, discard, or forget about the items. Having the items offers to the vulnerable group the opportunity to "try on the image of a smoker."[23(p124)] Doing so is likely part of a longer-term process of accepting the image and eventually the smoking behavior associated with it.

The Multistate Master Settlement Agreement with the major tobacco companies includes some restrictions on billboard and transit advertisements and some forms of promotional items.[55] However, tobacco advertising images will still be widely displayed inside and outside of stores, in magazines, in entertainment sections of newspapers, and at local sponsored events. Because these images hold the power to influence adolescent behavior, a more comprehensive restriction on image advertising is warranted. □

Contributors

L. Biener designed the baseline survey, oversaw the data collection, and analyzed the data. L. Biener and M. Siegel codesigned the follow-up survey and cowrote the paper.

Acknowledgments

This work was supported by grants from the Robert Wood Johnson Foundation Substance Abuse Policy Research Program (031587) and the Massachusetts Department of Public Health, Massachusetts Tobacco Control Program (Health Protection Fund).

The authors wish to thank Kenneth Warner, PhD, and Steven Sussman, PhD, for helpful comments on an earlier version of the paper.

References

1. *Preventing Tobacco Use Among Young People: A Report of the Surgeon General.* Atlanta, Ga: Centers for Disease Control and Prevention, National Center for Chronic Disease Prevention and Health Promotion, Office on Smoking and Health; 1994.
2. Cummings KM, Shah D, Shopland DR. Trends in smoking initiation among adolescents and young adults—United States, 1980–1989. *MMWR Morb Mortal Wkly Rep.* 1995;44:521–525.
3. Gilpin EA, Pierce JP. Trends in adolescent smoking initiation in the United States: is tobacco marketing an influence? *Tob Control.* 1997;6:122–127.
4. Pierce JP, Lee L, Gilpin EA. Smoking initiation by adolescent girls, 1944 through 1988: an association with targeted advertising. *JAMA.* 1994;271:608–611.
5. Pierce JP, Gilpin EA. A historical analysis of tobacco marketing and the uptake of smoking by youth in the United States: 1890–1977. *Health Psychol.* 1995;14:500–508.
6. Chapman S, Fitzgerald B. Brand preference and advertising recall in adolescent smokers: some implications for health promotion. *Am J Public Health.* 1982;72:491–494.
7. McNeill AD, Jarvis MJ, West RJ. Brand preferences among children who smoke. *Lancet.* 1985;2:271–272.
8. Aitken PP, Leathar DS, Scott AL, Squair SI. Cigarette brand preferences of teenagers and adults. *Health Promot.* 1987;2:219–226.
9. Goldstein AO, Fischer PM, Richards JW, Creten D. Relationship between high school student smoking and recognition of cigarette advertisements. *J Pediatr.* 1987;110:488–491.
10. Cummings KM, Hyland A, Pechacek TF, Orlandi M, Lynn WR. Comparison of recent trends in adolescent and adult cigarette smoking behaviour and brand preferences. *Tob Control,* 1997;6(suppl 2):S31–S37.
11. Aitken PP, Eadie DR. Reinforcing effects of cigarette advertising on under-age smoking. *Br J Addict.* 1990;85:399–412.
12. Pierce JP, Gilpin E, Burns DM, et al. Does tobacco advertising target young people to start smoking? Evidence from California. *JAMA.* 1991;266:3154–3158.

13. DiFranza JR, Richards JW, Paulman PM, et al. RJR Nabisco's cartoon camel promotes Camel cigarettes to children. *JAMA*. 1991;266: 3149–3153.
14. Hastings GB, Ryan H, Teer P, MacKintosh AM. Cigarette advertising and children's smoking: why Reg was withdrawn. *BMJ*. 1994;309: 933–937.
15. Centers for Disease Control and Prevention. Changes in the cigarette brand preferences of adolescent smokers—United States, 1989–1993. *MMWR Morb Mortal Wkly Rep*. 1994;43: 577–581.
16. Pollay RW, Siddarth S, Siegel M, et al. The last straw? Cigarette advertising and realized market shares among youths and adults, 1979–1993. *J Marketing*. 1996;60:1–16.
17. Charlton A. Children's advertisement-awareness related to their views on smoking. *Health Educ J*. 1986;45:75–78.
18. Botvin EM, Botvin GJ, Michela JL, Maker E, Filazzola AD. Adolescent smoking behaviour and the recognition of cigarette advertisements. *J Appl Soc Psychol*. 1991;21:919–932.
19. Unger JB, Johnson CA, Rohrbach LA. Recognition and liking of tobacco and alcohol advertisements among adolescents: relationships with susceptibility to substance use. *Prev Med*. 1995;24:461–466.
20. Evans N, Farkas A, Gilpin E, Berry C, Pierce JP. Influence of tobacco marketing and exposure to smokers on adolescent susceptibility to smoking. *J Natl Cancer Inst*. 1995;87:1538–1545.
21. Altman DG, Levine DW, Coeytaux R, Slade J, Jaffe R. Tobacco promotion and susceptibility to tobacco use among adolescents aged 12 through 17 years in a nationally representative sample. *Am J Public Health*. 1996;86:1590–1593.
22. Gilpin EA, Pierce JP, Rosbrook B. Are adolescents receptive to current sales promotion practices of the tobacco industry? *Prev Med*. 1997; 26:14–21.
23. Feighery E, Borzekowski DLG, Schooler C, Flora J. Seeing, wanting, owning: the relationship between receptivity to tobacco marketing and smoking susceptibility in young people. *Tob Control*. 1998;7:123–128.
24. O'Connell DL, Alexander HM, Dobson AJ, et al. Cigarette smoking and drug use in schoolchildren, II: factors associated with smoking. *Int J Epidemiol*. 1981;10:223–231.
25. Aitken PP, Leathar DS, Squair SI. Children's opinions on whether or not cigarette advertisements should be banned. *Health Educ J*. 1986; 45:204–207.
26. Aitken PP, Leathar DS, Squair SI. Children's awareness of cigarette brand sponsorship of sports and games in the UK. *Health Educ Res*. 1986;1:203–211.
27. Potts H, Gillies P, Herbert M. Adolescent smoking and opinion of cigarette advertisements. *Health Educ Res*. 1986;1:195–201.
28. Aitken PP, Leathar DS, O'Hagan FJ, Squair SI. Children's awareness of cigarette advertisements and brand imagery. *Br J Addict*. 1987;82: 615–622.
29. Klitzner M, Gruenewald PJ, Bamberger E. Cigarette advertising and adolescent experimentation with smoking. *Br J Addict*. 1991;86: 287–298.
30. Botvin GJ, Goldberg CJ, Botvin EM, Dusenbury L. Smoking behavior of adolescents exposed to cigarette advertising. *Public Health Rep*. 1993;108:217–224.
31. Gallup International Institute. *Teen-Age Attitudes and Behavior Concerning Tobacco*. Princeton, NJ: The George H. Gallup International Institute; 1992.
32. Roswell Park Cancer Institute. *Survey of Alcohol, Tobacco and Drug Use Among Ninth Grade Students in Erie County, 1992*. Buffalo, NY: Roswell Park Cancer Institute; 1993.
33. Slade J. Teenagers participate in tobacco promotions. Paper presented at: 9th World Conference on Tobacco and Health; October 10–14, 1994; Paris, France.
34. Biener L, Fowler FJ, Roman AM. *Results of the 1993 Massachusetts Tobacco Survey: Tobacco Use and Attitudes at the Start of the Massachusetts Tobacco Control Program*. Boston, Mass: Center for Survey Research, University of Massachusetts, Boston, and Massachusetts Department of Public Health; 1994.
35. Coeytaux RR, Altman DG, Slade J. Tobacco promotions in the hands of youth. *Tob Control*. 1995;4:253–257.
36. Schooler C, Feighery E, Flora JA. Seventh graders' self-reported exposure to cigarette marketing and its relationship to their smoking behavior. *Am J Public Health*. 1996;86:1216–1221.
37. Sargent JD, Dalton MA, Beach M, Bernhardt A, Pullin D, Stevens M. Cigarette promotional items in public schools. *Arch Pediatr Adolesc Med*. 1997;151:1189–1196.
38. Richards JW, DiFranza JR, Fletcher C, Fischer PM. RJ Reynolds' "Camel cash": another way to reach kids. *Tob Control*. 1995;4:258–260.
39. Lam TH, Chung SF, Betson CL, Wong CM, Hedley AJ. Tobacco advertisements: one of the strongest risk factors for smoking in Hong Kong students. *Am J Prev Med*. 1998;14: 217–223.
40. Alexander HM, Callcott R, Dobson AJ, et al. Cigarette smoking and drug use in schoolchildren, IV: factors associated with changes in smoking behaviour. *Int J Epidemiol*. 1983; 12:59–66.
41. Armstrong BK, deKlerk NH, Shean RE, Dunn DA, Dolin PJ. Influence of education and advertising on the uptake of smoking by children. *Med J Aust*. 1990;152:117–124.
42. Aitken PP, Eadie DR, Hastings GB, Haywood AJ. Predisposing effects of cigarette advertising on children's intentions to smoke when older. *Br J Addict*. 1991;86:383–390.
43. Pierce JP, Choi WS, Gilpin EA, Farkas AJ, Berry CC. Tobacco industry promotion of cigarettes and adolescent smoking. *JAMA*. 1998; 279:511–515.
44. Jackson C. Cognitive susceptibility to smoking and initiation of smoking during childhood: a longitudinal study. *Prev Med*. 1998;27:129–134.
45. Pierce JP, Farkas AJ, Evans N, Gilpin E. An improved surveillance measure for adolescent smoking? *Tob Control*. 1995;4(suppl 1):S47–S56.
46. Choi WS, Pierce JP, Gilpin EA, Farkas AJ, Berry CC. Which adolescent experimenters progress to established smoking in the United States. *Am J Prev Med*. 1997;13:385–391.
47. Pierce JP, Choi WS, Gilpin EA, Farkas AJ, Merritt RK. Validation of susceptibility as a predictor of which adolescents take up smoking in the United States. *Health Psychol*. 1996;15:355–361.
48. Biener L, Fowler FJ Jr, Roman AM. *Technical Report: 1993 Massachusetts Tobacco Survey*. Boston, Mass: Center for Survey Research, University of Massachusetts; 1994.
49. Tyas SL, Pederson LL. Psychosocial factors related to adolescent smoking: a critical review of the literature. *Tob Control*. 1998;7:409–420.
50. Santi SM, Cargo M, Brown KS, Best JA, Cameron R. Dispositional risk factors for smoking-stage transitions; a social influences program as an effect modifier. *Addict Behav*. 1994;19: 269–285.
51. Sussman S, Dent CW, Galaif ER. The correlates of substance abuse and dependence among adolescents at high risk for drug abuse. *J Subst Abuse*. 1997;9:241–255.
52. Richardson JL, Dwyer K, McGuigan K, et al. Substance use among eighth-grade students who take care of themselves after school. *Pediatrics*. 1989;84:556–566.
53. Radloff LS. The CES-D scale: a self-report depression scale for research in the general population. *Appl Psychol Meas*. 1997;1:385–401.
54. *SPSS* [computer program]. Version 8.0 for Windows. Chicago, Ill: SPSS Inc; 1997.
55. Kelder G, Davidson P. The Multistate Master Settlement Agreement and the future of state and local tobacco control: an analysis of selected topics and provisions of the Multistate Master Settlement Agreement of November 23, 1998. The Tobacco Control Resource Center, Inc, at Northeastern University School of Law; 1999. Available at: http://www.tobacco.neu.edu/msa/index.html.

Variation in Youthful Risks of Progression From Alcohol and Tobacco to Marijuana and to Hard Drugs Across Generations

Andrew Golub, PhD, and Bruce D. Johnson, PhD

ABSTRACT

Objectives. Much research has documented that youthful substance use typically follows a sequence starting with use of alcohol or tobacco or both and potentially proceeding to marijuana and then hard drug use. This study explicitly examined the probabilities of progression through each stage and their covariates.

Methods. A secondary analysis of data from the National Household Survey on Drug Abuse (1979–1997) was conducted with particular sensitivity to the nature of substance use progression, sampling procedures, and reliability of self-report data.

Results. Progression to marijuana and hard drug use was uncommon among persons born before World War II. The stages phenomenon essentially emerged with the baby boom and rose to a peak among persons born around 1960. Subsequently, progression risks at each stage declined. Progression risks were also higher among younger initiators of alcohol, tobacco, or marijuana use.

Conclusions. The recent increase in youthful marijuana use has been offset by lower rates of progression to hard drug use among youths born in the 1970s. Dire predictions of future hard drug abuse by youths who came of age in the 1990s may be greatly overstated. (*Am J Public Health.* 2001;91:225–232)

A central disconnect exists between the policy discussions about youthful substance use and empirical research. Much public policy rhetoric emphasizes how use of alcohol, tobacco, and marijuana by youths can lead to hard drug use and abuse. This perception evolved from Denise Kandel's findings in the 1970s that youths tended to start using alcohol or tobacco, or both, after which some (but not all) progressed to marijuana and then possibly hard drugs.[1,2] Much subsequent research has confirmed that this sequence has prevailed widely.[3–13] Only a few published studies have documented populations in which a substantial percentage of youths followed a different sequence; these studies examined high-risk populations within inner-city New York.[14–16] Consequently, many consider alcohol, tobacco, and marijuana to be *gateway drugs,* and 2 ideas have obtained political currency[17–19]: (1) reducing or postponing youthful initiation of alcohol, tobacco, and marijuana use can reduce subsequent hard drug abuse; and (2) recent increases in youthful tobacco and marijuana use may foreshadow an impending epidemic of hard drug use.

In contrast to this rhetorical perspective, survey programs typically monitor rates of use for various drugs but not rates of progression.[20,21] Moreover, no simple formula exists for calculating progression risks from prevalence rates. Two recent publications have attempted to bridge this gap with data from the National Household Survey on Drug Abuse (NHSDA). The Center on Addiction and Substance Abuse[22] reported that "[c]hildren 12–17 years old who use marijuana are 85 times more likely . . . to use cocaine than children who have never used [marijuana]." Zimmer and Morgan noted that "[f]or every 100 people who have tried marijuana . . . 28 have tried cocaine."[23(p36)] Both of these calculations had methodological shortcomings, among them the failure to adjust for the proportion of the youngest respondents who probably progressed to marijuana or cocaine use after the time of the interview. This article presents estimates that are sensitive to this and other serious methodological challenges.

Methods

In this article, we examine the risks of progression through 4 stages—(1) nonuse, (2) alcohol or tobacco, (3) marijuana, and (4) hard drugs—based on data from the NHSDA program, which were publicly available for surveys conducted in 1979, 1982, 1985, 1988, and 1990 to 1997. Each respondent's progression sequence was inferred from answers to the following question: "How old were you the first time you . . . [used *alcohol, cigarettes, marijuana,* and *various hard drugs*]?" Consistent with prior research on the gateway theory, the first stage was defined as use of alcohol or cigarettes, whichever occurred first.[1–13,15] The age at first use of hard drugs was defined by first use of cocaine powder, crack, or heroin. These street drugs can cause dependence, have been widely abused since the 1960s, and have been the focus of much public policy concern.[24] (The analysis did not examine the significance of using other psychoactive drugs such as inhalants, hallucinogens, and amphetamines; the careful expansion of the analysis to include these drugs is the subject of our next research effort.)

To ensure that respondents had completed their substance use progression, the analysis primarily focused on individuals who were at

The authors are with the National Development and Research Institutes, New York, NY.

Requests for reprints should be sent to Andrew Golub, PhD, National Development and Research Institutes, Two World Trade Center, New York, NY 10048 (e-mail: andygolub@worldnet.att.net).

This article was accepted March 24, 2000.

Note. The views and opinions expressed are those of the authors and do not necessarily reflect the positions of the Robert Wood Johnson Foundation or the National Development and Research Institutes.

least 26 years of age when interviewed. Prior research suggests that most individuals who do not initiate hard drug use by about 25 years of age never will.[2,25–27] Moreover, the nature of substance use progression after 25 years of age is almost certainly quite different from progression in adolescence. The study also analyzed the risk of progression by 17 years of age to examine more recent trends. In the remainder of this section, we describe the NHSDA, how the analyses accounted for survey errors, and the multivariate procedure used to study covariates of progression risks.

The NHSDA Program

The NHSDA has measured the use of illicit drugs, alcohol, and tobacco in the United States every 2 to 3 years since 1971 and annually since 1990.[21] Originally, the survey covered household residents 12 years and older living in the 48 contiguous states. Beginning in 1991, the target population was expanded to the entire US civilian noninstitutionalized population, including persons living in college dormitories, rooming houses, and shelters. (Interview year was included in the analysis of covariates risk to measure the effect of this methodological change.)

The NHSDA uses a stratified hierarchic sampling plan. The sample weights included in the data files were used to obtain unbiased estimates. The hierarchic structure generally reduces efficiency, even doubling standard errors for some estimates.[21] These design effects were not calculated because of the complexity of the analyses performed. Consequently, the standard errors reported should be viewed as lower bounds.

To ensure strong response rates, trained interviewers personally visit each selected residence to administer questionnaires. Self-administered answer sheets are used to ensure confidentiality and to facilitate disclosure of alcohol and drug use.

Four percent of the cases were excluded from analysis because information about birth year, substances ever used, or age at first use was lacking. This exclusion could bias estimates of progression rates to the extent that persons who had used more drugs also tended to provide incomplete information. Logistic regression was used to determine how the probability of exclusion varied with substances used (and respondent demographics) and to modify sample weights accordingly. Indeed, use of alcohol and use of hard drugs were modestly associated with exclusion (odds ratios [ORs] = 1.4 and 1.5, respectively). The primary sample included 100 282 NHSDA respondents 26 years and older.

Survey Errors

The NHSDA is prone to a variety of *sampling errors* related to not obtaining a representative sample and *response errors* related to obtaining less than completely accurate replies. The program tends to undersample many of the most serious drug abusers.[21] The progression rates would be underestimated to the extent that illegal drug users were less likely to remain in stable households and thus over time were increasingly less likely to be sampled by the NHSDA; we refer to this phenomenon as *attrition from the sampling frame.* An analysis of responses to the NHSDA across survey years by persons born in 1968 through 1973 yielded initially troubling findings.[26] When interviewed at 12 years of age, 19% of the cohort reported having initiated alcohol use by 11 years of age. However, when members of the same birth cohort (but not the same persons) were interviewed at 25 years, only 5% reported initiation by 11 years. This finding is consistent with the idea that many early alcohol initiators had become unavailable to the NHSDA.

However, data from the Rutgers Health and Human Development Project, in which the same persons were asked their age at first use on 2 occasions separated by 3 years, found a similar decline in early initiators.[26] This suggested that what seemed like attrition from the NHSDA sampling frame may have actually been caused by individuals inflating their age at first use over time. Prior research has identified several potential response biases that can cause an upward shift:[28,29]

1. *Forward telescoping:* respondents might underestimate the time since first use.
2. *Redefinition:* younger respondents might remember first use of alcohol as taking a few sips from a parent's drink, but older respondents might remember or redefine first use as sharing a 6-pack with friends.
3. *Deception:* older respondents might report an older age at first use to appear more socially acceptable.

This unreliability raised questions about using self-reports of age at first use to study substance use progression. However, further analysis with the Rutgers data suggested that the general order of initiation (as used in this article) *can* be reliably inferred from age at first use when alcohol and tobacco are grouped together into a single stage[9]; the inferred order involving alcohol and tobacco was not reliable. Inflation raised an additional concern with regard to estimating the risk of progression by 17 years of age. Many older respondents would have inflated their age at first use beyond 17 years of age. Consequently, that analysis was restricted to respondents aged 18 and no older.

In general, the research reviewed suggests that an accurate estimate of the risk of substance use progression faced by members of the general population can be inferred from self-reports of age at first use to the extent that NHSDA respondents disclosed lifetime use. Research suggests that individuals underreport the use of illegal drugs, although the amount of nondisclosure varies with recent and lifetime use, individual characteristics, and survey procedures.[30–32] This analysis could not accurately correct for nondisclosure because of a lack of highly specific information about the covariates of underreporting.

Analysis of Covariates

Logistic regression was used to examine systematic variation in progression risks from (1) nonuse to alcohol or tobacco use, (2) alcohol or tobacco to marijuana use, and (3) marijuana to hard drug use. A few cases did not conform precisely to the gateway sequence: 3.8% of the sample initiated alcohol or tobacco and marijuana use in the same year; 1.4% initiated marijuana use before alcohol or tobacco use; 0.7% initiated marijuana and hard drug use in the same year; 0.2% initiated hard drug use before marijuana; and 0.1% initiated hard drugs, alcohol or tobacco, and marijuana in the same year. These 6.2% of the cases presented a dilemma. Not including them in the analysis of covariates led to underestimates of the progression risks. However, including them confounded different sequences. We estimated the covariation both ways: (1) excluding cases that did not conform to the gateway sequence and (2) modifying cases to conform (e.g., adding use of alcohol or tobacco to sequences that had started with marijuana). Both approaches produced similar results. In this article, we present the results based on excluding nonconforming cases.

Research has identified numerous factors associated with the etiology of substance use, leading to many theories and metatheories.[33,34] One such explanation, *primary socialization theory,* provides a particularly useful framework for understanding the social context possibly underlying the gateway sequence.[35] This theory contends that individuals learn social norms and behaviors from 3 primary sources: family, school, and peer clusters (small groups of close friends). As a result, the sequence of substances youths tend to use reflects the age-based behavior norms of prevailing youth subcultures. Differences in such norms could lead to different sequences.

This general perspective guided the following selection of possible covariates of progression risks from the extremely limited choices recorded by the NHSDA. Each independent variable was coded as a set of dummy variables to identify the extent to which progression risk varied with deviation from a reference category. Thus, the base odds provided an estimate of the risk for respondents whose attributes matched all the reference categories. The total variation for each variable (after control for other independent variables) was measured with a Wald statistic.[36]

Birth year. What is "in" tends to shift across generations.[24,37] Prior research documented that the use of marijuana and hard drugs increased in popularity during the 1960s.[38] Thus, youths born since World War II (who came of age in the 1960s and later) were hypothesized to have been more likely to have progressed to marijuana and hard drug use. The popularity of heroin started declining in the 1970s, the popularity of cocaine (especially as crack) started declining in the late 1980s, and the popularity of marijuana has been increasing in the mid-1990s.[39,40] Thus, the risk of progression to hard drug use was hypothesized to have declined, whereas the risk of progression to marijuana use either held steady or even increased. Because of limited subsample sizes, birth years before 1910 were grouped into a single category, and birth years from 1910 through 1949 were grouped into 5-year cohorts. The NHSDA data included substantially more individuals born since 1950. These birth years were grouped into 2-year cohorts.

Region and metropolitan statistical area size. Substance use tends to vary by location and urbanicity. Individuals growing up in the Northeast and the West and in larger metropolitan areas were hypothesized to be more likely to progress at each stage. These variables were measured at the time of the interview and not while growing up. Consequently, a positive association could occur if marijuana and hard drug users disproportionately relocated to larger cities in the Northeast and the West.

Race/ethnicity. Peer group homophyly based on race/ethnicity is common, as are subcultural differences across these groups.[41] Blacks and Hispanics have been disproportionately represented at all stages of the criminal justice system for charges of drug-related offenses. Paradoxically, Whites typically have reported the highest rates of substance use.[42] Thus, Blacks and Hispanics were hypothesized to have lower progression risks than were Whites. The interpretation of this potential variation was heavily limited because only broad categories of race/ethnicity were provided by the NHSDA; individual differences in intensity of racial/ethnic identification were not measured; and numerous social, economic, and political factors correlated with race/ethnicity were not available.

Sex. Historically, behavior norms for boys and girls have differed greatly. It was hypothesized that these differences would result in males being more likely than females to progress at each stage of substance use.[41]

Age at first alcohol or tobacco and marijuana use. Several studies indicated that early initiation of substance use is associated with further substance use progression and subsequent problems.[2,22,43–45] Young adolescents (in their preteens or early teens) tend to be highly susceptible to peer influences.[46] It was hypothesized that these influences would lead to further progression. In contrast, young adults tend to be more autonomous and might be less likely to progress.

Interview year. Because of increasing political concern and increasing disapproval of drugs, individual willingness to report progression may have declined with time. Changes in NHSDA procedures—especially the expansion of the NHSDA target population in 1991 and the questionnaire redesign in 1994—also may have resulted in changes in reporting rates.[47]

Results

Figure 1 confirms that most NHSDA respondents followed the gateway sequence. In this transition diagram, each respondent's substance use history is characterized as a series of stages (cumulative set of substances ever used) and transitions through them. The number on each arrow indicates the weighted percentage of the sample that progressed through the designated transition. The horizontal linkages from nonuse to hard drugs correspond to the gateway sequence.

All individuals started on the far left with nonuse. Most of the sample (84.7%) first initiated alcohol or tobacco use, although some (9.9%) never used any substances. A majority of the sample (62.1%) ended their progression with alcohol or tobacco use. Others proceeded to marijuana (21.7%), and some of those progressed to hard drugs (7.7%). A few individuals reported initiation of multiple substances in a single year (3.8%, alcohol or tobacco and marijuana; 0.7%, marijuana and hard drugs; and 0.1%, all 3 substances). These multistage transitions are reported at the top of Figure 1. Very few cases deviated from the gateway sequence

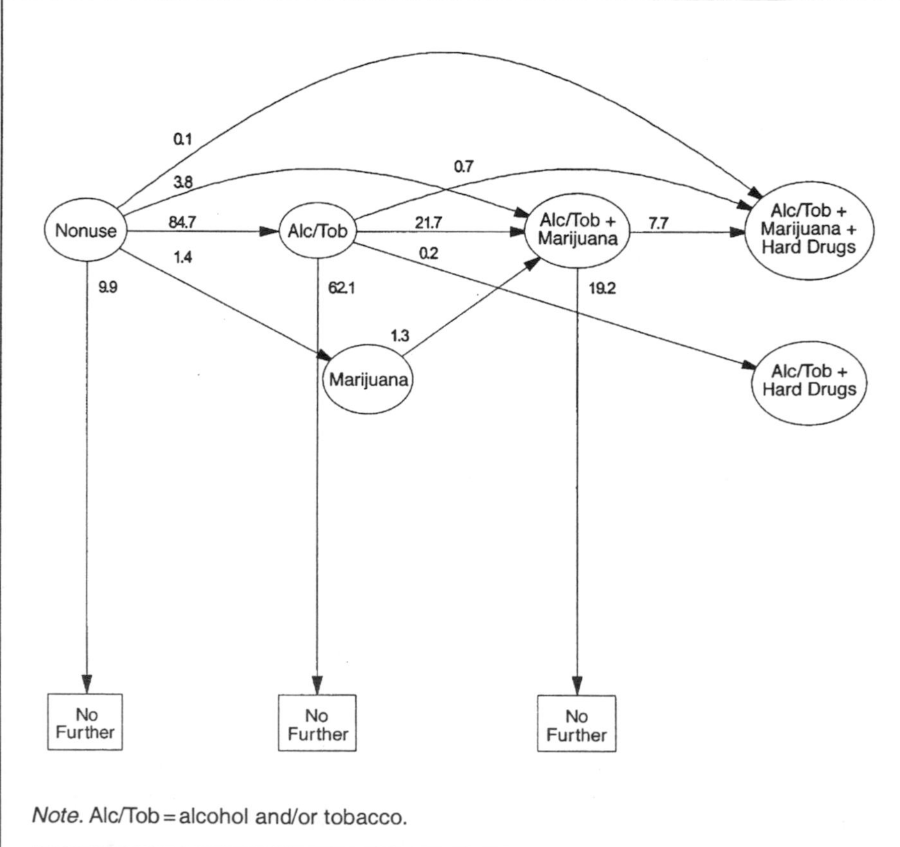

FIGURE 1—Variation in substance use sequences by 25 years of age: National Household Survey on Drug Abuse interviewees 26 years and older, 1979–1997 (N=100282).

(1.4% of the sample progressed directly from nonuse to marijuana use, and 0.2% progressed directly from alcohol or tobacco to hard drug use).

Table 1 presents an analysis of covariates of progression at each stage. The wide range of odds ratios indicates that individual progression risks varied substantially. Birth year had the largest Wald statistic (3684.7) in the model of progression from nonuse to alcohol or tobacco use, indicating that it explained the most variation after control for all other variables included in the analysis. Similarly, birth year explained the most variation in risk of progression from alcohol or tobacco to marijuana use (Wald = 10620.6), followed by age at first use of alcohol or tobacco (Wald = 4191.1). The most variation in risk of progression to hard drugs was explained by age at first marijuana use (Wald = 1312.5), followed by birth year (Wald = 282.2). The variation in risks associated with birth year and age at first use is examined at length subsequently in this report.

The amounts of variation explained by race/ethnicity and sex was similar to that for birth year with respect to risk of alcohol or tobacco use but much smaller with regard to subsequent progression risks. Blacks were less likely to progress to alcohol or tobacco use (OR = 0.43) than were otherwise similar Whites. Those Blacks who did progress were just as likely to proceed to marijuana use but slightly less likely to use hard drugs (OR = 0.83) than were Whites. Hispanics and females were much less likely to progress to alcohol or tobacco use (OR = 0.24 each). Their rates of subsequent progression approached but remained below those for Whites and males.

The variation associated with region was modest at each stage. Respondents from the South were slightly less likely to progress at each stage than those from the North. Respondents from the North Central region were about as likely to progress to alcohol or tobacco and marijuana use and slightly less likely to progress to hard drug use than were those from the North. Respondents from the West were slightly less likely to progress to alcohol or tobacco use, but those who did were slightly more likely to progress to marijuana and hard drug use.

The variation associated with metropolitan statistical area size also was small. Respondents from smaller metropolitan statistical areas (population < 1 million) were slightly less likely to progress to alcohol or tobacco and marijuana use than were those from larger metropolitan statistical areas. Respondents from non–metropolitan statistical areas were somewhat less likely to progress at each stage.

Respondents became steadily less likely to report progression to alcohol or tobacco use from 1979 to 1996. The variation in reported

TABLE 1—Variation in the Conditional Odds of Substance Use Progression by 25 Years of Age: National Household Survey on Drug Abuse (NHSDA) Interviewees 26 Years and Older, 1979–1997

	Estimated Odds Ratio by Transition		
	Nonuse to Alcohol/Tobacco	Alcohol/Tobacco to Marijuana	Marijuana to Hard Drugs[a]
Birth year			
Wald (19)	(3684.7**)	(10620.6**)	(282.2*)
<1910	0.09**	0.01**	
1910–1914	0.14**	0.01**	
1915–1919	0.22**	0.01**	
1920–1924	0.32**	0.01**	
1925–1929	0.43**	0.01**	
1930–1934	0.52**	0.02**	
1935–1939	0.59**	0.02**	0.28[c]**
1940–1944	0.75**	0.09**	0.13**
1945–1949	0.94	0.34**	0.48**
1950–1951	0.85*	0.63**	0.65**
1952–1953	0.98	0.75**	0.92
1954–1955	1.09	0.83**	0.81**
1956–1957	1.08	0.93	0.97
1958–1959	0.95	1.04	1.00
1960–1961[b]	1.00	1.00	1.00
1962–1963	0.99	0.98	1.15*
1964–1965	0.83*	0.91	1.00
1966–1967	0.83	0.76**	0.86
1968–1969	0.76*	0.74**	0.64**
1970–1971	0.74	0.72**	0.56**
Race/ethnicity			
Wald (3)	(2930.9**)	(640.3**)	(32.8**)
White[b]	1.00	1.00	1.00
Black	0.43**	1.04	0.83**
Hispanic	0.24**	0.40**	0.72**
Other	0.13**	0.43**	0.67**
Sex			
Wald (1)	(2782.0**)	(444.1**)	(114.5**)
Male[b]	1.00	1.00	1.00
Female	0.24**	0.65**	0.68**
Region			
Wald (3)	(264.7**)	(381.6**)	(121.1**)
Northeast[b]	1.00	1.00	1.00
North Central	1.03	0.98	0.77**
South	0.67**	0.81**	0.84**
West	0.88**	1.42**	1.27**
Metropolitan statistical area size			
Wald (2)	(151.4**)	(259.6**)	(57.8**)
>1 million[b]	1.00	1.00	1.00
<1 million	0.92**	0.94**	0.95
Non–metropolitan statistical area	0.70**	0.66**	0.70**
Alcohol/tobacco age, y			
Wald (4)	...	(4191.1**)	(15.1**)
0–11		2.13**	1.08
12–14		2.00**	1.06
15–17[b]		1.00	1.00
18–20		0.33**	0.74**
21–25		0.08**	0.34
Marijuana age, y			
Wald (4)	...	...	(1312.5**)
0–11			6.76**
12–14			2.43**
15–17[b]			1.00
18–20			0.46**
21–25			0.15**
Interview year			
Wald (11)	(177.7**)	(50.1**)	(21.1*)
1979	2.05**	1.22**	1.18
1982	1.67**	1.22**	1.29*
1985	1.61**	1.13	1.03
1988	1.41**	1.05	0.96
1990	1.20**	1.23**	1.02

Continued

TABLE 1—*Continued*

1991	1.30**	1.09	0.97
1992	1.22**	1.04	0.85**
1993	1.34**	1.17**	1.05
1994a[d]	1.55**	1.16	0.90
1994b[d]	1.31**	1.06	1.03
1995	1.15**	0.95	1.07
1996	1.02	1.03	1.00
1997[b]	1.00	1.00	1.00
Base odds	61.5:1	1.5:1	0.9:1
N	91464	78597	27216

Note. SEs for the log of parameter estimates were typically about 0.05. Ellipses indicate that data are not applicable.
[a]Hard drugs included cocaine powder, crack, and heroin.
[b]Reference category.
[c]Birth year < 1939.
[d]The NHSDA performed a split-sample analysis in 1994. Some respondents were given the old survey (1994a), and others received the new instrument (1994b).
*Significant at $\alpha = .05$ level.
**Significant at $\alpha = .01$ level.

progression to marijuana and hard drug use was much less substantial and statistically significant in only a few years. The estimates of progression risk generally were unaffected by the 2 most dramatic changes in the NHSDA program. The variation from 1990 to 1991 (when the NHSDA target population was expanded) and the variation across the split sample in 1994 (when the NHSDA questionnaire was revised) were not statistically significant for each model of progression except one (based on additional *t* tests not reported in Table 1). That model, the modest decline in risk of progression to marijuana use from 1990 to 1991, was statistically significant at the $\alpha =$ .05 but not at the more rigorous $\alpha = .01$ level.

Variation With Birth Year

Figure 2 presents the bivariate trends in transition probabilities by birth year. Alcohol or tobacco use was always popular; 80% or more of the respondents born since 1915 reported use by 25 years of age. The gateway linkages to marijuana and hard drug use, however, did not emerge until the generations born since World War II. Fewer than 5% of the alcohol or tobacco users born before 1940 ever progressed to marijuana use. This resulted in too few respondents to accurately calculate rates of progression to hard drugs by birth cohort. Among the 348 marijuana users born before 1940, only 9% progressed to hard drug use. Starting with birth years in the 1940s, the rate of progression to marijuana rose steadily to a peak of 55% (1958–1959 birth cohort) and then steadily declined to 43% (1970–1971 birth cohort). The conditional probability of progression from marijuana to hard drug use rose to 39% (1962–1963 birth cohort) and then declined to 24% (1970–1971 birth cohort).

Figure 3 extends the analysis of variation across birth cohorts by examining progression rates for 18-year-old respondents. Overall, respondents born in the 1970s were less likely than those born in the 1960s to progress at each stage, although some may yet progress by 25 years of age. The progression risk from nonuse to alcohol or tobacco use declined from 93% (1961–1967 birth years) to 83% (1979 birth year). The progression risk from alcohol or tobacco to marijuana use declined from 47% (1961–1967 birth years) to 26% (1974 birth year) and subsequently increased to 36% (1979 birth year). The progression risk from marijuana to hard drug use declined from 20% (1961–1967 birth years) to 6% (1979 birth year).

Variation With Age at First Use

Risks of progression by 25 years of age were substantially higher for individuals who initiated alcohol or tobacco and marijuana use at the earliest ages (Table 1). Figure 4 presents the bivariate association between age at first alcohol or tobacco use and progression to marijuana use, as well as the association between age at first marijuana use and progression to hard drug use for individuals born from 1956 to 1971. (These birth years were combined on the basis of the relative similarity in prevailing

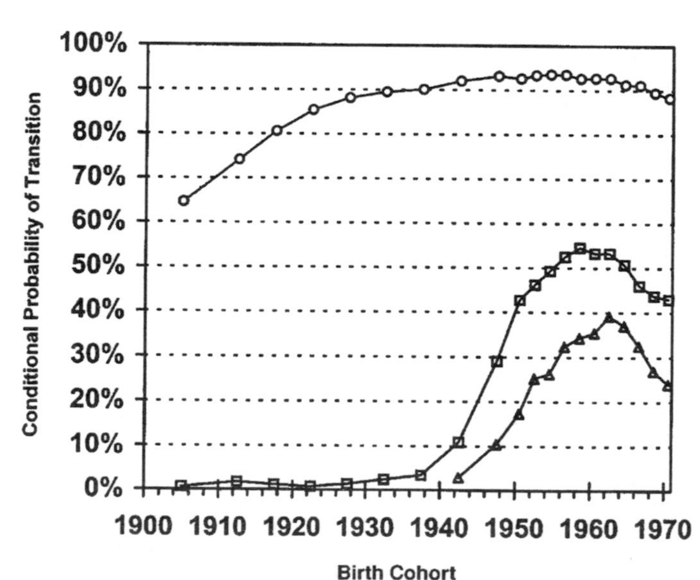

FIGURE 2—Variation across birth years in the conditional probabilities of substance use progression by 25 years of age: National Household Survey on Drug Abuse interviewees 26 years and older, 1979–1997 (N = 91464).

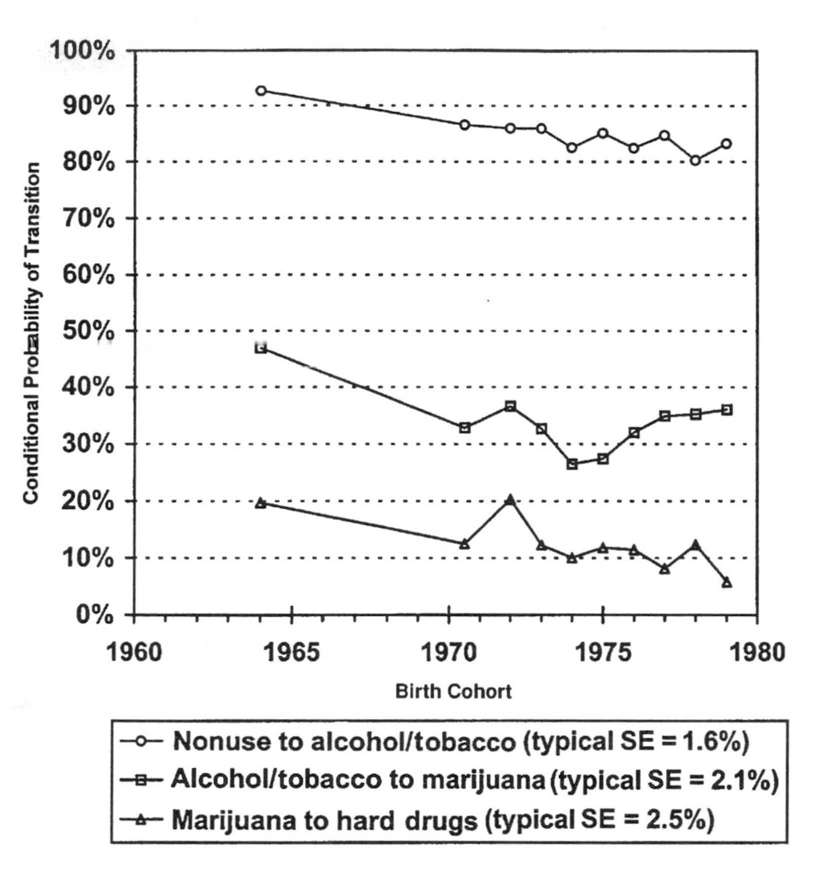

Note. 1961–1967 and 1970–1971 birth years were combined.

FIGURE 3—Variation across birth years in the conditional probabilities of substance use progression by 17 years of age: National Household Survey on Drug Abuse interviewees aged 18 years, 1979–1997 (N=6484).

transition rates identified in Table 1.) Those reporting initiation of alcohol or tobacco (or marijuana) use before 15 years of age were dramatically more likely to have progressed to marijuana (or hard drug) use than those who reported first use of alcohol or tobacco (or marijuana) after 17 years of age.

Discussion

The preponderance of studies replicating the gateway phenomenon suggests that the gateway theory might be a reliable foundation for guiding prevention policy and practice. This study identifies a way in which the gateway phenomenon appears to be unreliable; the probabilities of progression between stages have shifted dramatically across birth cohorts. Persons born before World War II who used alcohol or tobacco rarely tried marijuana, and the few who did use marijuana infrequently advanced to hard drug use. The gateway phenomenon emerged in the 1960s as the baby boom generation came of age. However, persons born since the early 1960s, who came of age in the 1980s, were substantially less likely to progress to marijuana, cocaine powder, crack, and heroin use.

Starting in the mid-1990s, youthful marijuana use started to increase.[20,21] A superficial application of the gateway theory would suggest that a new epidemic of hard drug use is imminent. However, a more careful analysis of all the data suggests that this might *not* happen. The probability of progression from alcohol or tobacco to marijuana use has increased in recent years, but the risk of progression by 17 years of age to cocaine powder, crack, or heroin has so far remained at relatively low levels. These youthful marijuana users may never progress to hard drug use. Indeed, ethnographic studies have documented cultural norms that encourage marijuana use but strongly discourage use of hard drugs among youths in inner-city New York.[40,48]

These findings suggest that the gateway phenomenon reflects norms prevailing among youths at a specific place and time and that the linkages between stages are far from causal. They further suggest that simply restricting youth's access to gateway drugs will not necessarily reduce subsequent hard drug abuse. A more effective strategy might be to try to understand and influence the prevailing norms, especially those affecting early initiators of alcohol, tobacco, and marijuana use.

Several policy analysts contend that substance use is merely one behavior caused by and contributing to problems in adolescence.[49,50] Their insights caution against viewing the complex challenges facing youths, their psychologic and emotional reactions, their social interactions, and their resulting behaviors as the product of a simple stages model. Rather, the prevailing stages, progression risks, and variations over time and across locations provide one window into youths' experiences. Public policy should be based on continuing observation of the rich and changing context in which the stages of youthful substance use prevail and the empirically verified effectiveness of alternative measures.

In this article, we advanced the methodology for analyzing stages of substance use within the context of adolescent development. Because NHSDA data collection is ongoing, this procedure provides a method for continually monitoring changes in youthful substance use progression to confirm prevailing shifts in norms of youth culture. This model should eventually be expanded to analyze the use of other fairly common illicit substances (e.g., inhalants, methamphetamine, lysergic acid diethylamide or "LSD," and methylenedioxymethamphetamine or "Ecstasy"), any of which could emerge as the hard drug of choice for youths coming of age in the 1990s and beyond. The model also should be extended to monitor the rates of progression from first use to regular, long-term, and problem use. In addition, further research into nondisclosure, response bias, and the covariates of each could potentially identify improvements to increase the accuracy of the calculations. □

Contributors

A. Golub and B. D. Johnson planned the study, interpreted the results, and wrote the paper. A. Golub performed the analysis.

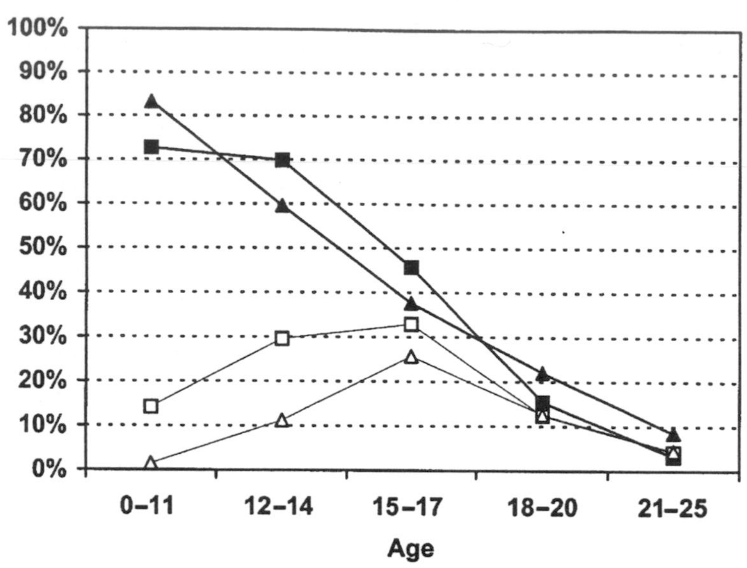

FIGURE 4—Variation in the conditional probability of substance use progression with age at first alcohol or tobacco use and first marijuana use: National Household Survey on Drug Abuse interviewees 26 years and older, born in 1956–1971 (N=22217).

Acknowledgments

Preparation of this paper was supported by a grant from the Robert Wood Johnson Foundation Substance Abuse Policy Research Program (033027).

References

1. Kandel DB. Stages in adolescent involvement in drug use. *Science.* 1975;190:912–914.
2. Kandel DB. Convergence in prospective longitudinal surveys of drug use in normal populations. In: Kandel DB, ed. *Longitudinal Research on Drug Use: Empirical Findings and Methodological Issues.* Washington, DC: Hemisphere Publishing; 1978:3–38.
3. Andrews JA, Hops H, Ary D, Lichtenstein E, Tildesley E. The construction, validation and use of a Guttman scale of adolescent substance use: an investigation of family relationships. *J Drug Issues.* 1991;21:557–572.
4. Blaze-Temple D, Kai Lo S. Stages of drug use: a community survey of Perth teenagers. *Br J Addict.* 1992;87:215–225.
5. Brook JS, Whiteman M, Gordon AS. Qualitative and quantitative aspects of adolescent drug use: the interplay of personality, family and peer correlates. *Psychol Rep.* 1982;51:1151–1163.
6. Donovan JE, Jessor R. Problem drinking and the dimension of involvement with drugs: a Guttman scalogram analysis of adolescent drug use. *Am J Public Health.* 1983;73:543–552.
7. Elliott DS, Huizinga D, Menard S. *Multiple Problem Youth: Delinquency, Substance Use, and Mental Health Problems.* New York, NY: Springer-Verlag; 1989.
8. Fleming R, Leventhal H, Glynn K, Ershler J. The role of cigarettes in the initiation and progression of early substance use. *Addict Behav.* 1989;14:261–272.
9. Golub AL, Labouvie E, Johnson BD. Response reliability and the study of adolescent substance use progression. *J Drug Issues.* 2000;30: 103–118.
10. Hays D, Ellickson PL. Guttman scale analysis of longitudinal data: a methodology and drug use applications. *Int J Addict.* 1991;25: 1341–1352.
11. Kandel DB, Yamaguchi K, Chen K. Stages of progression in drug involvement from adolescence to adulthood: further evidence for the gateway theory. *J Stud Alcohol.* 1992;53:447–457.
12. Mills CJ, Noyes HL. Patterns and correlates of initial and subsequent drug use among adolescents. *J Consult Clin Psychol.* 1984;52:231–243.
13. Welte JW, Barnes GM. Alcohol: the gateway to other drug use among secondary-school students. *J Youth Adolescence.* 1985;48:329–336.
14. Golub A, Johnson BD. The shifting importance of alcohol and marijuana as gateway substances among serious drug abusers. *J Stud Alcohol.* 1994;55:607–614.
15. Golub AL, Johnson BD. Substance use progression and hard drug abuse in inner-city New York. In: Kandel DB, ed. *Stages and Pathways of Involvement in Drug Use: Examining the Gateway Hypothesis.* New York, NY: Cambridge University Press. In press.
16. Mackesy-Amiti ME, Fendrich M, Goldstein PJ. Sequence of drug use among serious drug users: typical vs atypical progression. *Drug Alcohol Depend.* 1997;45:185–196.
17. Office of National Drug Control Policy. *The National Drug Control Strategy: 1997.* Washington, DC: US Government Printing Office; 1997: iii, 23–24. Publication NCJ 160086.
18. Sloboda Z, David SL. *Preventing Drug Use Among Children and Adolescents: A Research Based Guide.* Washington, DC: US Government Printing Office; 1997:7. NIH publication 97-4212.
19. Gfroerer JC, Epstein JF. Marijuana initiates and their impact on future drug abuse treatment need. *Drug Alcohol Depend.* 1999;54:229–237.
20. Johnston LD, O'Malley PM, Bachman JG. *National Survey Results on Drug Use From the Monitoring the Future Study, 1975–1998.* Vol 1. Rockville, Md: National Institute on Drug Abuse; 1999. NIH publication 99-4660.
21. *National Household Survey on Drug Abuse: Population Estimates 1998.* Rockville, Md: Substance Abuse and Mental Health Services Administration; 1999. DHHS publication SMA 99-3328.
22. *Cigarettes, Alcohol, Marijuana: Gateways to Illicit Drug Use.* New York, NY: Center on Addiction and Substance Abuse; 1994:iii.
23. Zimmer L, Morgan JP. *Marijuana Myths, Marijuana Facts: A Review of the Scientific Literature.* New York, NY: The Lindesmith Center; 1997:32–37.
24. Johnson BD, Muffler J. Sociocultural determinants and perpetuators of substance abuse. In: Lowinson JH, Ruiz P, Millman RB, Langrod JG, eds. *Substance Abuse: A Comprehensive Textbook.* 3rd ed. Baltimore, Md: Williams & Wilkins; 1997:107–117.
25. Chen K, Kandel DB. The natural history of drug use from adolescence to the mid-thirties in a general population sample. *Am J Public Health.* 1995;85:41–47.
26. Golub AL, Johnson BD, Labouvie E. Correcting household survey responses of age at first use of alcohol, tobacco, marijuana, and hard drugs for inaccurate recall and sample selection biases. *J Quant Criminology.* 2000;16:45–68.
27. Johnston LD. Toward a theory of drug epidemics. In: Donohew DH, Sypher H, Bukoski W, eds. *Persuasive Communication and Drug Abuse Prevention.* Hillsdale, NJ: Lawrence Erlbaum; 1991:93–132.
28. Eisenhower D, Mathiowetz NA, Morganstein D. Recall error: sources and bias reduction techniques. In: Biemer PP, Groves RM, Lyberg LE,

Mathiowetz NA, Sudman S, eds. *Measurement Errors in Surveys.* New York, NY: John Wiley & Sons; 1991:127–144.

29. Johnson RA, Gerstein DR, Rasinski KA. Recall decay and telescoping in self reports of alcohol and marijuana use: results from the National Household Survey on Drug Abuse [NHSDA]. *Proc Am Assoc Public Opin Researchers.* 1997.
30. Fendrich M, Vaughn CM. Diminished lifetime substance use over time: an inquiry into differential underreporting. *Public Opin Q.* 1994;58: 96–123.
31. Harrison LD. The validity of self-reported data on drug use. *J Drug Issues.* 1995;25:91–111.
32. Johnston LD, O'Malley PM. The recanting of earlier reported drug use by young adults. In: Harrison L, Hughes A, eds. *The Validity of Self-Reported Drug Use: Improving the Accuracy of Survey Estimates.* Rockville, Md: National Institute on Drug Abuse; 1997:59–80. NIDA Research Monograph 167.
33. Anderson TL. A cultural-identity theory of drug abuse. In: *Sociology of Crime, Law, and Deviance.* Vol 1. Greenwich, Conn: JAI Press; 1998:233–262.
34. Petraitis J, Flay BR, Miller TQ, Torpy EJ, Greiner B. Illicit substance use among adolescents: a matrix of prospective predictors. *Subst Use Misuse.* 1998;33:2561–2604.
35. Oetting ER, Donnermeyer JF. Primary socialization theory: the etiology of drug use and deviance, I. *Subst Use Misuse.* 1998;33: 995–1026.
36. Hosmer DW, Lemeshow S. *Applied Logistic Regression.* New York, NY: John Wiley & Sons; 1989.
37. Musto D. *The American Disease: Origins of Narcotic Control.* New York, NY: Oxford University Press; 1987.
38. Johnson RA, Gerstein DR. Initiation of use of alcohol, cigarettes, marijuana, cocaine, and other substances in US birth cohorts since 1919. *Am J Public Health.* 1998;88:27–33.
39. Golub AL, Johnson BD. Cracks decline: some surprises across US cities. In: *National Institute of Justice Research in Brief.* Washington, DC: National Institute of Justice; 1997. NCJ 165707.
40. Golub AL, Johnson BD. Cohort changes in illegal drug use among arrestees in Manhattan: from the Heroin Injection Generation to the Blunts Generation. *Subst Use Misuse.* 1999;34: 1733–1763.
41. Oetting ER, Donnermeyer JF, Trimble JE, Beauvais F. Primary socialization theory: culture, ethnicity, and cultural identification: the links between culture and substance use, IV. *Subst Use Misuse.* 1998;33:2075–2107.
42. Kandel DB. Ethnic differences in drug use: patterns and paradoxes. In: Botvin GJ, Schinke S, Orlandi MA, eds. *Drug Abuse Prevention With Multiethnic Youth.* Newbury Park, Calif: Sage Publications; 1995:81–104.
43. Grant BF, Dawson DA. Age at onset of alcohol use and its association with DSM-IV alcohol abuse and dependence: results from the National Longitudinal Alcohol Epidemiologic Survey. *J Subst Abuse.* 1997;9:103–110.
44. Robins LN, Przybeck TR. Age of onset of drug use as a factor in drug and other disorders. In: Jones CL, Battjes RJ, eds. *Etiology and Drug Abuse: Implications for Prevention.* Washington, DC: US Government Printing Office; 1985: 178–192. NIDA Research Monograph 56.
45. Yamaguchi K, Kandel DB. Patterns of drug use from adolescence to young adulthood, III: predictors of progression. *Am J Public Health.* 1984;74:673–681.
46. Kimmel DC, Weiner IB. *Adolescence: A Developmental Transition.* 2nd ed. New York, NY: John Wiley & Sons; 1995:286–299.
47. Substance Abuse and Mental Health Services Administration. *The Development and Implementation of a New Data Collection Instrument for the 1994 National Household Survey on Drug Abuse.* Rockville, Md: Substance Abuse and Mental Health Services Administration; 1996. DHHS publication SMA 96-3084.
48. Furst RT, Johnson BD, Dunlap E, Curtis R. The stigmatized image of the crackhead: a sociocultural exploration of a barrier to cocaine smoking among a cohort of youth in New York City. *Deviant Behav.* 1999;20:153–181.
49. Currie E. *Reckoning: Drugs, the Cities, and the American Future.* New York, NY: Hill & Wang; 1993.
50. Dryfoos JG. *Safe Passage: Making It Through Adolescence in a Risky Society.* New York, NY: Oxford University Press; 1998.

Are the Sales Practices of Internet Cigarette Vendors Good Enough to Prevent Sales to Minors?

| Kurt M. Ribisl, PhD, Annice E. Kim, MPH, and Rebecca S. Williams, MHS

With the emergence of Web sites selling tobacco products, there is concern that they may be selling tobacco products to minors. A 1997 report identified 13 Internet cigarette vendors and found that few asked or attempted to verify the buyer's age.[1] Similarly, a study of 108 Internet cigar vendors found that only one third featured minimum age-of-sale warnings.[2] The goal of the present study was to examine whether Internet vendors take adequate precautions to avoid selling cigarettes to minors.

Data were collected as part of a larger study on the sales practices of 88 Internet cigarette vendors that is described elsewhere.[3] Trained raters examined all pages of each Web site for minimum age-of-sale warnings and age verification and payment methods.

TABLE 1—Presence of Health Warnings and Minimum Age Verification Procedures for Internet Cigarette Vendors (N=88)

	No. (%)
No. of age warning(s)	
0	16 (18.2)
1	30 (34.1)
2	19 (21.6)
3-5	8 (9.1)
≥6	15 (17.0)
Location of age warning(s)[a]	
Home page	43 (59.7)
Product description page	26 (36.1)
Order form page	24 (33.3)
Both home and order form pages	16 (22.2)
Other page	38 (52.8)
Age verification method	
Self-verification of legal age[b]	43 (48.9)
Type in birthdate	13 (14.8)
Type in driver's license number	8 (9.1)
Provide photographic age identification at delivery	6 (6.8)
Other verification method	5 (5.7)
Enter credit card information	1 (1.1)
Site registered with parent-controlled filtering and blocking software	0 (0.0)
Method of payment	
Credit card	80 (90.9)
Money order or certified check	60 (68.2)
Personal check	51 (58.0)
Automated teller machine card	2 (2.3)
Other	9 (10.2)

[a]Of the 72 sites with age warning(s).
[b]Buyers must check a box on the ordering page that confirms that they are of legal age to purchase cigarettes, or buyers are warned that by submitting the order, they certify that they are of legal age.

Table 1 shows that 82% of the sites (n=72) featured one or more age warnings that the buyer must be 18 years or older to purchase cigarettes. Age warnings appeared mostly on the home pages of the Web sites (n=43); only one third featured a warning on the ordering page. The most common age verification method was self-verification, whereby potential buyers clicked a box stating that they were of legal age to purchase tobacco products (n=43) or typed in their birthdate (n=13). Only 8 sites featured the more rigorous age verification method of requiring a driver's license number that could be verified by the vendor. Only 6 Internet cigarette vendors stated that they required photographic age identification at point of delivery, the prevailing standard at retail outlets.

The results of our study suggested that most Internet cigarette vendors use inadequate procedures for age verification. Youths who misrepresent their age and obtain a money order could potentially purchase cigarettes on-line without difficulty. According to the State Youth Tobacco Surveys, 1.0% was the medium percentage of middle school and 1.4% was the medium percentage of high school current smokers who reported purchasing their last pack of cigarettes on the Internet.[4] Similar findings were described in a study of California high school students.[5]

One limitation of this study was that we assessed the specified age verification methods, but these may differ markedly once orders are placed. Some sites may verify age on delivery, even though this information is not explicitly stated on their Web site. Likewise, some sites that mentioned having age verification procedures may not actually impose them.

Substantial efforts have been made to prevent youth access to tobacco products from retail outlets,[6–8] including laws requiring in-person photographic age verification at the point of sale.[9] However, no federal laws ban the sale of tobacco products to minors through the Internet, and only a few states have attempted regulation. Rhode Island, for instance, banned Internet and mail-order sales of cigarettes without age verification at delivery.[10,11] Parent-controlled filtering and blocking software is not a viable solution for restricting youth access to Internet cigarette vendors because most of these programs do not block tobacco sites[12] and because none of the sites in this study were registered with parent-controlled access-filtering software sites. The findings of this study, combined with new data showing that youths are beginning to buy cigarettes via the Internet, emphasize the need for the passage and enforcement of policies to restrict youth access to tobacco products through this venue. ■

About the Authors

The authors are with the Department of Health Behavior and Health Education, University of North Carolina at Chapel Hill School of Public Health, Chapel Hill, NC. Kurt M. Ribisl is also with the Lineberger Comprehensive Cancer Center, University of North Carolina School of Medicine.

Requests for reprints should be sent to Kurt M. Ribisl, PhD, University of North Carolina at Chapel Hill, School of Public Health, Department of Health Behavior and Health Education, Chapel Hill, NC 27599-7440 (e-mail: kurt_ribisl@unc.edu).

This brief was accepted December 18, 2001.

Contributors

K.M. Ribisl conceived the idea for the research, directed the study, contributed to the interpretation of the data, and wrote the first draft of the report. A.E. Kim and R.S. Williams contributed to the study design and measurement and collected the data. A.E. Kim contributed to the writing and editing of the report, and R.S. Williams analyzed the data.

References

1. *Alcohol and Tobacco on the Web: New Threats to Youth.* Washington, DC: Center for Media Education; March 1997.

2. Malone RE, Bero LA. Cigars, youth, and the Internet link. *Am J Public Health.* 2000;90:790–792.

3. Ribisl KM, Kim AE, Williams RS. Web sites selling cigarettes: how many are there in the USA and what are their sales practices? *Tob Control.* 2001;10: 352–359.

4. Centers for Disease Control and Prevention. Youth tobacco surveillance, United States, 2000. *MMWR Morb Mortal Wkly Rep.* 2001;50(SS-4):1–84.

5. Unger JB, Rohrbach LA, Ribisl KM. Are adolescents attempting to buy cigarettes on the Internet? *Tob Control.* 2001;10:360–363.

6. Feighery E, Altman DG, Shaffer G. The effects of combining education and enforcement to reduce tobacco sales to minors: a study of four northern California communities. *JAMA.* 1991;266: 3168–3171.

7. Forster JL, Wolfson M. Youth access to tobacco: policies and politics. *Annu Rev Public Health.* 1998;19: 203–235.

8. Jason LA, Ji PY, Anes MD, Birkhead SH. Active enforcement of cigarette control laws in the prevention of cigarette sales to minors. *JAMA.* 1991;266: 3159–3161.

9. Fishman JA, Allison H, Knowles SB, et al. State laws on tobacco control–United States, 1998. *MMWR Morb Mortal Wkly Rep.* 1999;48(SS-03): 21–62.

10. Lehourites C. R.I. restricts Internet tobacco sales. *Associated Press.* October 26, 2000.

11. Scherer R. States crack down on Web tobacco sales. *Christian Science Monitor.* November 8, 2000:2.

12. *Youth Access to Alcohol and Tobacco Web Marketing: The Filtering and Rating Debate.* Washington, DC: Center for Media Education; 1999.

Cigar Use in New Jersey Among Adolescents and Adults

| Cristine D. Delnevo, PhD, MPH, Eric S. Pevzner, MPH, Michael B. Steinberg, MD, MPH, Charles W. Warren, PhD, and John Slade, MD

More than 3000 youths become daily smokers each day.[1] Millions of youths will die from a tobacco-caused disease,[2] and tobacco use remains the single leading preventable cause of death in the United States.[3] However, recent data indicate that the prevalence of cigarette smoking among youths nationally has declined since 1998.[4] Although the decline in cigarette use among youths is encouraging, the emergence of other tobacco products, such as cigars, as alternative forms of tobacco use by youths is alarming. The purpose of this report is to compare cigar use among adolescents and adults on the basis of data from New Jersey and the United States.

We used 3 sources of data in this report. For adolescents, data for New Jersey are from the 1999 New Jersey Youth Tobacco Survey, and national data are from the 1999 National Youth Tobacco Survey. For adults, data for New Jersey are from the 1998 Behavioral Risk Factor Surveillance System (BRFSS)[5]; cigar data were not collected in the 1999 BRFSS. Comparable adult cigar use data were not nationally available.

The methodology of the Youth Tobacco Survey, a school-based questionnaire, is described in detail elsewhere.[6] In brief, the New Jersey Youth Tobacco Survey used a 2-stage cluster sample design to obtain a representative statewide sample of students (N=15 871) in grades 7 through 12. Likewise, the National Youth Tobacco Survey used a 3-stage cluster sample design to produce a nationally representative sample of students (N=15 061) in grades 6 through 12. Both surveys were conducted during the fall school semester. For the purposes of this report, we excluded sixth-grade students from the National Youth Tobacco Survey middle-school sample to standardize comparisons.

TABLE 1—Ever and Current Cigar Use by Middle-School Students, High-School Students, and Adults in New Jersey and the United States

	Ever Cigar Use				Current Cigar Use			
	New Jersey[a]	95% CI	United States[b]	95% CI	New Jersey[a]	95% CI	United States[b]	95% CI
Middle school								
Male	26.0	(23.7, 28.3)	24.3	(21.4, 27.2)	11.0	(9.6, 12.4)	9.6	(7.9, 11.3)
Female	17.6	(15.1, 20.1)	13.5	(11.1, 15.9)	7.5	(6.3, 8.7)	5.3	(3.8, 6.8)
Total	21.8	(19.9, 23.7)	18.9	(16.6, 21.2)	9.3	(8.3, 10.3)	7.4	(6.1, 8.7)
High school								
Male	48.6	(45.6, 51.6)	51.1	(48.0, 54.2)	24.2	(22.1, 26.3)	20.3	(18.4, 22.2)
Female	33.0	(30.8, 35.2)	31.9	(29.1, 34.7)	12.6	(10.8, 14.4)	10.2	(8.6, 11.8)
Total	40.5	(38.7, 42.3)	41.6	(39.0, 44.2)	18.4	(17.1, 19.7)	15.3	(13.9, 16.7)
Adult								
Male	54.3	(50.6, 58.0)	NA		12.5	(10.1, 14.9)	NA	
Female	15.1	(12.9, 17.3)			1.3	(0.6, 2.0)		
Total	33.8	(31.6, 36.0)			6.6	(5.4, 7.8)		

Note: NA = not available.
Source. [a]New Jersey Youth Tobacco Survey 1999 (adolescents) and Behavioral Risk Factor Surveillance System 1998 (adults). [b]National Youth Tobacco Survey 1999.

Operational definitions of "current cigar use" were comparable in the 1999 Youth Tobacco Survey (i.e., smoked a cigar on 1 day or more in preceding 30 days) and the 1998 BRFSS (i.e., smoked a cigar in past month), offering a unique opportunity to compare youth and adult cigar smoking prevalence. Differences between prevalence estimates were considered to be statistically significant if the 95% confidence intervals did not overlap.

Last, note that data from the Youth Tobacco Survey and the BRFSS are based on self-reports, which are subject to underreporting or overreporting. The extent of this response bias cannot be determined, but school-based surveys may tend toward overreporting, whereas telephone surveys like the BRFSS tend toward underreporting of tobacco use behaviors.

Comparisons across groups documented remarkably high levels of cigar use among youths in New Jersey and the United States (Table 1). Sex differences were apparent in both adolescents and adults, with males reporting significantly higher rates of ever and current cigar use than females. Rates of ever and current cigar smoking were similar in New Jersey and the United States among high-school students; however, the prevalence of current cigar smoking in New Jersey (18.4; 95% confidence interval (CI)=17.1, 19.7) exceeded the national rate (15.3; CI=13.9, 16.7) by 25%.

The prevalence of cigar smoking in youths relative to adults, especially among females, in New Jersey is troublesome. Ever cigar use in New Jersey was highest among high-school students (40.5; CI=38.7, 42.3), followed by adults (33.8; CI=31.6, 36.0) and middle-school students (21.8; CI=19.9, 23.7). Furthermore, current cigar use was higher among middle-school (9.3; CI=8.3, 10.3) and high-school students (18.4; CI=17.1, 19.7) in New Jersey than it was among New Jersey adults (6.6; CI=5.4, 7.8). The disparity between adolescent and adult current cigar use was most dramatic among females. Middle-school (7.5; CI=6.3, 8.7) and high-school (12.6; CI=10.8, 14.4) females had a current cigar smoking rate 5 and 10 times higher, respectively, than that in adult women (1.3; CI=0.6, 2.0) in New Jersey.

After decades of stagnant consumption, cigar use surged during the 1990s, coinciding with increased cigar marketing, most notably the use of cigars by celebrities. By featuring celebrities such as Madonna, Michael Jordan, and supermodel Elle McPherson using cigars, the cigar industry has successfully marketed their products to adult women and adolescents of both sexes. Advertising and promotional activities have increased the visibility of cigar smoking,[7] thereby "normalizing" cigar use.[8,9] As is evident in New Jersey's data, the "new cigar users" are young people, including adolescent females. The effect of increased cigar marketing on young girls and women is considerable.

Casual cigar use is often dismissed as a non–health issue. However, even moderate cigar use carries significant health risks, including increased risk for oral, oropharyngeal, and laryngeal cancers. And as is the case with other carcinogenic products, risk increases with consumption (i.e., number of cigars smoked) and depth of inhalation. Furthermore, cigars have higher total nicotine content than cigarettes do and can deliver nicotine both through smoke and through direct oral contact with the tobacco wrapper. Consequently, a special concern is that adolescent cigar use may increase vulnerability for nicotine dependence, predisposing youths to initiation of and continued use of cigarettes and other tobacco products.[8]

The emergence of widespread cigar use among adult women and among adolescents of both sexes—combined with cigar use among men—is a significant public health threat. As funding for tobacco control increases and national rates of cigarette use appear to be declining, we must remain diligent in monitoring all forms of tobacco use. The Youth Tobacco Survey allows states such as New Jersey to monitor multiple forms of tobacco use and to examine emerging patterns among youth. However, even the most responsive surveillance system is rendered ineffectual if data are not disseminated and translated into public health policies and programs. The higher-than-expected levels of youth cigar use in New Jersey and the United States indicate that effective tobacco control programs must focus on all tobacco products, not just cigarettes. ■

About the Authors

Cristine D. Delnevo, Michael B. Steinberg, and John Slade are with University of Medicine and Dentistry of New Jersey–School of Public Health, New Brunswick, NJ. Eric S. Pevzner and Charles W. Warren are with the Centers for Disease Control and Prevention, Office on Smoking and Health, Atlanta, Ga.

Requests for reprints should be sent to Cristine D. Delnevo, PhD, MPH, University of Medicine and Dentistry of New Jersey–School of Public Health, 335 George St, Liberty Plaza, Suite 2200, PO Box 2688, New Brunswick, NJ 08903-2688 (e-mail: delnevo@umdnj.edu).

This brief was accepted January 19, 2002.

Contributors

C. D. Delnevo directed the New Jersey Youth Tobacco Survey, wrote drafts of the brief, and conducted analyses. E. S. Pevzner provided technical assistance on the New Jersey Youth Tobacco Survey and wrote drafts of the brief. M. B. Steinberg formulated the concept for the brief and wrote drafts of the brief. C. W. Warren provided technical assistance on the New Jersey Youth Tobacco Survey and contributed to the interpretation of results and editing of the brief. J. Slade provided content expertise in cigar use, health effects, and marketing and contributed to the editing of the brief.

Acknowledgments

Completion of this work was partially supported by a contract from the New Jersey Department of Health and Senior Services through funding from the Master Settlement Agreement.

We would like to thank Dawn Berney and Shyamala Muthurajah for their critical contributions to the 1999 New Jersey Youth Tobacco Survey. We also would like to thank Mary Hrywna for her review of an earlier version of the report.

References

1. Centers for Disease Control and Prevention. Incidence of initiation of cigarette smoking—United States, 1965–1996. *MMWR Morb Mortal Wkly Rep.* 1998; 47:837–840.

2. Centers for Disease Control and Prevention. Projected smoking-related deaths among youth—United States. *MMWR Morb Mortal Wkly Rep.* 1996;45: 971–974.

3. McGinnis MJ, Foege WH. Actual causes of death in the United States. *JAMA.* 1993;270:2207–2212.

4. Johnston LD, O'Malley PM, Bachman JG. *The Monitoring the Future National Survey Results on Adolescent Drug Use: Overview of Key Findings, 2001.* Bethesda, Md: National Institute on Drug Abuse; 2002: 61. NIH publication 02-5105.

5. Centers for Disease Control and Prevention. State-specific prevalence of current cigarette and cigar smoking among adults—United States, 1998. *MMWR Morb Mortal Wkly Rep.* 1999;48:1034–1039.

6. Centers for Disease Control and Prevention. Youth tobacco surveillance—United States, 1998–1999, CDC Surveillance Summaries. *MMWR Morb Mortal Wkly Rep.* 2000;49(SS-10):1–94.

7. Wenger L, Malone R, Bero L. The cigar revival and the popular press: a content analysis, 1987–1997. *Am J Public Health.* 2001;91:288–291.

8. National Cancer Institute. *Cigars: Health Effects and Trends.* Bethesda, Md: Public Health Service; 1998. Smoking and Tobacco Control Monograph, No. 9. NIH publication 98-4302.

9. Feit MN. Exposure of adolescent girls to cigar images in women's magazines, 1992–1998. *Am J Public Health.* 2001;91:286–288.

Validation of School Nurses to Identify Severe Gingivitis in Adolescents

| David Cappelli, DMD, MPH, and John P. Brown, PhD, BDS

This project created a mechanism to identify adolescents with marked gingival disease with a visual screening instrument that can be administered by a school nurse or health care worker. The prevailing paradigm in management of periodontal disease is that plaque removal controls gingivitis,[1] and gingival inflammation is a prerequisite for development of destructive periodontal disease.[2] Prior investigation[3] of a similar population in San Antonio, Tex, showed a high prevalence of severe gingival inflammation. Because school-based interventions are effective in oral health promotion,[4] establishment of an intervention strategy focused on (1) identification of the health problem; (2) referral for diagnosis, treatment, and follow-up; (3) education and counseling about risk behaviors and impediments to access to care; and (4) evaluation of the intervention methods.

Examinations were conducted in a mobile dental van at a middle school located in a predominantly Hispanic and dentally underserved community in the greater San Antonio area. Following a training session in which dentist and nurse were in agreement on the indices, a school nurse visually screened each student with a penlight, tongue depressor, and photographic reference that pictorially identified each visual index category to score the gingival health of each student. Descriptions of the Visual Periodontal Index and the Visual Oral Hygiene Index categories are presented in Table 1. The dentist screened each student independently of the school nurse and conducted a routine dental diagnostic examination. For this study, supragingival plaque,[5] gingival index,[1] and probing depth data were collected on Ramjford teeth[6] with a mirror and Michigan 'O' probe.

This project addressed 3 issues: (1) agreement of the nurse and dentist in the outcome of the visual examination, (2) effectiveness of the screening tool in detecting marked gingival disease, and (3) effectiveness of the screening process determined by referral for treatment. Of the 84 seventh-grade students who were screened, 92.8% were Hispanic and 56.6% were female. One third of the students presented with edematous gingival tissue with gross loss of contour and bleeding along the gingival margin corresponding to a Visual Periodontal Index of 2.

For the Visual Periodontal Index, the level of agreement was 83.33% (P=.00), and for the Visual Oral Hygiene Index, the level of agreement was 87.70% (P=.00), and both κ values indicated good reproducibility (Visual Periodontal Index=0.5794, P<.00; Visual Oral Hygiene Index=0.5006, P<.00), despite the subjectivity of the indexes (Table 2). Comparison of the dentist's visual screening to the clinical examination (Visual Periodontal Index to gingival index[1]; Visual Oral Hygiene Index to supragingival plaque[5]) showed a high level of sensitivity (Visual Periodontal Index=96.23%; Visual Oral Hygiene Index=98.44%) but less specificity (Visual Periodontal Index=50.00%; Visual Oral Hygiene Index=40.00%). Positive predictive value (Visual Periodontal Index=80%; Visual Oral Hygiene Index=66.67%) and negative predictive value (Visual Periodontal Index=86.44%; Visual Oral Hygiene Index=95.45%) indicated that this test was effective in detecting gingivitis in this population. False-negative findings were low (Visual Periodontal Index=3.77%; Visual Oral Hygiene Index=1.56%). The strength of the sensitivity of both visual tests increased the inclusion of cases, although individuals without gingival disease were being referred. Because the outcome of the screening was referral to a dental professional, maximization of the sensitivity at the expense of the specificity was considered an optimal end point.

To determine whether the visual screening examination could accurately identify those individuals who were diagnosed as requiring treatment, the nurse's visual examination was compared with referrals. Both of the nurse's scores were associated with referral (odds ratio [OR] for Visual Periodontal Index=

TABLE 1—Visual Periodontal Index and Visual Oral Hygiene Index Criteria[a]

Category	Description
	Visual Periodontal Index
0	Gum tissue healthy, appearing pink and firm.
1	Swelling and redness of gums next to the tooth surface(s) either localized or generalized.
2	Gum tissue appears bright red, gross loss of contour (form), and/or visible bleeding along gum margin.
	Visual Oral Hygiene Index
0	No plaque or tartar present.
1	Visible plaque and/or tartar in a thin line along the gums, or plaque on a few (isolated) teeth.
2	Visible plaque and/or tartar along the gum line of many teeth. Plaque appears as a thick line.
3	Visible plaque and/or tartar on more than half the surface (copious) of many teeth.

[a]Along with the description, each code was accompanied by a color photographic reference.

TABLE 2—Kappa Statistic Comparing the Accuracy of the School Nurse and Dentist With Visually Identified Gingival Disease

	Agreement, %	Expected Agreement, %	κ	z	P
Visual Periodontal Index	83.33	60.37	0.5794	6.99	.00
Visual Oral Hygiene Index	87.70	75.37	0.5006	6.65	.00

5.94; P=.00; OR for Visual Oral Hygiene Index=5.75; P=.05).

Of the 25 students referred for emergent needs, 5 (20%) either had scheduled an appointment or were seen by a dental professional after 4 months. Seven of the parents or guardians did not intend to schedule a dental visit, and the remainder were lost to follow-up.

Ultimately, the referral of patients with disease is a primary criterion determining the success of any screening program. Correlation to referral suggested that this visual screening examination was successful in the identification of patients with plaque accumulation resulting in gingivitis. The response rate of the parent or guardian to seek additional treatment was low because of the lack of oral health education of both adolescents and parents associated with the screening and other barriers but consistent with previous studies indicating that between 19% and 22% of referred patients seek treatment after screening.[7] Almost all of the parents who did not seek treatment noted access to and availability of a dentist and finances as primary reasons to not obtain treatment. These barriers are high for Mexican American populations.[8] Although a list of low-cost clinics was provided, access for the working parent was problematic because most clinics operate during daytime hours and have prolonged waiting times for appointments.

This screening tool provides the school nurse with defined criteria to identify students with severe gingival inflammation. The surgeon general's report cited disparities in oral health care among minority groups and recommended that nondental professionals participate in oral health promotion.[9] Screening and successful referral, not only for caries but also for early-onset gingival disease, can eliminate progression to frank periodontal disease. With demonstrable associations between periodontal disease and diabetes[10] and the increased prevalence of diabetes in adolescent Hispanic populations, this tool may be even more significant in maintaining overall health into adulthood. ■

About the Authors

The authors are with The University of Texas Health Science Center at San Antonio, Department of Community Dentistry.

Requests for reprints should be sent to David Cappelli, DMD, MPH, The University of Texas Health Science Center at San Antonio, Department of Community Dentistry, 7703 Floyd Curl Dr, San Antonio, TX 78229-3900 (e-mail: cappelli@uthscsa.edu).

This brief was accepted January 10, 2002.

Contributors

D. Cappelli organized the study, conducted the research, analyzed the data, and wrote the paper. J. P. Brown provided administrative and scientific support.

Acknowledgments

This research was supported by a grant from the Health Education Training Center at Texas.

Appreciation is expressed to Julia Garcia, RN, District Health Officer/Edgewood Independent School District, and Rose Garcia, RN, Brentwood Middle School, for their cooperation and support in the accomplishment of this project and the administration of the Edgewood Independent School District, San Antonio, Tex, for their unwavering dedication to the health of their children. Jane Steffensen, MPH, CHES, and Karen Holt, RDH, MS, The University of Texas Health Science Center at San Antonio, are acknowledged for their input and advice, as is Diana Saenz, who assisted with the implementation of this project. Dennis MacMahon, MS, provided statistical advice.

References

1. Loe H, Theilade E, Jensen SB. Experimental gingivitis in man. *J Periodontol.* 1965;36:177–187.

2. Schroeder HE, Attstrom R. Pocket formation: a hypothesis. In: Lehner T, Cimasoni G, eds. *Borderland Between Caries and Periodontal Disease II.* London, England: Academic Press; 1980:99–123.

3. Cappelli D, Ebersole JL, Kornman KS. Early onset periodontitis in Hispanic-American adolescents associated with *A. actinomycetemcomitans. Community Dent Oral Epidemiol.* 1993;22:116–121.

4. Centers for Disease Control and Prevention. Promoting oral health: interventions for preventing dental caries, oral and pharyngeal cancers, and sports-related craniofacial injuries: a report on recommendations of the Task Force on Community Preventive Services. *MMWR Morb Mortal Wkly Rep.* 2001;50(RR-21):11.

5. Silness J, Loe H. Periodontal disease in pregnancy, II: correlation between oral hygiene and periodontal condition. *Acta Odontol Scand.* 1964;22:121–135.

6. Silness J, Reynstrand T. Partial mouth recording of plaque, gingivitis, and probing depth in adolescents. *J Clin Periodontol.* 1988;15:189–192.

7. Harding M, Taylor G. The outcome of school dental screening in two suburban districts of Greater Manchester, UK. *Community Dent Health.* 1993;10: 269–275.

8. Anderson RM, Davidson PL. Ethnicity, aging and oral health outcomes: a conceptual framework. *Adv Dent Res.* 1997;11:203–209.

9. *Oral Health in America: A Report of the Surgeon General.* Rockville, Md: National Institute of Dental and Craniofacial Research, National Institutes of Health; 2000.

10. Loesche WJ. Association of oral flora with important medical diseases. *Curr Opin Periodontol.* 1997;4: 21–28.

Maternal Smoking During Pregnancy and Severe Antisocial Behavior in Offspring: A Review

| Lauren S. Wakschlag, PhD, Kate E. Pickett, PhD, Edwin Cook Jr, MD, Neal L. Benowitz, MD, and Bennett L. Leventhal, MD

Objectives. Recent research suggests that in utero exposure to maternal smoking is a risk factor for conduct disorder and delinquency. We review evidence of causality, a controversial but important public health question.

Methods. We analyzed studies of maternal prenatal smoking and offspring antisocial behavior within a causal framework.

Results. The association is (1) independent of confounders, (2) present across diverse contexts, and (3) consistent with basic science. Methodological limitations of existing studies preclude causal conclusions.

Conclusions. Existing evidence provides consistent support for, but not proof of, an etiologic role for prenatal smoking in the onset of antisocial behavior. The possibility of identifying a preventable prenatal risk factor for a serious mental disorder makes further research on this topic important for public health. (*Am J Public Health.* 2002;92: 966–974)

Smoking during pregnancy represents a major public health problem. Nearly half of all women who smoke continue to do so throughout their pregnancies.[1] As a result, in the United States alone, more than half a million infants per year are prenatally exposed to maternal smoking.[2] It has long been established that maternal smoking during pregnancy has adverse perinatal consequences. Newer evidence suggests that it may have consequences that extend far beyond the perinatal period.[3,4]

Recently, associations between maternal smoking during pregnancy and subsequent mental health problems in offspring have been reported. Specifically, youths whose mothers smoked during pregnancy are significantly more likely to develop severe antisocial behavior, including conduct disorder and delinquency.[5–12] The consistency of findings in studies to date is striking, but their interpretation is less clear. Exposure during pregnancy may play a causal role in the onset of severe antisocial behavior via teratological effects on the fetus. Alternatively, these data may represent a spurious association in that women who smoke during pregnancy have other risk factors that could lead to the development of psychiatric morbidity in their children. This issue bears more careful examination, because modifying the prevalence of exposure could present a rare opportunity to prevent serious psychopathology and reduce the social burden of severe antisocial behavior.[13]

Antisocial behavior, defined as chronic violation of social rules and norms, can have both violent and nonviolent manifestations.[14] When it occurs in a pattern that is severe, chronic, and pervasive, antisocial behavior is categorized as a mental disorder. In youths, severe antisocial behavior is diagnosed as conduct disorder; the adult diagnosis is antisocial personality disorder.[15] Delinquency, in contrast, is the legal system's way of conceptualizing antisocial behavior that is subject to adjudication. Delinquency involves commission of an illegal act, at times including criminal conviction. Delinquent behavior and conduct disorder symptoms are viewed as manifestations of the same underlying difficulty in modulating behavior and conforming to social norms.[14] However, as with criteria for any behaviorally defined disorder (and in contrast to disorders for which a biological marker exists), diagnostic criteria and criminal records are imperfect proxies for severe antisocial behavior.

Severe antisocial behavior is a substantial public health problem because of its prevalence, the significant associated economic and social costs, and the increased morbidity and mortality of individuals with an antisocial history.[13,16,17] Conduct disorder is one of the most severe mental disorders of childhood and the most frequent reason for referral to mental health clinics for mental health assessment and treatment. Prevalence estimates from a review of international studies range from 1% to 16%, and prevalence is higher in boys.[18]

The idea that an individual's long-term mental health and social adjustment might be constrained by exposure to maternal smoking prenatally may seem overly deterministic. However, increasing evidence shows that early life events, such as prenatal trauma, exposures, and deprivations, have a long-lasting influence on development and health.[19–24] The evidence linking maternal smoking during pregnancy with antisocial behavior in adolescent and adult offspring, which has been reported largely within the psychiatric and teratological literature, has not been critically examined from a public health perspective. Our objective in this article is to analyze existing studies within an epidemiological framework.

METHODS

MEDLINE and PsychINFO were searched to identify all studies published before June 2001 that examined the association between maternal smoking during pregnancy and severe antisocial behavior in offspring. Search terms were *maternal smoking, pregnancy,* and *prenatal exposure* and either *child behavior disorders, behavior problems, conduct disorder, delinquency,* or *antisocial personality disorder or behavior.* Relevant articles also were identified via consultation with experts in the field and review of references cited in all published studies. For the causal analysis, *severe antisocial behavior* was defined as either (1) presence of conduct disorder symptoms or receipt of a conduct disorder diagnosis, reflecting a clinically significant pattern of antisocial

TABLE 1—Review of Studies of Maternal Smoking During Pregnancy and Severe Antisocial Behavior in Offspring

Study[a]	Design	Sample	Measurement of Exposure	Exposed, %	Measurement of Outcome	Main Outcomes (Adjusted)
			Studies of conduct disorder (CD)			
Wakschlag et al.[9]	Clinic-based case-control	177 males (7–17 y), Georgia and Pennsylvania	Retrospective, self-report: "How much did you smoke during pregnancy?"	37	CD by diagnostic interview, multiple time points	OR for CD in boys = 3.3 (> ½ pack/day)
Fergusson et al.[6]	Population-based prospective cohort	1265 males and females (18 y), New Zealand	Self-report at birth: "How much did you smoke during pregnancy (each trimester)?"	32	CD symptoms by diagnostic interview	Linear increase in boys' mean CD score as exposure increased: 0.48 for nonexposed, 0.76 for < ½ pack/day, 1.04 for ≥ ½ pack/day, 1.32 for ≥ pack/day
Weissman et al.[12]	Offspring of case-control study of maternal depression	147 males and females (17–36 y), New York	Retrospective, self-report: "Did you ever smoke more than ½ pack/day during pregnancy?"	34	CD by diagnostic interview	RR for male early-onset CD = 4.1 (≥ ½ pack/day)
Wakschlag and Keenan[10]	Clinic-based case-control	129 males and females (2-5 y), Chicago, Ill	Retrospective, self-report: "How much did you smoke during pregnancy?"	23	ODD and CD symptoms by diagnostic interview	Mean ODD and CD score was 1.54 higher for exposed vs nonexposed
			Studies of criminal offending			
Brennan et al.[5]	Population-based prospective cohort	4169 males (34 y), Denmark	Prospective, self-report, while pregnant: "How much have you been smoking daily during the third trimester?"	51	Arrest history from national criminal register	OR for male persistent offending = 1.5, OR for male violent offending = 1.7 (> ½ pack/day)[b]
Rasanen et al.[8] (see also Rantakallio et al.[104])	Population-based prospective cohort	3883 males (16 y), Finland	Prospective, self-report, while pregnant: "Have you been smoking daily during pregnancy?"	16	Criminal offense from national criminal register	OR for male recidivism = 2.4, OR for male violent offending = 2.1 (any exposure)
Gibson et al.[33] (see also Gibson and Tibbetts[7,100])	Population-based prospective cohort	200 males and females (17 y), Philadelphia, Pa	Prospective, self-report: "How much have you been smoking daily during pregnancy?"	50	Age at first police contact from city police records	OR for early-onset offending = 2.6 for boys and 3.5 for girls (> ½ pack/day)[b]

Note. OR = odds ratio; RR = relative risk; ODD = oppositional defiant disorder.
[a]Related findings from the same cohort that have been reported in multiple articles are represented only once in this review.
[b]Calculated from data presented by the authors.

behavior based on diagnostic measures, or (2) a history of delinquency or antisocial behavior as measured via records of criminal offending. Table 1 summarizes studies that met inclusion criteria. The findings of studies that used nonspecific checklist ratings of child behavior problems rather than measures of more severe antisocial behavior are generally consistent with those presented here and are reviewed elsewhere.[3,25]

RESULTS OF CRITICAL ANALYSIS OF STUDIES

Temporality

Because fetuses do not develop conduct disorder in utero, intrauterine cigarette smoke exposure clearly precedes the disorder. Although this sequence is a necessary condition for causality, recognizing it adds little to our understanding of possible causal pathways, because the exposure precedes the outcome by a period of many years and may involve the interaction of exposure-related vulnerabilities with multiple other perinatal and postnatal risk factors.

Strength of Association

The association between maternal smoking during pregnancy and severe antisocial behavior is moderate. The odds of developing severe antisocial behavior are approximately 1.5 to 4 times greater for exposed than for nonexposed youths (Table 1).

Accurate estimation of the strength of this association is significantly constrained, however, by limitations of exposure measurement in research to date. Virtually no studies have used repeated, prospective measures of exposure. Many women stop smoking spontaneously when they learn that they are pregnant, but others quit, reduce, and relapse multiple times during pregnancy.[26] Thus, relying on measurement of exposure at a single time point often will not accurately characterize history of exposure. Furthermore, as can be seen in Table 1, characterization of exposure has varied widely in existing studies (e.g., "ever smoked" vs "smoked ½ pack/day or more"). Existing studies also have relied exclusively on self-reported smoking. In the absence of biological measurement of exposure, error is likely because of nondisclosure and underreporting. Self-reported cigarettes per day is also a relatively crude measure of exposure, because variations in smoking topography and metabolism result in differential exposure for the same "amount smoked."[27–29] Cotinine (a biomarker of tobacco exposure detectable in plasma, urine, and saliva) is a more precise measure of fetal exposure than maternal report.[30–32]

For these reasons, substantial misclassification of exposure in existing studies is likely, although the effects of such misclassification are unclear. The reported association may be underestimated because social sanctions against smoking during pregnancy increase the likelihood that smokers will not report truthfully. Such nondisclosure would tend to attenuate the effect, because it would lead to misclassification of exposed youth as nonexposed. Conversely, pregnant smokers with an antisocial history may be more likely to report smoking, because they presumably are less concerned about social norms than are pregnant smokers without an antisocial history. In this case, lack of inhibition might lead to artificial inflation of the association, because youths classified as exposed would be more likely to have other risk factors (e.g., hereditary factors) for conduct disorder.

Consistency

Studies of male offspring of mothers who smoked during pregnancy are notable for the consistency of their findings despite differing designs and populations. These studies have included clinic and community populations as well as populations at high risk for psychiatric disorders.[6,9,12,33] Because conduct disorder and criminal offending are overlapping constructs, we would expect—and, indeed, we observe—a similar pattern of effects for both types of outcomes. This consistency is in contrast to the absence of a systematic pattern of behavioral effects of exposure to illicit drugs, particularly cocaine.[34,35]

The apparent consistency may be due to the presence of similar methodological flaws in all of the existing studies. For example, although some of the studies controlled for maternal antisocial behavior, the extent to which maternal antisocial behavior overlaps with smoking status was not reported. If all of the mothers with an antisocial history were smokers, statistical control alone would be inadequate to separate these effects.

Studies are inconsistent in regard to possible behavioral effects in female offspring. Prenatal exposure to maternal smoking is not associated with increased relative risk (RR) of conduct disorder in girls.[6,11,12] However, several limitations of outcome measurement in studies to date make these negative findings difficult to interpret. First, conduct disorder is less prevalent in girls, and as a result, existing studies may have inadequate power to detect effects. In addition, the *Diagnostic and Statistical Manual of Mental Disorders, Fourth Edition (DSM-IV)*, diagnoses of conduct disorder and antisocial personality disorder capture only the extreme end of the spectrum of antisocial behavior, especially in girls.[36] Because rates of offending are much lower in females than in males, sample size issues also have led to the exclusion of females in all but 1 existing study of offending.[33] In this study, the odds of early-onset offending were actually comparable in boys and girls.[33] A second limitation of outcome measurement in existing studies is that whereas behavioral effects may manifest differently in boys and girls, sex differences in the pattern of effects have not been systematically examined. For example, conduct problems may take different forms for males and females (e.g., rape vs early unprotected sex), but *DSM-IV* criteria for conduct disorder are based primarily on male manifestations.[37,38]

Possible support for differential manifestations by sex may be found in the inconsistent findings to date on the relation of prenatal nicotine exposure to subsequent development of attention deficit–hyperactivity disorder.[9,39,40] Some of the studies in which exposure was found to be associated with attention deficit–hyperactivity disorder included girls[12,40] (e.g., RR of attention deficit–hyperactivity disorder in girls=2.16 vs RR=0.44 in boys),[12] whereas several of the studies in which attention deficit–hyperactivity disorder was not found to be associated with exposure consisted of boys only.[9,41]

Exposure may have a *lesser or minimal effect* on girls. Some evidence from animal studies indicates that males are more vulnerable to negative effects of prenatal exposure to nicotine.[42] Also, there may be no sex differences in the *original* behavioral vulnerabilities associated with exposure, but the *long-term* effect of these vulnerabilities may differ for girls and boys.[11] Clearly, more systematic examination of sex differences is needed, including use of large, population-based samples and measurement of a wide range of outcomes.

Specificity

In boys, the association of prenatal exposure to maternal smoking with psychiatric morbidity appears to be specific to antisocial behavior. Such exposure is unrelated to other disturbances of mental health and adjustment, such as mood or anxiety disorders.[6,9,12] In both clinic and community samples, studies that have examined the association between maternal smoking during pregnancy and conduct disorder relative to other psychiatric disorders in offspring found that exposure was specifically associated with conduct disorder.[6,9,12]

A major shortcoming of existing studies is that measurement of outcomes has been cross-sectional. As a result, we do not know anything about the developmental progression of conduct symptoms in youths with prenatal exposure. Existing diagnostic studies of exposed youths either have been clinic-based or have used samples of older children, who are already in the risk period for the development of conduct disorder. Most children who develop early-onset conduct disorder have a long history of behavior problems (e.g., temperamental difficulties as infants, oppositional defiant disorder as younger children) before manifesting a full-blown disorder or committing a delinquent act.[43,44] Thus, a specific causal pathway might include early symptoms of oppositional defiant disorder followed by the development of conduct disorder in adolescence. Recently, maternal smoking during pregnancy has been linked with oppositional defiant disorder symptoms in young children.[10,41,45] Also, preliminary evidence from studies of older youths shows that exposure is associated with early- rather than adolescent-onset conduct problems.[12,33] However, longitudinal research is needed to establish whether there is a specific and coherent pathway of exposure-related behavioral effects over time. Longitudinal data are also critical for testing whether there are specific behavioral effects of exposure or whether these are secondary to other perinatal and neurodevelopmental effects of maternal smoking.[46,47]

Dose–Response Relationship

There is preliminary evidence of a dose–response relationship from studies that have shown a linear relationship between number of cigarettes smoked and percentage of offspring with severe antisocial behavior.[5] There is also evidence of dose–response effects from animal studies.[48] To adequately confirm evidence of a dose–response relationship, precision in measurement of exposure is critical. The possibility that the shape of the dose–response curve is nonlinear has not been examined. No existing studies of the association between smoking during pregnancy and severe antisocial behavior in offspring have used measures of exposure sufficient to establish the existence—much less the shape—of a dose–response curve. Current evidence is insufficient to allow us to establish a threshold above which adverse behavioral effects might become clinically relevant.

Cessation of Exposure (Experimental Evidence)

Although exposure cannot be experimentally manipulated in humans, proving that cessation or reduction of exposure decreases risk to offspring would add substantial weight to a causal argument. One approach would be to compare outcomes of children whose mothers have a smoking history but did not smoke during pregnancy ("spontaneous quitters") with those of children whose mothers are persistent smokers.[49] One limitation of this approach is that women who are able to quit are likely to differ from women who are not, along precisely those psychological and psychiatric dimensions that may underlie the apparent exposure effect. For example, persistent smokers are more likely to have a history of conduct symptoms, less likely to have stable home environments, and more likely to have problematic relationships.[50]

Although women cannot be randomized to smoking and nonsmoking conditions, another strategy would be to follow the offspring of participants randomized to receive prenatal smoking cessation interventions.[51] However, current smoking cessation interventions are successful in only a minority of women.[52] The types of factors that reduce the likelihood that a woman will benefit from the intervention are the same factors that increase the risk of offspring conduct problems.[53] As a result, such studies cannot fully separate cessation effects from maternal characteristics that influence smoking behavior and, therefore, may provide biased estimates.

Biological Plausibility

Because true experimental evidence in humans cannot be obtained, findings from basic science are critically important for establishing causality.[25,54] Substantial evidence indicates that nicotine crosses the placental barrier and that smoking during pregnancy is associated with fetal neurotoxicity.[55] Neurotoxic effects are hypothesized to occur via (1) hypoxic effects on the fetal–placental unit (e.g., reduction of fetal blood flow) and (2) teratological effects on the developing fetal nervous system.[42] Animal research has established that in utero exposure to nicotine has enduring effects on neural function.[54] Although intrauterine exposure to maternal smoking involves exposure to many toxins, most evidence points to carbon monoxide and nicotine as the key neurobehavioral teratogens.[56–59]

Nicotine acts primarily through its action on nicotinic acetylcholine receptors.[25] Nicotinic receptors are present early in gestation, which suggests that nicotinic signaling plays a key role in neural development.[25] The fetal brain is protected against many neurotoxins, but it is exquisitely vulnerable to exogenous nicotine because it contains specific nicotine-sensitive receptors.[54] Continuous patterns of maternal smoking behavior (i.e., the tendency to smoke in a manner that maintains plasma nicotine levels at a steady state) also are likely to heighten the adverse effects of exogenous nicotine on the fetal brain, in contrast to the more episodic pattern of illicit drug use, which allows for central nervous system recovery.[54] This exogenous stimulation of nicotinic acetylcholine receptors in the immature nervous system interacts with the genes that direct differentiation of cells, thereby causing permanent alterations in cell functioning.[25,54] Exposure also has been shown to disrupt developmental actions of hormones and to interfere with processes related to sexual dimorphism of the brain, which may explain apparent sex differences in effects.[12,42]

In animals, demonstrated effects of prenatal exposure to nicotine and carbon monoxide include structural (e.g., abnormalities of cell differentiation), neuroregulatory (e.g., disruptions in neurotransmitter activity), and neurobehavioral (e.g., hyperactivity, deficits in arousal modulation) deficits.[48,54,60–62] In human infants, prenatal exposure to cigarette smoke also has been associated with early neurotoxic effects.[63]

The evidence that cigarette smoke constituents are behavioral teratogens fulfills the criterion of biological plausibility but is not sufficient proof that exposure to cigarette smoke in humans *causes* a disorder as complex and multifaceted as conduct disorder.

Consideration of Alternative Explanations

The greatest challenge in establishing whether prenatal exposure actually has a teratological effect is ruling out the possibility that the apparent effects are caused by confounding. Many obvious potential confounders have been statistically controlled in published studies (Table 2). Statistical control for a wide range of empirically and theoretically derived confounders has not appreciably al-

TABLE 2—Testing of Primary Alternative Explanations in Existing Studies

Study	Sociodemographic Factors	Parental Psychiatric Factors[a]	Parenting and Quality of Home Environment Factors[b]	Perinatal and Child Factors
Wakschlag et al.[9]	Maternal age SES Marital status Ethnicity	Antisocial personality Substance abuse	Discipline, communication, supervision	Exposure to illicit drugs or alcohol Pregnancy or birth complications Low birthweight
Fergusson et al.[6]	Maternal age SES Maternal education	Offending Substance abuse	Responsiveness (age 3) Parental conflict Youth report of: Parental physical discipline History of child abuse	Exposure to illicit drugs or alcohol Unplanned pregnancy
Weissman et al.[12]	Maternal age SES Marital status Ethnicity No. of children	Antisocial personality Substance abuse Depression Anxiety	Parental conflict Marital adjustment Youth report of: Family cohesion	Exposure to alcohol or caffeine Pregnancy or birth complications Low birthweight Environmental tobacco smoke
Wakschlag and Keenan[10]	Maternal age Public aid recipient Marital status Ethnicity	Maternal antisocial personality Offending Maternal depression	Observed responsiveness Harsh discipline Parenting stress and support	Low birthweight IQ
Brennan et al.[5]	Maternal age SES	Paternal offending Psychiatric hospitalization	Rejection (age 1)	Exposure to prescription drugs Pregnancy or birth complications
Rasanen et al.[8]	Maternal age SES Marital status	Maternal depression	...	Exposure to illicit drugs or alcohol Pregnancy or birth complications Unplanned pregnancy Infant developmental status
Gibson et al.[33]	Maternal age SES	...	Unstable home environment	Pregnancy or birth complications Low birthweight IQ

Note. SES = socioeconomic status.
[a]Measured for both parents, unless noted.
[b]Measured concurrently with outcome and by maternal report, unless noted.

tered associations between smoking during pregnancy and offspring antisocial behavior. However, in addition to the potential for as-yet-unmeasured confounders,[64–66] statistical control alone does not rule out the possibility of residual confounding.[67]

Three primary alternative explanations have been proposed:

1. *Confounding by social class.* Women who smoke are more likely than nonsmokers to be of low socioeconomic status,[68] which is associated with increased risk of antisocial behavior.[69] Although virtually all existing studies have controlled for some socioeconomic factors, socioeconomic status is likely to be both a strong confounder and poorly measured. The potential for residual confounding is therefore great. The association of maternal smoking during pregnancy and offspring behavior problems has been reported in Yugoslavia, a country where smoking and social class are positively associated, the reverse of the situation in the United States.[70] The association also has been replicated in samples with more uniform socioeconomic status distributions.[10,11,33]

2. *Confounding by parental psychiatric history.* Women with mental health problems are more likely to smoke than are healthy women, and their children are at increased risk for antisocial behavior.[71] This increased risk is the result of both genetic and environmental factors. In terms of possible genetic confounding, parental antisocial history has been controlled in all clinical studies but in only 1 of the existing studies of offending. Even in those studies that controlled for antisocial history, there may be substantial error in these measures because of (1) heavy reliance on maternal report of *paternal* antisocial behavior, (2) underestimation of parental antisocial behavior when measures of parental offending are used, and (3) limitations of diagnostic measures for capturing manifestations of conduct problems in women.[37]

Broadening assessment of familial risk to a wider range of traits might address some of these methodological issues.[72] However, even robust and varied measures of antisocial behavior may contain substantial error, because there are still no pathognomonic markers by which conduct disorder and antisocial personality disorder can be diagnosed with certainty.[73,74] For this reason, statistical control alone is insufficient to rule out the hypothesis of genetic confounding. Family studies that more directly assess contributions of heritability and environment (e.g., comparisons of siblings discordant for in utero exposure or twin-study designs in which some twin pairs have been exposed and some have not) would more clearly disaggregate contributions of exposure and of genetic factors in the development of offspring antisocial behavior.[64,74,75]

However, examining the question of genetic and teratological contributions to the development of antisocial behavior in offspring as an "either/or" issue is probably too simplistic. One possibility is that the "true" effect is neither wholly teratological nor solely genetic, but rather an interaction of these 2 processes. Current evidence on the genesis of psychiatric disorders supports a model in which susceptibility genes increase vulnerability but lead to disorder only in interaction with other environmental and biological factors (e.g., prenatal toxins).[74,76]

Parental psychiatric history also may be an environmental confounding factor because of the deleterious effects of parental psychopathology on the family environment.[77,78] For example, smoking and depression are associated, and depression is a barrier to quitting, particularly for women.[79,80] Women who are depressed are more likely to provide problematic parenting and to have marital discord, both of which are associated with increased risk of offspring behavior problems.[78] Several studies of maternal smoking and offspring conduct problems (including 1 study in which clinically depressed women were oversampled) have controlled for maternal depression.[9,12]

3. *Confounding by quality of family environment.* Women who smoke are more likely to provide inconsistent, harsh discipline and unresponsive parenting.[49,81,82] These same factors have been associated with the development of antisocial behavior in youth.[77,83] Virtually all of the existing studies have controlled for the quality of parenting and the home environment in some way. This control has not appreciably altered the association. However, a major limitation is that parenting generally has been measured via self-report, often concurrently with conduct problems. Proxy measures of poor-quality care, which are likely to contain substantial error, also have been used.[5] Observational measures of parenting provide a more objective assessment of the caregiving environment, and we have recently shown that exposure effects are independent of the observed quality of parenting.[10,11] Paternal behavior has not been directly assessed. Future studies should consider a wider range of family environmental factors (e.g., parenting stress, exposure to family violence).

One other important issue that has been examined only cursorily in these studies is that of separating the effects of prenatal smoking from the effects of postnatal exposure to environmental tobacco smoke. This is difficult to do, because prenatal smoking and environmental tobacco smoke are highly collinear. Environmental tobacco smoke exposure has been associated with neurodevelopmental and milder behavior problems (for a review, see Eskenazi and Castorina[84]) but not with severe antisocial behavior.

Consistency With Other Knowledge (Coherence)

The possibility that maternal smoking may play a causal role in the development of antisocial behavior in offspring is consistent with existing knowledge that prenatal insults and exposures have long-term adverse effects on health.[20,24,85] For example, exposure to wartime famine during pregnancy has been associated with increased risk of antisocial personality disorder,[86] and long-term behavioral effects have been found in the case of prenatal alcohol and lead exposure.[87] On the other hand, as discussed earlier, long-term behavioral effects of fetal exposure to cocaine have not been seen.

DISCUSSION

The body of existing evidence is consistently supportive, but certainly not definitive proof, of an etiologic role for prenatal exposure to nicotine in the onset of severe antisocial behavior in offspring. Published studies yield no evidence that is incompatible with a causal explanation for this association. These studies must be viewed as preliminary (because of the methodological limitations detailed above), but the cumulative evidence is provocative and sufficiently compelling to make further research in this area a matter of public health interest. Estimates of smoking-attributable risk for conduct problems suggest that if a causal relationship were established, the public health burden would be substantial.[4,88] Even if a modest effect were to be established, this would be significant because of the high prevalence of conduct disorder and delinquency.

Cigarette smoke is a powerful toxin for a broad spectrum of the population. There is little doubt that it is a risk factor for cancer and cardiovascular disease.[89] Similarly, it is widely accepted that intrauterine exposure to the constituents of cigarette smoke adversely affects fetal development, including birthweight and respiratory function.[89] This knowledge leads to the obvious question: Why is it important to invest further effort in establishing yet another problematic outcome of maternal smoking? We would answer this question by noting that once antisocial behavior has developed, it is highly persistent and difficult to treat.[90] Identified risk factors (e.g., low socioeconomic status, unstable family structure, and parental psychopathology) are often chronic and difficult to modify.

Future research must move beyond replication of these findings in different samples[91] toward more explicit attempts at refutation in studies specifically designed to test causality. Most critical for answering the question posed at the outset of this article—*Does maternal smoking during pregnancy cause severe antisocial behavior in offspring?*—is a program of research that (1) measures exposure with precision; (2) uses study designs that can separate risk factors associated with being a maternal smoker from exposure per se; (3) follows up exposed youths from infancy through adolescence to identify early exposure-related behavioral vulnerabilities and factors that determine whether these result in adverse behavioral outcomes over time; and (4) combines both observational and basic science approaches. Fundamental to this endeavor is the modeling and testing of specific causal pathways. A teratological effect may be direct or indirect. For example, a direct effect might occur via alterations in neurotransmitter systems that interfere with modulation of arousal (e.g., dopaminergic systems).[25] In contrast, the increased risk of antisocial behavior in exposed youths may be secondary to other exposure-related problems. For example, the increased risk of conduct problems in exposed youths might occur indirectly via effects of maternal smoking on birthweight and perinatal problems[46] and neuropsychological difficulties,[47] all of which increase the risk for later antisocial behavior.[92,93]

This article highlights the challenges and complexities of establishing a causal path from a perinatal event to a disorder that emerges sometimes decades later.[20] These challenges are not specific to prenatal exposure to maternal smoking and offspring antisocial behavior. Rather, they reflect the more general challenges of establishing causal pathways from risk factors operative during the first few years of life to pathological processes manifesting decades later.[94]

Most psychiatric syndromes are the result of complex causal chains involving genetic and other biological factors, proximal environmental factors, and distal social risk factors.[95] The lengthy time from perinatal exposure to the development of disorder makes it particularly difficult to establish causal pathways, especially because the ways in which risk factors work together are very complex, and the many intervening factors make it difficult to isolate effects of a single, specific factor. In addition, children are born with behavioral susceptibilities to a psychiatric disorder rather than the disorder itself.[74,96] Thus, establishing coherent temporal pathways is fundamental to establishing for whom and how these susceptibilities actually lead to disorder. This objective requires articulating developmental models that identify age-specific manifestations of vulnerabilities and dysfunction,[97] an area of science that is just emerging.[98,99]

Accurate identification of "caseness" is fundamental to establishing etiologic pathways, yet existing methods of classification do not fully capture the wide variation in phenotypic expression of psychiatric disorder.[74] In addition, potential effect modifiers must be identified and tested,[5,11,100] a daunting task because of the vast array of relevant risk factors and the fact that salient risks may be different in different developmental periods.[101]

The importance of this area of research extends far beyond the specific question at hand, which in turn provides a unique opportunity to develop and test etiologic pathways that can serve as a paradigm for broader research, because (1) there are well-quantified methods for measuring prenatal exposure to maternal smoking,[102] (2) a consistent association to a specific psychiatric disorder has been established, and (3) early manifestations of conduct problems emerge in the first few years of life.[103] For these reasons, the study of the long-term effects of maternal smoking holds much promise for informing our understanding of how insults to the developing brain affect early behavior and how the effects of such insults interact with contextual factors over time in the etiology of psychiatric disorders. ■

About the Authors

Lauren S. Wakschlag, Edwin Cook, and Bennett L. Leventhal are with the Department of Psychiatry, University of Chicago, Chicago, Ill. Kate E. Pickett is with the Departments of Health Studies and Obstetrics and Gynecology, University of Chicago, Chicago, Ill. Neal L. Benowitz is with the Division of Clinical Pharmacology and Experimental Therapeutics, Department of Medicine and Biopharmaceutical Sciences, University of California, San Francisco.

Requests for reprints should be sent to Lauren S. Wakschlag, PhD, University of Chicago, Department of Psychiatry, MC3077, 5841 S Maryland, Chicago, IL 60637 (e-mail: laurie@yoda.bsd.uchicago.edu).

This article was accepted December 14, 2001.

Contributors

L.S. Wakschlag and K.E. Pickett conducted the review of studies and placed them within the causal framework. All authors contributed to the conceptualization and writing of the article.

Acknowledgments

The writing of this article was supported in part by grants from the National Institute on Drug Abuse (K08 DA00330 to L.S. Wakschlag; DA02277 and DA01696 to N.L. Benowitz), the National Institute of Mental Health (K02 MH01389 to E. Cook), and the Walden and Jean Young Shaw Foundation and the Irving B. Harris Center for Developmental Studies to the Department of Psychiatry, University of Chicago.

References

1. Ebrahim S, Floyd L, Merritt R, Decoufle P, Holtzman D. Trends in pregnancy-related smoking rates in the United States, 1987–1996. *JAMA.* 2000;283:361–366.

2. Smith B, Martin J, Ventura S. *Births and Deaths: Preliminary Data for July 1997–June, 1998.* Hyattsville, Md: National Center for Health Statistics; 1999. Report 25.

3. Olds D. Tobacco exposure and impaired development: a review of the evidence. *Ment Retard Dev Disabil Res Rev.* 1997;3:257–269.

4. Wakschlag L, Leventhal B, Cook E Jr, Pickett K. Intergenerational health consequences of maternal smoking. *Econ Neurosci.* 2000;2:47–54.

5. Brennan P, Grekin E, Mednick S. Maternal smoking during pregnancy and adult male criminal outcomes. *Arch Gen Psychiatry.* 1999;56:215–219.

6. Fergusson D, Woodward L, Horwood L. Maternal smoking during pregnancy and psychiatric adjustment in late adolescence. *Arch Gen Psychiatry.* 1998;55:721–727.

7. Gibson C, Tibbetts S. Interaction between maternal cigarette smoking and Apgar scores in predicting offending behavior. *Psychol Rep.* 1998;83:579–586.

8. Rasanen P, Hakko H, Isohanni M, Hodgins S, Jarvelin MR, Tiihonen J. Maternal smoking during pregnancy and risk of criminal behavior among adult male offspring in the Northern Finland 1966 Birth Cohort. *Am J Psychiatry.* 1999;156:857–862.

9. Wakschlag L, Lahey B, Loeber R, Green S, Gordon R, Leventhal B. Maternal smoking during pregnancy and the risk of conduct disorder in boys. *Arch Gen Psychiatry.* 1997;54:670–676.

10. Wakschlag L, Keenan K. Clinical significance and correlates of disruptive behavior symptoms in environmentally at-risk preschoolers. *J Clin Child Psychol.* 2001;30:262–275.

11. Wakschlag L, Hans S. Maternal smoking during pregnancy and conduct problems in high-risk youth: a developmental framework. *Dev Psychopathol.* 2002;14:351–369.

12. Weissman M, Warner V, Wickramaratne P, Kandel D. Maternal smoking during pregnancy and psychopathology in offspring followed to adulthood. *J Am Acad Child Adolesc Psychiatry.* 1999;38:892–899.

13. Potter L, Mercy J. Public health perspectives on interpersonal violence among youth in the United States. In: Stoff D, Breiling R, Maser J, eds. *Handbook of Antisocial Behavior.* New York, NY: John Wiley & Sons; 1997:3–11.

14. Hinshaw S, Zupan B. Assessment of antisocial behavior in children and adolescents. In: Stoff D, Breiling J, Maser J, eds. *Handbook of Antisocial Behavior.* New York, NY: John Wiley & Sons; 1997:36–50.

15. *Diagnostic and Statistical Manual of Mental Disorders, Fourth Edition.* Washington, DC: American Psychiatric Association; 1994.

16. Bardone A, Moffitt T, Caspi A, Dickson N, Silva P. Adult mental health and social outcomes of adolescent girls with depression and conduct disorder. *Dev Psychopathol.* 1996;8:811–830.

17. Pajer K. What happens to "bad" girls? A review of the adult outcomes of antisocial adolescent girls. *Am J Psychiatry.* 1998;155:862–870.

18. Lahey B, Miller T, Gordon R, Riley A. Developmental epidemiology of the disruptive behavior disorders. In: Quay H, Hogan A, eds. *Handbook of Disruptive*

Behavior Disorders. New York, NY: Plenum Press; 1999:23–48.

19. Anand K, Scalzo F. Can adverse neonatal experiences alter brain development and subsequent behavior? *Biol Neonate*. 2000;77:69–82.

20. Gillman MW, Rich-Edwards JW. The fetal origin of adult disease: from sceptic to convert. *Paediatr Perinat Epidemiol*. 2000;14:192–193.

21. Glaser D. Child abuse and neglect and the brain—a review. *J Child Psychol Psychiatry*. 2000;41:97–116.

22. Graham Y, Heim C, Goddman S, Miller A, Nemeroff C. The effects of neonatal stress on brain development: implications for psychopathology. *Dev Psychopathol*. 1999;11:545–567.

23. Osmond C, Barker D. Fetal, infant and childhood growth are predictors of coronary heart disease, diabetes, and hypertension in adult men and women. *Environ Health Perspect*. 2000;108(suppl 3):545–553.

24. Watson J, Mednick S, Huttunen M, Wang X. Prenatal teratogens and the development of adult mental illness. *Dev Psychopathol*. 1999;11:457–466.

25. Ernst M, Moolchan E, Robinson M. Behavioral and neural consequences of prenatal exposure to nicotine. *J Am Acad Child Adolesc Psychiatry*. 2001;40:630–642.

26. Pickett K, Wakschlag L, Leventhal B. Maternal smoking during pregnancy: not a stable phenomenon. *Paediatr Perinat Epidemiol*. 2001;15:A27.

27. Dempsey D, Jacob III P, Benowitz NL. Accelerated metabolism of nicotine and cotinine in pregnant smokers. *J Pharmacol Exp Ther*. In press.

28. Haddow H, Knight G, Palomaki G. Measuring serum cotinine to aid in smoking cessation during pregnancy and to enhance assessment of smoking-related fetal morbidity. In: Poswillo D, Alberman E, eds. *Effects of Smoking on the Fetus, Neonate and Child*. Oxford, England: Oxford University Press; 1992:207–222.

29. Zacny JP, Stitzer ML. Cigarette brand-switching: effects on smoke exposure and smoking behavior. *J Pharmacol Exp Ther*. 1988;246:619–627.

30. Benowitz N. Biomarkers of environmental tobacco smoke exposure. *Environ Health Perspect*. 1999;107(suppl):349–355.

31. Dempsey D, Hanjnal B, Partridge J, et al. Tone abnormalities are associated with maternal smoking during pregnancy in in utero cocaine-exposed infants. *Pediatrics*. 2000;106:79–85.

32. Wang X, Tager I, Van Vunakis H, Sperizer F, Hanrahan J. Maternal smoking during pregnancy, urine cotinine concentrations, and birth outcomes. A prospective cohort study. *Int J Epidemiol*. 1997;26:978–987.

33. Gibson C, Piquero A, Tibbets S. Assessing the relationship between maternal cigarette smoking during pregnancy and age at first police contact. *Justice Q*. 2000;17:519–542.

34. Frank D, Augustyn M, Grant K, Pell T, Zuckerman B. Growth, development and behavior in early childhood following prenatal cocaine exposure: a systematic review. *JAMA*. 2001;285:1613–1625.

35. Hans S. Prenatal drug exposure: behavioral functioning in late childhood and adolescence. In: Wetherington C, Smeriglio V, Finnegan L, eds. *Behavioral Studies of Drug-Exposed Offspring: Methodological Issues in Human and Animal Research*. Rockville, Md: US Dept of Health and Human Services; 1996;164:261–276. Research Monograph 114, National Institute on Drug Abuse Monograph Series.

36. Zoccolillo M, Tremblay R, Vitaro F. DSM-III-R and DSM-III criteria for conduct disorder in preadolescent girls: specific but insensitive. *J Am Acad Child Adolesc Psychiatry*. 1996;35:461–470.

37. Wakschlag L, Gordon R, Lahey B, Loeber R, Green S, Leventhal B. Maternal age at first birth and boys' risk of conduct disorder. *J Res Adolescence*. 2000;10:417–441.

38. Zoccolillo M. Gender and the development of conduct disorder. *Dev Psychopathol*. 1993;1–2:65–78.

39. Milberger S, Biederman J, Faraone SV, Chen L, Jones J. Is maternal smoking during pregnancy a risk factor for attention deficit hyperactivity disorder in children? *Am J Psychiatry*. 1996;153:1138–1142.

40. Milberger S, Biederman J, Faraone S, Jones J. Further evidence of an association between maternal smoking during pregnancy and attention deficit hyperactivity disorder: findings from a high-risk sample of siblings. *J Clin Child Psychol*. 1998;27:352–358.

41. Pickett K, Wakschlag L, Loeber R, Stouhamer-Loeber L, Lahey B, Leventhal B. Multigenerational effects of maternal smoking during pregnancy. Paper presented at: Annual Meeting of the American Public Health Association; November 2000; Boston, Mass.

42. Lichtensteiger W, Schlumpf M. Prenatal nicotine exposure: biochemical and neuroendocrine bases of behavioral dysfunction. *Dev Brain Dysfunct*. 1993;6:279–304.

43. Lahey B, Waldman I, McBurnett K. The development of antisocial behavior: an integrative causal model. *J Child Psychol Psychiatry*. 1999;40:669–682.

44. Loeber R, Farrington D. Young children who commit crime: epidemiology, developmental origins, risk factors, early interventions and policy implications. *Dev Psychopathol*. 2000;12:737–763.

45. Day NL, Richardson GA, Goldschmidt L, Cornelius MD. Effects of prenatal tobacco exposure on preschoolers' behavior. *J Dev Behav Pediatr*. 2000;21:180–188.

46. Walsh R. Effects of maternal smoking on adverse pregnancy outcomes: examination of the criteria of causation. *Hum Biol*. 1994;66:1059–1092.

47. Fried P, Watkinson B, Gray R. Differential effects on cognitive functioning in 9 to 12 year olds prenatally exposed to cigarettes and marijuana. *Neurotoxicol Teratol*. 1997;20:293–306.

48. Ankarberg E, Fredriksoon A, Eriksson P. Neurobehavioral defects in adult mice neonatally exposed to nicotine: changes in nicotine-induced behavior and maze learning performance. *Behav Brain Res*. 2001;123:185–192.

49. Brook J, Brook D, Whiteman M. The influence of maternal smoking during pregnancy on the toddler's negativity. *Arch Pediatr Adolesc Med*. 2000;154:381–385.

50. Wakschlag L, Pickett K, Leventhal B. Smoking during pregnancy: problem behavior or behavior problem? 2001 Congress of Epidemiology; a joint meeting of the American College of Epidemiology, American Public Health Association (Epidemiology Section), Canadian Society for Epidemiology and Biostatistics, and Society for Epidemiologic Research. Toronto, Canada, June 13-16, 2001. Abstracts. *Am J Epidemiol*. 2001;153(suppl 11):S1–274. *Am J Epidemiol*. 2001;153:S244.

51. Quing Li C, Windsor R, Perkins L, Goldenberg R, Lowe J. The impact on infant birth weight and gestational age of cotinine-validated smoking reduction during pregnancy. *JAMA*. 1993;269:1519–1524.

52. Orleans CT, Barker DC, Kaufman NJ, Marx JF. Helping pregnant smokers quit: meeting the challenge in the next decade. *Tob Control*. 2000;9(suppl 3):III6–III11.

53. Pritchard C. Depression and smoking in pregnancy in Scotland. *J Epidemiol Community Health*. 1994;48:377–382.

54. Slotkin T. Fetal nicotine or cocaine exposure: which one is worse? *J Pharmacol Exp Ther*. 1998;285:931–945.

55. Benowitz N, ed. *Nicotine Safety and Toxicity*. New York, NY: Oxford University Press; 1998.

56. Navarro HA, Seidler FJ, Schwartz RD, Baker FE, Dobbins SS, Slotkin TA. Prenatal exposure to nicotine impairs nervous system development at a dose which does not affect viability or growth. *Brain Res Bull*. 1989;23:187–192.

57. Richardson S, Tizabi Y. Hyperactivity in the offspring of nicotine-treated rats: role of the mesolimbic and nigostriatal dopaminergic pathways. *Pharmacol Biochem Behav*. 1994;47:331–337.

58. Singh J. Early behavioral alterations in mice following prenatal carbon monoxide exposure. *Neurotoxicology*. 1986;7:475–481.

59. Storm JE, Valdes JJ, Fechter LD. Postnatal alterations in cerebellar GABA content, GABA uptake and morphology following exposure to carbon monoxide early in development. *Dev Neurosci*. 1986;8:251–261.

60. Ajarem J, Ahmad M. Prenatal nicotine exposure modifies behavior of mice through early development. *Pharmacol Biochem Behav*. 1998;59:313–318.

61. Thomas J, Garrison M, Slawecki C, Ehlers C, Riley E. Nicotine exposure during the neonatal brain growth spurt produces hyperactivity in preweanling rats. *Neurotoxicol Teratol*. 2000;22:695–701.

62. Tizabi Y, Popke EJ, Rahman M, Nespor S, Grunberg N. Hyperactivity induced by prenatal nicotine exposure is associated with an increase in cortical nicotine receptors. *Pharmacol Biochem Behav*. 1997;58:141–146.

63. Lackmann G, Angerer J, Tollner U. Parental smoking and neonatal serum levels of polychlorinated biphenyls and hexachlorobenzene. *Pediatr Res*. 2000;47:598–601.

64. Fergusson D. Prenatal smoking and antisocial behavior. *Arch Gen Psychiatry*. 1999;56:223–224.

65. Koren G. The association between maternal cigarette smoking and psychiatric diseases or criminal outcome in offspring: a precautionary note about the assumption of causation. *Reprod Toxicol*. 1999;13:345–346.

66. Wakschlag L, Pickett K, Leventhal B. Re: The association between maternal cigarette smoking and psychiatric diseases or criminal outcomes in the offspring [letter]. *Reprod Toxicol*. 2000;14:579–580.

67. Marshall J, Hastrup J, Ross J. Mismeasurement and the resonance of strong confounders: correlated errors. *Am J Epidemiol*. 1999;150:88–96.

68. Ventura S, Mathews J, Curtin S, Mathews T, Park M. *Births: Final Data for 1998.* Hyattsville, Md: National Center for Health Statistics; 2000. Report 48.

69. Loeber R, Stouthamer-Loeber M. Family factors as correlates and predictors of juvenile conduct problems and delinquency. In: Tonry M, Morris N, eds. *Crime and Justice: An Annual Review of Research.* Chicago, Ill: University of Chicago Press; 1986:29–149.

70. Wasserman G, Liu X, Pine D, Graziano J. Contribution of maternal smoking during pregnancy and lead exposure to early behavior problems. *Neurotoxicol Teratol.* 2001;23:13–21.

71. Fergusson D, Woodward L. Educational, psychosocial and early sexual outcomes of girls with conduct problems in early adolescence. *J Child Psychol Psychiatry.* 2000;41:779–792.

72. Goldman D. The search for genetic alleles contributing to self-destructive and aggressive behaviors. In: Stoff D, Cairns R, eds. *Aggression and Violence: Genetic, Neurobiological and Biosocial Perspectives.* Mahwah, NJ: Lawrence Erlbaum; 1996:23–41.

73. Carey G, Goldman D. The genetics of antisocial behavior. In: Stoff D, Breiling R, Maser J, eds. *Handbook of Antisocial Behavior.* New York, NY: John Wiley & Sons; 1997:243–254.

74. Merikangas K. Familial and genetic factors and psychopathology. In: Nelson C, ed. *The Effects of Early Adversity on Neurobehavioral Development.* Mahwah, NJ: Lawrence Erlbaum; 2000:281–316.

75. Cleveland HH, Wiebe RP, van den Oord EJ, Rowe DC. Behavior problems among children from different family structures: the influence of genetic self-selection. *Child Dev.* 2000;71:733–751.

76. Hyman S, Nestler E. *The Molecular Foundations of Psychiatry.* Washington, DC: American Psychiatric Press; 1993.

77. Capaldi D, Clark S. Prospective family predictors of aggression towards female partners for at-risk young men. *Dev Psychol.* 1998;34:1175–1188.

78. Fendrich M, Warner V, Weissman M. Family risk factors, parental depression and psychopathology in offspring. *Dev Psychol.* 1990;26:40–50.

79. Borrelli B, Bock B, King T. The impact of depression on smoking cessation in women. *Am J Prev Med.* 1996;12:378–387.

80. Breslau N, Kilbey M, Andreski P. Nicotine dependence and major depression: new evidence from a prospective investigation. *Arch Gen Psychiatry.* 1993;50: 31–35.

81. Chassin L, Presson C, Todd M, Rose J, Sherman D. Maternal socialization of adolescent smoking: the intergenerational transmission of parenting and smoking. *Dev Psychol.* 1998;34:1189–1202.

82. Kandel D, Wu P. The contributions of mothers and fathers to the intergenerational transmission of cigarette smoking in adolescence. *J Res Adolescence.* 1995; 5:225–252.

83. Wakschlag L, Hans S. Relation of maternal responsiveness during infancy to the development of behavior problems in high risk youths. *Dev Psychol.* 1999;37:569–579.

84. Eskenazi B, Castorina R. Association of prenatal maternal or postnatal child environmental tobacco smoke exposure and neurodevelopmental and behavioral problems in children. *Environ Health Perspect.* 1999;12:991–1000.

85. Olson J. Prenatal exposures and long-term health effects. *Epidemiol Rev.* 2000;22:76–81.

86. Neugebauer R, Hoek H, Susser E. Prenatal exposure to wartime famine and development of antisocial personality disorder in early adulthood. *JAMA.* 1999; 282:455–462.

87. Streissguth A. *Fetal Alcohol Syndrome: A Guide for Families and Communities.* Baltimore, Md: Paul H Brookes; 1997.

88. Williams GM, O'Callaghan M, Najman JM, et al. Maternal cigarette smoking and child psychiatric morbidity: a longitudinal study. *Pediatrics.* 1998;102:e11.

89. *The Health Benefits of Smoking Cessation.* Rockville, Md: Office on Smoking and Health; 1990.

90. Kazdin AE. Psychosocial treatments for conduct disorder in children. *J Child Psychol Psychiatry.* 1997; 38:161–178.

91. Buck C. Popper's philosophy for epidemiologists. *Int J Epidemiol.* 1975;4:159–168.

92. Moffitt T. The neuropsychology of conduct disorder. *Dev Psychopathol.* 1993;5:135–152.

93. Raine A, Brennan P, Mednick S. Birth complications combined with early maternal rejection at age one predispose to violent crime at age 18 years. *Arch Gen Psychiatry.* 1994;51:984–988.

94. Cicchetti D, Cannon T. Neurodevelopmental processes in the ontogenesis and epigenesis of psychopathology. *Dev Psychopathol.* 1999;11:375–394.

95. Kraemer H, Stice E, Kazdin A, Offord D, Kupfer D. How do risk factors work together? Mediators, moderators and independent, overlapping and proxy risk factors. *Am J Psychiatry.* 2001;158:848–856.

96. Rutter M. Nature-nurture integration: the example of antisocial behavior. *Am Psychol.* 1997;52:390–398.

97. Cannon T, Rosso I, Bearden C, Sanchez L, Hadley T. A prospective cohort study of neurodevelopmental processes in the genesis and epigenesis of schizophrenia. *Dev Psychopathol.* 1999;11:467–486.

98. Cole P, Michel M, Teti L. The development of emotion regulation and dysregulation: a clinical perspective. In: Fox N, ed. *The Development of Emotion Regulation: Biological and Behavioral Considerations.* Chicago, Ill: University of Chicago Press; 1994: 73–102.

99. Keenan K. Emotion dysregulation as a risk factor for psychopathology. *Clin Psychol Sci Pract.* 2000;7: 418–434.

100. Gibson CL, Tibbetts SG. A biosocial interaction in predicting early onset of offending. *Psychol Rep.* 2000; 86:509–518.

101. Shaw D, Winslow E. Precursors and correlates of antisocial behavior from infancy to preschool. In: Stoff D, Breiling R, Maser J, eds. *Handbook of Antisocial Behavior.* New York, NY: John Wiley & Sons; 1997: 148–158.

102. Benowitz N, SRNT Subcommittee on Biochemical Verification. Biochemical verification of tobacco use and cessation. *Nicotine Tob Res.* In press.

103. Keenan K, Wakschlag L. More than the terrible twos: the nature and severity of behavior problems in clinic-referred preschool children. *J Abnorm Child Psychol.* 2000;28:33–46.

104. Rantakallio P, Laara E, Isohanni M, Moilanen I. Maternal smoking during pregnancy and delinquency of the offspring: an association without causation? *Int J Epidemiol.* 1992;21:1106–1113.

Tobacco Industry Youth Smoking Prevention Programs: Protecting the Industry and Hurting Tobacco Control

| Anne Landman, BA, Pamela M. Ling, MD, MPH, and Stanton A. Glantz, PhD

Objectives. This report describes the history, true goals, and effects of tobacco industry–sponsored youth smoking prevention programs.

Methods. We analyzed previously-secret tobacco industry documents.

Results. The industry started these programs in the 1980s to forestall legislation that would restrict industry activities. Industry programs portray smoking as an adult choice and fail to discuss how tobacco advertising promotes smoking or the health dangers of smoking. The industry has used these programs to fight taxes, clean-indoor-air laws, and marketing restrictions worldwide. There is no evidence that these programs decrease smoking among youths.

Conclusions. Tobacco industry youth programs do more harm than good for tobacco control. The tobacco industry should not be allowed to run or directly fund youth smoking prevention programs. (*Am J Public Health.* 2002;92:917–930)

The tobacco industry is aggressively promoting its "youth smoking education and prevention" programs worldwide, modeled on ones it introduced in the United States in the 1980s,[1–3] nominally to reduce youth smoking.[4–9] R.J. Reynolds Tobacco (RJR) reported that by 1999 it had distributed materials to millions of young Americans through amusement parks, video arcades, theaters, schools, Boys and Girls Clubs, and baseball camps.[9] In 2001, Philip Morris announced that it was "actively involved in more than 130 [youth smoking prevention] programs in more than 70 countries."[8] The few studies that have compared industry programs with public health campaigns found that industry programs were less appealing and convincing to youths[10–14] and that industry programs neglected the health effects of tobacco use and subtly promoted smoking.[15] Public health advocates have questioned the appropriateness of industry-sponsored youth smoking prevention programs.[16–19]

Previously-secret tobacco industry documents provide an important source of information on industry activities.[20] Academic studies of industry documents and youths have focused on proving that the tobacco industry targeted youths in its advertising.[21–24] We analyzed tobacco industry documents to determine why the industry developed youth programs, to describe the themes that were pursued and how these programs were used, and to find evidence of whether these programs reduce youth smoking. The purpose of the industry's youth smoking prevention programs is not to reduce youth smoking but rather to serve the industry's political needs by preventing effective tobacco control legislation, marginalizing public health advocates, preserving the industry's access to youths, creating allies within policymaking and regulatory bodies, defusing opposition from parents and educators, bolstering industry credibility, and preserving the industry's influence with policymakers.

METHODS

We searched the following tobacco industry document archives made available by tobacco litigation during the 1990s: the University of California–San Francisco's Mangini collection of RJR and British American Tobacco marketing documents (http://www.library.ucsf.edu/tobacco), tobacco industry document Web sites (Philip Morris: http://www.pmdocs.com; Brown and Williamson: http://www.brownandwilliamson.com; RJR: www.rjrtdocs.com; Lorillard: http://www.lorillarddocs.com; Tobacco Institute: www.tobaccoinstitute.com), Tobacco Documents Online (http://www.tobaccodocuments.org), and the Minnesota Select Set (outside.cdc.gov:8080/BASIS/ncctld/web/mnimages). Search terms included the following: "youth," "youth smoking prevention," "YSP," "prevention," "access," "youth programs," "evaluation," "tracking," and the names of individual youth programs, such as Action Against Access and Helping Youth Decide. We extended the searches by using the names of key organizations and individuals identified in relevant documents, their office locations, project dates, and reference (Bates) numbers. Searches were conducted between June and December 2001. Initial searches yielded thousands of documents; these were read, and those relevant to tobacco industry–sponsored youth smoking prevention efforts were selected, yielding a collection of 496 documents, which were analyzed in detail. We sought to be exhaustive in our searching to ensure that, to the best of our ability, the documents discussed in this report fairly and accurately represent the material we located.

RESULTS

Origins and Goals of the Tobacco Industry's Programs

The tobacco industry implements 4 types of youth smoking prevention programs (Table 1): programs that speak directly to youths, programs that speak to parents, programs directed toward retailers, and programs that fund mainstream youth organizations. These programs stress several common themes: (1) smoking is an "adult choice," (2) children start smoking because of peer pressure and a lack of proper role modeling and guidance from their parents, and (3) an emphasis of "the law" as the reason not to smoke. Each type of program offers unique benefits for the industry. None discusses the fact that nicotine is addictive, that smoking or passive smoking causes disease, or that tobacco marketing has a role in promoting

TABLE 1—Tobacco Industry-Sponsored Youth Programs and How They Benefit the Industry

Program Characteristics	Benefits Sought by Tobacco Industry	Examples	How Program Has Been Used by Industry
		Programs That Speak Directly to Youth	
Spread through media campaigns. Portray smoking as an "adult choice" and an "adult decision." Sample themes: "Kids Don't Smoke" "Smoking Isn't Cool" "Wait Until You're Older"	Marginalize opposition to make it appear extreme. Reinforce smoking as an adult choice. Undermine campaigns: weaker messages, target inappropriately young teens. Gain credibility by working with educators. Maintain access to youth.	"Right Decisions, Right Now" (RJR, 1991). Can I Do It? (Czech). "Juveniles Should Not Smoke" (Finnish, 1992). "Smoking Can Wait" (Russian, 1994–95). MTV campaign in Europe.	Promoted weakly "antismoking" messages. Generated good PR. Built alliances with educators. Used to fight legislation in Iowa, California, New Hampshire, Wisconsin, and other states (arguing it's not necessary). Successfully fought restrictive legislation overseas. Used to collect marketing data on youth.
		Programs That Speak to Parents	
Spread through brochures, booths at festivals, and public gatherings. Sample themes: "Talk to your kids" Assist youth with decisionmaking. Parental empowerment.	Marginalize opposition. Blame parents and society (not marketing) for youth smoking. Gain credibility by working with parent groups.	"Responsible Living Program" (TI), which included "Helping Youth Decide" (TI, 1984) and "Helping Youth Say No" (TI, 1990; PM, 1994).	Program promoted to legislators in many states. Generated good PR outreach to minority community parents.
		Programs for Retailers to Nominally Decrease Youth Access	
Spread through stickers and posters in retail shops and visits by cigarette representatives. Sample themes: Check identification. Smoking is for adults only. Retailer has responsibility for youth access in stores.	Marginalize opposition. Imply age is the only reason not to smoke. Keep industry abreast of local legislative activity. Build alliances with retailers. Shift attention away from industry's contribution to, and responsibility for, youth smoking.	"Action Against Access" (PM, 1995). "We Card" (Coalition for Responsible Tobacco Retailing). "It's the Law" (TI, 1990; PM, 1994). "Support the Law" (RJR, 1992).	Implemented in ASSIST states to fight legislation and used retailers to alert industry about local ordinance efforts. Got Tobacco Industry representation on Nevada governor's youth smoking group. Undermined attempts by FDA to regulate tobacco. Used to fight strict access legislation in Iowa.
		Direct Funding of Youth Organizations	
Spread through reputable, credible youth organizations, often with the promise that programs were designed or executed independently of tobacco companies.	Gain credibility, attain aura of legitimacy. Build alliances with reputable youth groups.	NASBE. 4-H "Health Rocks." US Junior Chamber of Commerce. Seeking alliances with Scouts, YMCA/YWCA, Boys and Girls Clubs, Junior Achievement.	Built alliances, attempted to use NASBE as mouthpiece for industry rhetoric. NASBE president used for extensive media tours. Undermined first anti-tobacco media campaign in Minnesota.

Note. TI = Tobacco Institute; PM = Philip Morris; RJR = R. J. Reynolds; NASBE = National Association of State Boards of Education; ASSIST = American Stop Smoking Intervention Study; FDA = Food and Drug Administration; PR = public relations.

smoking. The tobacco industry first introduced programs aimed at youths and their parents (such as Helping Youth Decide) in the mid-1980s, programs aimed at retailers in the early 1990s, and funding of mainstream youth organizations and worldwide expansion of these programs in the late 1990s.[25,26]

Youth programs were developed as a response to 2 major industry concerns: public scrutiny of industry marketing practices and the threat of legislation or regulation. In 1978, US Secretary of Health, Education, and Welfare Joseph Califano accused the tobacco industry of marketing to children,[27,28] the nonsmokers' rights movement emerged, and the Federal Trade Commission considered the regulation of tobacco advertising. In 1982, the industry failed to defeat a federal excise tax bill, generating concern about its eroding public position and lobbying power. In a December 9, 1982, speech to the Tobacco Institute Executive Committee's annual meeting, institute President Samuel Chilcote observed that the industry's "image as an unbeatable lobby has been punctured."[29] A confidential Tobacco Institute presentation, "The Development of Tobacco Industry Strategy" (probably written around 1982–1983), suggests:

> The potential positive outcomes of adopting programs of this nature [socially responsible programs] may be . . . a more sophisticated understanding by government regulators of the

> needs/behaviors of industry. *For example, a program to discourage teens from smoking (an adult decision) might prevent or delay further regulation of the tobacco industry.*[30] [italics added]

A youth smoking prevention program might help the industry deflect meaningful regulation of its marketing practices.

The purpose of the industry's youth programs was, from the beginning, to serve the industry's political needs. A November 27, 1984, memo from Tobacco Institute Vice President Anne Duffin to Dave Henderson and Roger Mozingo (also of the Tobacco Institute) shows that the institute promoted its youth prevention programs to legislative audiences with the expectation that doing so would help "to discourage [restrictions on free] sampling and other legislation and to solicit quotable comment from community leaders."[31] A 1986 "Presentation to the Communications Committee" about the institute's Helping Youth Decide program, probably written by Duffin, puts the new youth program in the broadest political context:

> Note I say "project" because that is exactly what "Helping Youth Decide"—HYD for short—is. *What it should be . . . is a legislative program* . . . and it is now ready to be that. The need for this legislative resource is greater than it ever has been. The cigarette advertising issue has been right smack at center state [sic] now since late spring . . . on Capitol Hill . . . and, increasingly, in states and cities.[32] [italics added]

Likewise, in 1991 Philip Morris restated that the success of the "youth initiatives" would be determined by whether they led to a "reduction in legislation introduced and passed restricting or banning our sales and marketing activities" as well as "passage of legislation favorable to the industry" and "greater support from business, parent and teacher groups."[33]

The youth strategy repeatedly played a key role in the industry's efforts to undermine state tobacco control initiatives. A 1985 progress report for the Tobacco Institute reported that its Responsible Living program (which included Helping Youth Decide and Helping Youth Say No) was used to defeat legislation in New Hampshire, Maryland, Wisconsin, and California. The program also won the industry endorsements from state legislators in California, Illinois, Michigan, New Hampshire, and Missouri.[34] In addition, the industry used youth programs as part of its unsuccessful 1988 bid to defeat a California initiative to increase the tobacco tax to fund a tobacco control program (Proposition 99), arguing that because it had its own youth programs, the tax was "unnecessary."[35] Youth programs played a part in the industry's attempts to defeat a 1991 Iowa ban on cigarette vending machines and free samples,[36] a 1996 ingredients disclosure bill in Vermont,[37] and other state efforts to regulate tobacco.[38]

Industry Programs Directed at Youths and Parents Complement Tobacco Advertising

In designing its youth campaigns, the industry took care not to contradict or interfere with tobacco advertising.[39,40] In 1985, Duffin wrote John Rupp and Lee Stafford of the industry's law firm Covington & Burling, seeking advice on how to draft a brochure on Helping Youth Decide to avoid mentioning the health consequences of smoking:

> Because of criticism from the antis [anti-smokers] on HYD [Helping Youth Decide], I'd like to get our own scenario in on cigarettes—*not touching on any health implications,* but positing that youngsters don't need to smoke to look "grown up," needn't blindly follow the examples of others, etc.
> I'm toying with consulting with the likes of Dan Horn [a psychologist who had been a leader in smoking research in the federal government until he retired in 1978], if he could be persuaded of our good intentions and give us the psychologist's view of how to approach this *without mentioning health.*[41] [italics added]

Presenting smoking as an "adult choice," a "forbidden fruit," and an act of rebellion are common industry marketing themes.[42–45] A 1977 Imperial Tobacco marketing research report from Canada, "Subject: Project 16 English Youth," typifies how the industry uses "forbidden fruit" messages to interest youth:

> Of course, one of the very things that are attractive is [the] mere fact that cigarettes are forbidden fruit. Everywhere they [Canadian teenagers] turn are admonitions to stay away from it. School lectures and teachers may [sic] not to smoke. Parents (even smoking ones) say not to smoke. Therefore, when the adolescent is looking for something that at the same time makes them feel different and also makes them feel that they are old enough to ignore this weight of authority *so as to feel that they have made their own choice,* what better could be found than a cigarette? It is not just a smoke. It is a statement, a naughty adventure, a milestone episode.[45] [italics added]

These themes send mixed messages when used in "smoking prevention."[15,46] Philip Morris ran literal "forbidden fruit" messages in a 1999 series of full-page advertisements in news magazines aimed at parents that featured a bowl of fruit (or a glass of milk with cookies) and the questions, "What else are you leaving out for your kids?" and "What else is within your kids' reach?"[47–49]

One of the motivations behind the Tobacco Institute's youth programs was to displace educational programs developed by public health groups because these "almost all consist of wrongful 'scare' tactics" and "present smoking as repugnant and unhealthy."[40,50] A 1991 Tobacco Institute "Discussion Paper" shows how youth programs helped place responsibility for youth smoking on parents' inability to control peer pressure, a strategy that allowed the industry to shift the focus away from its advertising practices while portraying tobacco control advocates as "extremist":

> The youth program and its individual parts support The Institute's objective of discouraging unfair and counterproductive federal, state and local restrictions on cigarette advertising, by:
>
> • Providing ongoing and persuasive *evidence* that the industry is actively discouraging youth smoking and independent *verification* that the industry's efforts are valid.
> • Reinforcing the belief that peer pressure—not advertising—is the cause of youth smoking.
> • Seizing the political center and forcing the anti-smokers to an extreme.
>
> The strategy is fairly simple:
>
> 1. Heavily promote industry opposition to youth smoking.
> 2. Align the industry with broader, more sophisticated view of the problem, i.e., parental inability to offset peer pressure.
> 3. Work with and through credible child welfare professionals and educators to tackle the "problem."
> 4. Bait anti-tobacco forces to criticize industry efforts. Focus media on anti's extremism. Anticipate and blunt antis strongest points . . . for positioning purposes. Broad-based advertising . . . has the important effect of making the public aware that the industry *says* it is trying to do the right thing."[51] [italics in original]

Whereas the industry was aggressive in *saying* that it was doing the "right thing," we were not able to locate any "persuasive evidence" verifying that the industry's youth smoking prevention programs actually reduced youth smoking.

Tobacco Industry Retailer Programs Help Fight Tobacco Control

In 1990, the Tobacco Institute launched the "It's the Law" program, which urged retailers to post signs and stickers and to wear lapel buttons stating that they did not sell tobacco to persons under 18.[52] Philip Morris took over management of the "It's the Law" program in 1994[26] and made it part of its Action Against Access program in 1995. The retailer portion, named "Ask First—It's the Law," included training to ask for proof of age.[53] A series of e-mails in 1996 between high-level Philip Morris executives reveal that Philip Morris heavily advertised the Action Against Access campaign in locations where legislators, not children, would be sure to see them.[54] Philip Morris used the presence of these programs to argue against the government's funding further tobacco control efforts.[55]

In addition, the industry has used its youth access programs to recruit a network of retailers as an "early warning system" to detect and defeat local tobacco control ordinances.[56–58] The tobacco industry funded its retail allies to perform these actions, and the retailer training program "It's the Law" helped facilitate the contact. A confidential 1992 report by Kurt Malmgren, senior vice president of state activities at the Tobacco Institute, to Chilcote makes this clear:

> For monitoring purposes, we fund our allies in the convenience store groups to regularly report on ordinance introductions and assist in campaigns to stop unreasonable measures. Promotion of the Institute's "It's the Law" program and other industry programs play a helpful role as well.[57]

A 1994 speech by Ellen Merlo, senior vice president of corporate affairs at Philip Morris, reveals that Philip Morris also enlisted the assistance of retailers to help defeat local ordinance efforts:

> . . . with . . . local activity rampant, we realized we had to have some way to control the bleeding. We needed an effective system to let us know when and where local laws were being proposed, either at town meetings, in the local city councils or by Boards of Health. Working with the New England Convenience Store Association and other tobacco companies, we developed a network whereby local retailers could assist us by providing information on legislative activities in every Massachusetts Community. We've discovered that if we have enough advance notice . . . and get somebody there for the public hearing, we can make a difference.[56]

The industry used this network to detect and fight not only youth access measures and advertising restrictions but also clean-indoor-air laws.[59–63]

In 1994, the US Food and Drug Administration (FDA) announced its intent to pursue regulations to protect children from tobacco promotion and nicotine addiction. The regulations would have ended tobacco advertisements within 1000 feet of schools, eliminated self-service tobacco displays, and required "tombstone" advertising for tobacco products (advertisements that consist only of black print on a white background, without pictures).[64] Philip Morris used its Action Against Access youth program as part of its argument that the FDA's proposal was unnecessary.[65] A 1996 RJR press release argued that the FDA regulation was unnecessary because the industry's We Card program was "now making a measurable difference."[66] The release gave no details about the relative size of this claimed "difference" or how it was measured, nor any verification that it was measured at all.

Working Through Third Parties: The National Association of State Boards of Education

The tobacco companies recognize that they lack credibility with the public and policymakers.[67,68] This situation makes representation by credible third parties an indispensable tool for the tobacco industry to achieve its goals, particularly in dealing with politicians.[69] A speaker in a 1984 Philip Morris Corporate Affairs World Conference explained this bluntly: "So the whole question of . . . enlisting this whole third-party concept in our defense structure is to give us clout, to give us power, to give us credibility, to give us leverage, to give us access where we don't ordinarily have access ourselves."[69]

In 1984, the Tobacco Institute recruited a credible third party on youth by formalizing an alliance with the National Association of State Boards of Education (NASBE). The Tobacco Institute solicited NASBE to disseminate its Helping Youth Decide program, a component of the institute's Responsible Living youth program (Table 1). The Tobacco Institute carefully considered the political value of NASBE's partnership. An April 12, 1984, Tobacco Institute memorandum from Tom Humber, chair of the Tobacco Institute's Communications Committee, to the institute's Executive Committee about recommendations for the Responsible Living program summarizes the "distinct advantages to working with NASBE":

> • NASBE will provide us with an established, clear link to all levels of government: federal, state and local.
> • NASBE's members tend not to be educators, but members of the business–political community elected or appointed to serve on their respective State Boards of Education. They are not "cause" oriented and are, for the most part, politically savvy and supportive of business perspectives. There is no evidence of anti-tobacco bias at NASBE. . . . potential critics within the educational establishment will be cautious about raising objections to this program. . . . At the direction of the Executive Committee, exploratory discussions have been held with NASBE.[70]

The Tobacco Institute hired NASBE's past president, Jolly Ann Davidson, to tour the country with Walker Merryman, the institute's vice president for communication, to promote the program to the media and legislators.[71–73] The first places the institute planned to send Davidson and Walker were states considering legislation that would limit or ban promotions that offered free samples of cigarettes.[74,75]

Shortly after joining with the Tobacco Institute, NASBE found itself criticized by health advocates.[76–79] James A. Swomley, managing director of the American Lung Association, wrote to NASBE, pointing out that the institute was using NASBE as a legislative tool.[80–82] Tobacco Institute Vice President Anne Duffin noted NASBE's troubles in her 1986 memorandums and presentation to the institute's Communications Committee[32,83] and assisted in drafting NASBE's responses to critics.[84]

Conflict emerged between NASBE and the Tobacco Institute as they tried to find common acceptable wording for their joint public statements. For example, Duffin questioned some of the objections that Phyllis Blaunstein, executive director of NASBE, had to claims in a draft brochure promoting Helping Youth Decide. Blaunstein wanted to remove a statement that "both organizations believe that postponing a decision is in itself making a decision," saying that the phrase was "inconsistent with our [the Tobacco Institute's] claim that we don't want kids to smoke."[85] Blaunstein also pushed the institute to remove the claim that "cigarette makers have received little credit for their efforts to avoid the youth market" from the brochure.[85] Mutual frustration with wording continued to be a persistent problem between NASBE and the institute[32,86–88]; in April 1985, after several exchanges, Lana Muraskin, director of the Helping Youth Decide program at NASBE, wrote a short letter to Duffin withdrawing permission for the institute to use NASBE's logo on a brochure touting the success of Helping Youth Decide.[89]

Soon, the institute started holding money over NASBE's head to try to force the organization to cooperate with its public relations goals. In a May 30, 1986, memorandum, Duffin stated her intent to remind a NASBE official that:

> (1) we have not got our money's worth in planned projects in any year so far
> (2) we certainly have not had the full time attention of the three staffers whose time we reportedly have been paying and
> (3) we will set up our 1986 payment based on completed projects delivered, not drafts, as has been our downfall.[90]

A handwritten February 2, 1987, memorandum by a NASBE employee reflects growing ill will between the 2 organizations, particularly Duffin's references to people "at T.I. who question whether they are getting their money's worth from our past and current efforts."[91]

In 1988, NASBE terminated its relationship with the institute by withdrawing its sponsorship of the youth programs.[92,93]

The Tobacco Institute then created its own "independent foundation" to replace NASBE. This foundation, the Family COURSE Consortium, was presented as a "not-for-profit organization comprised of educators, youth organization professionals and other interested parties."[94] The "single goal" of the Family COURSE Consortium was to promote youth programs in a manner responsive to the institute.[92] Early in 1989, the Tobacco Institute redirected the Responsible Living Program to focus solely on the distribution and promotion of the Helping Youth Decide booklet, noting that the institute's "Federal Relations Division feels that the legislative benefits of the HYD [Helping Youth Decide] program are great and have expressed their desire that the promotion of these booklets continue."[95]

Use of Third Parties in the Late 1990s: Philip Morris and 4-H

A 1999 Philip Morris internal presentation about youth programs states Philip Morris's intent to pursue "strategic partnership outreach" to 4-H Clubs, Boys and Girls Clubs, the Junior Achievement, Kids Café, the YMCA, and the YWCA with a youth nonsmoking program.[96] However, Philip Morris sought more pervasive influence in these organizations than simply making presentations to their members. Philip Morris intended to place its own representatives on the boards of these organizations and to provide money in the form of grants of $10 000 to $100 000.[96]

The national 4-H program is the youth education branch of the US Department of Agriculture's Cooperative Extension Service, an agricultural information service that maintains offices in counties throughout the United States. (4-H stands for "Head, Heart, Hands, and Health.") 4-H Club participants range in age from 5 to 21. The program has a long-standing reputation as a respected youth service organization and emphasizes "learning-by-doing."

In 1998, Philip Morris approached representatives of 4-H and offered a $4.3 million grant to design and implement a youth antismoking program. 4-H, which previously had not dealt with cigarette manufacturers to any significant extent, agreed to move forward with "planning the new Philip Morris USA initiative."[97] On March 18, 1999, Philip Morris sent the national 4-H office the first installment check for $1.7 million,[98] and on March 24, the National 4-H Council publicly announced its new alliance with Philip Morris.[99]

The 4-H Clubs of America immediately became the target of intense protest from the public health community. The American Lung Association, American Heart Association, American Cancer Society, Americans for Nonsmokers Rights, American Medical Association, and National Center for Tobacco Free Kids wrote to 4-H, citing the industry's history of aligning itself with various respectable organizations to polish its public image and shore up its legislative clout. (4-H shared the resulting correspondence with Philip Morris.[100–104]) As a result, 27 of 50 state 4-H organizations rejected involvement in the partnership with Philip Morris. The national 4-H organization, however, continued its partnership with Philip Morris.

The Health Rocks program that evolved out of 4-H's tobacco funding in 2001 has the nominal goal of reducing youth smoking and tobacco use.[105] The program's Web site states, "the [Health Rocks] evaluation also showed a need for the program to focus more on life skills in general—not just tobacco use prevention."[105] Like earlier tobacco industry–created programs, the Health Rocks program seeks to broaden and diffuse youth tobacco prevention efforts into a program aimed at "develop[ing] life skills, with a special emphasis on youth smoking prevention" and to "engage youth and adults as partners in developing and implementing community strategies to prepare young people to make healthy lifestyle choices."[106]

In justifying the alliance, Richard Sauer, head of the National 4-H Council, responded to organizations that had criticized 4-H by repeating the themes of Philip Morris's public relations campaign, stating that Philip Morris was a "new," more responsible company:

> We continue to see old references from 20 or more years ago about what Philip Morris is or another tobacco company did or did not do. None of us today can do anything about the past. I believe that Philip Morris, USA, which is under new corporate leadership, has recognized its responsibility to prevent underage smoking and has made a commitment to fulfill that responsibility by funding this program for two years.[107]

Evaluation: The Criterion for "Success" Is Not Preventing Smoking

We searched industry document sites by using an extensive list of terms, including "evaluation," "assessment," "tracking," "outcome," "research," "result," and the names of every youth program we had identified, in an attempt to find any industry research on the effectiveness of tobacco companies' "youth smoking" programs. We did not find any evidence that these programs had been evaluated in terms of effect on the rates of youth smoking. Instead, tobacco companies studied the reach and effectiveness of these programs as though they were public relations campaigns, tracking the number of "media hits," awareness of the program among adults, and the effect of the program on their corporate image.[108–112]

A 1986 evaluation report written by NASBE for the Tobacco Institute's Helping Youth Decide program concentrates on describing the audience, the reasons people request the educational booklet, the circumstances in which the booklet has been used, and users' feedback on the attractiveness, helpfulness, or usefulness of booklet elements.[113,114] The section of the evaluation dealing with the efficacy of the program fails to define any criteria for "success."[114] A 1994 RJR report on youth campaigns states that a retailer program in the United Kingdom was "very successful," simply because 80% of retailers there were using point-of-sale materials provided by the National [tobacco] Manufacturers Association. No mention was made of success related to an actual reduction in youth smoking rates.[115]

Although the industry conducted surveys and focus groups while developing its youth smoking prevention programs to select appealing advertisements with clear messages, we did not find any research evaluating the advertising's effect on teen smoking. Most of the formative research focuses on demonstrating teens' ability to identify the main message of the advertisements. Philip Morris's advertising agency, Young & Rubicam, conducted surveys testing youth smoking prevention billboard advertisements with groups of teenagers in New York in 1992.[116] Young & Rubicam also tested television advertisements with children aged 10 to 14 and their parents in 1998.[117] In both cases, the firm monitored teens' ability to identify the main message of the advertisement and various other responses to the advertising, such as liking, attention, ability to relate, interest, ability to understand, and uniqueness.[116] The main result reported to television stations in 1998 was that nearly all of the children studied could identify the main message of the advertisements to be "Don't smoke/Not to Smoke."[117]

Philip Morris's vice president in charge of youth smoking prevention in 2000, Carolyn Levy, had formerly conducted marketing research,[118] including research on teens.[119,120] As part of its research on reactions to its television advertising campaign, Philip Morris did ask parents how much the commercial would convince their child not to smoke. In responding to a television network's questions about evidence for the effectiveness of the advertisements, Levy combined 3 divergent response categories ("very much," "somewhat," and "very little"), thus counting any response but the most negative as a positive assessment of the effectiveness of the commercials.[117]

Philip Morris complained when the media pointed out the apparent lack of measures of the effectiveness of the company's advertising campaign in actually preventing teen smoking.[121] In an interview with ABC television news in 1999, Levy admitted that Philip Morris did not ask its study group children whether the advertisements would have any influence on their decision of whether to smoke.[122] Continuing this pattern, Philip Morris ran a series of youth antismoking advertisements during the 2000 Super Bowl football games called "My Reasons." The sole basis of Philip Morris's claim of the advertisements' effectiveness apparently was an informal survey asking 400 youths and their parents whether they understood the basic message in the advertisement. Aside from reporting that 97% of parents and 98% of children understood that the message in the advertisements was against smoking, Philip Morris did not indicate whether the advertisements had any effect on the children's intent to smoke.[123] Philip Morris has sophisticated methods of testing cigarette advertisements and assessing relevance, imagery, and intent to purchase the advertised brand,[124,125] but the company did not appear to use these to assess how its youth smoking prevention advertisements would affect purchasing behavior.

In contrast, the industry assessed in great detail the public relations and legislative outcomes associated with its youth smoking prevention programs. In 1986, the Tobacco Institute asked its lobbyists to rate the Helping Youth Decide programs' value to the company as a legislative tool.[108] In 1995, Philip Morris added a module to its consumer tracking surveys, which tracked approximately 700 smokers per week, to monitor the effect of its Action Against Access program.[109,111] The module asked smokers whether they were aware that Philip Morris (as opposed to the government or politicians) started the Action Against Access program, whether they had noticed changes in signage and identification checking, and whether and how the program affected their feelings about Philip Morris.[110] Both the reported results of this survey tracking and the original questionnaires neglect any assessment of youth smoking or reduction in youth access to tobacco. Philip Morris's September 1995 National Visibility Study audited 3729 stores for visible signage for the company's "Ask First–It's the Law" program, and also measured the visibility of RJR's underage signage. There was no mention of measurement of actual youth access to cigarettes in the study.[109]

A 2001 youth program evaluation plan for Lorillard Tobacco's new youth smoking prevention program states, "Objective: Communicate the news of the launch of Lorillard's new Youth Smoking Prevention Program. Strategy: Build as much 3rd party credibility as possible. Make the story national news. . . ."[126] The evaluation document does not say that an objective is to measurably reduce youth smoking rates. Like all of the other industry youth smoking programs, the outcomes are evaluated not in terms of influencing teen smoking but rather in terms of the effects on adult response and Lorillard Tobacco's corporate image.

"Youth Smoking Prevention" Legitimizes Tobacco Industry Research on Teens

The tobacco industry has been criticized for directing its marketing efforts at young children.[21–24,127–131] Indeed, evidence that it did so seriously undercut the industry's political and legal position during the 1990s. Practices such as the use of cartoon characters to advertise cigarettes brought the tobacco industry as a whole under closer scrutiny.[132–136] It became dangerous for the industry to even study teenagers, and thus the industry invented code words to avoid explicit mention of teens in its marketing research.[24] The industry's new "teen smoking prevention" programs beginning in the late 1990s have provided cover

TABLE 2—Comparison of Marketing Research for "Youth Smoking Prevention" and "Young Adult Marketing" by Philip Morris

"Youth Smoking Prevention" Research[137]	"Young Adult" Marketing Research[140]
Key question areas to include	Profiling the young adult male smoker
· Lifestyle	· Leisure time activities
· Pop culture	· General attitudes
· Dating	· Social circles
· Aspirations	· Aspirations and objectives
· Not smoking in the context of things that most concern teens today	· Attitudes about smoking
	· Brand image

for the industry to begin aggressive studies of teenage attitudes toward smoking.

Although these data nominally are collected as part of a "youth smoking prevention" effort, they contain precisely the same information tobacco marketers need to sell their products to young people. In fact, Philip Morris used the same advertising agency, Young & Rubicam, to develop both its "youth smoking prevention" advertisements[116,137] and its cigarette advertisements.[138,139] A comparison of the topics of a Philip Morris "youth smoking prevention" study and a "young adult smoker" cigarette marketing study reveals great similarity (Table 2).[137,140]

Even if tobacco industry research on teens were legitimately used to deter rather than encourage smoking, the same research could also be used to design programs with little or no impact on smoking initiation. In 1992 and 1993, Young & Rubicam conducted research with teens in New York City schools to "understand the underlying dynamics of how youths aged 12–17 resist or succumb to social pressures, particularly as it [sic] relates to the decision not to smoke."[116,137] Rather than focusing on older teens, who are at the highest risk for smoking initiation and who would be sensitive to messages aimed at young adults, Philip Morris found that it could tailor a smoking prevention advertisement specifically to younger teens.[116]

These messages would leave older teens vulnerable to "young adult" cigarette advertising.[141] Indeed, Young & Rubicam's research indicated that New York City "teens think of themselves more as 'young adults' than kids."[137] In 1992, Young & Rubicam's research on New York teenagers revealed that younger and older teens reacted differently to advertisements and that teens were more responsive to advertisements depicting people their own age. Thus, one could tailor a message to younger teens (12–14 years old in this study) or to older teens (15–17 years old), depending on the age of the actor: "The quantitative study validates the appeal of this campaign. But it also points to the importance of casting younger for younger teens (currently the campaign shows older teens perhaps explaining why this execution is more attention-getting for the older teens)."[116]

The plans appear to involve modifying the campaign to appeal to the younger teens only. By 1998, Philip Morris was targeting even younger children (aged 10–14 years) for its "youth smoking prevention" advertisements. Young & Rubicam also conducted the research for these advertisements, and the firm did not survey older teens as it had in the past. Instead, it tested the advertisements on children aged 10 to 14 years and their parents.[117] Philip Morris's research on teenagers allowed it to develop advertisements that scored well with parents and appeared to target the youngest teens. By not making teenagers aged 15 to 18, who are at a substantially greater risk to start smoking, the intended audience for these messages, the company preserved the primary source of new smokers.

Lorillard Tobacco Company has also enjoyed new legitimate access to teens through its youth smoking prevention programs. Lorillard has been able to place its "Tobacco Is Whacko" advertisements in youth markets to which they would otherwise be denied legal access, including the most popular teen television shows on Warner Brothers Prime Time, ESPN, and MTV; the "Miss Teen USA Pageant" and "Billboard Music Awards"; sports events such as ESPN's "Summer X-Games"; wrestling shows on USA, UPN, and TNT; and in DC and Marvel comic books, *Seventeen* magazine, and *Teen People.*[142,143] Many of these advertisements encourage teens to visit Lorillard's Web site, where they can fill out surveys and enter sweepstakes. Not only does this information allow Lorillard to develop a mailing list of teens, it also allows the company to collect psychographic data (information about activities, interests, and opinions that can be used to develop consumer psychological profiles)[144] through inquiries about popular clothing trends, dream vacations, hot music groups, television and movie stars teens admire, computer games, favorite sports events and athletes, superheroes, and what they feel the president's priorities should be.[145] The "Tobacco Is Whacko" program provides Lorillard with cover for continuing to contact and study teens.

Tobacco Industry Youth Smoking Prevention Programs Outside the United States

During the 1990s, the tobacco industry repeated its pattern of implementing youth programs to boost its image and deflect public health legislation worldwide (Table 3), just as it has in the United States since the early 1980s. A 1993 memorandum, "Youth Campaigns for Latin America," by Cathy Lieber, Philip Morris's director of corporate affairs for the Latin American region, states that Philip Morris needs to implement youth programs to counteract negative publicity in Latin America:

> Increasing pressure from anti-tobacco forces in Latin America has created the need to explore various options to counter negative publicity. One theme that has recently surfaced in several markets is that multinational companies target children in ad campaigns.
> . . . Taking into consideration the emerging adverse legislative climate in the region, we have an opportunity to create good will for the tobacco industry by going public with a campaign to discourage juvenile smoking. *Our objective is to communicate that the tobacco industry is not interested in having young people smoke and to position the industry as a "concerned corporate citizen" in an effort to ward off further attacks by the anti-tobacco movement.*[146] [italics added]

In non–English-speaking countries, the tobacco industry has used translations of its

TABLE 3—Examples of Worldwide Expansion of Tobacco Industry Youth Smoking Prevention Programs

Year	Place	Slogan/Message	Media	Tobacco Company	Source
1981	UK	Campaign for retailers regularly updated until 1989	Stickers, leaflets	TAC	Philip Morris[3]
1983	Australia	"It's the law—cigarettes cannot be sold to those under 18"	Brochure, stickers	PM Australia	
1987	Australia	Campaign on prohibition of cigarette sales to minors	Signs	TI Australia	
1989	Canada	"We don't sell tobacco products to minors"	Stickers	Can Tob Man Council	
1989	Japan	"You may not smoke until you are 20 years old"	Posters	TI Japan	
1990	Ecuador	"Smoking is an adult decision"	Television	Proesa	
1990	Hong Kong	"If you're not old enough to drive, you're not old enough to smoke"	Posters	TI Hong Kong	
1990	Malta	"We don't sell cigarettes to children"	Stickers, leaflets	Malta TIAC	
1990	Mauritius	Campaign to discourage minors from smoking	Stickers	BAT	
1990	Singapore	"Children, don't smoke"	Posters	Tob Man Importers Assn.	
1991	Canada	Information kit update: "We don't sell tobacco products to minors"	Information kit	Can Tob Man Council	
1992	Finland	"Amer does not want youngsters to smoke"	Posters, ads	Amer Group/Amer Tupakka	
1992	Japan	Stickers for vending machines updated	Stickers	TI Japan	
1992	Sweden	"Advantage smoke free"	Stickers	BAT	
1993	Australia	"It's the law" campaign aimed at educating retailers	Badges, booklet, stickers kit	PM Australia	
1993	Hong Kong	"If you're not old enough to drive..."	Posters	TI Hong Kong	
1993	GCC	Warning of trademark use, particularly regarding goods for children	Ads	PM Services, PM Europe SA	
1993	Mauritius	Sticker campaign to discourage minors from smoking	Stickers	BAT	
1993	Taiwan	Campaign for retailers	Stickers	TI Taiwan	
1994	Australia	Campaign for retailers in South Australia and Victoria	Portfolio, stickers, brochure	US TI	
1994	EEC	PMCS draft campaign	Posters	PMCS	
1994	Japan	Leaflet to retailers regarding discouraging smoking among young people	Leaflet	TI Japan	
1994	Russia	PM Moscow no-smoking campaign, part 1	Posters, brochure	PM EEMA	
1995	Puerto Rico	"Right Decisions—Right Now"	Brochure	RJR and PM Latin America	
1996	Finland	Juvenile integrity campaign	Stickers, posters	Finnish NMA and Daily Goods Retailers Association	
2001	France	"Children under 18 must not smoke; tobacco consumption by children is a problem for all of us; smoking must be for adults only"	Posters	PM	E-mail communications obtained through GLOBALink
2001	Europe	"You can be cool without cigarettes"	MTV ads	PM, BAT, Japan Tobacco	
2001	Germany	14-year-old boy saying, "I don't smoke"	Cinema ads, school computers	PM	
1999	France	"Minors should not smoke"	Cigarette pack labels, retail signs	PM	
1998–2001	New Zealand	"I've got the power"	School program	PM	
2001	New Zealand	"It's the law"	Retail signs	PM	
2001	Romania	"It's your choice" (with approval of health, education, and sports ministers)	PM, BAT		
2001	Brazil	"It's the law"	Retail signs	PM	S. A. Bialous, written communication, April 18, 2001
2001	Mexico	"We don't want minors to smoke, and we are avoiding it" (endorsed by Health Ministry)	media unknown	Tobacco companies	E-mail communications obtained through GLOBALink
2001	Romania	"Action YSP—youth smoking prevention," "Be cool, be yourself" (Ministry of Health & Family also sponsors)	Video ads, shows, arts events, skateboard contest	JTI (RJR)	

Note. GCC = Gulf Cooperation Council; EEMA = Eastern Europe, Middle East, and Africa; EEC = European Economic Community; TI = Tobacco Institute; PM = Philip Morris; RJR = R. J. Reynolds; BAT = British American Tobacco; MTV = MusicTelevision Network. Other abbreviations are taken from reference 3.

messages that can be interpreted as ambiguous, sending a "forbidden fruit" message to youngsters, or that focus on decisionmaking rather than on the health effects of smoking. A Philip Morris Russian slogan had the connotation of "feel it, experience it,"[147] and a slogan in Hong Kong associated smoking with being old enough to drive.[148,149]

A 1994 planning document for a youth smoking campaign circulated for comments to Philip Morris employees in marketing and legal departments for the Scandinavia, Finland, and Eastern European regions reveals that Philip Morris planned to extend a US-originated "Kids Don't Smoke" campaign into Poland to counter what it called a "very vocal and visible small group of [anti-tobacco] militant extremists" who were "attacking the tobacco industry."[150–152] Philip Morris's campaign was to tell Polish children aged 10 to 15 years that they are not mature or educated enough to decide to smoke, without mentioning the health effects of smoking.[152]

In 2001, the "corporate responsibility" section of Philip Morris's commercial Web site[8] described a youth smoking prevention program in the Czech Republic called "Can I Do It?" The Web site states that the program was "piloted in 70 Czech schools and has the support of the Minister of Education" and that it has "the support of other project partners including the Parents Union of the Czech Republic." Philip Morris predicted that by 2004, its "Can I Do It?" program will have spread to more than 90% of the schools in the Czech Republic.[8] Philip Morris International's commercial Web site also states that its youth smoking prevention initiatives have won the company the support of international federal, state, and municipal governments, noting that these programs have allowed Philip Morris to forge alliances with government branches that might otherwise stay at arm's length from the tobacco industry: national ministries of health, education, youth and sports, and environment and justice, and commissioners of television and entertainment.[8]

Beginning in the mid-1990s, Philip Morris began using its Action Against Access program to head off restrictive legislation around the world. Philip Morris's 1995 plan for "Juvenile Integrity Campaign EEMA (Eastern Europe/Middle East/Asia)" shows that the company was deeply concerned that increased public awareness of the industry practice of marketing to youths was eroding its credibility and possibly leading to advertising bans.[153] The plan's author observed that Philip Morris's 1992 Finnish "Juveniles Should Not Smoke" campaign "successfully halted extreme legislation to pass"[153] and that its 1994–1995 Russian "Smoking Can Wait" campaign "significantly added to efforts to create a balanced atmosphere for a tobacco advertising debate in the Russian (Moscow) society."[153] Philip Morris also sought to enact legal age limits for cigarette sales to deflect blame from itself for youth smoking, saying that such age limits "signal [that] the ultimate responsibility [for youth smoking] belongs to parents and society" rather than tobacco companies. As in the United States, Philip Morris also sought to enact legal age limits to "eliminate anti-tobacco groups' demands for ad bans on the basis of "protection of youth."[153]

DISCUSSION

Tobacco industry "youth smoking prevention" programs began to emerge in the 1980s as a political response to increased public scrutiny of industry marketing tactics aimed at youths. After introducing these programs, the industry discovered and began exploiting their utility as effective public relations tools to deflect regulation. During the late 1990s, the industry rapidly expanded these programs worldwide, often with the assistance of educational authorities and governments. This expansion has occurred in the absence of any objective evidence from the tobacco industry or other sources that these programs actually reduce youth smoking and despite the fact that the few studies that do exist in the academic literature suggest that they do not prevent—and may even encourage—youth smoking.[13,15]

The tobacco industry's youth smoking prevention programs do not implement the strategies that have been demonstrated to influence youth smoking: aggressive media campaigns that denormalize tobacco use and stress the industry's dishonesty,[154,155] tax (price) increases that reduce the affordability of cigarettes,[156,157] and smoke-free workplaces[158,159] and homes[160–162] that reduce the social acceptability of smoking and reinforce the nonsmoking norm.[163–169]

The industry's programs consistently fail to address the health consequences of tobacco use and never mention that nicotine is addictive.[15] In particular, the "truth" youth smoking prevention campaign advertisements that stress industry deception were more memorable and convincing to more teens than the Philip Morris "Think. Don't Smoke." campaign.[10–12] "Think. Don't Smoke." advertisements have also been associated with an increase in the intention to smoke in the next year.[170] Even Philip Morris's own focus groups, created to gauge public opinion regarding its youth campaigns, reveal that tobacco industry–led campaigns are "universally rejected as not credible" and that people believe that these such campaigns are "contradictory to industry interests."[171]

Although the industry has generally been successful in introducing its programs, there have been some exceptions. Despite substantial financial inducement and the support of the National 4-H Council, 27 state 4-H branch organizations refused to participate in Philip Morris's program. In 2000, when Philip Morris distributed book covers that said "Think. Don't Smoke." to schools in California without prior authorization, the effort was resoundingly rejected on the advice of the California Departments of Education and Justice.[172] The departments distributed a joint memorandum warning schools that Philip Morris was attempting to promote its corporate identity among children by distributing the book covers and asking that Philip Morris stop the campaign and recall the book covers (Rosaedit Villasenor, Pomona Public Schools; Personal communication; January 11, 2000). This statewide rejection represented a significant improvement in the understanding of tobacco industry motives by the Department of Education, which 10 years earlier had been distributing Tobacco Institute programs.[38]

Citizens and policymakers should reject any "educational" programs by the tobacco industry. If the tobacco industry were sincere in its stated desire to contribute to reducing youth smoking, it would stop opposing policies and programs that have been demonstrated to be effective. Policymakers who believe that the industry would do anything that would negatively affect recruitment of new smokers are ignoring history and fooling themselves. ■

About the Authors

Anne Landman is with the American Lung Association of Colorado, Denver. Pamela M. Ling is with the Traineeships in AIDS Prevention Studies, Center for AIDS Prevention Studies, University of California, San Francisco. Stanton A. Glantz is with the Center for Tobacco Control Research and Education, Institute for Health Policy Studies, Cardiovascular Research Institute, University of California, San Francisco.

Requests for reprints should be sent to Stanton A. Glantz, PhD, Professor of Medicine, Box 0130, University of California, San Francisco, CA 94143 (e-mail: glantz@medicine.ucsf.edu).

This article was accepted February 14, 2002.

Contributors

All authors contributed to the conception and writing of the manuscript. A. Landman and P.M. Ling located most of the industry documents.

Acknowledgments

This work was supported by the American Lung Association of Colorado, the National Institutes of Health (grant T32 MH-19105), and the National Cancer Institute (grant CA-87472).

References

1. Philip Morris [inferred]. Juvenile integrity initiative draft proposal, EEMA region 950809. Philip Morris. August 9, 1995. Bates No. 2501078368/8403. Available at: http://www.pmdocs.com. Accessed December 11, 2001.

2. Philip Morris International [corporate author]. A global commitment to responsible marketing. Philip Morris. 19950200/E, 1995. Bates No. 2501047433/7437. Available at: http://www.pmdocs.com. Accessed December 11, 2001.

3. MEV. Youth campaigns [chart listing tobacco industry youth campaigns 1981–1996]. Philip Morris Tobacco Company. March 4, 1996. Bates No. 2501109041/9042. Available at: http://www.pmdocs.com. Accessed July 13, 2001.

4. Philip Morris [inferred]. Philip Morris USA embarks on a long term, comprehensive youth smoking prevention effort [press release announcing youth smoking prevention initiative]. Philip Morris. December 3, 1998. Bates No. 2063663124/3126. Available at: http://www.pmdocs.com. Accessed December 11, 2001.

5. Lorillard Tobacco Company [corporate author]. The Lorillard Tobacco Company unveils youth smoking prevention program—cutting edge ads to be broadcast [company press release]. Lorillard Tobacco Company. October 12, 1999. Bates No. 80319052/9054. Available at: http://www.lorillarddocs.com. Accessed December 11, 2001.

6. R.J. Reynolds. Right decisions right now. Working together to discourage youth smoking [advertisement]. R.J. Reynolds Tobacco Company. 1993. Bates No. 512538753 -8753. Available at: http://www.rjrtdocs.com. Accessed December 11, 2001.

7. Levy C. Smoking by young people. Philip Morris USA also wants to reduce incidence of smoking by young people. *BMJ.* 1999;319:1268–1269.

8. Philip Morris International. Corporate responsibility—youth smoking prevention: Philip Morris International; 2001. Available at: http://www.pmintl.com. Accessed December 12, 2001.

9. R.J. Reynolds Tobacco Company. Right decisions right now fact sheet; 2001. Available at: http://www.rightdecisionsrightnow.com/facttex.htm. Accessed December 18, 2001.

10. Farrelly M, Healton C, Davis K. Truth and videotapes: reactions to truth campaign ads by smoking status. Abstract presented at: 129th Annual Meeting of the American Public Health Association; October 21–25, 2001; Atlanta, Ga.

11. Haviland ML. Comparison of Legacy's truth with the Philip Morris Campaign. Abstract presented at: 129th Annual Meeting of the American Public Health Association; October 21–25, 2001; Atlanta, Ga.

12. Moon-Howard J, Arnold E, Haviland ML. Assessing the efficacy of anti-smoking messages for urban youth at risk: a comparison of the American Legacy Foundation and Philip Morris ad campaigns. Abstract presented at: 129th Annual Meeting of the American Public Health Association; October 21–25, 2001; Atlanta, Ga.

13. DeBon M, Klesges RC. Adolescents' perceptions about smoking prevention strategies: a comparison of the programmes of the American Lung Association and the Tobacco Institute. *Tob Control.* 1996;5:19–25.

14. Teenage Research Unlimited. Counter-tobacco advertising exploratory [copy of a research report originally prepared for the Arizona, California, and Massachusetts public health anti-tobacco media campaigns]. Philip Morris Tobacco Company. January–March 1999. Bates No. 2069512053/2063. Available at: http://www.pmdocs.com. Accessed October 10, 2000.

15. DiFranza JR, McAfee T. The Tobacco Institute: helping youth say "yes" to tobacco [editorial; see comments]. *J Fam Pract.* 1992;34:694–696.

16. National Center for Tobacco Free Kids. A long history of empty promises: the cigarette companies' youth anti-smoking programs. Washington, DC; March 2, 2000. Available at: http://tobaccofreekids.org/research/factsheets/pdf/0010.pdf. Accessed March 18, 2002.

17. National Center for Tobacco Free Kids. Philip Morris and targeting kids. Washington, DC; August 28, 2001. Available at: http://tobaccofreekids.org/research/factsheets/pdf/0011.pdf. Accessed March 18, 2002.

18. Bates C, Watkins P, McNeill A, Hammond R. Danger! PR in the playground: action on smoking and health, UK. October 2000. Available at: http://www.ash.org.uk/html/advspo/html/prmenu.html. Accessed November 14, 2001.

19. Chapman S. The pied pipers of puffing. *Tob Control.* 1999;8:14–16.

20. Malone RE, Balbach ED. Tobacco industry documents: treasure trove or quagmire? [comments in: *Tob Control.* 2000;9:261–262]. *Tob Control.* 2000;9:334–338.

21. Perry CL. The tobacco industry and underage youth smoking: tobacco industry documents from the Minnesota litigation. *Arch Pediatr Adolesc Med.* 1999;153:935–941.

22. Pollay RW. Targeting youth and concerned smokers: evidence from Canadian tobacco industry documents. *Tob Control.* 2000;9:136–147.

23. Hastings G, MacFadyen L. A day in the life of an advertising man: review of internal documents from the UK tobacco industry's principal advertising agencies [see comments]. *BMJ.* 2000;321:366–371.

24. Cummings KM, Morley C, Horan J, Steger C, Leavell N. Marketing to America's youth: evidence from corporate documents. *Tob Control.* 2002;11(suppl 1):i5–i17.

25. Author unknown. No title [graphic timeline of events pertaining to industry youth program activities]. Philip Morris. May 1996. Bates No: 2501211400A/1401. Available at: http://www.pmdocs.com. Accessed December 11, 2001.

26. Author unknown. Timelines [5-page timeline of industry youth program activities]. Philip Morris Tobacco Company. May [estimated] 1996. Bates No. 2501211402/1406. Available at: http://www.pmdocs.com. Accessed July 13, 2001.

27. Califano JA. Untitled [from Legal Department file room]. Lorillard Tobacco Company. June 15, 1979. Bates No. 03642229. Available at: http://www.lorillarddocs.com. Accessed December 11, 2001.

28. Goldsmith CH, Grefe EA. Untitled [letter from president of Philip Morris to president of the United States requesting apology for Califano's remarks]. Philip Morris. April 28, 1978. Bates No. 1005129063/9065. Available at: http://www.pmdocs.com. Accessed December 11, 2001.

29. Chilcote SJ. Comments of Samuel D. Chilcote Jr. Executive Committee. December 9, 1982. Tobacco Institute. December 9, 1982. R.J. Reynolds Tobacco Company. Bates No. 503907679 -7698. Available at: http://www.rjrtdocs.com. Accessed December 11, 2001.

30. Author unknown. The development of tobacco industry strategy [confidential speech/presentation/report]. Tobacco Institute. Undated. Bates No. TIMN0018970/8979. Available at: http://www.tobaccoinstitute.com. Accessed December 11, 2001.

31. Duffin AH. Promotion of NASBE/TI youth program before legislative and other audiences [confidential memo]. Tobacco Institute. November 27, 1984. Bates No. TIMN0174394. Available at: http://www.tobaccoinstitute.com. Accessed December 11, 2001.

32. AHD [AHD is Anne H. Duffin in many other Tobacco Institute documents]. "Helping youth decide." A presentation for Communications Committee, October 30, 1986. Tobacco Institute. October 27, 1986. Bates No. TIMN0174182/4192. Available at: http://www.tobaccoinstitute.com. Accessed July 14, 2001.

33. Slavitt JJ. TI youth initiative. Philip Morris. February 12, 1991. Bates No. 2500082629. Available at: http://www.pmdocs.com. Accessed December 11, 2001.

34. AHD [probably Anne H. Duffin]. Progress report on the Responsible Living Program. Tobacco Institute. June 10, 1985. Tobacco Documents Online. Bates No. TIMN0174575–4601. Available at: http://

www.tobaccodocuments.org. Accessed December 28, 2000.

35. Harris TC. Planning meeting on impending "Prop 99" efforts. R.J. Reynolds Tobacco Company. December 20, 1991. Bates No. 511999020. Available at: http://www.rjrtdocs.com. Accessed December 11, 2001.

36. Cornell WA, Lispen Whitten. Youth program mailing [memo]. Tobacco Institute. November 28, 1990. Bates No. TIMN0195117/5118. Available at: http://www.tobaccoinstitute.com. Accessed December 11, 2001.

37. Author unknown. Vermont ingredients disclosure plan [file name: Ingredients disclosure]. Philip Morris. August 16, 1996. Bates No. 2062398753/8756. Available at: http://www.pmdocs.com. Accessed December 11, 2001.

38. Glantz S, Balbach E. *Tobacco War: Inside the California Battles.* Berkeley: University of California Press; 2000.

39. Chilcote SD, Kornegay HR. New directions implementation [discussion of "new directions" plan for Tobacco Institute]. October 19, 1981. Bates No. TIMN0067411/7421. Available at: http://www.tobaccoinstitute.com. Accessed December 11, 2001.

40. Tobacco Institute [organizational author]. Responsible living for teenagers a public service proposal for the tobacco industry [report]. Tobacco Institute. May 1982. Bates No. 04210397/0441. Available at: http://www.tobaccoinstitute.com. Accessed December 11, 2001.

41. Duffin AH. Legal advice from John Rupp and Lee Stanford regarding youth program workshop guide [Bliley collection No. 19618]. Tobacco Institute. November 8, 1985. Bates No. TIMN0167402. Available at: http://www.tobaccodocuments.org. Accessed December 11, 2001.

42. Author unknown. FUBYAS Social Group Spectrum. R.J. Reynolds Tobacco Company. 1984. Bates No. 502762721 -2726. Available at: http://www.rjrtdocs.com. Accessed December 11, 2001.

43. Author unknown. Younger adult smokers lifestyles and attitudes [Minnesota selected document]. Brown and Williamson Tobacco Company. Undated. Bates No. 170052241/2255. Available at: http://www.bw.aalatg.com/public.asp. Accessed December 11, 2001.

44. Kwechansky Marketing Research I. Report for: Imperial Tobacco Limited—subject project plus/minus [Minnesota selected document]. Imperial Tobacco. May 7, 1982. Bates No. 566627751/7824. Available at: http://www.tobaccodocuments.org. Accessed December 11, 2001.

45. Kwechansky Marketing Research I. CPY5—subject: project 16 English youth. Imperial Tobacco. October 18, 1977. Bates No. 566627826–7935. Available at: http://www.tobaccodocuments.org. Accessed December 11, 2001.

46. Glantz SA. Preventing tobacco use—the youth access trap [editorial; see comments]. *Am J Public Health.* 1996;86:156–158.

47. PD. Youth access prevention message points 2/18/00. Philip Morris Tobacco Company. February 18, 2000. Bates No. 2071788874/8879; actual ads are Bates Nos. 2071788856/8857, 8862/8863/8902/8903. Available at: http://www.pmdocs.com. Accessed December 7, 2001.

48. Philip Morris [corporate author]. What else is within your kids rich? [sic]. Philip Morris. February [estimated] 2000. Bates No. 2071788856. Available at: http://www.pmdocs.com. Accessed December 11, 2001.

49. Philip Morris [corporate author]. What else are you leaving out for your kids? Philip Morris. February [estimated] 2000. Bates No. 2071788857. Available at: http://www.pmdocs.com. Accessed December 11, 2001.

50. Chilcote SD, Kornegay HR. New directions implementation [discussion of "new directions" plan for Tobacco Institute and how it will be implemented]. Tobacco Institute. October 19, 1981. Bates No. TIMN0067411/7421. Available at: http://www.tobaccoinstitute.com. Accessed December 11, 2001.

51. Author unknown. Discussion paper [confidential report; source: public affairs files, Susan Stuntz]. Tobacco Institute. January 29, 1991. Bates No. TIMN0164422/4424. Available at: http://www.tobaccoinstitute.com. Accessed December 11, 2001.

52. Merryman W. "It's the Law" program helps DC retailers. Tobacco Institute. May 31, 1991. Bates No. TIMN0380101. Available at: http://www.tobaccoinstitute.com. Accessed November 19, 2001.

53. Philip Morris. Philip Morris USA announces initiative against youth smoking. Philip Morris Tobacco Company. June 26, 1995. Bates No. 2501210841/0843. Available at: http://www.pmdocs.com. Accessed November 19, 2001.

54. Merlo E. RE: Icon ad. Philip Morris. April 1, 1996. Bates No. 2046945003B; e-mail also includes Bates Nos. 2046945002, 2046945002B, and 2046945003C–E. Available at: http://www.pmdocs.com. Accessed December 11, 2001.

55. Slavitt JJ. Counter ASSIST plan. Philip Morris. January 17, 1992. Bates No. 2023916866/6867. Available at: http://www.pmdocs.com. Accessed December 11, 2001.

56. Merlo E. No title [speech given by Ellen Merlo]. Philip Morris Tobacco Company. October 24, 1994. Bates No. 2040236685/6706. Available at: http://www.pmdocs.com. Accessed November 13, 2001.

57. Malmgren K, Chicolte S. Draft local program. Tobacco Institute. November 30, 1992. Bates No. 2023959567/9579; cover letter is Bates No. 2023959566. Available at: http://www.pmdocs.com. Accessed December 7, 2001.

58. Walls T, Daragan K, Pontarelli J. CAC presentation #4. Philip Morris Tobacco Company. July 8, 1994. Bates No. 2041183751/3790. Available at: http://www.pmdocs.com. Accessed December 6, 2001.

59. Welsh-Huggins A. Lawmakers try again to stop health boards from banning smoking. *Associated Press State & Local Wire.* October 11, 2001.

60. Riskind J, Bradshaw J. Tobacco forces, foes to butt heads on smoking. *Columbus Dispatch.* February 4, 1995:1C.

61. Philip Morris. An important message about your board of health. 1995. Bates No. 2063417286/7294. Available at: http://www.pmdocs.com. Accessed December 3, 2001.

62. Author unknown. Organizations in support of House Bill 299. Philip Morris Tobacco Company. March 26, 1996. Bates No. 2063422603/2604. Available at: http://www.pmdocs.com. Accessed December 6, 2001.

63. The Hannah Report. "Under 18 No Tobacco" program commences. Philip Morris Tobacco Company. August 13, 1996. Bates No. 2062905640/5641. Available at: http://www.pmdocs.com. Accessed December 6, 2001.

64. Food and Drug Administration. Regulations restricting the sale and distribution of cigarettes and smokeless tobacco products to protect children and adolescents. *Federal Register.* 1995;60:41314–41451.

65. Parrish SC. Presentation to the board: FDA issues update. Philip Morris. August 30, 1995. Bates No. 2047690071/0090. Available at: http://www.pmdocs.com. Accessed December 11, 2001.

66. Tobacco Institute [organizational author]. FDA regulations called ineffective and illegal. Industry shares goal of reducing youth smoking, joins with others in opposition to FDA rules [published press release]. Tobacco Institute. August 23, 1996. Bates No. 514853473/3474. Available at: http://www.rjrtdocs.com. Accessed December 11, 2001.

67. Blackman LCF. The credibility of the industry stance. British American Tobacco. May 22, 1980. Bates No. 100429169/9174. Available at: http://outside.cdc.gov:8080/BASIS/ncctld/web/mnimages/DDW?W=DETAILSID=762. Accessed December 13, 2001.

68. Author unknown. CH—perceived credibility of information sources on public health issues. Philip Morris Tobacco Company. 1991. Bates No. 2028464060/4063. Available at: http://www.pmdocs.com. Accessed December 19, 2001.

69. Blake J, Dowling J, Florio D, et al. Philip Morris Incorporated 840000 corporate affairs world conference Rye Brook, New York 840913 workshop—dealing with the issues indirectly: constituencies. Philip Morris. September 13, 1984. Bates No. 2025421934/2000. Available at: http://www.pmdocs.com. Accessed December 13, 2001.

70. Humber T. Memorandum. Committee recommendations on "Responsible Living" project. Lorillard Tobacco Company. April 12, 1984. Bates No. 04210444/0455. Available at: http://www.lorillarddocs.com. Accessed November 19, 2001.

71. Duffin A. Media schedule Walker Merryman/Jolly Ann Davidson. Tobacco Institute. September [estimated] 1984. Bates No. TIMN0208662. Available at: http://www.tobaccoinstitute.com. Accessed December 13, 2001.

72. AHD [probably Anne H. Duffin]. Jolly appearances on HYD. Tobacco Institute. April 4, 1985. Bates No. TIMN0053316. Available at: http://www.tobaccoinstitute.com. Accessed December 13, 2001.

73. Radio TV Reports Inc. Davidson/Merryman interview: "Helping Youth Decide." Tobacco Institute. September 26, 1984. Bates No. TIMN0208145/8150. Available at: http://www.tobaccoinstitute.com. Accessed December 13, 2001.

74. Duffin AH. Fourth Quarter Jolly & Walker tour [memo to Walker Merryman]. Tobacco Institute. August 23, 1985. Bates No. TIMN0207998/7999. Available at: http://www.tobaccoinstitute.com. Accessed December 19, 2001.

75. AHD [probably Anne H. Duffin]. Youth program broadcast appearances. Tobacco Institute. March 6, 1985. Bates No. TIMN0053396. Available at: http://www.tobaccoinstitute.com. Accessed July 14, 2001.

76. McBeath WH, American Public Health Association. Untitled letter [to NASBE opposing their collaboration with Tobacco Institute and "Helping Youth Decide"]. Tobacco Institute. July 8, 1985. Bates No. TIMN0207986/7987. Available at: http://www.tobaccoinstitute.com. Accessed December 19, 2001.

77. Whelan EM, American Council on Science and Health. Untitled letter [to NASBE opposing "Helping Youth Decide" and collaboration with Tobacco Institute]. Tobacco Institute. January 11, 1985. Bates No. TIMN0207984/7985. Available at: http://www.tobaccoinstitute.com. Accessed December 19, 2001.

78. Seffrin JR. Hypocrisy—by default or by design? Tobacco Institute. April 1985. Bates No. TIMN0202006. Available at: http://www.tobaccoinstitute.com. Accessed December 19, 2001.

79. National Association of State Boards of Education (NASBE). Untitled letter [response to C. Everett Koop's letter regarding "Helping Youth Decide"]. Tobacco Institute. January 8, 1985. Bates No. TIMN0202005. Available at: http://www.tobaccoinstitute.com. Accessed December 19, 2001.

80. Swomley JA. Untitled [letter to NASBE Board of Directors regarding "Helping Youth Decide"]. Tobacco Institute. August 1985. Bates No. 505090599–0599; the first page of this letter is probably Bates No. 505090596; NASBE's reply (in part) can be found at Bates No. 505090598. Available at: http://www.rjrtdocs.com. Accessed December 19, 2001.

81. Blaunstein PL, National Association of State Boards of Education. Untitled letter [reply to James Swomley's letter regarding "Helping Youth Decide"]. Tobacco Institute. September 3, 1985. R.J. Reynolds Tobacco Company. Bates No. 505090598–0598; the letter this refers to is Bates No. 505090599 and probably No. 505090596. Available at: http://www.rjrtdocs.com. Accessed December 19, 2001.

82. Swomley JA. Untitled letter [opposing NASBE participation in "Helping Youth Decide"]. Tobacco Institute. August 20, 1985. Bates No. TIMN0207979/7980; this document contains the complete letter and is identical to Nos. 505090596 and 505090599 on the R.J. Reynolds Web site. Available at: http://www.tobaccoinstitute.com. Accessed December 19, 2001.

83. Duffin A. National Association of State Boards of Education. Tobacco Institute. December 16, 1986. Bates No. TIMN0174177/4178. Available at: http://www.tobaccoinstitute.com. Accessed July 14, 2001.

84. Duffin AH. Untitled letter [suggestions for new form letter NASBE is using to answer critical mail]. Tobacco Institute. March 11, 1985. Bates No. TIMN0053386/3388; copies of the draft letters are Bates Nos. TIMN0053389 and TIMN0053390. Available at: http://www.tobaccoinstitute.com. Accessed July 14, 2001.

85. AHD [probably Anne H. Duffin]. Youth program success story folder. Tobacco Institute. April 11, 1985. Bates No. TIMN0053306/3307. Available at: http://www.tobaccoinstitute.com. Accessed July 14, 2001.

86. AHD. Untitled [note probably written by Anne Duffin to "Nancy" about NASBE changes on HYD success story folder]. Tobacco Institute. April 11, 1985. Bates No. TIMN0053300. Available at: http://www.tobaccoinstitute.com. Accessed July 14, 2001.

87. AHD [probably Anne H. Duffin]. Untitled [NASBE logo off success story folder]. Tobacco Institute. April 24, 1985. Bates No. TIMN0167515/7520; p. 7515 is filed separately from 7516–7520. Available at: http://www.tobaccoinstitute.com. Accessed July 14, 2001.

88. Author unknown. Opening new doors [success of "Helping Youth Decide" booklet]. Tobacco Institute. 1985. Bates No. TIMN0053302/3304. Available at: http://www.tobaccoinstitute.com. Accessed July 14, 2001.

89. Muraskin L. Untitled [letter requesting NASBE logo not to appear on success story brochure]. Tobacco Institute. April 24, 1985. Bates No. TIMN0177963. Available at: http://www.tobaccoinstitute.com. Accessed July 14, 2001.

90. AHD. Untitled [note probably written by Anne Duffin planning negotiations with NASBE over money]. Tobacco Institute. May 30, 1986. Bates No. TIMN0318906. Available at: http://www.tobaccoinstitute.com. Accessed July 14, 2001.

91. Karen. Memorandum re: HYD project [memo is to "Phyllis"—probably Phyllis Blaunstein, executive director of NASBE]. Tobacco Institute. February 2, 1987. Bates No. TIMN0170082/0084. Available at: http://www.tobaccoinstitute.com. Accessed July 14, 2001.

92. Stuntz S. Memorandum [to Samuel D. Chilcote, outlining Tobacco Institute's efforts to replace NASBE as Responsible Living program sponsor]. Tobacco Institute. December 15, 1988. Bates No. TIMN0182254/2255. Available at: http://www.tobaccoinstitute.com. Accessed July 4, 2001.

93. Stuntz S. Efforts to replace NASBE on Responsible Living program. Tobacco Institute. December 15, 1988. Bates No. TIMN0182245/2246. Available at: http://www.tobaccoinstitute.com. Accessed December 13, 2001.

94. Sparber P, Blaunstein P. Family COURSE Consortium program offering. Tobacco Institute. 1991. Bates No. TIMN0166619/6621. Available at: http://www.tobaccoinstitute.com. Accessed December 13, 2001.

95. Stuntz S. Continuation of HYD program. Tobacco Institute. March 3, 1989. Bates No. TIMN0193575/3577. Available at: http://www.tobaccoinstitute.com. Accessed July 14, 2001.

96. Author unknown. Model YSP plant communities youth smoking prevention model communities plan. Philip Morris. June 2, 1999. Bates No. 2070740693/0707. Available at: http://www.pmdocs.com. Accessed December 13, 2001.

97. Tyler BY. Untitled letter. Philip Morris. October 1, 1998. Bates No. 2069554227. Available at: http://www.pmdocs.com. Accessed December 13, 2001.

98. Daragan K. Untitled letter. Philip Morris. March 18, 1999. Bates No. 2069554281. Available at: http://www.pmdocs.com. Accessed December 13, 2001.

99. National 4-H [organizational author]. Media alert—press conference Thurs 000325 9AM draw communities together, stop youth smoking. Philip Morris. March 24, 1999. Bates No. 2070740823. Available at: http://www.tobaccoinstitute.com. Accessed December 13, 2001.

100. Shields D. Untitled letter. Philip Morris. February 1, 1999. Bates No. 2069500522. Available at: http://www.pmdocs.com. Accessed December 13, 2001.

101. Nenno M. Untitled letter. Philip Morris. February 15, 1999. Bates No. 2069500521. Available at: http://www.pmdocs.com. Accessed December 13, 2001.

102. Garrison JR. Untitled letter. Philip Morris. January 21, 1999. Bates No. 2069500520. Available at: http://www.pmdocs.com. Accessed December 13, 2001.

103. Wheeler MC. Untitled letter. Philip Morris. March 3, 1999. Bates No. 2069500517/0518. Available at: http://www.pmdocs.com. Accessed December 13, 2001.

104. Houston TP. Untitled letter. Philip Morris. April 20, 1999. Bates No. 2069500498. Available at: http://www.pmdocs.com. Accessed December 13, 2001.

105. National 4-H Council. Health, wellness, and safety programs: health rocks! 2001. Available at: http://www.fourhcouncil.edu/programs/category.asp?scatid=36&catid=1&subid=11. Accessed December 19, 2001.

106. National 4-H Council. Health rocks! 2001. Available at: http://www.healthrocks.org/resource/showquestion.asp?fldAuto=33&fid=14. Accessed December 19, 2001.

107. Sauer RJ. Untitled letter [to William Novelli responding to opposition of their Youth Smoking Prevention program]. Philip Morris. March 23, 1999. Bates No. 2069500509/0510. Available at: http://www.pmdocs.com. Accessed November 13, 2001.

108. Author unknown. Field staff evaluation of resources (1985 through 1986). Tobacco Institute. August 1986. Bates No. TIMS0025751/5782. Available at: http://www.tobaccoinstitute. Accessed December 13, 2001.

109. Author unknown. AAA measurement methodologies. Philip Morris Tobacco Company. 1995. Bates No. 2045191320. Available at: http://www.pmdocs.com. Accessed September 15, 2000.

110. Author unknown. Action Against Access. Philip Morris Tobacco Company. August 15–November 26, 1995. Bates No. 2045191191/1315. Available at: http://www.pmdocs.com. Accessed July 9, 2001.

111. Author unknown. Action Against Access module. Philip Morris Tobacco Company. August 15, 1995. Bates No. 2045191316/1318. Available at: http://www.pmdocs.com. Accessed July 9, 2001.

112. Divall L. National survey annotated questionnaire. Philip Morris Tobacco Company. July 21, 1995. Bates No. 2045175251/5261. Available at: http://www.pmdocs.com. Accessed September 29, 2000.

113. National Association of State Boards of Education. Helping Youth Decide. An evaluation of its use. Tobacco Institute. March 1986. Bates Nos. TIMN0169494/9518 and TIFL0306374 –6398. Available at: http://www.tobaccoinstitute.com. Accessed July 13, 2001.

114. Author unknown. Evaluation design: Helping Youth Decide. Tobacco Institute. August 20, 1985. Bates No. TIMN0168465/8471. Available at: http://www.tobaccoinstitute.com. Accessed December 13, 2001.

115. Author unknown. Campaigns to discourage juve-

nile smoking (by date launched). R.J. Reynolds. October 4, 1994. Bates No. 512572963/2969. Available at: http://www.rjrtdocs.com. Accessed December 13, 2001.

116. Young & Rubicam. Philip Morris youth no smoking effort advertising research. Philip Morris Tobacco Company. September 1992. Bates No. 2046522325/2397. Available at: http://www.pmdocs.com. Accessed July 10, 2001.

117. Levy CJ. RE: Philip Morris USA youth smoking prevention TV execution clearance. Philip Morris Tobacco Company. November 11, 1998. Bates No. 2069512288/2294. Available at: http://www.pmdocs.com. Accessed October 13, 2001.

118. Dunn WL. Proposed study by Levy. Philip Morris Tobacco Company. November 3, 1977. Bates No. 1003293588. Available at: http://www.tobaccodocuments.org. Accessed June 4, 2001.

119. Ryan F, Levy C. 1600—smoker psychology behavioral research annual report. Philip Morris Tobacco Company. June 13, 1977. Bates No. 1000369089/9121. Available at: http://www.pmdocs.com and tobaccodocuments.org. Accessed August 8, 2001.

120. Johnston M. Trends in smoking among high school seniors. Philip Morris Tobacco Company. August 15, 1985. Bates No. 2040282066/2092. Available at: http://www.tobaccodocuments.org. Accessed September 24, 2001.

121. Merlo E. Untitled [letter from Ellen Merlo to ABC News]. Philip Morris Tobacco Company. March 30, 1999. Bates No. 2069512083/2084. Available at: http://www.pmdocs.com. Accessed July 9, 2001.

122. Claiborne R. No title [letter to Ellen Merlo regarding ABC News story on youth smoking advertisements]. Philip Morris Tobacco Company. March 31, 1999. Bates No. 2069512081/2082; the letter this responds to can be found at Bates No. 2069512083/2084. Available at: http://www.pmdocs.com. Accessed July 9, 2001.

123. Author unknown. YSP Superbowl ad: my reasons message points 990102. Philip Morris. January 10, 2000. Bates No. 2071787255/7260. Available at: http://www.pmdocs.com. Accessed December 13, 2001.

124. Author unknown. Copy testing program. Philip Morris Tobacco Company. June 1992. Bates No. 2040712964/3059. Available at: http://www.pmdocs.com. Accessed February 13, 2002.

125. Author unknown. Copy testing. Philip Morris Tobacco Company. March 20, 1984. Bates No. 2500002208/2252. Available at: http://www.pmdocs.com. Accessed February 13, 2002.

126. BMSG Worldwide. Lorillard youth smoking prevention program opinion PR/ad launch program results summary. Lorillard Tobacco Company. January 20, 2000. Bates No. 81760962/0971. Available at: http://www.lorillarddocs.com. Accessed December 13, 2001.

127. University of California San Francisco, The Library & Center for Knowledge Management, Tobacco Control Archives. Joe Camel Campaign: Mangini v R.J. Reynolds Tobacco Company Collection: University of California San Francisco; 2001. Available at: http://www.library.ucsf.edu/tobacco/mangini. Accessed December 13, 2001.

128. William Esty, McCain JH. NFO preference share data—"youth" market. R.J. Reynolds Tobacco Company. March 8, 1973. Bates No. 501167049–7051. Available at: http://www.rjrtdocs.com. Accessed December 12, 2001.

129. Marketing Innovations I. Title: Project report. Youth cigarette—new concepts. Brown and Williamson. September 1972. Bates No. 170042014. Available at: http://www.bw.aalatg.com. Accessed December 14, 2001.

130. Achey TL. Product information. Lorillard Tobacco Company. August 30, 1978. Bates No. 03537131/7132. Available at: http://www.lorillarddocs.com. Accessed December 14, 2001.

131. Johnston M. Young smokers—prevalence, trends, implications and related demographic trends. Philip Morris. March 31, 1981. Bates No. 1000390805/0806. Available at: http://www.pmdocs.com. Accessed December 14, 2001.

132. Pierce JP, Choi WS, Gilpin EA, Farkas AJ, Berry CC. Tobacco industry promotion of cigarettes and adolescent smoking [see comments; published erratum appears in *JAMA*. 1998;280:422]. *JAMA*. 1998;279:511–515.

133. Breo DL. Kicking butts—AMA, Joe Camel, and the "black-flag" war on tobacco. *JAMA*. 1993;270:1978–1984.

134. Fischer PM, Schwartz MP, Richards JW Jr, Goldstein AO, Rojas TH. Brand logo recognition by children aged 3 to 6 years. Mickey Mouse and Old Joe the Camel [see comments]. *JAMA*. 1991;266:3145–3148.

135. DiFranza JR, Richards JW, Paulman PM, et al. RJR Nabisco's cartoon camel promotes Camel cigarettes to children [see comments; published erratum appears in *JAMA*. 1992;268:2034] *JAMA*. 1991;266:3149–3153.

136. Pierce JP, Gilpin EA, Choi WS. Sharing the blame: smoking experimentation and future smoking-attributable mortality due to Joe Camel and Marlboro advertising and promotions. *Tob Control*. 1999;8:37–44.

137. Young & Rubicam. Youth initiative campaign launch. Philip Morris Tobacco Company. March 1993. Bates No. 2023588507/8546. Available at: http://www.pmdocs.com. Accessed July 10, 2001.

138. Young & Rubicam. Chesterfield. Philip Morris Tobacco Company. March 24, 1994. Bates No. 2500096977/7024. Available at: http://www.pmdocs.com. Accessed June 7, 2001.

139. Young & Rubicam. Brand X: a qualitative exploratory among young adult male smokers. Philip Morris Tobacco Company. February 1994. Bates No. 2040174998/5045. Available at: http://www.pmdocs.com. Accessed August 30, 2000.

140. Philip Morris Tobacco Company. Profile of the young adult Marlboro smoker part I: males, 18 to 24 years old. Philip Morris Tobacco Company. August 1994. Bates No. 2061804612/4673. Available at: http://www.pmdocs.com. Accessed August 30, 2000.

141. Ling PM, Glantz SA. Why and how the tobacco industry sells cigarettes to young adults: evidence from industry documents. *Am J Public Health*. 2002;92:908–916.

142. Author unknown. Lorillard Tobacco Youth Smoking Prevention program national television 991014–991031/991115–991205. Lorillard Tobacco Company. October 14, 1999. Bates No. 80318200/8206. Available at: http://www.lorillarddocs.com. Accessed December 21, 2001.

143. Author unknown. Lorillard Youth Smoking Prevention program full year 2000 continuity with impact. Lorillard Tobacco Company. 2000. Bates No. 83688941. Available at: http://www.lorillarddocs.com. Accessed December 21, 2001.

144. Ling PM, Glantz SA. Using tobacco industry marketing research to design more effective tobacco control campaigns. *JAMA*. In press.

145. Lorillard Tobacco Company. TeenH.I.P. Survey; 2001. Available at: http://www.buttoutnow.com. Accessed November 15, 2001.

146. Lieber CL. Youth campaign for Latin America. Philip Morris Tobacco Company. September 23, 1993. Bates No. 2503007040/7041. Available at: http://www.pmdocs.com. Accessed November 15, 2001.

147. Author unknown. Translation of posters Moscow youth no smoking campaign. Philip Morris Tobacco Company. 1994. Bates No. 2500082593; the actual advertisements are found at Bates No. 2500082586/2594. Available at: http://www.pmdocs.com. Accessed November 15, 2001.

148. Tobacco Institute of Hong Kong. The Tobacco industry is launching a programme to deter Hong Kong children and minors from smoking or purchasing cigarettes. Philip Morris Tobacco Company. May 29, 1990. Bates No. 2501109205; the advertisement is Bates No. 2501109206. Available at: http://www.pmdocs.com. Accessed December 12, 2001.

149. Tobacco Institute Hong Kong [inferred]. If you're not old enough to drive . . . you're not old enough to smoke. Philip Morris Tobacco Company. May 29, 1990. Bates No. 2501109206; the press release crediting the Tobacco Institute of Hong Kong is Bates No. 2501109205. Available at: http://www.pmdocs.com. Accessed November 15, 2001.

150. Philip Morris [inferred]. Untitled [organizational charts for Philip Morris Europe/EEMA]. Philip Morris Tobacco Company. 1992. Bates No. 2025602554/2563. Available at: http://www.pmdocs.com. Accessed December 12, 2001.

151. Mandato JA. Untitled [memo outlining Philip Morris Eastern Europe Middle East Africa regional restructuring]. Philip Morris Tobacco Company. May 1990. Bates No. 2501389902/9915. Available at: http://www.pmdocs.com. Accessed December 12, 2001.

152. Philip Morris. "Juveniles shouldn't smoke" campaign brief. Philip Morris Tobacco Company. October 4, 1994. Bates No. 2501047671/7673. Available at: http://www.pmdocs.com. Accessed April 19, 2001.

153. Philip Morris [inferred]. Juvenile integrity initiative draft proposal, EEMA region. Philip Morris Tobacco Company. August 11, 1995. Bates No. 2501241404/1444; 2501241401 is an attached e-mail from R. P. Reavey to Stig Carlson in Corporate Affairs for Philip Morris. Available at: http://www.pmdocs.com. Accessed November 15, 2001.

154. Goldman LK, Glantz SA. Evaluation of antismoking advertising campaigns [see comments]. *JAMA*. 1998;279:772–777.

155. Healton C. Who's afraid of the truth? *Am J Public Health*. 2001;91:554–558.

156. Chaloupka FJ. Macro-social influences: the effects of prices and tobacco-control policies on the demand for tobacco products. *Nicotine Tob Res*. 1999;1(suppl 1):S105–S109.

157. Biener L, Aseltine RH Jr, Cohen B, Anderka M.

Reactions of adult and teenaged smokers to the Massachusetts tobacco tax. *Am J Public Health.* 1998;88: 1389–1391.

158. Chapman S, Borland R, Scollo M, Brownson RC, Dominello A, Woodward S. The impact of smoke-free workplaces on declining cigarette consumption in Australia and the United States. *Am J Public Health.* 1999; 89:1018–1023.

159. Fichtenberg CM, Glantz SA. Smokefree workplaces substantially reduce smoking: a systematic review. *BMJ.* In press.

160. Farkas AJ, Gilpin EA, Distefan JM, Pierce JP. The effects of household and workplace smoking restrictions on quitting behaviours. *Tob Control.* 1999;8: 261–265.

161. Gilpin EA, White MM, Farkas AJ, Pierce JP. Home smoking restrictions: which smokers have them and how they are associated with smoking behavior. *Nicotine Tob Res.* 1999;1(2):153–162.

162. Pierce JP, Gilpin EA, Farkas AJ. Can strategies used by statewide tobacco control programs help smokers make progress in quitting? *Cancer Epidemiol Biomarkers Prev.* 1998;7:459–464.

163. Institute of Medicine. *State Programs Can Reduce Tobacco Use.* Washington, DC: National Cancer Policy Board, Institute of Medicine, National Research Council; 2000. Available at: http://www.nap.edu. Accessed November 2, 2001.

164. Glantz SA, Jamieson P. Attitudes toward secondhand smoke, smoking, and quitting among young people. *Pediatrics.* 2000;106:E82.

165. *Preventing Tobacco Use Among Young People: A Report of the Surgeon General.* Atlanta, Ga: US Dept of Health and Human Services; July 1994.

166. Kaplan RM, Ake CF, Emery SL, Navarro AM. Simulated effect of tobacco tax variation on population health in California. *Am J Public Health.* 2001;91: 239–244.

167. Centers for Disease Control and Prevention. *Best Practices for Comprehensive Tobacco Control Programs.* Atlanta, Ga: National Center for Chronic Disease Prevention and Health Promotion, Office on Smoking and Health; August 1999.

168. Johnston M. Handling and excise tax increase. Philip Morris USA. September 3, 1987. Bates No. 2022216179/6180. Available at: http://www.pmdocs.com. Accessed November 15, 2001.

169. Johnston M. Teenage smoking and the federal excise tax on cigarettes. Philip Morris USA. September 17, 1981. Bates No. 2001255224/5227. Available at: http://www.pmdocs.com. Accessed November 15, 2001.

170. Farrelly MC, Healton CG, Davis KC, Messeri P, Hersey JC, Haviland ML. Getting to the truth: evaluating national tobacco countermarketing campaigns. *Am J Public Health.* 2002;92:901–907.

171. Murray S. Focus groups country reports draft report–Germany. Philip Morris Tobacco Company. February 1, 1994. Bates No. 2501631336/1341; cover letter with author is No. 2501361335. Available at: http://www.pmdocs.com. Accessed November 15, 2001.

172. Lockyer B, Eastin D. Attorney General Lockyer and Schools Chief Eastin warn of misleading Philip Morris anti-smoking campaign [press release]. Sacramento: California Departments of Justice and Education; April 16, 2001.

Coverage of Tobacco Dependence Treatments for Pregnant Women and for Children and Their Parents

Jennifer K. Ibrahim, PhD, Helen Halpin Schauffler, PhD, Dianne C. Barker, MHS, and C. Tracy Orleans, PhD

In 2000, 36% of the 32 million Medicaid recipients and 25% of pregnant Medicaid recipients were smokers.[1,2] Rates of tobacco use in the general population were considerably lower: 23% of the general population in 2000[2] and 12% of pregnant women in 1999.[3] Helping pregnant women to quit smoking would have enormous health benefits, including reducing tobacco-related spontaneous abortions, rates of low-birthweight infants, admissions to neonatal intensive care units, infant deaths from perinatal disorders, and sudden infant death syndrome.[4,5]

In addition, 9.2% of youths in grades 6 through 8 and 28.5% of youths in grades 9 through 12 reported being current smokers in 2000.[6] Reduction in tobacco use by youths and their parents would also have important health benefits. Not only are children and adolescents harmed by exposure to secondhand smoke, but they also underestimate the addictiveness of nicotine and its future health consequences; 73% of teen daily smokers who think they won't be smoking in 5 years are still smoking 5 to 6 years later.[7] Nearly 90% of adult smokers had their first cigarette before they were 18 years old.[7]

The 2000 Public Health Service (PHS) clinical practice guideline *Treating Tobacco Use and Dependence* recommends health insurance payment for services demonstrated to be effective in helping smokers to quit, thereby reducing the barrier of cost.[8] Nonmedication counseling interventions, including individual face-to-face, group, and telephone counseling, are recommended as the first line of treatment for pregnant smokers at the initial prenatal visit and throughout pregnancy, given the uncertain risks and benefits of pharmacotherapy for maternal and fetal health outcomes.[8]

For adolescents, the PHS guideline recommends assessing tobacco use and offering cessation counseling[8] that increases quit rates above naturally occurring levels.[9] The guideline also recommends that pediatricians "offer smoking cessation advice and interventions to parents to limit children's exposure to secondhand smoke."[8] Medicaid requires states to cover specific preventive services, including prenatal care and Early and Periodic Screening, Detection, and Treatment (EPSDT) services for youths younger than 21 years.[10] Coverage for additional preventive services, such as treatments for tobacco use and dependence, is optional and decided by each state.

The purpose of this research was to determine the extent to which guidline-based tobacco dependence treatments are covered by state Medicaid programs for pregnant women, and under EPSDT for children and their parents who smoke.

METHODS

In the fall of 2000, we faxed a 10-page survey to the directors of all states plus the District of Columbia Medicaid programs (n=51) to obtain information on Medicaid coverage of tobacco dependence treatments.[11] One-third of the directors responded within 2 weeks of the initial fax; we followed up by telephone, e-mail, and fax for a 100% response rate. Survey questions addressed coverage for pharmacotherapy, counseling services, and screening practices under EPSDT, as well as special cessation programs, home visits, and counseling for pregnant women.

RESULTS

Coverage for Pregnant Women

Ten state Medicaid programs offer benefits specifically for the treatment of tobacco dependence in pregnant women, with all but 1 of these including some form of counseling (Table 1). Additionally, of the 21 states that reported covering home visit programs for pregnant women, 13 include coverage of counseling for tobacco dependence. In all, 16 state programs cover some form of counseling for pregnant smokers.

Coverage and Services Under EPSDT

Under EPSDT, 7 states cover smoking cessation counseling for children, and 4 cover counseling for their smoking parents. Sixteen state Medicaid programs cover some form of pharmacotherapy for treating tobacco use under EPSDT for youths and their parents who smoke. The most commonly covered pharmacological treatment is bupropion SR (including Zyban and Wellbutrin). Fewer than 10 states cover the nicotine patch, inhaler, nasal spray, or gum under EPSDT.

Fifteen state Medicaid programs require EPSDT providers to screen youths younger than 18 years for tobacco use. Six of these states also require EPSDT providers to screen parents. Seventeen states require Medicaid providers to conduct health education with youths during routine visits; 6 of those states require providers to conduct health education with the children's parents.

Validation

Because data were collected by self-report, we asked each state Medicaid director to submit a written copy of his or her state's tobacco dependence treatment policies for validation; 20 provided written documentation validating what they had reported, 11 reported having no specific benefit language for tobacco dependence treatments (indicating that pharmacotherapy was covered under their standard drug benefit), and 3 did not respond to our request for documentation. We observed no contradictions when we compared the survey responses with the documentation.

DISCUSSION

The PHS guideline for treating tobacco dependence—as it pertains to pregnant women, children, and adolescents—is not being followed by the majority of state

TABLE 1—State Medicaid Tobacco Dependence Treatment Programs and Benefits for Pregnant Women and Children, 2000[a]

	Pregnant Women Who Smoke, Covered Under Medicaid			Children and Their Parents Who Smoke, Covered Under EPSDT			
State	Offers Special Program	Covers Counseling	Covers Home Visit Counseling	Covers Drugs	Covers Counseling	Requires Providers to Conduct Health Education	Requires Providers to Screen for Tobacco Use
Alabama							Parents and children
Arizona				Children only	Children only	Children only	Children only
Arkansas				Parents and children			
California	Yes	Yes	Yes	Parents only	Parents and children	Parents and children	Parents and children
Colorado	Yes	Yes		Children only			
Connecticut				Children only	Children only	Children only	Children only
Delaware				Parents and children			
Hawaii				Parents and children	Children only		
Idaho							
Illinois			Yes	Parents and children		Children only	
Indiana							
Iowa						Parents and children	
Kansas				Parents only	Parents only	Children only	Parents and children
Louisiana	Yes					Parents and children	Parents and children
Maine	Yes	Yes					Children only
Maryland						Children only	Children only
Massachusetts	Yes	Yes	Yes			Children only	Children only
Minnesota			Yes				
Nevada			Yes	Children only		Children only	
New Hampshire	Yes	Yes	Yes	Parents and children	Parents and children	Parents and children	Parents and children
New Jersey				Parents and children			Children only
New Mexico			Yes	Parents and children		Parents and children	Children only
North Carolina			Yes				
North Dakota			Yes				
Oregon	Yes	Yes	Yes				
Rhode Island			Yes		Children only	Children only	Children only
South Dakota				Children only			
Texas						Parents and children	Parents and children
Utah						Children only	
Vermont				Parents and children	Parents and children	Children only	
Virginia	Yes	Yes	Yes	Parents and children			
Washington	Yes	Yes	Yes			Children only	Children only
West Virginia	Yes	Yes					
Total no. (%)	10 (20%)	9 (18%)	13 (26%)	16 (32%)	8 (16%)	17 (34%)	15 (30%)

Note. EPSDT = Early and Periodic Screening, Detection, and Treatment programs.
[a]Eighteen state Medicaid programs (in Alaska, Florida, Georgia, Kentucky, Michigan, Mississippi, Missouri, Montana, Nebraska, New York, Ohio, Oklahoma, Pennsylvania, South Carolina, Tennessee, Washington, DC, Wisconsin, and Wyoming) did not cover any special programs or benefits for tobacco users who were pregnant or who received services under EPSDT.

Medicaid and EPSDT programs, despite strong evidence that health insurance coverage for tobacco dependence treatments increases both the use of these services and quit rates.[12,13] Adding coverage for effective tobacco dependence treatments to the federally mandated Medicaid benefits package for pregnant women and for children and parents under EPSDT would eliminate the disparities in coverage across the states and make a significant difference in the health of low-income pregnant women and their children, 2 of our most vulnerable populations. ■

About the Authors

Jennifer K. Ibrahim and Helen Halpin Schauffler are with the Center for Health and Public Policy Studies, University of California, Berkeley. Dianne C. Barker is with Barker Bi-Coastal Health Consultants, Calabasas, Calif. C. Tracy Orleans is with the Robert Wood Johnson Foundation, Princeton, NJ.

Requests for reprints should be sent to Jennifer K. Ibrahim, PhD, University of California, San Francisco, Center for Tobacco Control Research and Education, 530 Parnassus Ave, Suite 366, San Francisco, CA 94143-1390 (e-mail: ibrahim@itsa.ucsf.edu).

This brief was accepted April 23, 2002.

Contributors

J. K. Ibrahim is the primary author and was responsible for analyzing the survey data from the 50 state Medicaid programs, conducting background research, and writing the brief. H. Halpin Schauffler is the second author and was responsible for obtaining funding for the state Medicaid surveys, creating the framework, reviewing and revising the analysis of the survey data, and writing the brief. Both D. C. Barker and C. T. Orleans participated in creating the framework for the brief, as well as reviewing and revising drafts.

Acknowledgments

This research was conducted by the Center for Health and Public Policy Studies at the University of California, Berkeley, and funded by grant 022246 from the Robert Wood Johnson Foundation.

Human Participant Protection

No protocol approval was needed for this study.

References

1. Kaiser Family Foundation. *Medicaid Enrollment: Kaiser Commission on Medicaid and the Uninsured.* Washington, DC: Kaiser Family Foundation; 2000.

2. Centers for Disease Control and Prevention. Behavioral Risk Factor Surveillance System 2000 survey data. Available at: http://www.cdc.gov/brfss/ti-surveydata2000.htm. Accessed September 9, 2002.

3. Mathews TJ. Smoking during pregnancy in the 1990s. National Vital Statistics Report. 2001:49(7):1–16.

4. Melvin CL. Pregnant women, infants, and the cost savings of smoking cessation. *Tob Control.* 1997; 6(suppl 1):S89–S91.

5. *Women and Smoking: A Report of the Surgeon General.* Atlanta, Ga: Centers for Disease Control and Prevention, National Center for Chronic Disease Prevention and Health Promotion, Office on Smoking and Health; 2001.

6. Centers for Disease Control and Prevention. *Investment in Tobacco Control: State Highlights, 2001.* Atlanta, Ga: Centers for Disease Control and Prevention, National Center for Chronic Disease Prevention and Health Promotion, Office on Smoking and Health; 2001.

7. *Preventing Tobacco Use Among Young People: A Report of the Surgeon General.* Atlanta, Ga: Centers for Disease Control and Prevention, National Center for Chronic Disease Prevention and Health Promotion, Office on Smoking and Health; 1994.

8. Fiore MC, Bailey WC, Cohen SJ, et al. *Treating Tobacco Use and Dependence. Clinical Practice Guideline.* Rockville, Md: US Dept of Health and Human Services, Public Health Service; 2000.

9. Sussman S, Lichtman K, Ritt A, Pallonen UE. Effects of thirty-four adolescent tobacco use cessation and prevention trials on regular users of tobacco products. *Subst Use Misuse.* 1999;34:1469–1503.

10. Centers for Medicare and Medicaid Services. *Medicaid: A Brief Summary.* Available at: http://cms.hhs.gov/publications/overview-medicare-medicaid/default4.asp. Accessed September 9, 2002.

11. Schauffler HH, Mordavsky J, Barker D, Orleans CT. State Medicaid coverage for tobacco dependence treatments—United States, 1998 and 2000. *MMWR Morb Mortal Wkly Rep.* 2001;50:979–982.

12. Schauffler HH, McMenamin S, Olsen K, Boyce-Smith G, Rideout JA, Kamil J. Variations in treatment benefits influence smoking cessation: results of a randomised controlled trial. *Tob Control.* 2001;10:175–180.

13. Curry SJ, Grothaus LC, McAfee T, Pabiniak C. Use and cost effectiveness of smoking-cessation services under four insurance plans in a health maintenance organization. *N Engl J Med.* 1998;339:673–679.

| SECTION V |

Disparities in Tobacco Use

Smoking Among Chinese Americans: Behavior, Knowledge, and Beliefs

Elena S. H. Yu, PhD, MPH, Edwin H. Chen, PhD, Katherine K. Kim, PhD, RN, and Sawsan Abdulrahim, MPH

Objectives. This report describes and examines factors significantly associated with smoking among Chinese Americans, using multiple logistic regression methods.

Methods. We conducted a population-based survey (n=644, age=40–69 years) in Chicago's Chinatown using a Chinese questionnaire based on the National Health Interview Survey (NHIS).

Results. Smoking prevalence was 34% for males and 2% for females. Some 93% of current smokers had smoked regularly for 10 or more years. Low education (odds ratio [OR]=2.41; 95% confidence interval [CI]=1.31, 4.46), use of a non-Western physician or clinic for health care (OR=2.64; 95% CI=1.46, 4.80), and no knowledge of early cancer warning signs and symptoms (OR=2.52; 95% CI=1.35, 4.70) were significantly associated with smoking among men.

Conclusions. The male prevalence of smoking is higher than those reported in California, the NHIS, and the Behavioral Risk Factor Surveillance System (BRFSS); exceeds the rate for African Americans aged 18 years and older; is comparable with the rate for African American males aged 45 to 64 years; and is far above the Healthy People 2010 target goal of less than 12%. Multisite surveys and smoking cessation campaigns in Chinese are needed. (*Am J Public Health.* 2002;92:1007–1012)

Each year, 4 million deaths—nearly equally divided between developed and developing countries—are attributable to smoking.[1] China alone has almost a million smoking-associated deaths per year,[2,3] while in the United States the figure is 430000,[4] estimated to exceed deaths due to AIDS, car accidents, alcohol, suicides, homicides, firearms, and illegal drugs combined.[5] Overall, in developed nations, tobacco use contributes to the death of about one third of those aged 35 to 69 years,[1] resulting in a premature loss of 20 to 25 years of life.[1,6,7]

Cigarette-smoking status and patterns of use among adults in the United States have been systematically monitored through programmatic surveys,[8–11] analysis of birth certificates,[12] and funded research. The National Health Interview Survey (NHIS) derives annual estimates of health characteristics (including smoking status) through a probability sample of noninstitutionalized civilian adults,[8] while the Behavioral Risk Factor Surveillance System (BRFSS) provides state-based estimates of cigarette users among persons aged 18 years and older living in the 50 states and the District of Columbia.[4] However, data are limited for Asian Americans and Pacific Islanders (AAPIs), now counted at more than 11 million[8,13]—the fastest-growing ethnic minority group in the United States.

The Surgeon General's Report of 1998 is the latest nationwide review of the diverse tobacco control needs of major racial/ethnic minority groups, including AAPIs.[14] The information conveyed by the aggregation of numbers masks important subgroup and regional differences. An understanding of the heterogeneity of cigarette use among AAPI subpopulations is crucial for the formulation of useful health policies and the development of sound intervention programs. The objectives of this report are to describe smoking behavior, knowledge, and beliefs among Chinese Americans and to better understand the factors associated with their knowledge and continuing use of cigarettes despite the known harmful effects.

In prevalence studies, "current smoking" (or cigarette use) is defined as having smoked at least 100 cigarettes in one's lifetime and currently smoking. The prevalence of cigarette use in China has been reported to be 33.8% for both sexes,[15–17] 61% for men aged 15 years and older,[1,3,7] and 73% for men aged 40 years and older.[3] Three fifths of Chinese male smokers started smoking at 15 to 20 years of age.[15] The target goal in China is to reduce the smoking rate for men aged 15 years and older to below 58%.[18] Obviously, the smoking epidemic in China is on a different order of magnitude than that found in the United States today, where the goal for 2010 is to reduce the prevalence of smoking to less than 12%.[19] For the general US population aged 18 years and older, the prevalence of cigarette smoking has declined from 29% in 1987[20] to 26% in 1994[21] and 24.7% in 1997.[11]

Although data on smoking are available from BRFSS and NHIS interviews conducted in English, the small sample size of AAPIs has hampered precise estimates. Researchers often have to pool data sets across years or concatenate disparate samples from different locations in order to obtain crude estimates for AAPIs, as was done in the Surgeon General's Report on tobacco use in 1998.[14] The report showed a smoking rate for AAPIs of 23.8% from 1978 to 1980, which dropped to 15.3% in the period 1994 to 1995,[14,21] only to increase to 16.9% in 1997.[11] These results differ from that based on a recent BRFSS survey of AAPIs in the 10 states where they are most populous; this revealed a smoking prevalence of 10.7%,[22] with sevenfold variation by state (4.7% in Maryland, 36.1% in Oregon). The sample size was too small to produce meaningful statistics for AAPI subpopulations, but studies in several localities showed heterogeneous smoking prevalence for different subgroups, ranging from 9.1% among Chinese Americans[23] to 23.1% among Southeast Asians.[24]

Nearly 1 of every 4 AAPIs is of Chinese descent. Despite the high prevalence of tobacco use in China and the fact that the overwhelming majority (83%) of Chinese Americans aged 18 years and older are foreign born,[25] the smoking prevalence reported for Chinese Americans is low—between 9.1%

and 10.9%.[23,25,26] Below, we review some important factors that have been reported to be associated with cigarette use among AAPIs and, specifically, Chinese Americans.

Sex

Some 27.6% of men and 22.1% of women in the United States are current smokers.[11] Among AAPIs, population-based estimates mask a two- to fivefold sex difference—from 32.5% for men vs 14.7% for women in the 1978–1980 NHIS to 25.1% for men vs 5.8% for women in the 1994–1995 NHIS.[14] Reported rates of smoking among AAPI men include 32.8% for Cambodians,[24] 38.5% for Koreans,[27] 39% for Chinese,[28] 41.7% for Vietnamese, and 51.2% for Laotians.[24] Intragroup sex variation is especially dramatic for Chinese Americans—28.1% for men vs 1.2% for women in Oakland[29] and 16.5% for men vs 2.6% for women in San Francisco.[23]

Age

NHIS trend data show that smoking tends to be higher among persons younger than 55 years and lower among older adults. Prevalence tends to be highest in the 25- to 44-year age group for the general US population, AAPIs, and Chinese.[14] However, among Chinese men in California, only a minimal age difference in smoking prevalence exists for persons aged 25 years and older.[14,30]

Education

Cross-sectional surveys in the United States have established an inverse relationship between education level and smoking.[14,30–32] Data from China have shown a similar gradient (43% prevalence among the college educated, 53% for high school graduates, 68% for illiterates).[33] In the United States, an inverse association in the prevalence of smoking among AAPIs by level of education was reported in the California survey.[14,31] Data on AAPIs from the 1994–1995 NHIS, however, do not strongly support the inverse association between education and smoking prevalence (less than high school education, 13.3% prevalence; education beyond high school, 14.4% prevalence), and in the 1989–1991 Oakland BRFSS survey the association is inconsistent, with no smokers at the "some college" level.[14,29]

Spoken English Fluency

Among immigrants, the ability to speak English varies inconsistently with smoking status.[32,34] The 1990–1991 BRFSS in California found that 31.8% of Chinese not fluent in English were smokers, a rate somewhat lower than that found for Vietnamese (36.6%).[29] Just how strongly associated spoken English fluency is with smoking among Chinese Americans living outside of California remains to be studied.

Usual Source of Health Care

Lack of access to mainstream health care systems has been a problem for underserved populations. Low smoking prevalence has been reported from an analysis of patients at the Kaiser Permanente Health Plan in California,[26,31] but past studies on Chinese American smoking[23,24] did not examine the net effect of source of care.

Knowledge of Early Cancer Warning Signs and Symptoms

Studies on Chinese American smoking behavior have apparently not examined the association between smoking status and early cancer warning signs and symptoms (i.e., change in bowel or bladder habits, a sore that does not heal, unusual bleeding or discharge, thickening or lump in breast or elsewhere, indigestion or difficulty swallowing, obvious change in wart or mole, nagging cough or hoarseness). We examined them as part of our objectives.

METHODS

Sample

This study is part of a larger Asian American Cancer Control Developmental Project.[27,35] A list of Chicago's Chinatown residents was generated by merging several files, including compiled surnames, telephone directories, and Chinese newspaper subscribers. A 2-stage probability sampling method was used to randomly select Chinese households from the defined sampling frame.[36] Of all eligible individuals enumerated by telephone, one person from each household was randomly selected for an interview. Eligibility was defined by age (40–69 years), self-classified ethnicity (Chinese), and residence within the defined boundary of Chinatown. Budgetary constraints restricted eligibility criteria to the age group most likely to benefit from the use of cancer screening tests.

Instrument

We constructed both Mandarin and Cantonese Chinese versions of the Cancer Control Supplement Questionnaire used in the 1987 NHIS. Several translators independently produced parallel translations, which were back-translated for verification of accuracy and comprehension of technical terms. Differences in meanings were identified, discussed, and resolved. In-depth probes, think-aloud methods, and focus groups were used to ensure the conceptual equivalence and comprehensibility of the final survey instrument.[37] We conducted mock interviews and pretests to finalize the survey instrument using subjects whose sociodemographic characteristics resembled those of Chinatown residents but who resided elsewhere in Chicago. Photographs of tobacco products (type, size, brand) were prepared for use during interviews.

Data Collection

The major Chinese-language newspapers in Chicago provided media publicity about a forthcoming health study. No mention was made of cancer or smoking so as not to taint responses. Letters were mailed out to introduce the project and to explain the random sample selection process, the voluntary nature of survey participation, the confidentiality of the interview, and a phone number to call if householders had questions. Trained interviewers conducted the survey in Chinese at each respondent's home after written informed consent was obtained.

Statistical analysis was performed with SAS (SAS Institute Inc, Cary, NC) and SPSS (SPSS Inc, Chicago, Ill). Group differences were compared by χ^2 test. Multiple logistic regression analysis was performed to evaluate the factors associated with smoking behavior, knowledge, and beliefs in order to take into account the effects of potential confounding variables.

RESULTS

Sample Characteristics

A total of 644 Chinese completed the survey, representing a response rate of 80%. Sex

TABLE 1—Demographic Characteristics of Study Sample of Chinese Americans Living in Chicago's Chinatown, by Sex

Characteristic	Male (n = 312)	Female (n = 332)
Age, y		
Mean	53.3	54.5
SD	9.1	9.0
Range	40–69	40–69
Education, %		
≤6 y	30.4	53.9
>6 y	69.6	46.1
Marital status, %		
Married	93.6	80.4
Not married	6.4	19.6
Usual source of health care, %		
No care	55.4	49.4
Traditional Chinese medicine	4.8	6.9
Western-style pharmacy	2.9	2.4
Clinics	14.4	16.0
Western MD's office	22.4	25.3
Spoken English fluency, %		
Not at all/poorly	59.9	77.4
Makes do/can speak moderately or well	40.1	22.6
Length of residence in US, y		
Mean	11.4	10.7
SD	10.2	10.3
Median	8.0	7.0

Note. Total percentage may not add to 100 due to rounding.

TABLE 2—Cigarette Smoking Status Among Chinese Americans Living in Chicago's Chinatown and Among 1997 National Health Interview Survey (NHIS) Respondents, by Sex

Sample and Sex	% Never Smokers[a]	% Former Smokers[b]	% Current Smokers[c]
Chinese Americans			
Men (n = 312)	40.1	26.3	33.6
Women (n = 332)	96.1	1.8	2.1
NHIS respondents			
Men	15.5	20.9	27.0 (27.6)[d]
Women	58.9	19.0	22.1 (21.5)[d]

Note. Data on NHIS respondents are from the 1997 NHIS of adults aged 18 years or older from all racial/ethnic groups.[11] Despite changes in the 1997 NHIS, questions on smoking remained unchanged.
[a]Never smokers were respondents who had not smoked at least 100 cigarettes in their lifetime.
[b]Former smokers were persons who had smoked at least 100 cigarettes but no longer smoked at the time of interview.
[c]Current smokers were persons who reported having smoked at least 100 cigarettes during their lifetime and who smoked every day or some days at the time of the interview.
[d]Numbers in parentheses are for persons 45 to 64 years old as reported in reference 8. Corresponding figures for former and never smokers were not published. Data for persons aged 40 to 69 years were not tabulated.

differences by age were minimal but quite substantial in terms of education (Table 1). About half of each sex did not have a regular source of health care. The vast majority could not speak any English or spoke it poorly; most (males, 65.3%; females, 56.9%) did not have any religious affiliation (data not shown).

Comparison With NHIS Data

We compared our findings with those reported for the general US population in the 1997 NHIS[11] using comparable criteria of defining smoking status (Table 2). The prevalence of current smoking was higher among men in Chicago's Chinatown (33.6%) than in the NHIS sample (27.6% among men aged 45 to 64 years, the group closest in age to our sample). Since Chinese American women were predominantly nonsmokers (96.1%, vs 58.9% of women in the NHIS), only data for males are presented below.

Smoking Behavior of Chinese Males

The percentage of Chinese American men who had smoked a pipe or cigar at least 50 times in their lifetime was 11% and 3%, respectively. Only 1 man was a current pipe smoker; 2 were current cigar smokers. Five percent of Chinese men had used chewing tobacco at least 20 times in their lifetime; only 2 were current chewers. Three persons reported that they had used snuff or betel nut (another addictive substance commonly used in Asia) at least 20 times in their lives and were still using them. Betel nut is the fruit of *Areca catechu*; it is usually sprinkled with calcium oxide, salt, and powdered root of liquorice and served wrapped in a tobacco leaf, which is chewed and then spat out.

On average, current smokers started smoking at 19 years of age (former smokers at 19.9 years). For current and former smokers combined, the starting age ranged from 7 to 52 years (median = 18.5). The most common reasons given for smoking (multiple responses allowed) were habit (40%), addiction (36%), enjoyment (14%), and social functions (11%). Among the current smokers, 93% had smoked cigarettes regularly for more than 10 years; only 5% had smoked for 10 years or less. About 39% of the smokers reported lighting up a cigarette immediately after awakening, 28% within an hour of awakening, and 25% within 1 to 5 hours of waking up. Marlboro (29.5%) and Viceroy (25.7%), followed by Winston (14.3%) and Kent (12.4%), were the preferred brands; some 4.8% smoked the brand 555 and 3.8% reported having no brand loyalty. Smokers tended to favor nonmentholated (93.3%), filter-tipped (97.1%), and soft-pack (79%) cigarettes. Preference for regular-size cigarettes ran high (83.8%). Most popular were regular cigarettes (61%), followed by light cigarettes (36.2%). Some (44%) smoked half a pack to a pack of cigarettes a day, and 42% smoked less than half a pack a day.

Quitting Attempts

Among current smokers, 47% had made at least one serious attempt to quit; of these, 59% had tried more than once. The most commonly used method for quitting was "cold turkey" (76%), followed by reduced smoking (25%) and using Nicorette, a nonprescription gum used as nicotine replacement therapy (PharmacieAB, Stockholm, Sweden) (14%). Unsuccessful quitting attempts were attributed to addiction (20%), the fact that "others smoke so [they] go along" (18%), and social functions (10%). Forty-eight percent of current smokers claimed that they could quit any time if they really wanted to, but a large percentage (42%) admitted that they could not quit. Nearly half of the current smokers (47.6%) reported having been advised by their doctors to stop smoking.

TABLE 3—Frequency and Percentage of Never Smokers and Current Smokers Among Chinese American Men Living in Chicago's Chinatown, by Selected Demographic Variables (n = 230)

		Never Smoker		Current Smoker	
Characteristics	n	(n = 125)	%	(n = 105)	%
Age, y					
40–54	129	77	61.6	52	49.5
55–69	101	48	38.4	53	50.5
Education,** y					
≤6	68	25	20.0	43	41.0
>6	162	100	80.0	62	59.0
Spoken English fluency*					
Not at all/poorly	132	61	48.8	71	67.6
Makes do/speaks moderately or well	98	64	51.2	34	32.4
Length of residence in US, y					
<10	131	74	59.2	57	54.3
≤10	99	51	40.8	48	45.7
Usual source of health care**					
None/Eastern medicine/Western pharmacy	148	68	54.4	80	76.2
Clinics/Western MD's office	82	57	45.6	25	23.8
Knowledge of cancer warning signs**					
No knowledge	157	73	58.4	84	80.0
Knowledge of 1 or more signs	73	52	41.6	21	20.0

*P < .01; **P<.001, based on χ^2 test for comparing 2 categories of each characteristic by smoking status.

TABLE 4—Relationship Between Selected Demographic Variables and Current and Never Smoking Status Among Chinese American Men Living in Chicago's Chinatown[a] (n = 230)

	Current vs Never Smokers OR (95% CI)
Education (elementary or less = 1)	2.41 (1.31, 4.46)*
Usual source of health care (not using clinics or Western MD's office = 1)	2.64 (1.46, 4.80)*
Knowledge of cancer warning signs (no knowledge = 1)	2.52 (1.35, 4.70)*

Note. OR = adjusted odds ratio; CI = confidence interval.
[a]Multiple logistic regression analysis using stepwise selection. Current smoker is coded as 1. Variables not selected into the model are age, spoken English fluency, and years of residency in the United States. Hosmer–Lemeshow goodness-of-fit test P = .9653.
*P < .01.

Contrast Between Never and Current Smokers

Being a current smoker was significantly associated with low level of education, poor spoken English fluency, not using clinics or a Western doctor's office as a usual source of health care, and having no knowledge of even 1 early cancer warning sign or symptom (Table 3). About 14% of both smokers and never smokers had an immediate family member who had had cancer. Age and years of residence in the United States were not significantly associated with smoking status. Only 27% of smokers owned their homes, compared with 46% of never smokers (data not shown).

Factors Associated With Smoking Status

We used multiple logistic regression analysis to evaluate the effects of selected independent variables on smoking status (current vs never), after adjusting for the presence of other variables considered important from our literature review. Age, education, spoken English fluency, years in the United States, usual source of care, and knowledge of early cancer warning signs and symptoms were dichotomized. Only education, usual source of care, and knowledge of early cancer warning signs and symptoms were statistically significant when stepwise selection using log-likelihood criteria was applied (Table 4). Interaction terms were examined and did not substantially improve the model fit.

Our final model indicates that Chinese American men with less than an elementary school education were more than twice as likely as those with a higher level of education to be current smokers, after the effects of usual source of health care and knowledge of cancer signs and symptoms are taken into consideration (odds ratio [OR] = 2.41; 95% confidence interval [CI] = 1.31, 4.46). Likewise, those who did not use clinics or a Western physician's office for their usual source of health care were more than twice as likely to be current smokers, other things equal (OR = 2.64; 95% CI = 1.46, 4.80). The magnitude of effect was similar for knowledge of early cancer warning signs and symptoms, after the other 2 variables were controlled for (OR = 2.52; 95% CI = 1.35, 4.70).

Smoking and Alcohol Use

About 70% of the 125 male never smokers were never drinkers; 12% were former drinkers and 18.4% were current drinkers. Among the 105 current smokers, the corresponding percentages of drinkers were as follows: never, 53.3%; former, 19.1%, current, 27.6% (data not shown). The association between smoking and alcohol use is statistically significant (χ^2_2 = 6.436; P<.05).

Knowledge of Smoking and Major Diseases

We asked questions about the association of smoking with 5 major diseases by using a true–false response format. For 3 diseases—bronchitis, lung cancer, and emphysema—more than three quarters of Chinese men (80%, 78%, and 75%, respectively) knew that smoking is a causal factor. For the other 2 diseases—throat or mouth cancer and heart disease—only about half of the respondents were knowledgeable (52% for throat or mouth cancer and 50% for heart disease). However, knowledge of the association between smoking and throat or mouth cancer, bronchitis, and heart disease by smoking status was not significant (data not shown). For lung cancer and emphysema, knowledge of the disease was significantly associated with the 3 levels of smoking status (current, former, and never). The percentage of those who were aware that smoking causes lung cancer and emphysema was lower among current smokers (69.5% and 71.4%, respectively) than among never smokers (87.2% and 76.8%, respectively), with former smokers showing little variation (75.6% and 76.8%, respectively).

Beliefs About Smoking

We added 2 items to the 5 smoking-belief questions in the NHIS, one designed to capture fatalism and the other to inquire about chewing betel nut. Statistically significant differences in smoking beliefs by smoking status were found only for the following items: (1) "Everything causes cancer, so it does not matter whether one smokes or not" (agreed with by 48% of current smokers, 12% of former smokers, and 13% of never smokers); (2) "Chewing betel nut is harmful to one's health" (27% of current smokers, 29% of former smokers, and 44% of never smokers); (3) "Most deaths from lung cancer are caused by cigarette smoking" (61% of current smokers, 67% of former smokers, and 79% of never smokers).

Useful Sources of Information

When asked to name their most useful sources of health information, the most often mentioned sources were newspapers (34%), books (25%), doctors (23%), magazines (18%), friends (16%), television (14%), family (10%), and radio (5%). Fewer than 2% of Chinese men named pamphlets and workplace. Asked about what location would be most convenient to them if they were to be offered a 2-hour class on how to reduce their chances of getting cancer, 3 of every 5 Chinese men identified the community center, followed by a local school (28%), church (18%), clubs (4%), and home (4%). Only about 2% named another site (e.g., hospital, senior center, workplace).

DISCUSSION

Several of our findings are noteworthy. First, previous studies have reported low smoking prevalence for Chinese Americans, befitting the image of a "model minority."[38] In reality, their rates vary considerably by nativity, location, and other factors. Our study shows a smoking prevalence for men that is between the low rates reported for Chinese aged 18 years and older[12,14,23,30] and the high rate reported for Chinese men aged 60 to 96 years.[28] The prevalence is not quite half of what is found in China. By US norms, the smoking prevalence of the Chinese American men in our study is high; it exceeds the reported rates for the last decade among African American men aged 18 years and older[8,11,14] and is comparable to the rate (39.4%) found for African American men aged 45 to 64 years in the 1997 NHIS.[8,11] Current smoking prevalence among Chicago's Chinatown Chinese men aged 40 to 69 years is more than double the desired Healthy People 2010 target goal of less than 12%.

Second, age and cohort effects are confounded in the variation of smoking status by age. Since the overwhelming majority of older Chinese are foreign-born non–English speakers, their smoking prevalence is higher than the rate reported for younger cohorts of English-speaking, mostly US-born, Chinese Americans who respond to BRFSS telephone interviews. Studies with extraordinarily large samples are needed to monitor the smoking prevalence of different age cohorts by nativity.

Third, the following methodological differences between our study and others most likely contributed to the differences in the results: (a) we conducted a population-based survey in Chinatown; (b) we sampled adults aged 40 to 69 years; (c) we met face-to-face, not over the telephone, with interviewees; (d) we interviewed in Chinese languages; (e) our survey instrument was standardized—the kind and number of explanations provided to the respondents were rehearsed during training.

Clearly, replication studies are very much needed. However, in designing intervention programs, some thought should be given to the immediately controllable factors (source of health care and knowledge of early cancer warning signs and symptoms). Smokers and the community at large can benefit from the establishment of smoking cessation programs in Chinese languages.

Except for the NHIS and the BRFSS, which surveyed mostly English-speaking AAPIs, we have found only 2 population-based studies aimed at estimating tobacco use among Chinese Americans, both conducted in California.[23,29] Given the geographic variability in immigrant compositions, coordinated multisite, large-sample surveys of smoking focused on Chinese Americans—the largest subgroup in the AAPI community—in states or areas where they are most populous is necessary to obtain precise estimates of smoking prevalence, health risks, and health status.

Proclaimed as the single most preventable and controllable factor in morbidity and mortality reduction,[39] smoking is one of the important risk factors or causal agents in at least 6 of the top 10 leading causes of death for the nation—heart diseases, cancer, cerebrovascular diseases, chronic obstructive pulmonary diseases, diabetes mellitus, and atherosclerosis, which together account for 69.7% of all deaths.[40] Among Chinese Americans, heart disease and cancer combined account for 58.3% of all deaths. Cerebrovascular diseases add another 8.4%, bringing the total proportional mortality from tobacco-related deaths for just the 3 leading causes of death up to 66.7%. In the 25- to 64-year age range, cancer is the leading cause of death for Chinese Americans,[41] and cancer of the lung and bronchus is the leading cause of cancer deaths for all ages. Hence, even a small decline in smoking prevalence among Chinese Americans will have a significant beneficial public health impact in reducing morbidity and mortality among AAPIs.

CONCLUSIONS

This is the first population-based study of Chinese American smoking behavior, knowledge, and beliefs, conducted in Chinese and using a standardized instrument that mirrors the NHIS format, to be implemented outside of California. We found that the overall smoking prevalence in our sample of Chicago Chinatown Chinese aged 40 to 69 years was 17.4% (men, 34%; women, 2%). Results of multiple logistic regression analyses show that the 3 major variables significantly associated with smoking status were education, usual source of health care, and knowledge of early cancer warning signs and symptoms. After these 3 variables were adjusted for, factors identified as important in previous studies (i.e., age, spoken English fluency, and years in the United States) were not significantly associated with being a current smoker. Moreover, nearly half of the current smokers had already been advised by their physicians to stop smoking. "Cold turkey" was the most common quitting method. Future plans for multisite studies on smoking and health should include the development of Chinese-language instruments and interventions for Chinese-speaking Chinese Americans. ■

About the Authors

Elena S.H. Yu and Sawsan Abdulrahim are with the Division of Epidemiology and Biostatistics, Graduate School of Public Health, San Diego State University, San Diego, Calif. Edwin H. Chen is with the Division of Epidemiology and Biostatistics, School of Public Health, University of Illinois at Chicago. Katherine K. Kim is with the Kirkhof School of Nursing, Grand Valley State University, Allendale, Mich.

Requests for reprints should be sent to Elena S.H. Yu, PhD, MPH, Division of Epidemiology and Biostatistics, School of Public Health, San Diego State University, San Diego, CA 92182 (e-mail: eyu@mail.sdsu.edu).

This article was accepted February 23, 2001.

Contributors

The Chinese American substudy of the project was conceptualized, designed, and implemented by E.S.H. Yu with the collaboration of E.H. Chen. E.S.H. Yu led the writing of the paper with statistical support from E.H. Chen. K.K. Kim contributed to some aspects of the study and the writing of the paper. S. Abdulrahim performed preliminary analysis on the entire sample, examined the consistency of the responses, and explored factors for smoking behavior.

Acknowledgments

The study was supported by National Cancer Institute grant RO1 CA 49569.

We thank P.S. Levy for technical advice on sampling and W.T. Liu for translation assistance. We owe a debt of gratitude to our respondents, bilingual interviewers, project staff, and innumerable community leaders.

References

1. Peto R. Smoking and death: the past 40 years and the next 40. *Br Med J.* 1994;309:937–939.

2. Liu BQ, Peto R, Chen ZM, et al. Emerging tobacco hazards in China, I: retrospective proportional mortality study of one million deaths. *Br Med J.* 1998; 317:1411–1422.

3. Niu SR, Yang GH, Chen ZM, et al. Emerging tobacco hazards in China, II: early mortality results from a prospective study. *Br Med J.* 1998;317:1423–1424.

4. Centers for Disease Control and Prevention. State-specific prevalence of current cigarette and cigar smoking among adults—United States, 1998. *MMWR Morb Mortal Wkly Rep.* 1999;48:1034–1039.

5. Lynch BS, Bonnie RJ. *Growing up Tobacco Free: Preventive Nicotine Addiction in Children and Youths.* Washington, DC: Institute of Medicine, National Academy Press; 1994.

6. Peto R, Lopez AD, Boreham J, Thun M, Heath C. Mortality from tobacco in developed countries: indirect estimation from national vital statistics. *Lancet.* 1992; 339:1268–1278.

7. Peto R, Lopez AD, Boreham J, Heath C, Thun M. *Mortality From Tobacco in Developed Countries, 1950–2000.* Oxford, England: Oxford University Press; 1994.

8. *Health United States 2000.* Hyattsville, Md: National Center for Health Statistics; 2000.

9. Kann L, Kinchen SA, Williams BI, et al. Youth risk behavior surveillance—United States, 1999. *MMWR Morb Mortal Wkly Rep.* 2000;49(SS-5):1–18.

10. Centers for Disease Control and Prevention. Surveillance for selected tobacco-use behaviors—United States, 1990–1994. *CDC Surveill Summ.* 1994;43(SS-3): 925–929.

11. Centers for Disease Control and Prevention. Cigarette smoking among adults—United States, 1997. *MMWR Morb Mortal Wkly Rep.* 1999;48:993–996.

12. Mathews TJ. Smoking during pregnancy, 1990–96. *Natl Vital Stat Rep.* 1998;47(10):1–12.

13. *Resident Population Estimates of the United States by Sex, Race, and Hispanic Origin: April 1, 1990 to July 1, 1999, With Short-Term Projection to March 1, 2000.* Washington, DC: Population Estimates Program, Population Division, US Census Bureau. Available at: http://www.census.gov/population/estimates/nation/infile3-1.txt. Accessed April 11, 2000.

14. *Tobacco Use Among US Racial/Ethnic Minority Groups—African Americans, American Indians and Alaska Natives, Asian Americans and Pacific Islanders, and Hispanics: A Report of the Surgeon General.* Atlanta, Ga: National Center for Chronic Disease Prevention and Health Promotion, Office on Smoking and Health; 1998.

15. Weng XZ. Smoking—a serious health problem in China. *Chin Med J (Engl).* 1988;101:371–372.

16. Weng XZ, Hong ZG, Chen DY. Smoking prevalence in Chinese aged 15 and above. *Chin Med J (Engl).* 1987;100:886–892.

17. Yu JJ, Mattson ME, Boyd GM, et al. A comparison of smoking patterns in the People's Republic of China with the United States: an impending health catastrophe in the Middle Kingdom. *JAMA.* 1990;264:1575–1579.

18. Cheng TO. Teenage smoking in China. *J Adolescence.* 1999;22:607–620.

19. *Healthy People 2010: Understanding and Improving Health.* 2nd ed. Washington, DC: Dept of Health and Human Services; 2000.

20. Schoenborn CA, Boyd GM. Smoking and other tobacco use. *Vital Health Stat 10.* 1989;No. 169.

21. *Healthy People 2000 Review, 1995–96.* Hyattsville, Md: Public Health Service; 1996. DHHS Publication PHS 96-1256.

22. Bolen JC, Rhodes L, Powell-Griner EE, Bland SD, Holtzman D. State-specific prevalence of selected health behaviors, by race and ethnicity—Behavioral Risk Factor Surveillance System, 1997. *MMWR Morb Mortal Wkly Rep.* 2000;49(SS-2):1–60.

23. Thridandam M, Fong W, Jang M, Louie L, Forst M. A tobacco and alcohol use profile of San Francisco's Chinese community. *J Drug Educ.* 1998;28:377–393.

24. Centers for Disease Control and Prevention. Cigarette smoking among Southeast Asian immigrants—Washington State, 1989. *MMWR Morb Mortal Wkly Rep.* 1992;41:854–855, 861.

25. Kuo J, Porter K. Health status of Asian Americans: United States, 1992–94. *Adv Data Vital Health Stat.* August 7, 1998;298:1–16.

26. Klatsky AL, Tekawa I, Armstrong MA, Sidney S. The risk of hospitalization for ischemic heart disease among Asian Americans in Northern California. *Am J Public Health.* 1994;84:1672–1675.

27. Kim K, Yu ESH, Chen EH, Kim J, Brintnall R, Vance S. Smoking behavior, knowledge, and beliefs among Korean Americans. *Cancer Pract.* 2000;8: 223–230.

28. Choi ES, McGandy RB, Dallal GE, et al. The prevalence of cardiovascular risk factors among elderly Chinese Americans. *Arch Intern Med.* 1990;150:413–418.

29. Center for Disease Control. Cigarette smoking among Chinese, Vietnamese, and Hispanics—California, 1989–1991. *MMWR Morb Mortal Wkly Rep.* 1992;41: 362–367.

30. Burns D, Pierce JP. *Tobacco Use in California, 1990–1991.* Sacramento: California Dept of Health Services; 1992.

31. Escobedo LG, Zhu BP, Giovino GA, Erickson MP. Educational attainment and racial differences in cigarette smoking. *J Natl Cancer Inst.* 1995;87:1552–1553.

32. Samet JM, Howard CA, Coultas DB, Skipper BJ. Acculturation, education, and income as determinants of cigarette smoking in New Mexico Hispanics. *Cancer Epidemiol Biomarkers Prev.* 1992;1:235–240.

33. Chen MZ. Smoking in China. *World Health Forum.* 1995;16:10–11.

34. Chen MS Jr, Guthrie R, Moeschberger M, et al. Lessons learned and baseline data from initiating smoking cessation research with Southeast Asian adults. *Asian Am Pac Isl J Health.* 1993;1:194–214.

35. Yu ESH, Kim KK, Chen EH, Brintnall RA. Breast and cervical cancer screening among Chinese American women. *Cancer Pract.* 2001;9:81–91.

36. Levy PS, Lemeshow S. *Sampling of Population: Methods and Applications.* New York, NY: John Wiley & Sons; 1991.

37. Jobe JB, Mingay DJ. Cognitive laboratory approach to designing questionnaires for surveys of the elderly. *Public Health Rep.* 1990;105:518–524.

38. Chen MS, Hawks BL. A debunking of the myth of healthy Asian Americans and Pacific Islanders. *Am J Health Promot.* 1995;9:261–268.

39. Novello AC. From the Surgeon General, US Public Health Service. Tobacco control. *JAMA.* 1993;270:806.

40. Hoyert DL, Kochanek KD, Murphy SL. Deaths: final data for 1997. *Natl Vital Stat Rep.* 1999;47: 1–104.

41. Hoyert DL, Kung HC. Asian or Pacific Islander mortality, selected states, 1992. *Month Vital Stat Rep.* 46(suppl 1):1–63.

Prevalence and Predictors of Tobacco Use Among Asian Americans in the Delaware Valley Region

| Grace X. Ma, PhD, CHES, Steve Shive, PhD, MPH, Yin Tan, MD, MPH, and Jamil Toubbeh, PhD

Objectives. This study examined tobacco use rates and potential predictors of use among Asian Americans residing in the Delaware Valley region.

Methods. A cross-sectional survey design was used. The sample consisted of 1174 Chinese, Koreans, Vietnamese, and Cambodians.

Results. Findings indicated that the mean age at initiation of tobacco use was 18.3 years. Among the respondents, 40.2% had a history of tobacco use, and 29.6% were current users. Men were more likely than women to smoke. There were significant differences between never smokers, current smokers, and ex-smokers in sex, ethnicity, educational attainment, and marital and employment status.

Conclusions. The findings suggest that tobacco use is still a serious public health problem among Asian Americans, especially men. (*Am J Public Health.* 2002;92:1013–1020)

Tobacco use is the single most important preventable cause of illness and death in the United States, accounting for more than 430 000 deaths annually.[1] In the states of Pennsylvania and New Jersey in 1999, for example, cigarette smoking accounted for 36 000 deaths, and death rates attributed to smoking were 346/100 000 and 372/100,00, respectively.[2] In the same year, New Jersey ranked 14th among the states in number of deaths from smoking, whereas Pennsylvania ranked 21st. Approximately 480 368 years of potential life were lost in the 2 states in 1999, or an average of 13.3 years for each death due to smoking, and the estimated cost of tobacco use in regard to related medical expenses was $4.7 billion.[2]

In 2000, the US Behavioral Risk Factor Surveillance Survey (BRFSS) revealed that median smoking prevalence rates were 24.4% among men and 21.2% among women.[3] State-specific versions of the 2000 survey showed that adult smoking prevalence rates were 24.3% in Pennsylvania (25.4% of men and 23.3% of women) and 21% in New Jersey (23.5% of men and 18.6% of women).[3]

Asian Americans and Pacific Islanders, the fastest growing US ethnic/racial group, represent approximately 3% of the residents of the greater Philadelphia region of Pennsylvania and New Jersey (the site of the present study).[4] By and large, city and state tobacco prevention programs are failing to reach members of the Asian American community, whose smoking behaviors remain largely unchanged. In turn, the community lacks an understanding of the health risks associated with tobacco use.[5]

Analysis of data on Pennsylvania's 2.3 million smokers reveals that nicotine addiction is associated with early smoking initiation.[6] Data on male high school seniors derived from the Monitoring the Future Survey indicates that Asian youth smoking rates increased from a moderately low 16.8% in 1989 to a high of 20.6% in 1994.[7,8] A study conducted in an ethnically and racially diverse section of Philadelphia showed that 18.2% of White adolescents, 9.0% of African American adolescents, and 14.1% of Asian American adolescents had smoked daily since they began smoking.[9] In general, however, Asian Americans begin smoking later in life than members of other racial/ethnic groups, and this is particularly true for Asian American men.[10–12]

It has long been asserted that sociodemographic characteristics have a significant impact on tobacco use prevalence patterns. This relationship has been the subject of scrutiny in the general population[13–15] but not in the Asian American population.[11,16–18] Studies on the latter, substantiated by data from the Centers for Disease Control and Prevention,[19–21] show that smoking prevalence rates among Asian Americans vary by sex.

Despite conclusive evidence of a relationship between age and smoking behaviors among Asian Americans, current studies indicate variability in smoking prevalence rates among men. For example, a study of Vietnamese men in Massachusetts conducted by Wiecha et al.[11] indicated that the highest smoking rates were among men aged 25 to 44 years.

It has been shown that smoking rates among Asian American men also vary according to ethnic subgroup: 35% to 56% among Vietnamese, 33% among Koreans, 71% among Laotians, 71% among Cambodians, and 55% among Chinese.[22,23] A more recent national study found that 34% of Vietnamese American men and 31% of Korean American men were current smokers.[24] Collectively, these findings clearly indicate significantly higher smoking rates for Southeast Asian men than among men in other racial or ethnic groups studied to date.[7,10,11,16–19,25,26]

Research on the relationship between smoking and educational level has led to the conclusion that smoking rates decrease as a function of educational attainment. That is, the highest prevalence rates have been observed among those with a high school education or less, and the lowest rates have been observed among those with a graduate school education.[11,17,18]

Recent studies have found a high prevalence of certain types of cancer among Asian Americans and Pacific Islanders. According to Chen and Hawks,[27] lung cancer, the leading cause of death among Asian Americans and Pacific Islanders, is 18% more prevalent among Southeast Asian men than among White men, and rates are expected to increase as a result of this group's smoking patterns.

Doong[28] pointed out that cancer is the leading cause of death among Asian American women, and Chu[29] concluded that cancer is highly associated with smoking in both male and female Chinese Americans. Chu noted that Chinese American men and women have high rates of nasopharyngeal cancer relative to other racial/ethnic groups (e.g., 14 and 11 times higher, respectively, than their counterparts in the White population).

In response to the need for tobacco control and prevention and in an attempt to reduce the incidence of and risk for cancer among Asian Americans in the Delaware Valley region of Pennsylvania and New Jersey, the Asian Tobacco Education, Cancer Awareness, and Research (ATECAR) project was established at Temple University in Philadelphia. The goal of ATECAR is to form a sustainable public health infrastructure by building strategic partnerships between health service agencies and Asian community organizations. A comprehensive needs assessment questionnaire was developed as a preliminary step toward initiation of tobacco control, prevention, and intervention programs.

The primary purpose of the study described in this article, conducted in 2000, was to determine tobacco use rates among the Asian American community in the Delaware Valley region. A secondary purpose was to determine the demographic variables that are potential predictors of current tobacco use among members of this ethnically and racially diverse community.

METHODS

We used a cross-sectional survey design because of the advantages provided by this method[30–33]; also, we adapted a stratified-cluster proportional sampling technique.[34] Initially, we identified Asian American community organizations (n=52) located in the 7 counties of the Delaware Valley region of Pennsylvania and southern New Jersey using information provided by the Asian Community Cancer Coalition, a health service agency, and ATECAR project staff. These community organizations were located throughout the 7 counties thereby maximizing the opportunity to obtain a representative sample of Asian Americans across ethnic subgroups, ages, and socioeconomic status.

From the list of 52 organizations, 26 were randomly selected and divided into clusters. The selected organization clusters were stratified according to 4 race/ethnicity or language groups (Chinese, Korean, Vietnamese, Cambodian). A proportional allocation procedure was used in which sample sizes were assigned proportionally to subgroups.[33]

Instrument

A 77-item questionnaire was developed for the survey. Some of the questionnaire items were modified from other instruments, including the 2000 National Health Interview Survey, the 1998 National Household Survey on Drug Abuse, the 1999 Youth Risk Behavior Survey, the Florida Youth Tobacco Survey, and the American Indian Cancer Control Project instrument. Average time required to complete the questionnaire was 20 to 25 minutes.

A pilot test was conducted to establish the reliability and validity of the instrument and to verify data collection methods. Appropriateness of questionnaire format, validity of content, level of difficulty, and length of time required to complete the survey were also determined. The face validity and content validity of the questionnaire were tested with 50 Asian American adults who did not participate in the study. The Guttman split-half reliability coefficient was 0.67, indicating that, overall, participants responded consistently to questionnaire items.

Data Collection Procedures

Surveys were administered in both one-to-one and group formats. ATECAR staff, in conjunction with community organization leaders, administered the self-report survey to Asian American participants on site in the community organizations' facilities. Participants had the option of responding in English or in Chinese, Korean, Cambodian, or Vietnamese. Translators were provided when needed for individual or group translations.

Data Analysis

Data were analyzed with SPSS 10.0 Chicago, IL: SPSS, Inc.; 1999. We used descriptive statistics to summarize data collected for demographic variables (described subsequently). The χ^2 test for independence was used to determine Asian subgroup differences in demographic characteristics and smoking rates. This test was also used to determine significant differences between smoking status and demographic variables. A one-way analysis of variance was used to determine mean differences between the subgroups in age and age at initiation of tobacco use.

Logistic regression analyses were used to identify the potential predictor variables of current tobacco use. Independent variables included sex, age, country of birth, length of time residing in the United States, educational attainment, occupation, marital status, children younger than 18 years living at home, employment status, and immigration status. The dependent variable was current tobacco use, defined as "having used tobacco within the last 30 days."

RESULTS

Sample Characteristics

The overall sample consisted of 1174 respondents, distributed as follows: Chinese, 34.9%; Korean, 37.1%; Vietnamese, 16.7%; Cambodian, 8.4%; and "other," 2.7% (Table 1). This last category consisted of Laotian, Hmong, Filipino, and Japanese Americans. There were more men (55.2%) than women (44.8%; χ^2_4= 15.6, $P<.01$) in the 4 Asian American subgroups. The mean age was 41.4 years. Approximately 70% of the sample was between 23 and 60 years of age. About 16% of the respondents were younger than 22 years; 14% were older than 60 years. Significant age differences were found between the groups ($F_{4,1133}$=73.4, $P<.001$).

Overall, 8.8% of Chinese, 1.2% of Koreans, 6.8% of Vietnamese, and 9.4% of Cambodians were born and had spent their entire lives in the United States. Substantial percentages of Chinese (36.6%), Korean (64.9%), Vietnamese (43.8%), and Cambodian (58.6%) respondents had lived in the United States for more than 10 years. Approximately 52% of respondents reported US citizenship, 31.8% reported permanent residency, and 16.3% reported that they were not US citizens.

In terms of education, 10.1% of respondents had less than a high school education, 37.3% had graduated from high school, and 42.5% had a college education. There were significant differences in educational attainment between the groups (χ^2_{20}=209.8, $P<.001$). Chinese (31.5%) exhibited the highest rate of professional or graduate education, followed by Cambodians (18.8%), Koreans (12.0%), and Vietnamese (4.8%).

Approximately 53% of the respondents were employed full-time, 17.0% were employed part-time, and 29.7% were unemployed. We observed significant subgroup differences in employment status as well (χ^2_8= 50.1, $P<.001$). Koreans (60.6%) were more

TABLE 1—Demographic Characteristics of the Sample

	Chinese (n = 410)	Korean (n = 436)	Vietnamese (n = 196)	Cambodian (n = 100)	Other (n = 32)	χ^2	*df*	Total (n = 1174)
Sex, %						15.6*	4	
Male	53.8	51.4	67.3	56.6	46.9			55.2
Female	46.2	48.6	32.7	43.4	53.1			44.8
Country of birth, %						2374.4*	16	
China	77.2	0.2	0	1.3	6.9			26.8
Korea	0	98.1	2.4	0	0			38.8
Vietnam	8.6	0.7	95.9	16.5	0			20.0
Cambodia	.08	0	0	40.5	0			3.3
Other	13.4	1.0	1.8	41.8	93.1			11.0
Length of time in US, %						148.9**	12	
≤2 y	24.8	13.9	10.9	8.1	40.6			17.5
3-5 y	13.5	7.4	8.3	4.0	9.4			9.5
6-10 y	16.2	12.7	30.2	14.1	12.5			16.9
>10 y	36.6	64.9	43.8	58.6	28.1			50.0
Entire life	8.8	1.2	6.8	15.2	9.4			6.2
Level of education, %						209.8**	20	
High school or less	10.5	5.2	12.8	23.5	12.5			10.1
High school	32.3	35.5	44.4	54.1	31.3			37.3
Trade school	3.5	4.0	3.7	4.1	3.1			3.8
Associate degree	5.3	4.5	15.0	5.1	0			6.4
College	17.0	38.8	19.3	13.3	34.4			25.7
Graduate/professional	31.5	12.0	4.8	0	18.8			16.8
Occupation, %						113.8**	16	
Student	19.9	19.0	37.1	62.7	47.6			27.2
Executive, professional	24.5	10.2	0.8	0	9.5			13.1
Businessperson, manager	29.5	37.6	25.0	13.7	28.6			29.9
Manual laborer	11.1	12.2	21.2	11.8	9.5			13.4
Semiskilled laborer	14.9	21.0	15.9	11.8	4.8			16.4
Marital status, %						143.4**	16	
Married	70.5	79.9	59.8	33.3	32.3			68.6
Separated	2.0	1.7	1.6	1.3	3.2			1.8
Divorced	1.5	2.0	1.6	1.3	3.2			1.7
Widowed	3.0	5.7	0.5	1.3	3.2			3.5
Never married	22.9	10.8	36.4	62.7	58.1			24.4
Children <18 y at home, %	55.6	45.3	46.6	45.8	21.9	18.7**	4	48.3
Employment status, %						50.1**	8	
Full time	51.8	60.6	52.8	36.8	31.3			53.4
Part time	21.1	12.4	18.1	10.5	37.5			17.0
Unemployed	27.1	27.0	29.0	52.6	31.3			29.7
Immigration status, %						80.5**	8	
US citizen	49.5	49.9	68.4	42.7	35.5			51.9
Permanent resident	25.3	36.8	28.9	43.8	25.8			31.8
Noncitizen	25.3	13.3	2.6	13.5	38.7			16.3
Age, y, %								
14-17	7.5	2.1	5.7	37.1	13.8			7.9
18-22	6.0	3.1	11.5	29.9	24.1			8.3
23-40	37.7	24.6	47.4	24.7	44.8			33.6
41-60	35.7	48.0	27.6	4.1	13.8			35.6
≥60	13.2	22.2	7.8	4.1	3.4			14.6
Age, y, mean (SD)[a]	41.4 (15.8)	48.5 (15.1)	36.9 (13.9)	23.9 (12.7)	28.7 (11.7)			41.4 (16.5)

[a]Group differences were significant ($F = 66.6$, $P < .001$).
*$P < .01$; **$P < .001$.

likely to be employed full-time than were Chinese (51.8%), Vietnamese (52.8%), or Cambodians (36.8%). In regard to type of occupation, 29.9% of respondents reported that they were employed in a business; 29.8% reported that they were manual or semiskilled laborers, 27.2% reported that they were students, and 13.1% reported that they were executives or professionals. Significant differences between the groups were observed in regard to occupation (χ^2_{16}=113.8, P<.001).

In terms of marital status, 68.6% of respondents were married, 3.5% were divorced or separated, 3.5% were widowed, and 24.4% had never been married. We observed significant subgroup differences in this area as well (χ^2_{16}=143.4, P<.001). Koreans (79.9%) were more likely to be married than were Chinese (70.5%), Vietnamese (59.8%), or Cambodians (33.3%). In addition, there were significant differences among Chinese (55.6%), Koreans (45.3%), Vietnamese (46.6%), and Cambodians (45.8%) in regard to children younger than 18 years living at home (χ^2_4=18.7, P<.001).

Smoking Prevalence

Approximately 40% of respondents reported ever having used tobacco, and 30% reported current tobacco use. Rates of lifetime use varied among the subgroups: Chinese, 33%; Koreans, 43%; Vietnamese, 47%; and Cambodians, 50% (χ^2_1=21.1, P<.001). Current tobacco use rates reflected similar variations: Chinese, 24.1%; Koreans, 26.8%; Vietnamese, 40.3%; and Cambodians, 42.4% (χ^2_4=27.9, P<.001).

We observed significant differences among ever smokers by sex and ethnicity. A larger proportion of men than of women reported tobacco use (odds ratio [OR]=4.30; 95% confidence interval [CI]=3.21, 5.74). Among those who had ever smoked, 81.4% were men, and rates varied according to ethnic group, ranging from 75% to 87%. Among ever smokers, 18.6% were women, ranging from 13% to 25% according to ethnic subgroup.

Similar trends were observed for current smokers. Men were more likely to use tobacco than were women (χ^2_1=105.1, P<.001). Approximately 78% of current smokers were men, and subgroup rates among men ranged from 71% to 85%. Overall, 21.8% of current smokers were female, ranging from 15% to 29% according to ethnic subgroup.

Also, we observed significant differences between current smokers, never smokers, and ex-smokers in ethnicity, educational attainment, marital status, and employment status (Table 2). The differences in smoking status between ethnic subgroups were significant (χ^2_8=47.1,

TABLE 2—Demographic Characteristics, by Smoking Status

	Never smokers (n=700), %	Current smokers (n=345), %	Ex-smokers (n=127), %	χ^2	*df*
Sex				223.5*	2
Male	37.6	78.3	89.8		
Female	62.4	21.7	10.2		
Country of birth				3.91	2
United States	5.5	7.7	9.7		
Other	94.5	92.3	90.3		
Length of time in US				12.1	8
≤2 y	18.3	17.7	12.8		
3-5 y	9.1	10.8	8.0		
6-10 y	17.4	18.3	10.4		
>10 y	49.8	46.2	60.8		
Entire life	5.5	7.0	8.0		
Ethnicity				47.1*	8
Chinese	39.2	28.7	28.3		
Korean	35.5	33.9	55.1		
Vietnamese	14.8	22.9	10.2		
Cambodian	7.1	12.5	5.5		
Other	3.4	2.0	0.8		
Level of education				33.9*	10
High school or less	10.7	11.0	4.8		
High school	38.8	39.0	24.8		
Trade school	4.0	3.9	2.4		
Associate degree	5.6	8.6	4.8		
College	23.1	25.0	40.8		
Graduate/professional	17.9	12.5	22.4		
Occupation				12.8	8
Student	27.3	28.6	23.5		
Executive, professional	15.2	7.8	15.3		
Businessperson, manager	28.9	29.2	36.5		
Manual laborer	11.6	18.2	10.6		
Semiskilled laborer	17.0	16.1	14.1		
Marital status				28.0*	8
Married	66.5	65.6	87.5		
Separated	1.5	2.8	0.8		
Divorced	1.4	2.8	0.8		
Widowed	4.3	3.1	0.8		
Never married	26.3	25.6	10.0		
Children <18 y at home	49.6	46.0	48.4	1.1	2
Employment status				22.9*	4
Full time	48.5	58.8	65.6		
Part time	18.0	18.0	8.2		
Unemployed	33.5	23.2	26.2		
Immigration status	2.0	4		2.0	4
US citizen	52.0	50.0	56.8		
Permanent resident	32.1	32.8	27.2		
Noncitizen	15.9	17.2	16.0		

*P<.001.

$P<.001$). Southeast Asians (Cambodians and Vietnamese) were more likely to be current smokers or ex-smokers than were Chinese and Koreans. Never smokers and ex-smokers were more likely to have a higher level of education than current smokers. Never smokers (66.5%) and ex-smokers (87.5%) were more likely to be married than current smokers (65.6%). Furthermore, never smokers were more likely to be female, to never have been married, to be foreign born, and to be unemployed.

Current Tobacco Use

Among current cigarette smokers, 31.6% reported daily use. We observed a significant difference in frequency of tobacco use among the ethnic subgroups ($\chi^2_{12}=33.8$, $P<.001$; Table 3). Koreans (85.3%) were more likely to report daily use than were Chinese (73.8%), Vietnamese (70.0%), or Cambodians (62.1%). Cigarettes were the most popular type of tobacco used (90.2%), followed by cigars (37.9%), pipes (30.8%), and chewing tobacco (20.5%). Koreans (96.3%) were more likely to be cigarette smokers than were Vietnamese (90.7%), Chinese (86.9%), or Cambodians (81.0%; $\chi^2_4=9.9$, $P<.05$).

Approximately 29% of current smokers were businesspeople; 28.6% were students. We observed significant group differences in occupation among current smokers ($\chi^2_{16}=23.7$, $P<.05$). Cambodian students (61.1%) were more likely to be smokers than were Chinese (28.1%), Vietnamese (36.0%), or Korean (13.1%) students. Among those who reported business-related or managerial occupations, Koreans (34.4%) were more likely than Chinese (29.8%), Vietnamese (26.0%), or Cambodians (16.7%) to be smokers.

We also found significant differences in employment status between the subgroups ($\chi^2_8=21.8$, $P<.01$), with Cambodians exhibiting the greatest likelihood of being unemployed. Finally, there were significant group differences among smokers in marital status ($\chi^2_{16}=45.2$, $P<.001$). Korean smokers were more likely to be married (75.9%) than were Vietnamese (71.8%), Chinese (60.8%), or Cambodian (44.1%) smokers.

Tobacco Initiation

A Tukey test revealed significant differences between the subgroups in age at initiation of smoking ($F_{4,412}=9.7$, $P<.001$). Cambodians (mean = 14 years, SD = 4.3) began using cigarettes at a significantly earlier age than did Chinese (mean = 18.1 years, SD = 5.3). Koreans (mean = 19.8 years, SD = 6.4) initiated use significantly later than did Vietnamese (mean = 16.9 years, SD = 5.1) and Cambodians. As shown in Table 4, friends (64.0%) were the most frequently reported initial source of tobacco, followed by stores (23.5%), family members (4.0%), and vending machines (0.4%). Differences in initial source of tobacco across subgroups were not significant.

Acculturation and Prevalence

We also observed significant differences between subgroups in regard to immigration status, length of time residing in the United States, and country of birth (Table 3). Current smokers were more likely to be foreign born. Vietnamese smokers (67.1%) were significantly more likely to be US citizens than were smokers in the other 3 subgroups. Across all subgroups, the majority of smokers had resided in the United States for 6 or more years.

Correlates of Current Tobacco Use

A logistical regression analysis was undertaken to determine the independent variables that best predicted current tobacco use after consideration of the effects of the other variables (Table 4). The following variables were not associated with current tobacco use and were eliminated from the regression model: country of birth, length of time in the United States, educational attainment, children younger than 18 years of age living at home, employment status, and immigration status. Nagelkerke's "max-rescaled" R^2 value, an estimate of variations in outcome variables explained by a logistic regression model, was calculated. The max-rescaled R^2 was 0.21, indicating that 21% of the variance in current tobacco use was explained by the logistic regression model.

The following variables were positively associated with current tobacco use: sex, occupation, marital status, and age. Women, persons who had never been married, executives or professionals (vs students), and older respondents were less likely to be smokers.

DISCUSSION

Our findings revealed differences not only in tobacco use but also in demographic characteristics across the Asian American subgroups examined, including differences in sex, age, length of time residing in the United States, educational attainment, occupation, and marital, employment, and immigration status. Previous studies have shown that subgroups of Asian Americans and Pacific Islanders differ in language, religion, culture, immigration and generation histories, socioeconomic status, and the extent to which they are acculturated or assimilated into the White or Anglo-American culture.[35,36]

The overall smoking rate among our sample was 29.4%; rates among the ethnic subgroups ranged from 24.1% to 43.0%. This finding is consistent with results of previous studies revealing smoking prevalence rates of between 25.3% and 71%.[1,19,23–25,37] In the current study, the rate of lifetime smoking was 40.2%, ranging from 32.9% to 50.0% across the subgroups studied. This rate is substantially higher than overall smoking rates among adults in Pennsylvania, New Jersey,[3] and Philadelphia[38] and rates among White and Black adults, but it is comparable to the rate for Hispanic adults in Pennsylvania.[39]

Our results indicate that smoking may be as serious a problem among Asian Americans as it is in the general population, if not more so, especially when the ethnic subgroup differences presented here are taken into account. Considered in the light of the 2010 national goal of reducing the rate of tobacco use among adults to 12% or less,[40] these high rates may require the special attention of state public health agencies and an infusion of federal funds into local prevention, intervention, and cessation programs.

Mean age at initiation of tobacco use among the sample studied was 18.3 years, a finding that is also consistent with previous studies.[10,11,41] Subgroup differences, however, provide a more accurate assessment of needs. Cambodians and Vietnamese were oversampled to ensure their adequate representation in the Asian American population studied. Both of these subgroups exhibited low mean ages at smoking initiation—14 and 17 years, respectively—corroborating findings of earlier studies.[42]

TABLE 3—Demographic Characteristics of Current Tobacco Users by Ethnic/Racial Subgroup

	Chinese (n=99)	Korean (n=117)	Vietnamese (n=79)	Cambodian (n=43)	Other (n=7)	χ^2	*df*	Total (n=345)
Age of initiation, y, mean (SD)[a]	18.1 (5.3)	19.8 (6.4)	16.9 (5.1)	13.9 (4.3)	18.7 (3.8)			18.3 (5.9)
Sex, %						9.72*	4	
Male	70.7	79.5	84.8	81.0	71.4			78.2
Female	29.3	20.5	15.2	19.0	28.6			21.8
Frequency of smoking, %						33.8***	12	
Within the last year	4.6	6.3	13.3	3.4	20.0			7.5
Monthly	3.1	2.1	5.0	13.8	40.0			12.2
Weekly	18.5	6.3	11.7	20.7	0			75.2
Daily	73.8	85.3	70.0	62.1	40.0			31.6
Type of tobacco, %								
Cigarettes	85.5	96.1	90.1	80.0	85.7	9.97*	4	89.5
Pipe	26.9	25.7	53.8	25.0	0	8.14	4	31.9
Cigar	40.0	42.1	40.0	28.0	50.0	1.64	4	38.5
Chew	28.6	15.6	26.3	20.0	0	2.31	4	21.7
Country of birth, %						23.7***	4	
United States	11.7	1.8	8.2	13.5	14.3			7.7
Other	88.3	98.2	91.8	86.5	85.7			92.3
Level of education						89.6***	20	
High school or less	10.4	6.0	13.7	23.3	0			11.0
High school	34.4	32.8	47.9	53.5	14.3			38.8
Trade school	1.0	6.0	1.4	9.3	0			3.9
Associate degree	7.3	5.2	19.2	4.7	0			8.7
College	19.8	41.4	12.3	9.3	57.1			25.1
Graduate/professional	27.1	8.6	5.5	0	28.6			12.5
Length of time in US, %						37.5**	16	
≤2 y	26.3	19.0	7.6	14.0	14.3			17.7
3-5 y	12.1	12.1	8.9	7.0	14.3			10.8
6-10 y	13.1	13.8	34.2	11.6	28.6			18.3
>10 y	37.4	52.6	44.3	55.8	28.6			46.2
Entire life	11.1	2.6	5.1	11.6	14.3			7.0
Initial source of tobacco, %						23.7	16	
Friends	52.8	70.4	63.5	67.6	80.0			64.0
Family	9.7	3.1	1.6	0	0			4.0
Vending machine	1.4	0	0	0	0			0.4
Store	33.3	18.4	23.8	17.6	20.0			23.5
Other	2.8	8.2	11.1	14.7	0			8.1
Occupation, %						27.2*	16	
Student	28.1	13.1	36.0	61.1	33.3			28.6
Executive, professional	14.0	8.2	2.0	0	16.7			7.8
Businessperson, manager	29.8	34.4	26.0	16.7	33.3			29.2
Manual laborer	17.5	23.0	20.0	5.6	0			18.2
Semiskilled laborer	10.5	21.3	16.0	16.7	16.7			16.1
Marital status, %						45.2***	16	
Married	60.8	75.9	71.8	44.1	14.3			65.6
Separated	5.2	1.9	1.4	2.9	0			2.8
Divorced	2.1	4.6	1.4	0	14.3			2.8
Widowed	1.0	5.6	0	2.9	14.3			2.8
Never married	30.9	12.0	25.4	50.0	57.1			25.9

Continued

TABLE 3—*Continued*

Have children <18 y at home, %	46.1	45.6	50.7	45.0	0	6.6	4	45.8
Employment status, %						21.8**	8	
Full time	47.3	72.1	56.4	53.8	57.1			58.9
Part time	27.5	12.6	20.5	10.3	0			18.1
Unemployed	25.3	15.3	23.1	35.9	42.9			23.0
Immigration status						34.5***	8	
US citizen	48.9	43.4	67.1	37.5	42.9			49.8
Permanent resident	21.1	38.9	31.6	45.0	28.6			32.8
Noncitizen	30.0	17.7	1.3	17.5	28.6			17.3

[a]Group differences were significant ($F = 9.7$, $P < .001$).
*$P < .05$; **$P < .01$; ***$P < .001$.

TABLE 4—Final Logistic Regression: Predictor Variables of Current Smoking (n = 550)

	Coefficient (SE)	Odds Ratio	95% Confidence Interval
Male (vs female)	1.68 (0.26)***	5.36	3.21, 8.93
Executive/professional (vs student)	-1.28 (0.44)**	0.28	0.12, 0.66
Divorced (vs married)	1.74 (0.75)*	5.68	1.30, 24.85
Widowed (vs married)	2.26 (1.07)*	9.54	1.17, 77.79
Never married (vs married)	-0.89 (0.37)*	0.41	0.20, 0.84
Age	-0.03 (0.12)**	0.97	0.95, 0.99

*$P < .05$; **$P < .01$; ***$P < .001$.

Differences in tobacco use among the Asian American population and other ethnic groups and differences within Asian American subgroups lend support to the idea that cultural differences affect tobacco use patterns. For example, our study showed that current smokers were more likely to have been born outside the United States. Although it is generally assumed that immigrants' tobacco use will eventually conform to mainstream patterns of smoking, the current study clearly indicates that any prevention or intervention programs for immigrants must promote protective factors that the subculture provides and reduce factors that lead to heavy tobacco use.

Our findings suggest that intervention and prevention efforts need to focus on men and on the role of the family in influencing smoking behavior. The focus on men is particularly critical, because younger male Asians tend to emulate adult Asians' behaviors. For example, studies have shown that those who are heavy smokers are more likely to give cigarettes as gifts.[43] Because smoking among Asian men is more tolerated among Asian Americans than smoking among women, Asian male adolescents may perceive this exchange of cigarettes as gifts as both an acceptance of smoking as a cultural norm and a reflection of one's affection or respect for others inside and outside the family circle. These and similar cultural mores have a tangible influence on smoking behavior, especially among young people, and require special attention by prevention, intervention, and cessation program planners.

Cause and effect cannot be determined from the findings of this study. However, family structure, marital status, occupation, and age seem to be related to current tobacco use, a circumstance that affords opportunities for further exploration of the relative impact of these variables on smoking behavior as well as on program planning.

The comprehensive needs assessment questionnaire developed for the study further corroborated the findings of other studies regarding tobacco use in Asian American populations—in particular, lower perceived risks regarding smoking-related cancers and chronic diseases and a pervasive lack of readiness for change in smoking behavior among Asian American smokers.[44,45] The current findings prompted ATECAR to respond to these special needs by developing a series of community-based, culturally tailored comprehensive tobacco prevention, intervention, and cessation programs for the target Asian communities.

Among these programs are 2 research-based community tobacco prevention and intervention programs for adults and young people, a culturally adapted Asian youth smoking cessation program, a theory-based Asian adult smoking cessation intervention trial, a physician-based smoking intervention program to be provided in conjunction with intensive motivational behavior counseling, and a pilot study addressing cervical cancer among Vietnamese women, the group with the highest cervical cancer morbidity rate in the United States. This last component, although unrelated to the objectives of the study, was a by-product of the comprehensive assessment to which ATECAR felt obligated to respond. (ATECAR's experience in developing and implementing health surveys in Asian American communities is the subject of an upcoming article.)

Our study involved 3 major limitations. First, as a result of the cross-sectional design,[30–33] cause and effect relationships could not be determined. For example, it is difficult to determine cultural influences on tobacco use with such a design. Second, the self-report procedure did not allow determination of the relative veracity of cohort responses. Finally, certain cultural factors and characteristics of the sample made simple random sampling difficult. Most community organizations, for example, would not provide membership lists because of confidentiality issues, and Asian Americans are generally reluctant to provide researchers with personal information. Such obstacles mandated modifications of the simple random sampling design to facilitate greater access to these communities and subgroups. Despite these limitations, we consider our approach viable and the data appropriate for the design of more culturally appropriate prevention, intervention, and cessation programs for our study community. ■

About the Authors

Grace X. Ma, Yin Tan, and Jamil Toubbeh are with the Department of Health Studies, Center for ATECAR, Temple University, Philadelphia, Pa. Steve Shive is with the Department of Health and Community Services, California State University, Chico.

Requests for reprints should be sent to Grace X. Ma, PhD, CHES, Department of Health Studies, Temple University, 304A Vivacqua Hall, PO Box 2843, Philadelphia, PA 19122-0843 (e-mail: grace.xueqin.ma@temple.edu).

This article was accepted February 5, 2002.

Contributors

G.X. Ma made substantial contributions to the conception and design of the study, to analysis and interpretation of the data, and to revisions of the article. S. Shive contributed to analysis and interpretation of the data, assisted in the drafting of the article, and provided statistical expertise. Y. Tan contributed to the acquisition, analysis, and interpretation of the data and assisted in the drafting of the article. J. Toubbeh contributed to the conception and design of the study and to revisions of the article.

Acknowledgments

This research was funded by the National Cancer Institute.

We are grateful to members of the Asian Community Cancer Coalition for their contributions to data collection, to Xuefen Su and Nu Bui for assisting with data entry, to Frank Jackson and Dr Ken Chu for input on the study, and to Dr Shanyang Zhao for reviewing the article.

References

1. Centers for Disease Control and Prevention. Cigarette smoking among adults—United States, 1998. *MMWR Morb Mortal Wkly Rep.* 2000;49:881–893.

2. *State Tobacco Control Highlights—1999.* Atlanta, Ga: Centers for Disease Control and Prevention; 1999. CDC publication 99-5621.

3. Centers for Disease Control and Prevention. State-specific prevalence of current cigarette smoking among adults, and policies and attitudes about secondhand smoke—United States, 2000. *MMWR Morb Mortal Wkly Rep.* 2001;50:1101–1106.

4. *1990 Census of the Population.* 112th ed. Washington, DC: US Bureau of the Census; 1990.

5. Schneider Institute for Health Policy. *Substance Abuse: The Nation's Number One Health Problem.* Princeton, NJ: Robert Wood Johnson Foundation; 2001.

6. *Saving Lives and Money With Settlement Funds.* Narberth, Pa: Coalition for a Tobacco Free Pennsylvania; 1999.

7. *Tobacco Use Among US Racial/Ethnic Minority Groups—African Americans, American Indians and Alaska Natives, Asian Americans and Pacific Islanders, and Hispanics: A Report of the Surgeon General.* Atlanta, Ga: Centers for Disease Control and Prevention; 1998.

8. Sussman J, Burton D, Dent C, Stacy A, Flay B. *Developing School-Based Tobacco Use and Prevention and Cessation Programs.* Beverly Hills, Calif: Sage Publications; 1995.

9. Ma GX, Shive SE, Legos P, Tan Y. Ethnic differences in adolescent smoking behaviors, sources of tobacco, knowledge and attitudes toward restriction policies. *Addict Behav.* In press.

10. Wiecha JM. Differences in patterns of tobacco use in Vietnamese, African-American, Hispanic, and Caucasian adolescents in Worcester, Massachusetts. *Am J Prev Med.* 1996;12:29–37.

11. Wiecha JM, Lee V, Hodgkins J. Patterns of smoking, risk factors for smoking, and smoking cessation among Vietnamese men in Massachusetts (United States). *Tob Control.* 1998;7:27–34.

12. Chen X, Unger JB. Hazards of smoking initiation among Asian American and non-Asian adolescents in California: a survival model analysis. *Prev Med.* 1999; 28:589–599.

13. Escobedo LG, Peddicord JP. Smoking prevalence in US birth cohorts: the influence of gender and education. *Am J Public Health.* 1996;86:231–236.

14. Shopland DR, Niemcryk SJ, Marconi KM. Geographic and gender variations in total tobacco use. *Am J Public Health.* 1992;82:103–106.

15. Covey LS, Zang EA, Wynder EL. Cigarette smoking and occupational status: 1977 to 1990. *Am J Public Health.* 1992;82:1230–1234.

16. Moeschberger ML, Anderson J, Kuo Y, Chen MS, Wewers M, Guthrie R. Multivariate profile of smoking in Southeast Asian men: a biochemically verified analysis. *Prev Med.* 1997;26:53–58.

17. Thridandam M, Fong W, Jang M, Louie L, Forst M. A tobacco and alcohol use profile of San Francisco's Chinese community. *J Drug Educ.* 1998;28:377–393.

18. Jenkins CN, McPhee SJ, Ha N, Nam TV, Chen A. Cigarette smoking among Vietnamese immigrants in California. *Am J Health Promotion.* 1995;9:254–256.

19. Centers for Disease Control. Behavioral risk factor survey of Chinese—California, 1989. *MMWR Morb Mortal Wkly Rep.* 1992;41:266–270.

20. Centers for Disease Control and Prevention. Tobacco use among high school students—United States, 1997. *JAMA.* 1998;279:1250–1251.

21. Centers for Disease Control and Prevention. Cigarette smoking among adults—United States, 1995. *MMWR Morb Mortal Wkly Rep.* 1997;46:1217–1220.

22. Jenkins C. Response. *J Natl Cancer Inst.* 1996; 88:841.

23. Han FF, Kim SH, Lee MS, Miller JS, Rhee S, Song H. *Korean Health Survey: A Preliminary Report.* Los Angeles, Calif: Korean Health Education Information and Referral Center; 1989.

24. *Smoking Among Asian Americans: A National Tobacco Survey.* San Francisco, Calif: National Asian Women's Association; 1998.

25. Centers for Disease Control. Behavioral risk factor survey of Vietnamese—California, 1991. *MMWR Morb Mortal Wkly Rep.* 1992;41:69–72.

26. Centers for Disease Control. Cigarette smoking among Chinese, Vietnamese, and Hispanics—California, 1989–1991. *MMWR Morb Mortal Wkly Rep.* 1992;41: 362–367.

27. Chen MS, Hawks BL. A debunking of the myth of the healthy Asian American and Pacific Islander. *Am J Health Promotion.* 1995;9:261–268.

28. Doong T. A message on behalf of David Satcher, MD, PhD, surgeon general. *Asian Am Pac Islander J Health.* 1998;6:408–409.

29. Chu KC. Cancer data for Asian Americans and Pacific Islanders. *Asian Am Pac Islander J Health.* 1998;6: 130–139.

30. Babbie E. *Survey Research Methods.* 2nd ed. Belmont, Calif: Wadsworth Publishing Co; 1990.

31. Fink A, Kosecoff J. *How to Conduct Surveys: A Step-by-Step Guide.* Newbury Park, Calif: Sage Publications; 1985.

32. Fowler FJ. *Survey Research Methods.* Newbury Park, Calif: Sage Publications; 1988.

33. Sudman S, Bradburn NM. *Asking Questions.* San Francisco, Calif: Jossey-Bass; 1986.

34. Federer W. *Statistics and Society: Data Collection and Interpretation.* 2nd ed. New York, NY: Marcel Dekker Inc; 1991.

35. Sue D, Sue S. Cultural factors in the clinical assessment of Asian-Americans. *J Consult Clin Psychol.* 1987;55:479–487.

36. Kitano H, Daniels R. *Asian Americans: Emerging Minorities.* Englewood Cliffs, NJ: Prentice Hall; 1988.

37. *National Center for Health Statistics Public Use Data Tapes, 1978–1995.* Hyattsville, Md: National Center for Health Statistics; 1996.

38. Centers for Disease Control and Prevention. Cigarette smoking in 99 metropolitan areas—United States, 2000. *MMWR Morb Mortal Wkly Rep.* 2001;50: 1107–1113.

39. *Request for Proposals to Provide Statewide Comprehensive Tobacco Control Programs for the Department of Health.* Harrisburg, Pa: Commonwealth of Pennsylvania Dept of Health; 2001.

40. *Healthy People 2010.* Washington, DC: US Dept of Health and Human Services; 2000.

41. Chen X, Unger JB, Johnson CA. Is acculturation a risk factor for early smoking initiation among Chinese American minors? A comparative perspective. *Tob Control.* 1999;8:402–410.

42. *Preventing Tobacco Use Among Young People: A Report of the Surgeon General.* Atlanta, Ga: Centers for Disease Control and Prevention; 1994.

43. Wolfson M, Forster JL. Adolescent smokers' provision of tobacco to other adolescents. *Am J Public Health.* 1997;87:649–651.

44. Ma GX, Tan Y, Feeley R, Thomas P. Perceived risks of certain types of cancer and heart disease among Asian American smokers and non-smokers. *J Community Health.* In press.

45. Ma GX, Tan Y, Toubbeh JI. Differences in readiness for smoking behavior change among Asian American current smokers. *Addict Behav.* In press.

Do Sex and Ethnic Differences in Smoking Initiation Mask Similarities in Cessation Behavior?

| Gene A. McGrady, MD, MPH, and Linda L. Pederson, PhD

Objectives. This study compared success in smoking cessation by sex, ethnic status, and birth cohort.

Methods. African and European American respondents to the 1996 Current Population Survey (tobacco supplement) and the 1987 National Health Interview Survey (cancer control and cancer epidemiology supplements) constituted the study population. Elapsed time from smoking initiation to cessation was compared via nonparametric tests and survival analysis techniques.

Results. Findings showed that success in quitting was independent of ethnic status and sex and that population differences in smoking initiation age (assuming no differences in quitting behavior) could produce statistical associations between sex/ethnicity and smoking cessation.

Conclusions. Population differences in smoking initiation patterns can mask similarities in cessation rates. (*Am J Public Health.* 2002;92:961–965)

Cigarette smoking remains the most important contributor to preventable morbidity and mortality in the United States.[1] Promotion of smoking cessation is a public health priority, but it continues to be the case that most individuals who successfully quit smoking do so on their own, without the aid of formal programs.[2–7] Among individuals who have quit on their own, data from many epidemiological studies suggest that men are more likely to quit than are women,[5,8,9] and Whites more likely to quit than Hispanics or African Americans.[5,10–15] Results regarding sex and ethnic differences in cessation have not, however, been consistent.[16,17] Specifically, when duration of smoking has been taken into account,[16] no differences in quitting behavior have been found.

In this study, we examined ethnic and sex differences in successful quitting, taking duration of smoking into account. Elapsed time from smoking initiation to cessation ("time to quit") was defined as individuals' reported age at quitting minus their reported age at initiation. This quantity approximates duration of smoking (it does not adjust for time off smoking due to quit attempts) and serves as an individual-level measure of successful quitting. In the framework of survival analysis, time to quit (or duration) is considered a "failure time," a strategy that allows cessation to be viewed as a dynamic population process.

Conceptualizing cessation as a population process brings observational and measurement issues to attention. Specifically, it forces consideration of the possibility that the results of a process measurement taken at one point in time may differ from the results of the same measurement taken at a later time as a consequence of the time evolution of the process. We analyzed data sets collected in 1987 and 1996 in an effort to assess this possibility and its implications. We addressed the possibility of cohort differences in quitting behavior (generational trends) by constructing and comparing birth cohorts with respect to time-to-quit values.

METHODS

Data collected in 2 national surveys, the Current Population Survey (CPS) of January 1996 and the National Health Interview Survey (NHIS) of 1987, were used in analyzing smoking cessation. Both the CPS and the NHIS are ongoing surveys targeting the civilian, noninstitutionalized population of the United States.

The NHIS is conducted by the National Center for Health Statistics and serves as the principal source of information on the health of the US population. In this survey, a multistage probability design is used to select sample households representative of the target population. Within selected households, information on all adult members (18 years or older) is collected by trained interviewers.[18] In 1987, tobacco use and other cancer-related information was assessed at the national level via supplementary cancer control and cancer epidemiology questionnaires.

The CPS is conducted by the Bureau of the Census and serves as the source of official government statistics on employment and unemployment. This survey also involves the use of a multistage probability design in selecting nationally representative households. Within households, information on all members 15 years or older is collected.[19] In January 1996, a tobacco use survey was conducted as a supplement to the CPS.[20] Proxy responses were permitted in this supplement (as shown in the first 3 CPS questions described subsequently), but these data were excluded from the analyses described here.

Information of interest in analyzing cessation was assessed via self-reports in both surveys. Variables used were derived from respondents' answers to the following questions: (1) Have you smoked 100 cigarettes in your entire life? (NHIS) or Has [household member in question] smoked 100 cigarettes in his/her entire life? (CPS); (2) Do you currently smoke cigarettes? (NHIS) or Does [household member in question] now smoke cigarettes every day, some days, or not at all? (CPS); (3) How old were you when you first started smoking cigarettes fairly regularly? (NHIS) or How old was [household member in question] when he/she first started smoking cigarettes fairly regularly? (CPS); and (4) How long ago did you stop smoking? (NHIS) or About how long has it been since you completely stopped smoking cigarettes? (CPS).

Individuals responding yes to question 1 were classified as ever smokers. Those responding no (NHIS) or not at all (CPS) to question 2 were classified as former smokers. Age at initiation was determined by response to question 3. Finally, for question 4, time to quit was defined for each individual as reported length of time from initiation to cessation of smoking. Among former smokers, current age (in days) and reported elapsed time since quitting were used in computing age at cessation.

Among CPS respondents, age at survey completion was used to estimate year of birth (1995 minus age); NHIS respondents reported their year of birth. Ten-year birth cohorts (1896–1905, 1906–1915, . . ., 1966–1975, 1976 and later), selected for compatibility with our previous investigations,[21] were constructed according to birth year. Data for ethnic groups other than Black or White (CPS, n=2221; NHIS, n=1537) and data for which the time-to-quit variable was missing or unknown were not analyzed.

A successful quitter was defined as a former smoker who had maintained abstinence for 1 year or longer. Initially, we assessed sex and ethnic differences in successful quitting by comparing time-to-quit distributions using appropriate *k*-sample and 2-sample tests. These results did not, however, account for the complex sampling design used in the 2 surveys. Thus, another hypothesis-testing approach was taken to account for the complex design. The Kolmogorov–Smirnov statistic[22,23] was used in pairwise comparisons of time-to-quit distributions. *P* values associated with these tests were adjusted, via estimation of design effect and effective sample size,[24,25] to account for the survey design.

The adjustment procedure followed that of Kish.[24] For each birth cohort and each combination of 2 subdomains—race/ethnicity and sex—a weighted Kolmogorov–Smirnov statistic and associated *P* value were calculated. Because survey design variables were not published in the CPS data, we calculated the variances (accounting for sampling design) for Kolmogorov–Smirnov statistics estimated in that data set by considering these statistics as differences in proportions and using the generalized variance functions supplied in the documentation.

In the case of the NHIS data, we used bootstrap resampling in estimating variance.[26,27] Specifically, we produced 200 resamples by sampling with replacement from 62 pseudostrata; 3 (of 4) pseudo–primary sampling units were sampled independently in each pseudostratum. As a means of bias reduction,[27] the weight associated with each selected record was multiplied by the factor 1.33 (4/3).

We then calculated design effects[24] for the contrast by comparing the variance with the survey design taken into account and the simple random sampling variance. On the basis of these design effects, we calculated effective sample sizes and adjusted *P* values.[23,28]

RESULTS

Respondent characteristics are shown in Table 1. African Americans were oversampled in the 1987 NHIS. In those data, suc-

TABLE 1—Numbers of Respondents, by Birth Cohort, Sex, Ethnic Status, and Reported Smoking Status

	All Respondents				Ever Smokers				Successful Quitters[a]			
Birth Cohort	Black Males	White Males	Black Females	White Females	Black Males	White Males	Black Females	White Females	Black Males	White Males	Black Females	White Females
					Current Population Survey, 1996: tobacco supplement							
1896	3	53	13	165	2	22	0	19	0	19	0	16
1906	42	606	106	1315	14	351	16	331	8	309	11	262
1916	124	1929	240	3051	77	1268	66	1116	47	1063	50	775
1926	179	2590	337	3381	117	1763	123	1552	63	1233	82	901
1936	271	3119	451	3919	163	2004	171	1894	72	1218	73	918
1946	424	4675	713	6027	250	2571	268	2755	75	1209	84	1185
1956	454	5037	808	6510	182	2273	280	2810	43	710	61	959
1966	344	3514	690	4487	97	1268	129	1671	13	248	16	361
1976	139	1165	190	1340	13	282	14	287	0	16	1	23
					National Health Interview Survey, 1987: cancer epidemiology/control supplements							
1896	30	301	80	762	13	145	10	121	10	124	3	91
1906	156	1028	259	2107	97	699	67	627	58	523	39	367
1916	241	1771	403	2710	167	1290	153	1174	78	872	76	540
1926	261	1839	407	2322	189	1349	194	1146	74	712	61	452
1936	324	2215	499	2533	221	1550	242	1375	64	673	71	475
1946	478	3463	898	4308	287	2042	425	2065	65	772	77	688
1956	461	3443	1038	4433	216	1625	435	2128	24	401	47	540
1966	160	873	273	1040	32	271	51	351	3	26	4	49

[a]Former smokers reporting cessation lasting at least 1 year.

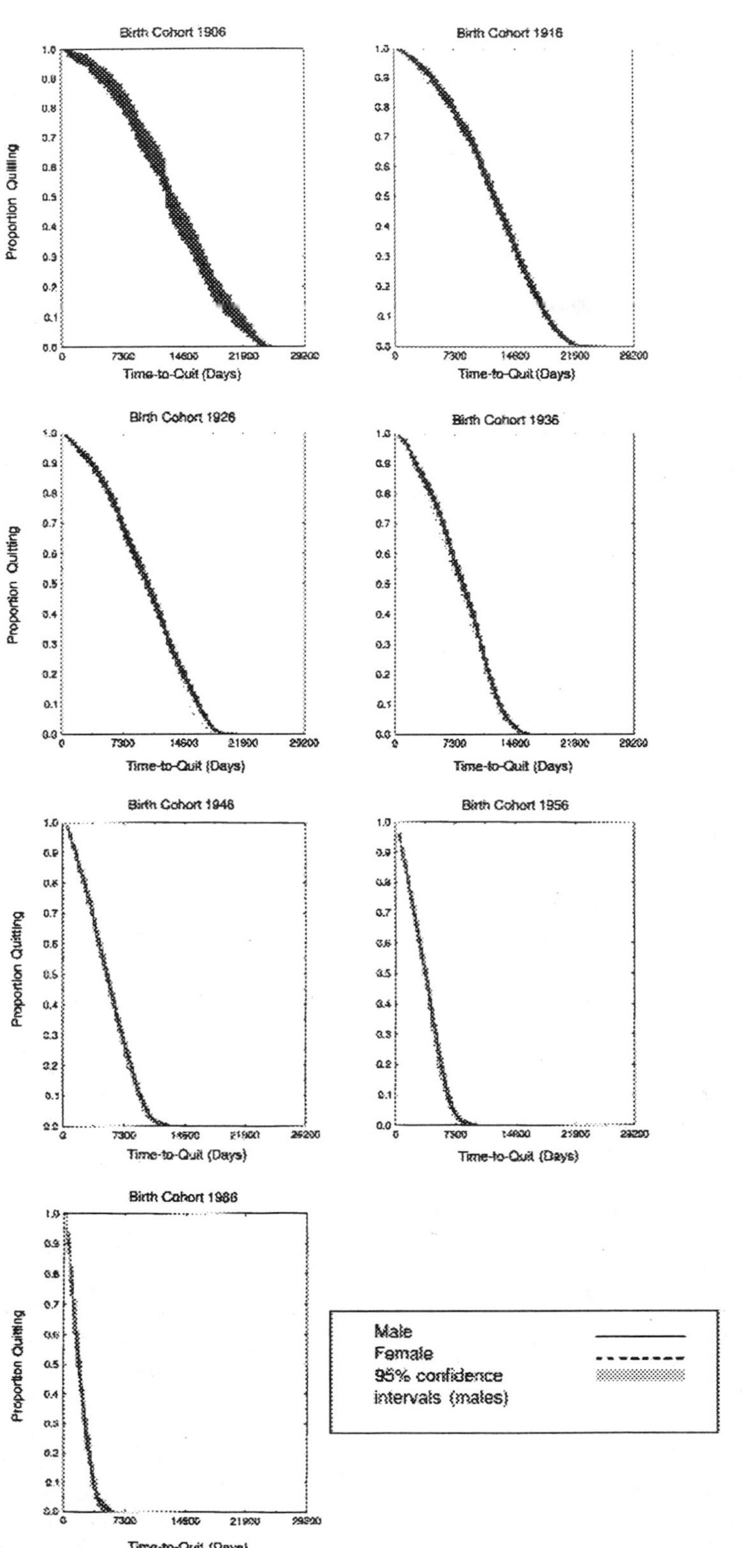

FIGURE 1—Male and female time-to-quit distributions, by birth cohort: Current Population Survey, 1996.

cessful quitters were represented in all birth cohorts, although the sample size was small for the 1896 birth cohort (Table 1). Fewer African Americans overall, and no successful quitters belonging to the 1896 cohort, were sampled in the 1996 CPS.

Figure 1 displays male and female time-to-quit distributions by birth cohort. Distributions are presented as survival curves; probabilities of successful cessation are shown on the y-axis, and time-to-quit values are shown on the x-axis. Pointwise confidence bands are included. The similarity of male and female cessation patterns is evident in all birth cohorts, with confidence bands indicating that the distributions are statistically indistinguishable. A similar conclusion held for the comparison of African American and European American cohorts (data not shown). In both cases, confidence bands were calculated with an assumption of simple random sampling. That is, the complex sampling design of the survey data was not accounted for in these results. As a remedy, hypothesis-testing procedures (as described earlier) were used, and results (available on request) confirmed that the compared distributions were statistically indistinguishable.

The quit ratio is a commonly used measure of smoking cessation in populations. We examined the proposition that 2 populations having identical time-to-quit distributions can display significantly different quit ratios if the pattern of initiation is different in the populations. If members of one group systematically initiate smoking at earlier ages than members of a comparison group, and both groups are equally likely to quit after a given duration of smoking, then the early-initiating group would be expected to contain a larger proportion of quitters at most observation times.

A Monte Carlo simulation experiment was performed to assess this proposed mechanism quantitatively. Mean prevalence rates of current smoking and quit ratios were generated for 2 populations under the assumption of identical time-to-quit distributions but differing initiation patterns. We compared quit ratios by computing a relative ratio representing the quit ratio of one group divided by the ratio of the other group.

The experiment revealed that lower mean age at initiation for one population results in relative ratios above 1.0 that decrease toward 1.0 as observation time increases; larger differences in mean age at initiation result in larger relative ratios. Variability in initiation age has an effect independent of mean age; other factors being equal, initiation occurring over shorter periods of time in one population increases the relative ratio. The simulated prevalence of smoking is initially larger in early-initiating groups but becomes smaller in comparison as cessation proceeds. The results of this experimental simulation confirm that statistical associations of sex and ethnic status with quit ratios on the order reported in the literature could be produced by differences in mean age at initiation of 1 or 2 years.

DISCUSSION

The analyses described here lead to 2 main conclusions. First, our findings contradict previous research results suggesting that success in quitting cigarette smoking is a function of ethnic status or sex and that women and African Americans lag behind in terms of smoking cessation. The validity of these findings is supported by 2 considerations: (a) the data examined are nationally representative; and (b) results were consistent over 2 separate observations (1987 and 1996) and for all cohorts examined, whose experiences span the history of mass cigarette use in the United States. Second, given that ethnic and sex differences in initiation age have been demonstrated for African American and European American populations,[29–32] use of the quit ratio to compare cessation rates in these populations is problematic. We suspect that any measure of cessation that does not account for an individual's duration of smoking may involve similar limitations.

Two possibilities may threaten the validity of these conclusions. First, comparison of time-to-quit distributions could lead to error if reported initiation age, smoking status, or age at cessation were systematically misclassified. In the literature of which we are aware,[33–35] evidence does not support the presence of sex or ethnic bias in reports of these variables. A second possibility is that time to quit may be misrepresented if quit attempts or time away from smoking resulting from such attempts differ systematically between populations (e.g., if number of quit attempts or time away from smoking during attempts is systematically greater in one population). Data relating to quit attempts among former smokers were not collected in the CPS, but such data *were* collected in the cancer control supplement of the 1987 NHIS. Analyses of these data indicate no significant male–female or Black–White differences in either number of quit attempts or duration of most recent (or only) quit attempt.

Implications of these conclusions for smoking cessation surveillance and research are clear. With respect to tobacco use surveillance, use of the quit ratio appears to be inadequate. It is important to measure and monitor both initiation and cessation if present status and trends in smoking are to be correctly interpreted. Similarly, with respect to smoking cessation research, measures of quitting that account for duration of smoking may be most appropriate, both in analyzing factors associated with cessation and in evaluating interventions. Additional research on the relation between number of quit attempts and duration of attempts might be helpful in connecting clinical trial results to long-term successful cessation. ■

About the Authors

Gene A. McGrady is, and at the time of the study Linda L. Pederson was, with the Department of Community Health and Preventive Medicine, Morehouse School of Medicine, Atlanta, Ga.

Requests for reprints should be sent to Gene A. McGrady, MD, MPH, Department of Community Health and Preventive Medicine, Morehouse School of Medicine, 720 Westview Dr, SW, Atlanta, GA 30310 (e-mail: genemc@gene.msm.edu).

This article was accepted December 6, 2001.

Contributors

Both authors participated in the initial conception and design of the study. G.A. McGrady was primarily responsible for the data analysis. Both authors contributed to interpretation of data and to drafting and revision of the article.

Acknowledgments

This research was supported in full by the National Cancer Institute (grant RO3-CA83337).

References

1. Centers for Disease Control and Prevention. Smoking-attributable mortality and years of potential life lost—United States, 1984. *MMWR Morb Mortal Wkly Rep.* 1997;46:444–451.

2. *Cancer Facts and Figures.* New York, NY: American Cancer Society; 1986.

3. Fiore MC, Novotny TE, Pierce JP, et al. Methods used to quit smoking in the United States: do cessation programs help? *JAMA.* 1990;263:2760–2765.

4. Lando HA, Pechacek TF, Fruetel J. The Minnesota Heart Health Program community Quit and Win contests. *Am J Health Promot.* 1994;9:85–87.

5. Coambs RB, Lis S, Kozlowski LT. Age interacts with heaviness of smoking in predicting success in smoking cessation. *Am J Epidemiol.* 1992;135:240–246.

6. Pederson LL. Smoking behavior of Canadians. In: *Canada's Health Promotion Survey 1990: Technical Report.* Ottawa, Ontario, Canada: Health and Welfare Canada; 1993:91–101.

7. Prochaska JO, DiClemente CC, Velicer WF, et al. Predicting change in smoking status for self-changers. *Addict Behav.* 1985;10:395–406.

8. Hymowitz N, Cummings M, Hyland A, et al. Predictors of smoking cessation in a cohort of adult smokers followed for five years. *Tob Control.* 1997;6(suppl 2):S57–S62.

9. Derby CA, Lasater TM, Vass K, et al. Characteristics of smokers who attempt to quit and those who recently succeeded. *Am J Prev Med.* 1994;10:327–334.

10. Gilpin E, Pierce JP, Goodman J, et al. Reasons smokers give for stopping smoking: do they relate to success in stopping? *Tob Control.* 1992;1:256–263.

11. Tunstall CD, Ginsberg D, Hall SM. Quitting smoking. *Int J Addict.* 1985;10:1089–1112.

12. Haire-Joshu D, Morgan G, Fisher EB. Determinants of cigarette smoking. *Clin Chest Med.* 1991;12:711–725.

13. Effectiveness of smoking-control strategies: editorial note from the Centers for Disease Control. *JAMA.* 1992;268:1645–1646.

14. Carmody TP. Affect regulation, nicotine addiction, and smoking cessation. *J Psychoactive Drugs.* 1992;24:111–122.

15. Centers for Disease Control and Prevention. Cigarette smoking among adults—United States, 1993. *MMWR Morb Mortal Wkly Rep.* 1994;43:925–930.

16. Freund KM, D'Agostino RB, Belanger AJ, et al. Predictors of smoking cessation: the Framingham Study. *Am J Epidemiol.* 1992;135:957–964.

17. Fiore MC, Novotny TE, Pierce JP, et al. Trends in cigarette smoking in the United States: the changing influence of gender and race. *JAMA.* 1989;261:49–55.

18. *Sample Design and Estimation Procedures for the National Health Interview Survey, 1985–1994.* Hyattsville, Md: National Center for Health Statistics; 1989. DHHS publication PHS 89-1384.

19. *The Current Population Survey Design and Methodology.* Washington, DC: US Bureau of the Census; 1985. Technical paper 40.

20. *Current Population Survey, January 1996: Tobacco Use Supplement* [machine-readable data file]. Washington, DC: US Bureau of the Census; 1998.

21. McGrady GA, Ahluwalia JS, Pederson LL. Smoking initiation and cessation in African Americans attending an inner-city walk-in clinic. *Am J Prev Med.* 1998;14:130–137.

22. Siegal S. *Nonparametric Statistics for the Behavioral Sciences.* New York, NY: McGraw-Hill Book Co; 1956: 127–136.

23. Kendall M, Stuart A. *The Advanced Theory of Statistics: Inference and Relationship.* Vol. 2. 4th ed. London, England: Charles Griffen & Co Ltd; 1979.

24. Kish L. *Survey Sampling.* New York, NY: John Wiley & Sons Inc; 1965.

25. Skinner CJ, Hold D, Smith TMF. *Analysis of Complex Surveys.* New York, NY: John Wiley & Sons Inc; 1989.

26. Efron B, Tibshirani RJ. *An Introduction to the Bootstrap.* New York, NY: Chapman & Hall; 1993.

27. Korn EG, Graubard BI. *Analysis of Health Surveys.* New York, NY: John Wiley & Sons Inc; 1999.

28. Press WH, Teukolsky SA, Vetterling WT, Flannery BP. *Numerical Recipes in C: The Art of Scientific Computing.* 2nd ed. New York, NY: Cambridge University Press; 1992.

29. Escobedo LG, Anda RF, Smith PF, Remington PL, Mast EE. Sociodemographic characteristics of cigarette smoking initiation in the United States: implications for smoking prevention policy. *JAMA.* 1990;264: 1550–1555.

30. Gilpin EA, Lee L, Evans N, Pierce JP. Smoking initiation rates in adults and minors: United States, 1944–1988. *Am J Epidemiol.* 1994;140:535–543.

31. Centers for Disease Control. Differences in the age of smoking initiation between blacks and whites—United States. *MMWR Morb Mortal Wkly Rep.* 1991; 40:754–757.

32. Faulkner DL, Escobedo LG, Zhu B, Chrismon JH, Merritt RK. Race and the incidence of cigarette smoking among adolescents in the United States. *J Natl Cancer Inst.* 1996;88:1158–1160.

33. Krall EA, Valadian I, Dwyer JT, Gardener J. Accuracy of recalled smoking data. *Am J Public Health.* 1989;79:200–206.

34. Means B, Habina K, Swan GE, Jack L. Cognitive research on response error in survey questions in smoking. *Vital Health Stat 6.* 1992;No. 5.

35. Clark P, Gautam SP, Hlaing WM, Gerson LW. Response error in self-reported current smoking frequency by black and white established smokers. *Ann Epidemiol.* 1996;6:483–489.

Burning Love: Big Tobacco Takes Aim at LGBT Youths

Secret tobacco industry documents lay bare the industry's targeting, seduction, and recruitment of minority groups and children. They also unmask Big Tobacco's disdain for its targets.

| Harriet A. Washington

A DECADE AGO, FORMER Winston honcho David Goerlitz sneered that the R.J. Reynolds Tobacco Company had built its fortune by marketing to "the young, poor, black, and stupid."[1] A tobacco executive who risked such candor today might add, "the lesbian, gay, bisexual, transgender, and Hispanic." But such loose talk is very unlikely today because a series of legal reversals and losses in the court of public opinion have created an acutely circumspect tobacco consortium.

Decades ago, flagrant, disrespectful stereotypes marked the industry's initial courting of African Americans. Sports sponsorships, cartoon characters, and trinkets clearly labeled yesterday's marketing efforts to children and youths. But by the late 1980s, tobacco firms could read the writing on the billboard. Public health advocates and African American activists joined to protest such egregious forms of targeted marketing as the saturation of urban communities with billboards. Even more vociferous protests castigated the design and marketing of cigarettes and tobacco blends targeted exclusively at African Americans.

By the mid-1990s, Minnesota Attorney General Hubert Humphrey III wrested a legal settlement from the nation's major tobacco companies into which he incorporated a brilliant public relations stealth bomb: He forced the release and publication of Big Tobacco's secret internal marketing and research documents on the Internet for all to read. These documents laid bare, in the industry's own damning words, the oft-denied targeting, seduction, and recruitment of minority groups and children. They also unmasked Big Tobacco's disdain for its targets.

The ensuing spate of state and federal legal victories over Big Tobacco has, among other things, specifically banned traditional means of marketing to young people, such as cartoons, billboards, and advertisements in periodicals with significant youth readership.

These developments, while public health successes, have also served to drive tobacco's youth recruitment efforts underground, where they continue, shrouded in coded language and the all-too-familiar denials. The tobacco industry still boasts a marketing budget of $8.4 billion per year for the United States alone,[2] and the hidden truth about today's targeted marketing of vulnerable groups such as lesbian, gay, bisexual, and transgender (LGBT) youths will be even harder to excavate than was yesterday's.

Big Tobacco's past approaches toward targeting minorities, especially African Americans, are illuminating and may prove instructive for detecting its current ploys toward forbidden markets such as youths, especially LGBT youths. For example, Big Tobacco made loyal customers (and defenders) of many African Americans by lavishing positive attention on them when the rest of corporate America still considered Blacks to be marketing pariahs. Tobacco firms hired African Americans before other elements of corporate America welcomed or even accepted them, and tobacco firms infused languishing African American media, cultural, and advocacy groups with desperately needed financial support (box on page 1091).

But as the targeted-marketing backlash in the African American community has limited and sometimes stymied tobacco firms' influence, these companies have sought out lucrative new markets. Internal marketing memos show that the tobacco industry has scoured the globe for new target communities as starved for corporate attention and acceptance today as African Americans were yesterday. These new targets include Hispanics, the fastest growing element of the population, and sexual minorities.

Today, tobacco firms are emerging from their corporate closets to openly engage in every type of marketing targeted at gay adults. Most alarmingly, the targeted marketing focuses on LGBT youths, but the cynical marketing snares for the young are carefully hidden and slyly labeled. Today, tobacco's corporate language is sanitized in a Newspeak of acronyms and is bowdlerized to delete any overt reference to youth marketing. The industry whose internal memos once blithely spoke of recruiting Black 14-year-olds is now careful to refer in print and in public only to "young smokers 18 and older."

> "Tobacco companies have always been aware of sexual minorities as customers who smoked at extremely high rates, but only in the last decade have they embraced marketing targeted at gays in earnest and in large numbers."

SLAUGHTER OF THE INNOCENTS

The tobacco industry has never admitted targeting LGBT youths or even targeting youths at all, despite Joe Camel, cartoons, logo-rich children's trinkets, and sponsorship of youth-oriented sporting and music events. In the face of denials and the recent absence of loose-lipped memos, how can one know that Big Tobacco markets to LGBT youths?

The first clue is a look at the fruits of that targeting, because the overwhelming majority of adult smokers were once underage smokers, and almost no smokers, gay or straight, take up the habit after age 20. Tobacco companies know that they must hook a smoker as a child or not at all, and the US tobacco industry invests $23 million *every day* to ensure that they do.[6–8] Twenty-eight percent of high school students smoke, as opposed to 23% of adults. Every day, 5000 children take their first puff; 2000 are unable to stop and thus swell the ranks of the nation's smokers. One third of the addicted will die from their smoking habits—and this doesn't count the 14% of boys who become addicted to the smokeless tobacco popularized by generations of sports heroes who chew, dip, and spit very publicly.[2]

A number of studies have determined that children are 3 times as susceptible to tobacco advertising than adults and that such advertising is a more powerful inducement than is peer pressure.[9,10]

Ugly as this picture is, the prospects of avoiding tobacco addiction are much bleaker for LGBT youths. The prevalence of smoking is around 46% for gay men and 48% for adult lesbians,[11,12] twice as high as for their peers. Data on bisexual and transsexual smoking behavior are sparse, as are data on the smoking behavior of sexual minorities who are also members of high-risk racial and ethnic minority groups. Still, smoking prevalence is likely to be disastrous at the intersection of such high-risk groups.

The smoking rates of LGBT youths are just as high as those of adults, which is hardly surprising. And not only do twice as many LGBTs as other Americans take up smoking; they find it harder to quit, although most want to. Eighty percent of the 1011 adult respondents in a 2001 American Medical Association (AMA)–Robert Wood Johnson (RWJ) Foundation poll said they had tried to stop smoking but could not.[13] Like African Americans, members of sexual minority groups pay a much

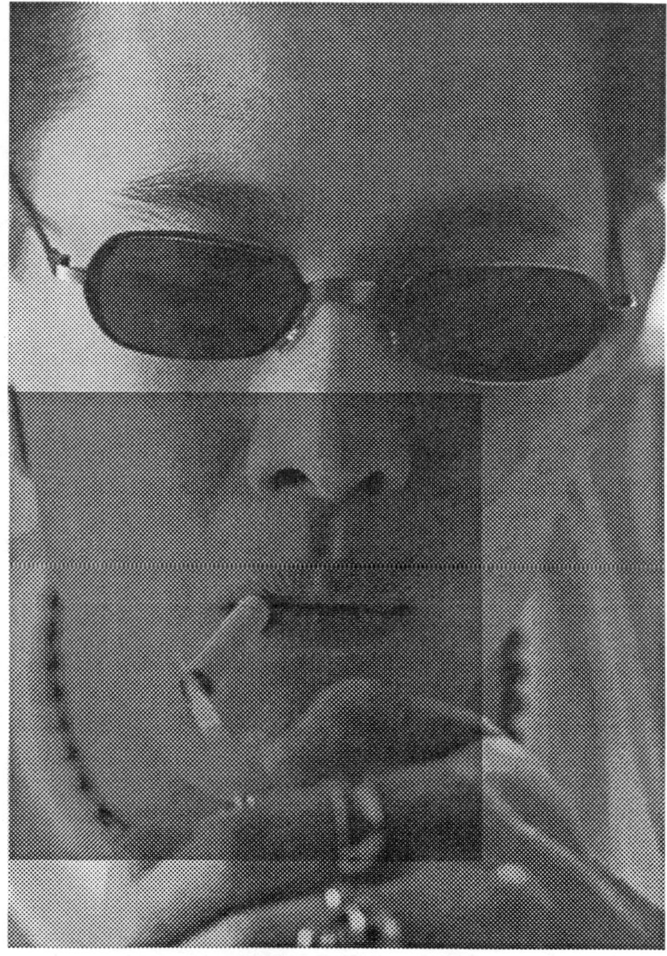

Gay and lesbian adults smoke twice as much as their peers.

The tobacco industry has scoured the globe for new target communities as starved for corporate attention and acceptance today as African Americans were yesterday. These new targets include Hispanics, the fastest growing element of the population, and sexual minorities.

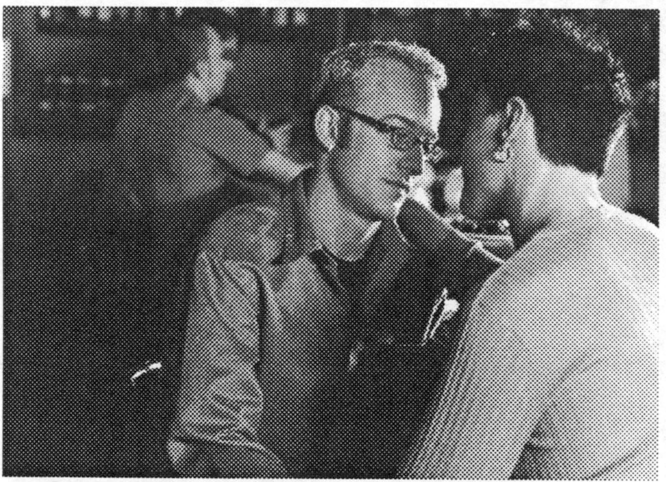

Linking cigarettes, alcohol, and the bar scene has been a staple of tobacco marketing strategies.

higher medical price for their tobacco addiction. The direct health effects of smoking for gays and lesbians are legion, although the exact figures are still a matter of debate.[11] Lesbians who use tobacco face risks of breast cancer, colorectal cancer, and other cancers 5 times higher than those of other women.[11] The Centers for Disease Control and Prevention (CDC) calculates that the life expectancy of a homosexual man is 8 to 20 years less than that of other men[14] and that high smoking rates contribute directly and indirectly to their early deaths. Some researchers fear that cigarette smoking may increase the risk of HIV infection and accelerate the progression to AIDS.[15] HIV-positive men have the highest smoking rates of all,[15] and heavy smoking triggers immune function changes that also worsen the prognosis for other infectious diseases such as sexually transmitted diseases and hepatitis C.[15,16]

Despite all these studies, surveys reveal that gay smokers do not believe that smoking a pack a day constitutes a health risk.[17] This is a dangerous attitude, because the health effects of smoking are not always related to the dose.

The scourge of tobacco addiction doesn't wait for adulthood to erode the mental and physical health of LGBT youths. These youths already face much higher vulnerabilities to violence, suicide, and risk-taking behavior (including risky sexual behaviors) than their peers. Young gay smokers are the greatest risk takers; their higher rates of alcohol and drug use[15] lead many experts to characterize tobacco as a "gateway drug" for gay youths.

LGBT youths also pay a high price in direct health effects of their smoking addiction, such as 30% to 87% higher rates of cancer. The synergistic effect of tobacco and alcohol encourages a constellation of other respiratory diseases and of ear, nose, and throat diseases; early smoking also inflates the lifetime risks not only of premature death but also of impairments such as blindness and infertility.

Ninety percent of smokers start in their teens,[17] and LGBT smokers start even younger; in one survey, 13 years was the median age for girls.[18] Tobacco firms therefore know that their efforts to target gays and lesbians will work only if they target gay youths younger than 18, the legal smoking age in most states.

The tobacco industry's targeting of the LGBT communities is a matter of record. Alcohol companies, many owned by tobacco firms, have targeted gays[12] as far back as the 1950s, when Joseph Cotton, with a hand resting on his double, slyly touted Smirnoff vodka, "mixed or straight."[19] Tobacco companies have always been aware of sexual minorities as customers who smoked at extremely high rates, but only in the last decade have they embraced marketing targeted at gays in earnest and in large numbers.

The secret tobacco documents placed on various Web sites afford revealing insights into the industry's changing perception of the LGBT communities. Internal memos reveal that tobacco companies sought gay voters' support as early as 1983,[2] when they wished to repeal workplace smoking bans in San Francisco.[12] An internal Philip Morris memo from 1985 reveals grudging admiration at how views of gays and lesbians as customers were changing: "It seems to me that homosexuals have made enormous progress in changing their image in this country. . . . A few years back they were considered damaging, bad and immoral, but today they have become acceptable members of society. . . .We should research this material and perhaps learn from it."[20]

A few years later, when African Americans were successfully protesting targeted community saturation by tobacco firms, the tobacco industry began openly contemplating sexual minorities as a less troublesome market. In the 1990s, just after the protests that aborted the marketing of Uptown to urban African Americans, a "Top Secret Operation Rainmaker" memo listed gays as a marketing "issue" to be discussed.[21] Paradoxically, this marketing attention was catalyzed by a concerted political attack mounted on the tobacco consortium by gays. When the AIDS Coalition to Unleash Power (ACT-UP) organized a 1990 boycott of Philip Morris over its support of Jesse Helms, tobacco companies responded by donating large funds to AIDS organizations in appeasement efforts,[17] just as they have showered politically pivotal African American organizations with money. Tobacco firms swiftly followed these overtures to gays and lesbians with national advertising campaigns. In 1991, a *Wall Street Journal* headline trumpeted, "Overcoming a deep-rooted reluctance, more firms advertise to [the] gay community." The story called gays and lesbians "a dream market" and focused on the tobacco industry's courtship of LGBT media giants such as *Genre*.[22]

Between 1990 and 1992, a series of ads for American Brands' Montclair featured an aging, nattily dressed man sporting an ascot, a pinky ring in lieu of a wedding ring, a captain's hat, and an orgiastic expression. This was perceived as a gay or effeminate persona by many readers and media analysts, a reading that American Brands denies. Benson & Hedges, for its part, touted a series of gay-themed ads for its Kings brand in *Genre*, a gay fashion and lifestyle magazine, as well as in *Esquire* and *GQ*, which have significant gay male readerships.

Recent marketers have not overlooked lesbian and bisexual women.[12] Philip Morris's Virginia Slims ads send messages of independence, camaraderie, and iconoclasm that appeal to feminists as well as lesbians. But the ads, appearing in such magazines as *Essence* and *Ms.*, have departed from women in lipstick and heels to feature more androgynous and sexually ambiguous portrayals of women. Women couples are shown fishing in plaid shirts, mesh vests, and hip boots; women duos in tailored clothes are captured in a tête-à-tête over coffee; women even throw appreciative glances at each other on the street over text that exhorts them not to "follow the straight and narrow."

Marlboro, the most popular cigarette brand among gay men, has flaunted the brand's rugged hypermasculine image in venues calculated to appeal to gays. For example, one large billboard features a close-up of a substantial male crotch clad in weathered jeans with a carton of Marlboros slung in front of it. The image hangs between 2 gay bars in San Francisco's Mission district.[12]

The health advocacy backlash to Big Tobacco's first flirtation with gay media was swift and sure. The Coalition of Lavender Americans on Smoking and Health (CLASH) issued a press release that read in part, "This is a community already ravaged by addiction: we don't need the Marlboro man to help pull the trigger."[12]

BEYOND BILLBOARDS

If the experiences of racial minorities—notably African Americans—serve as a guide, targeted advertising will be just the tip of the tobacco iceberg. The underwriting of key cultural institutions is another insidious route to the control of minority lungs. So is control over the specialized news media that minorities trust. Until 5 or 6 years ago, nearly all African American publishers retained, and sometimes defended, alcohol and tobacco advertisers. For example, in 1998, Dorothy Leavell, who was then president of the National Newspaper Publishers Association, said, "Adult African Americans are mature enough to make [their] own decisions unless government makes tobacco illegal." Leavell acknowledged that tobacco money provided key support for the 121 publications her group represented: "The tobacco-settlement negotiations have hurt our publications dollarwise." She lamented the fact that tobacco advertising revenues fell "from a peak of 12–20 million a year [in 1995] to less than 6 million [in 1998]" (D. Leavell, oral communication, 1998).

Many African American publications still embrace and defend tobacco advertising, not from choice, but out of desperation. Alcohol and tobacco corporations have long showered African American publications with advertising and philanthropic revenue while other national corporate advertisers shunned their pages, taking African American consumers' money but refusing to advertise in such important publications as *Ebony*, *Essence*, or *Jet*. Smaller magazines and newspapers found corporate support even more elusive and were often completely dependent upon the tobacco industry (which owns many alcohol companies). Curious news policies ensued; medical writers, for example, were ordered to avoid the topic of smoking, and articles about cardiovascular disease were published that did not mention tobacco use as a risk factor.

Key African American advocacy organizations such as the Urban League and the National Association for the Advancement of Colored People (NAACP) were gratified not only by large be-

Blacks and other racial/ethnic groups have been targeted by the tobacco industry through ads such as this Virginia Slims ad, with its suggestive undertones.

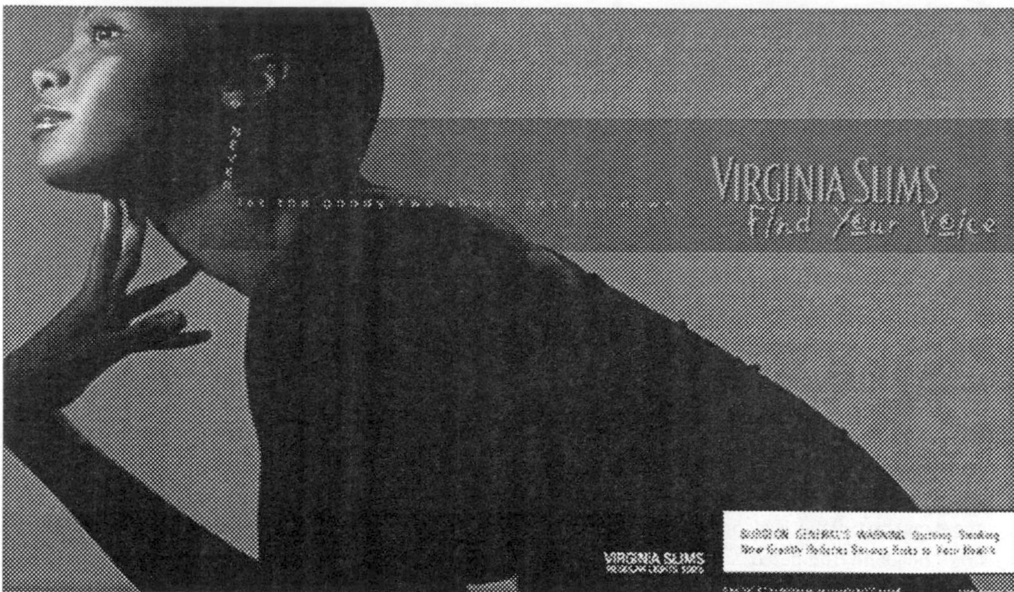

"Alcohol and tobacco corporations have long showered African American publications with advertising and philanthropic revenue while other national corporate advertisers shunned their pages."

quests but the presence of highly placed, highly visible African American tobacco company staff. For African Americans, tobacco has been a good corporate friend in a hostile corporate universe. In 1992, "R.J. Reynolds also decided "to improve [the employment] recruitment process by the development of an attractive corporate image to be systematically utilized in recruitment ads. . . . [F]eel-good 'social-responsibility' campaigns by tobacco companies help the industry not only to sway political and public opinion but to continue to recruit effective salespeople and boost employee morale." This thrust includes hiring more sexual minorities, supporting their organizations, and addressing issues of importance to LGBT communities.[23] In this context, consider the insights of Janelle Lavelle, whose gay advocacy group opposed Senator Jesse Helms's 1990 reelection. At that time, Lavelle told *The Advocate*, "The protests make working with other minority groups . . . harder because Philip Morris is one of the most labor-positive and minority-positive corporations in North Carolina." She added, "Philip Morris has openly gay people working at several places. As North Carolina companies go, Philip Morris is a jewel."[24]

Today, the targeting of gays and lesbians is escalating because gays constitute a very attractive consumer market. They boast a high disposable income and are "attention-starved and very loyal," according to Jeff Vitale, president of Overlooked Opinions, an LGBT marketing firm.[12] For example, 94% of gay readers in one survey said that they would support advertisers in gay magazines and contributors to gay organizations.[12]

And, of course, LGBTs have high smoking rates.

LGBT YOUTHS IN THE CROSSHAIRS

This supremely attractive LGBT market has an important feature in common with both heterosexuals and with the racial minorities on which Big Tobacco cut its targeted-marketing teeth: It can be captured and retained only by attracting potential smokers while they are very young.

A 1981 secret Lorillard memo asks rhetorically, "Where should our marketing thrust be?" and replies, "keep riding with Newport" because it is "heavily supported by Blacks and under-18 smokers. We are on somewhat thin ice should either of these two groups decide to shift their smoking habits."[15]

Unfortunately, federal and state lawsuits have not ended the seduction of children by Big Tobacco. By 1998, a flurry of successful state and federal lawsuits had snatched from the industry's bag of marketing tricks such options as advertising at sporting events and on billboards and in children's publications. However, Big Tobacco quickly replaced such traditional sponsorships with increased product placement in films, logo-rich announcements, sponsorship of alternative music clubs, and moving billboards on taxis. Such venues are more likely to reach and to appeal to some LGBT youths than traditional sporting events and ads in heterosexual women's and men's magazines. A 2002 University of Chicago report documents that despite the explicit 1998 prohibitions, the 3 largest US tobacco companies have selectively increased youth targeting.[26] "Cigarette companies had to become slightly more subtle about it, but they continue to aim their advertising at people under 18," avers Paul Chung, MD.[26]

Another reason for the tobacco industry's subtlety in targeting LGBT youths may be that it found young teens responded negatively to overtly sexual messages, according to secret docu-

Sold Down Tobacco Road

WHAT WERE AFRICAN AMERICANS' favorite radio stations in 1967—alphabetized, by city? How many owned automobiles, and where were these car owners most likely to live? What was the African American median income in 1971? How many hours of television did the average Black man watch that year? Did he prefer flavored, filtered, or menthol cigarettes? And exactly how cool a menthol cigarette did he like to smoke–to *the degree*?

Ask a tobacco company.

The marketing and biochemical research documents that were released as part of Minnesota's 1996 settlement with Big Tobacco reveal a staggeringly exhaustive research dossier on African American culture, habits, physiology, and biochemistry. This intimate portrait of Black America enabled the design of special tobacco products developed with African Americans in mind. The special blends were then painstakingly test marketed down to the smallest cynical details; these included packaging with an Afrocentric red, black, and green color scheme, an "X" logo that evokes political hero Malcolm X, and packs that opened from the bottom because demographic surveys revealed that this was a favored practice of Black men.

The evolution of marketing targeted at African Americans is too complex to describe in great detail here, but its history reveals some important parallels to the way in which Big Tobacco is making overtures to the LGBT communities.

Secret tobacco company documents available on the Internet reveal how the industry meticulously researched African American habits and manipulated corporate and media leadership. The early efforts of the 1950s, 1960s, and 1970s were crudely stereotypical. Newspapers were to be eschewed in favor of musical advertisements, because "The beat, the tempo, and the 'feeling' of the 'Soul' music is almost instinctively identifiable to the Negro ear, which is accustomed to this sound." [3]

"... 'Outdoors' (hunting, skiing, sailing) is not felt to be suitable, as these are considered unfamiliar to the Negro..."[3] The Montclair ads of the 1990s and the Project Scum campaign (see text) mirror such offensive stereotypes.

However, later documents revealed an appalling sophistication both in content and in quality as the targeted marketing became subtler. With the aid of hundreds of surveys, focus groups, and social and even biochemical studies of African Americans, tobacco companies researched and planned very effective marketing campaigns. They even launched special brands, mostly menthol, specifically targeted to African Americans, just as Marlboros, Virginia Slims, and Camels are marketed specifically to LGBT youths today, through marketing campaigns such as Project Scum.

African American communities have been saturated with billboards and placards featuring ethnically diverse smokers, frequent cigarette giveaways, and nefarious tobacco products such as "blunt wraps"—rolls of tobacco used to hold marijuana. For a quarter, children and the poor can buy "loosies," or illegal single cigarettes, much more frequently in communities of color than in other areas.

But Big Tobacco's siege of the African American community didn't stop there. It proceeded to kill with corporate kindness. In the 1950s, boardrooms and marketing plans tended toward the male and monochromatic. But the top 5 American tobacco companies had discovered that there was green in Black communities, and the tobacco industry offered African Americans influential work and well-paid careers when other companies barred Blacks from their boardrooms.

Just as tobacco companies today hire openly gay staff and pour funds into LGBT organizations, both local and national, they filled the cash-starved coffers of nearly every influential African American organization from the National Urban League to local churches. Tobacco has been the best corporate friend that Black America ever had, pouring so much money into political, social, artistic, and religious organizations that, like hooked smokers, these pivotal African American organizations cannot function without tobacco. Tobacco companies did not forget to invest in important politicians and to shower advertising and other financial support on influential African American news and entertainment media, which have become dependent on this habitual largess.

Today, the 28% smoking rate among African Americans is higher than the national norm. After dropping briefly during the antitargeting backlash of the 1990s,[4] smoking rates among African American youths are climbing again. What's worse, 75% of male African American smokers use menthol cigarettes. This is no coincidence, suggests Philadelphia lawyer William Adams, who has brought targeted marketing cases against Big Tobacco.[5] He recalls that "In 1957, only 5% of African Americans who smoked consumed menthol products. This represents fantastic growth. The taste for menthol was carefully cultivated by the tobacco industry itself" (W. Adams; oral communications; February 20, 1998, and May 14, 1999).

The 1990s saw a burgeoning African American opposition to targeted marketing, especially to cynically specialized cigarette brands such as Uptown, Camel Menthol, and X, and to the billboards and ads that target minority children. Such opposition has made African Americans increasingly difficult and expensive consumers. The first Surgeon General's Report to focus on the smoking habits of racial and ethnic groups further damaged the relationship between Big Tobacco and African Americans by documenting the persistent targeting of young African Americans.

But the African American community remains vitally important to the cigarette industry. African Americans represent nearly 14% of the population and 38% of its smokers (vs 31% for the total population). African Americans still constitute a large total market share of 8 top brands, especially Kool (20.5%).[4]

ments generated as early as 1978. A trial advertising campaign for Old Gold filters found that sexually referential advertising "produces no increase in brand switching or awareness and that it does not contribute to the success of Old Gold lights." The report cited children's negative reactions to "the whole sexual erection thing . . . 'get it on' . . . ugh . . . I wouldn't go for it. . . ."[27]

The news media made much of the high recognition of Joe Camel among young children and the plans to use sweet flavorings in cigarettes. More apropos to LGBT youths, however, are marketing strategies directed at youths who are beginning to recognize their sexual identities. For example, in one internal memo, tobacco companies muse how helpful it would be if they could discover that tobacco helps a common health concern such as acne.[28]

Access to cigarettes also remains easy for children. Although cheap "loosies" are more available in minority neighborhoods to African American children, children of all ethnicities can easily buy tobacco products from vending machines and the Internet. A 1983 study showed that 25% of children younger than 13 purchased cigarettes from vending machines.[29]

Big Tobacco's canon of Newspeak includes an important veiled reference to young smokers: FUBYAS, the acronym for First Usual Brand Younger Adult Smokers. The first brand smoked by a youth is tremendously important to marketers. Smokers are notoriously brand loyal, making it expensive and difficult to induce them to change brands. Therefore, tobacco companies seek to induce seduction by and loyalty to a brand, not to the smoking habit. The tobacco documents reveal a great deal of finely detailed research to tailor tobacco brands to very specific populations and their subgroups. "FUBYAS" are youths because youths constitute the vast majority of "first" smokers. Thus, targeting FUBYAS is, by definition, marketing to youths. For gay markets, this is marketing targeted at gay youths. We know this because tobacco companies do not target children in broad strokes but rather narrowly, by race, by income, and by personality, as illustrated by tobacco documents full of stereotyped descriptions. "The elements that FUBYAS know are their social groups. These are large, loosely knit but highly labeled sub-societies from which FUBYAS draw their identity. . . . The FUBYAS readily classifies others into the groups, and knows what his 'membership' is."[30] "This is good news, because therein lies differentiation and opportunity," concludes a tobacco company document cited in the *Washington Post*.[30]

For example, a June 1994 tobacco document observes, "research indicates that adult smokers are of different sexes, races and sexual orientations."[31] The descriptions of these targets are rarely flattering. For example, More brand cigarettes are targeted at women—but not just any women, according to internal marketing memos: "Woman—liberated, but not ball-busting." Users of generic cigarettes are described as "not mentally stable . . . imageless, hobos, tramps, rag pickers."[32,33]

Companies also target children by sexual orientation. As with lesbian Virginia Slims and gay male Montclair campaigns on the early 1990s, the targeting is covert, but it exists. Strategies by which tobacco companies have increased the targeting of LGBT youths include the following:

- *Exploiting the bar culture.* In one survey, 32% of lesbians and gays cited the bar culture as a factor in their nicotine addiction.[12] Drinking in bars fosters the smoking habit by lowering inhibitions and fuels LGBT alcoholism rates, which are 3 times the national average.[12] The synergy of alcohol and smoking is a special hazard for gays, as it multiplies the risks of cancer and other diseases.

The importance of the bar culture is not lost on the industry, whose documents show a heavy marketing investment in bar crowds, including "African American" and "alternative" bars

Cigarettes are sometimes packaged with free gifts that appeal to both young adults and youths.

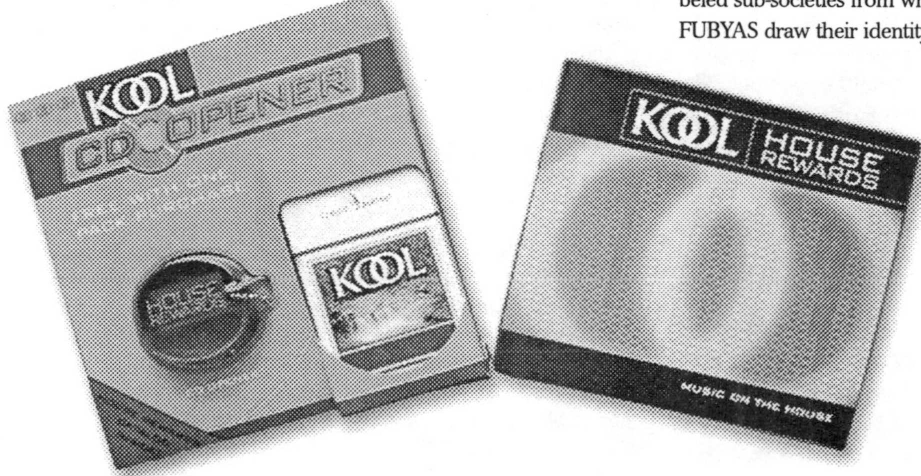

where tobacco company representatives distribute free cigarette samples, hold contests with tobacco premiums as prizes, and sometimes take over the bar to buy free drinks.

• *Exploiting drug use rates,* which are higher among LGBT youths, a fact that Big Tobacco has not hesitated to use to its advantage.

• *Targeting geographical areas* where many young LGBTs congregate socially, such as the Castro and Tenderloin districts of San Francisco.

PROJECT SCUM

The industry that has always denied that it targets youths, despite the detailed statements, reports, and youth marketing plans in its secret internal memos, today refuses to admit its targeting of LGBT youths. Unfortunately, in the absence of a confession, hard evidence is hard to come by. But hard evidence of plans to target LGBT youths can sometimes be excavated from internal tobacco marketing documents that were never meant for consumers' eyes.

Between 1995 and 1997, R.J. Reynolds internal documents recorded corporate-wide overtures to the young LGBT community in what must be one of the least flattering targeted marketing plans in history. In "Project Scum," R.J. Reynolds tried to market Camel and Red Kamel cigarettes to San Francisco area "consumer subcultures" of "alternative life style." R.J. Reynolds's special targets were gay people in the Castro district, where, as the company noted, "The opportunity exists for a cigarette manufacturer to dominate."[34] The gay Castro denizens were described as "rebellious, Generation X-ers," and "street people." Both the coded labeling of targets as "Generation X-ers" in the mid-1990s and as "rebellious" indicates their youth. Project Scum also planned to exploit the high rates of drug use in the "subculture" target group by saturating " 'head shops' and other nontraditional retail outlets with Camel brand." More telling than the guardedly worded report itself are the scrawled marginalia such as "Gay/Castro" and "Tenderloin." The observation "higher incidents [sic] of smoking in subcultures" has the phrase "and drugs" written in.[34–36]

In one copy, the word "Scum" is crossed out and the word "Sourdough" substituted by a belatedly cautious executive. After such careful sanitizing, the final document could have emerged as Project Sourdough with no clear written evidence that young LGBTs had ever been targeted.

The readiness such documents evinced to exploit the higher drug use rates among LGBT youths sheds marketing light on some dubious promotional devices. For example, Philip Morris has given away key rings with its Alpine Extra Light cigarettes that conceal a screw-top glass vial. Surveys by the smoking cessation group Quit, from Melbourne, Australia, suggest that most youths think these premiums are for holding drugs. Unprompted, 10 of the 13 groups surveyed suggested that the vials were meant to carry "drugs," "coke," "stash," and "speed." One youth summed it up: "It's a key ring, and it's what people typically use to carry drugs."[37]

STRANGE BEDFELLOWS

In the early 1990s, tobacco companies began forging legislative and political ties with the LGBT community, just as they had with many African American politicians, the African American news media, and with groups such as the National Urban League. The tobacco industry began introducing antidiscrimination bills that purported to offer protection against sexual-orientation bias but whose addenda and riders protected the rights of smokers—and of the companies that feed smokers' habits. According to the Tobacco Institute, by September 23, 1992, the industry had enlisted the help of local gay and lesbian alliances to pass smoker protection/"antidiscrimination" laws in 20 states.[38]

> *"Philip Morris sought to expand its pursuit of the US Hispanic community by sponsoring soccer events, Latin music events, and Hispanic festivals and by giving away cigarettes."*

Sometimes, however, tobacco companies knew that anti-tobacco LGBT groups troubled by high rates of LGBT addiction would not support them, so they formulated plans to cut these leadership groups out of the picture and appeal directly to gay voters.

In 1998, California voters were offered Proposition 10, a measure to substantially hike cigarette taxes. A concerned Tobacco Institute (an industry consortium) sought professional advice from marketers, researchers, and consultants on how best to garner the gay vote. Consultant David Mixner advised the Tobacco Institute "to bypass" gay organizations: "Since it is apparent that we are not going to have the endorsement of most Gay and Lesbian leadership, it is important to use these campaign tools to bypass that and go directly to the Gay and Lesbian voter with a message that will resonate."[39]

Just as struggling African American media tended to defend (or to conveniently ignore) targeted marketing by Big Tobacco, some LGBT media view tobacco's growing attention to gay and lesbian customers as a boon.

In response to a August 17, 1992, *Wall Street Journal* story by Joanne Lipman, Don Tuthill, the publisher of *Genre*, wrote, "The Philip Morris/Genre story is not a story of

> 'the tobacco industry . . . turning its marketing muscle on another minority'; it is a story of inclusion . . . a story about a major marketing company recognizing, including and supporting a frequently disenfranchised and overlooked segment of the U.S. population. . . . this is exactly the kind of support that gay media has sought for years."[40]

Joe Landry, publisher of *Out* and *The Advocate*, crowed that Big Tobacco's advertising "shows we're making progress. . . . Lots of companies are adding diversity marketing to their budgets, which used to mean money for advertising mainly to blacks and Hispanics, but now it's meant largely, and sometimes mainly, for gay and lesbian customers."[41]

However, the targeting of racial and ethnic groups is hardly a thing of the past; indeed, it is escalating and gaining precision. For example, a perusal of the online tobacco documents shows that tobacco companies have added surgically precise research on Hispanic markets to their ethnic marketing mix.

As early as 1988, Philip Morris sought to expand its pursuit of the US Hispanic community by sponsoring soccer events, Latin music events, and Hispanic festivals and by giving away cigarettes. The proposed budget for the Hispanic Marlboro campaign alone was $3.5 million.[42–44]

Recently, however, such targeting has achieved sophistication; it is no longer in broad strokes but rather surgical strikes. For example, although Lorillard market research details that African American men are the largest market for menthol cigarettes, in some Los Angeles and New York Hispanic communities, menthol is perceived as the choice of gay men. But in others menthol is seen as macho, and in still others as an acceptable choice for anyone, man or woman.[42]

In sum, one can see dramatic parallels between tobacco's courtship of the LGBT community today and its targeted marketing of African Americans decades ago. The industry gave African Americans the corporate attention and acceptance they craved, advertising in their media and neighborhoods. It became a generous and attentive corporate friend, investing heavily in African American organizations of every stripe. It hired many African Americans and non-White women in positions of responsibility in an era when boardrooms were male and monochromatic.

Behind the scenes, however, Big Tobacco's secret documents reveal that it slyly targeted children and knowingly sabotaged the health of a community already ravaged by high disease rates.

Today, tobacco companies view both racial and sexual minorities as key markets. Targeted marketing of tobacco to sexual minorities seems likely to mirror the process that worked so powerfully to addict and sicken African Americans.

Marketing targeted at LGBTs will probably accelerate, for several reasons:

- The LGBT community is an extremely attractive new consumer base, with high disposable income, a very brand-loyal culture, a tradition of tobacco use, and a hunger for corporate attention and acceptance.
- The Internet will make it irresistibly quick and easy to precisely target and survey specific demographic groups within the LGBT community for specific tobacco products, much easier than detailing racial minorities has been during the past 40 years.
- The Internet also offers a way to market and sell cigarettes to underage youths, including LGBT youths.

All this means that we may see marketing aimed at LGBTs—and, by implication if not definition, at *young* LGBTs—escalate in scope and directness. The wave of the future may be revealed by Germany's Reemstma tobacco company, whose advertisements have thrown yesterday's coded ambiguity to the winds. Ads for its New West brand have featured a gay male marriage and copy that exhorted, "Men! . . . taste how strong this one is."[12] Reemstma's Web sites include one labeled "Queer," which offers a dazzling cornucopia of advertisements, news, fashion, music, games, chat rooms, explicit gay pornography, and, of course, tobacco products, all tailored to the tastes and interests of LGBT consumers.[45]

What better illustration of how Big Tobacco increasingly views the LGBT community with lust rather than apprehension? As a growing number of companies court the gay market, analysts predict that this desirability will achieve widespread corporate acceptability. Then tobacco advertising may become omnipresent within the LGBT communities, just as tobacco billboards, ads, promotions, sponsorship, employees, and products did in African American communities by the 1970s, seducing new generations of smokers. ■

About the Author

Harriet A. Washington is with the Harvard Medical School, Boston, Mass.

Requests for reprints should be sent to Harriet A. Washington, 4049 Broadway, #123, New York, NY 10032 (e-mail: haw95@aol.com).

This article was accepted April 16, 2002.

References

1. Tobacco Institute memo from Samuel Chilcote, Jr, to Rep. Thomas Luken's Subcommittee on Transportation and Hazardous Materials [re: Protect Our Children From Cigarettes Act of 1989]. July 26, 1989. Bates No. 515687450. Available at: http://tobaccodocuments.org/rjr/515687449-7757.html. Accessed May 15, 2002.

2. The campaign for tobacco-free kids. Available at: http://tobaccofreekids.org/adgallery. Accessed April 21, 2002.

3. Holland G. A study of ethnic markets [by R. J. Reynolds marketing officials]. September 1969. Bates No. 501989230. Available at: http://www.tobaccodocuments.org. Accessed June 17, 1998.

4. Stolberg SG. Rise in smoking by young blacks erodes a success story. *New York Times.* April 4, 1998: A24.

5. Slobodzian J. Civil rights suit names tobacco. *Natl Law J.* November 2, 1998:A10.

6. DiFranza JR, Librett JJ. State and federal revenues from tobacco consumed by minors. *Am J Public Health.* 1999;89:1106–1108.

7. The toll of tobacco in the United States of America. Available at: http://tobaccofreekids.org/research/factsheets/pdf/0072.pdf. Accessed May 23, 2002.

8. Cummings KM, Pechacek T, Shopland D. The illegal sale of cigarettes to us minors: estimates by state. *Am J Public Health.* 1994;84:300–302.

9. Evans N, Farkas A, Gilpin E, Berry C, Pierce JP. Influence of tobacco marketing and exposure to smokers on adolescent susceptibility to smoking. *J Natl Cancer Inst.* 1995;87:1538-1545.

10. Pierce JP, Choi WS, Gilpin EA, Farkas AJ, Berry CC. Tobacco industry promotion of cigarettes and adolescent smoking [with erratum in *JAMA.* 1998; 280:422]. *JAMA.* 1998;279:511-505.

11. *Lesbians and Smoking Fact Sheet.* Washington, DC: NOW Foundation; October 16, 2001. Available at: http://www.nowfoundation.org/health/lybdkit/factsheet.html. Accessed March 4, 2002.

12. Goebel K. Lesbians and gays face tobacco targeting. *Tob Control.* 1994;3: 65-67.

13. Author unknown. Most smokers try to quit, but can't [poll]. September 11, 2001. Available at: http://www.umich.edu/~umtrn/websites.html. Accessed September 11, 2001.

14. Bosworth, Brandon. A last drag? *Am Enterprise Online.* November 15, 2001. Available at: http://www.theamericanenterprise.org/hotflash011115.htm. Accessed May 23, 2002.

15. Ardey DR, Edlin BR, Giovino GA, Nelson DE. Smoking, HIV infection and gay men in the United States. *Tob Control.* 1993;2:156–158.

16. Newell GR, Mansell PW, Wilson MB, Lynch HK, Spitz MR, Hersh EM. Risk factor analysis among men referred for possible acquired immune deficiency syndrome. *Prev Med.* 1985;14:81-91.

17. Paralusz KM. Ashes to ashes: why FDA regulation of tobacco advertising may mark the end of the road for the Marlboro Man. *Am J Law Med.* Spring 1998;24:89–122.

18. Rosario M, Hunter J, Gwadz M. Exploration of substance abuse among lesbian gay and bisexual youth: prevalence and correlates. *J Adolesc Res.* October 1997;12:454–476.

19. Steele BC. From pickups to SUVS: winking ads that appealed to gay men as early as the 1950's lead the way for today's bold appeals to lesbian and gay consumers. *The Advocate.* August 15, 2000:14.

20. Philip Morris marketing memo, March 29, 1985. Bates No. 2023268366/8374. Available at: http://www.pmdocs.com. Accessed March 1, 2002.

21. Top Secret Operation Rainmaker, Tuesday, 20 March 1990. Bates No. 2048302227–2048302230. Available at: http://tobaccodocuments.org/usc_tim/1251.html. Accessed May 20, 2002.

22. Rigdon JE. Overcoming a deep-rooted reluctance, more firms advertise to gay community. *Wall Street Journal.* July 16, 1991: B1.

23. Institute for Consumer Responsibility. Georgians Against Smoking Pollution newsletter. 1984 (est.). Bates No. 2045748385-8398. Available at: http://tobaccodocuments.org/usc_tim/2045748385-8398.html. Accessed March 6, 2002.

24. Institute for Consumer Responsibility. [No title]. 1984 (est.). Bates No. 2045748385-2045748398. Available at: http://tobaccodocuments.org/pm/2045748385-8398.html. Accessed March 28, 2002.

25. Replies to 5-year plan questionnaire. 1981. Bates No. 03490806-03490844. Available at: http://tobaccodocuments.org/youth/AmYoLOR00000000.Rm.html. Accessed May 20, 2002.

26. Cigarette ads target youth, violating $250 billion 1998 settlement [press release]. Chicago, Ill: University of Chicago Hospitals & Health System, Public Relations Office; March 12, 2002.

27. OGF Vitality Test WAVE II. Bates No. 91145517-91145643. Available at: http://tobaccodocuments.org/lor/91145517-5643.html. Accessed May 23, 2002.

28. Memo suggesting consideration of formation of a scientifically oriented group to review work made at tobacco industry expense. Tobacco Institute. June 19, 1974. Bates No. TIMN0068332. Available at: http://www.smokescreen.org. Accessed March 7, 2002.

29. Kessler DA, Witt AM, Barnett PS, et al. The Food and Drug Administration's regulation of tobacco products. *N Eng J Med.* 1996;335:988–994.

30. [Author unknown.] Cigarette marketers' decades-old stereotypes may threaten today's deal. *Washington Post.* January 19, 1998: A23.

31. Landman A. Confidential—recap of Hispanic meeting. Bates No. 2060286766. Available at: http://tobaccodocuments.org/landman/2060286766.html. Accessed March 8, 2002.

32. Bender G. Image attributes of cigarette brands. For Brown and Williamson Tobacco Corp. January 1982. Bates No. 670575136-670575158. Available at: http://tobaccodocuments.org/usc_tim/247684.html. Accessed April 1, 2002.

33. Mindset segments. January 3, 1991. Bates No. 510320848– 510320876. Available at: http://tobaccodocuments.org/landman/510320848-0876.html. Accessed April 1, 2002.

34. Simkins BJ. Project Scum. R. J. Reynolds Tobacco Co. December 12, 1995. Bates No. 518021121–518021129. Available at: http://tobaccodocuments.org/landman/518021121.html. Accessed April 4, 2002.

35. Project Scum. R. J. Reynolds Tobacco Co. April 2, 1996. Bates No. 519849940–519849948. Available at: http://tobaccodocuments.org/rjr/519849940-9948.html. Accessed April 4, 2002.

36. O'Conner LM. Project Scum. R. J. Reynolds Tobacco Co. 1997. Bates No. 517060265–517060272. Available at: http://tobaccodocuments.org/rjr/517060265-517060272.html. Accessed January 28, 2001.

37. Chapman S. Campaigners accuse tobacco firm of dubious ploy. *BMJ* 2000;320:1427.

38. Anti-discrimination measures. The Tobacco Institute. September 23, 1992. Bates No. TIMN0030964-TIMN0030965. Available at: http://tobaccodocuments.org/ti/TIMN0030964-0965.html. Accessed May 20, 2002.

39. Mixner D. Memo from DBM Associates [consultant to the Tobacco Institute] to Grant Gillham, Joe Shumate & Associates, Inc. Bates No. TCAL0404793. Available at: http://tobaccodocuments.org/landman/TCAL0404793.html. Accessed April 14, 2002

40. Letter to Joanne from Don Tuthill. August 17, 1992. Bates No. 2023439114. Available at: http://tobaccodocuments.org/pm/2023439114-9115.html. Accessed March 1 2002.

41. Pertman A. Gay market, ads target big dollars, not big change. *Boston Globe.* February 4, 2001:E1.

42. Marlboro Hispanic promotions 880000 marketing plan. 1988 (est). Bates No. 2048679289/294. Available at: http://www.tobaccodocuments.org/pm/2048679289-9294.html#images. Accessed April 21, 2002.

43. Hispanic market opportunity assessment. Progress update presentation. January 1985. Bates No. 504617452–504617507. Available at: http://tobaccodocuments.org/rjr/504617452-7507.html. Accessed April 21, 2002.

44. The Hispanic market. February 10, 1983. Bates No. 2042463401–2042463437. Available at: http://tobaccodocuments.org/pm/2042463401-3437.html. Accessed March 10, 2002.

45. Reemtsma West brand cigarettes "Queer" Web page. Available at: http://www.west.de/queer. Accessed May 15, 2002.

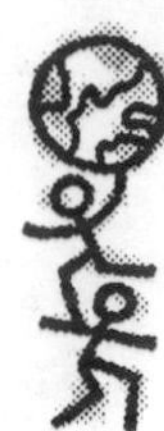

African American Women and Smoking: Starting Later

| Joyce Moon-Howard, DrPH

It is commonly accepted that adolescence is the period for initiation into smoking and other tobacco use behaviors. However, evidence is increasing that the set of presumptions about adolescent onset of tobacco use may not be true for all cultural or subpopulation groups.

Secondary analysis of data from the 2000 National Health Interview Survey (NHIS) was used to examine ethnic differences in smoking patterns among African American and White women. Results showed a striking racial/ethnic difference in age of onset; African American women initiate smoking later than White women at each age group.

Prevention interventions need to continue beyond adolescence well into the adult years, especially for African American women. Late onset for these women represents an often missed window of opportunity for prevention. (*Am J Public Health.* 2003;93:418–420)

IT IS COMMONLY ACCEPTED that tobacco use has an age-defined period of onset: adolescence is the period for initiation into smoking and other tobacco use behaviors.[1] Surveillance data show a relatively narrow age range for smoking onset, after which the presumed risk of initiation decreases. A number of studies conclude that very few people begin to use tobacco as

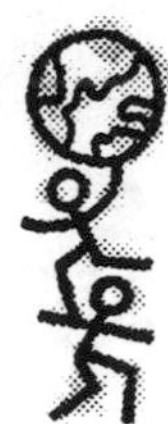

adults; they note that most adult smokers report that first use had occurred by the time they graduated from high school.[1,2] In addition, several studies have shown that adolescent onset is strongly associated with continued use throughout the life course.[1] Health problems associated with smoking are a function of the duration (years) and the intensity (amount) of use. Thus, earlier onset would provide more time and opportunity for the risk of more serious health consequences.[3,4]

These research findings have influenced tobacco control proponents who have strongly urged that prevention efforts be targeted at preadolescents and young teens (<18 years old), reasoning that postponing the onset of tobacco use in adolescence makes it less likely that initiation will occur. The overwhelming majority of tobacco education and prevention initiatives target youths aged younger than 18 years. These efforts include school-based education and prevention programs, banning billboard advertisement of tobacco within 1000 feet of schools, enforcing laws restricting minors' access to tobacco products, and youth-oriented mass media campaigns.[5]

However, there is increasing evidence that the set of presumptions about adolescent onset and duration of tobacco use may not be true for all cultural or subpopulation groups. It is encouraging that smoking prevalence has decreased in the United States.[2] However, a focus on overall prevalence masks important differences within racial/ethnic, sex, and age-specific groups.[6,7] A case in point is smoking patterns among White and Black women, especially at younger ages.

ETHNIC/RACIAL DIFFERENCES IN SMOKING PATTERNS FOR WOMEN

Several studies have shown that African Americans are more likely than not to begin smoking beyond the "typical" age of onset in early adolescence. Smoking rates among Black women continue to increase through the 20s and then plateau.[8] Rates of smoking are higher for White women than for Black women at each age group up to the mid-30s, after which rates for Black women rise above those for White women until the late 40s. For example, 28% of young White women aged 18 to 20 years reported current smoking in the 2000 National Health Interview Survey (NHIS), compared with 15% of Black women in this age group (Figure 1). In contrast, at ages 41 to 43, more Black women (36%) than White women (28%) are current smokers.

A number of factors could influence prevalence rates by age, including differences in quitting patterns as well as differences in age of onset. The racial/ethnic differences in quit rates and cessation efforts have been discussed at length elsewhere.[6,10–12,13] Less attention has been paid to racial/ethnic differences in age at onset of smoking.

The 2000 NHIS also collected data on age of smoking onset. The mean age of onset for Black women was 19.28 years (SD=5.60), more than a year older than the age of onset for White women, 18.21 years (SD=5.56). The difference in initiation rates shows that nearly two thirds (65%) of the White women who ever smoked began smoking by age 18, while slightly more than half (54%) of the Black women had begun smoking by 18.

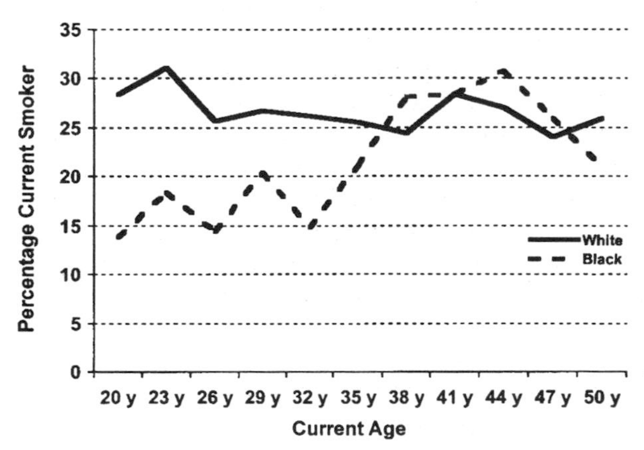

FIGURE 1—Smoking prevalence for women, by current age: 2000 National Health Interview Survey.[9]

As other researchers have pointed out, overall population prevalence rates can mask trends affecting younger age groups. Figure 2 shows the mean age of smoking onset by current age at time of interview for all women who ever smoked. As the trend line shows, there are striking racial/ethnic difference in age of onset; African American women initiate smoking later than White women at each age group. Clearly, age of onset is younger for women in more recent birth cohorts. However, at each age group, African American women report later age of smoking initiation.

IMPLICATIONS FOR TOBACCO PREVENTION

Different patterns in age of onset have implications for tobacco prevention and education. Age of initiation for Black women is well beyond the target of most prevention initiatives. School-based programs, for example, would not reach young women aged older than 18 years, which is past the age of high school completion. It is not clear what factors are associated with late smoking initiation among African American women. In general, little is known about adult smoking initiation, and very little attention has been given to prevention of adult smoking onset. However, understanding later onset among women is an especially urgent public health issue.

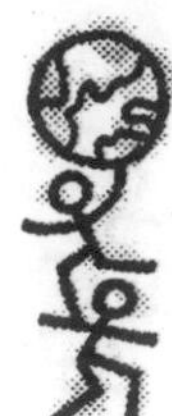

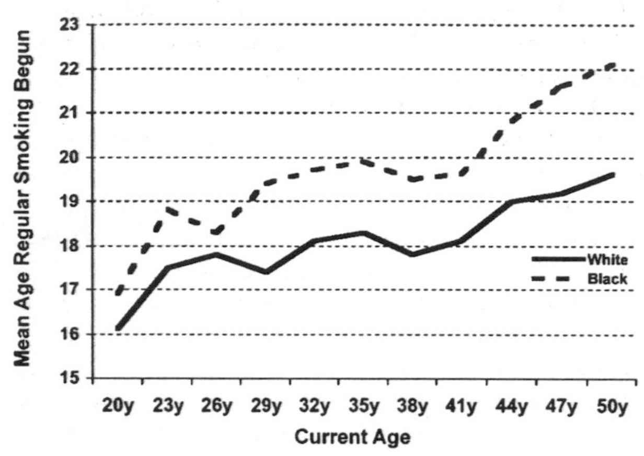

FIGURE 2—Mean age of smoking onset for women, by current age: 2000 National Health Interview Survey.[9]

Postadolescence onset occurs during peak childbearing and child-rearing ages, when the health risk from tobacco affects not only the women but their children as well.[2]

The assumptions of prevention campaigns focused on adolescents (i.e., smokers start in their teen years; teen smokers are more likely to continue) appear not to be valid for many, if not most, African American women. This raises the question of whether a "one size fits all" approach to prevention initiatives has more than limited utility for Black women. Indeed, prevention messages that target only youths may miss a significant at-risk population. Smoking and smoking-related cancers are major sources of excess mortality in African American communities,[10,12,13,15] and African Americans die disproportionately more from smoking-related cancers than any other population group in the United States.[8] Research is needed to further clarify not only patterns of smoking, including onset and cessation efforts, but also differential risks for smoking among different racial/ethnic, sex, and age groups.

Tobacco control efforts have made great strides, and we must take every opportunity to continue the progress. It is clear that prevention interventions need to continue beyond adolescence and well into the adult years, especially for African American women. Given that smoking is more persistent among African American women, preventing onset is critical. Late onset for these women represents an often missed window of opportunity for prevention. ■

About the Author

Requests for reprints should be sent to Joyce Moon-Howard, Department of Sociomedical Sciences, Center for Applied Public Health, Mailman School of Public Health, Columbia University, 722 West 168th Street, New York, NY 10032 (e-mail: jmh7@columbia.edu).

This article was accepted November 8, 2002.

References

1. Kandel DB, Warner LA, Kessler RC. The epidemiology of substance use and dependence among women. In: Wetherington CL and Roman AB, eds. *Drug Addiction Research and the Health of Women.* Rockville, MD: National Institute of Drug Abuse Research Monograph; 1998.

2. *Women and Smoking: A Report of the Surgeon General.* Atlanta, Ga: Office of Smoking and Health, National Center for Chronic Disease Prevention and Health Promotion; 2001.

3. *Preventing Tobacco Use Among Young People: A Report of the Surgeon General.* Atlanta, Ga: Office of Smoking and Health, National Center for Chronic Disease Prevention and Health Promotion; 1994.

4. Centers for Disease Control and Prevention (CDC). *Reducing the Health Consequences of Smoking: 25 Years of Progress. A Report of the Surgeon General.* Rockville, Md: US Dept of Health and Human Services; 1989. CDC publication 89-8411.

5. National Center for Tobacco Free Kids. Campaign for Tobacco Free Kids. Available at: http://tobaccofreekids.org/reports/tobacctoll.php3?stateID=ny. Accessed September 2002.

6. Geronimus AT, Neidert LJ. Age patterns of smoking in US black and white women of childbearing age. *Am J Public Health.* 1993;83:1258–1264.

7. Centers for Disease Control and Prevention. Current trends [and] differences in the age of smoking initiation between blacks and whites—United States. *MMRW Morb Mortal Wkly Rep.* 1991;44:754–757.

8. *Tobacco Use Among US Racial/Ethnic Minority Groups—African Americans, American Indians and Alaska Natives, Asian Americans and Pacific Islanders, and Hispanics: A Report of the Surgeon General.* Atlanta, Ga: Office of Smoking and Health, National Center for Chronic Disease Prevention and Health Promotion; 1998.

9. 2000 National Health Interview Survey. National Center for Health Statistics, Division of Data Services. Hyattsville, Md. Available at: http://www.cdc.gov/nchs/nhis.htm. Accessed February 4, 2003.

10. Robinson LA, Klesges. RC. Ethnic and gender differences in risk factors for smoking onset. *Health Psychol.* 1997;16:499–505.

11. Morabia A, Costanza MC. Ages at initiation of cigarette smoking and quit attempts among women: a generation effect. *Am J Public Health.* 2002;92:71–74.

12. Manfredi C, Lacey L, Warnecke R, Balch G. Method effects in survey and focus group findings: understanding smoking cessation in low-SES African American women. *J Health Educ Behav.* 1997;24:786–800.

13. Griesler PC, Kandel DB. Ethnic differences in correlates of adolescent cigarette smoking. *J Adolesc Health.* 1998;23:167–180.

14. McGrady GA, Pederson LL. Do sex and ethnic differences in smoking initiation mask similarities in cessation behavior? *Am J Public Health.* 2002;92:961–965.

15. Shervington DO. Attitudes and practices of African-American women regarding cigarette smoking: implications for interventions. *J Natl Med Assoc.* 1994;86:337–343.